CONTEMPORARY CLINICAL IMMUNOLOGY AND SEROLOGY

•

Kate Rittenhouse-Olson, Ph.D. S.I.^{CM} (ASCP)

Editor, Immunological Investigations
Professor, Director Biotechnology Undergraduate Program
Department of Biotechnical and Clinical Laboratory Sciences
School of Medicine and Biomedical Sciences
University of Buffalo

Ernesto De Nardin, M.S., Ph.D.

Associate Editor, Immunological Investigations
Professor, Department of Oral Biology
Department of Microbiology and Immunology
Schools of Medicine and Dentistry
University of Buffalo

Pearson

Boston Columbus Indianapolis New York San Francisco Upper Saddle River
Amsterdam Cape Town Dubai London Madrid Milan Munich Paris Montreal Toronto
Delhi Mexico City Sao Paulo Sydney Hong Kong Seoul Singapore Taipei Tokyo

Notice: The authors and the publisher of this volume have taken care that the information and technical recommendations contained herein are based on research and expert consultation, and are accurate and compatible with the standards generally accepted at the time of publication. Nevertheless, as new information becomes available, changes in clinical and technical practices become necessary. The reader is advised to carefully consult manufacturers' instructions and information material for all supplies and equipment before use, and to consult with a health care professional as necessary. This advice is especially important when using new supplies or equipment for clinical purposes. The authors and publisher disclaim all responsibility for any liability, loss, injury, or damage incurred as a consequence, directly or indirectly, of the use and application of any of the contents of this volume.

Publisher: Julie Levin Alexander
Publisher's Assistant: Regina Bruno
Executive Acquisitions Editor: John Goucher
Associate Editor: Melissa Kerian
Editorial Assistant: Erica Viviani
Development Editors: Laura Horowitz, Anne Seitz, and Gretchen Miller, Hearthside Publishing Services
Director of Marketing: David Gesell
Executive Marketing Manager: Katrin Beacom
Marketing Coordinator: Alicia Wozniak
Senior Managing Editor: Patrick Walsh
Project Manager: Christina Zingone-Luethje
Senior Operations Supervisor: Ilene Sanford

Operations Specialist: Lisa McDowell
Senior Art Director: Jayne Conte
Cover Designer: Suzanne Behnke
Cover Art: © Deco Images II / Alamy
Media Editor: Amy Peltier
Lead Media Project Manager: Lorena Cerisano
Full-Service Project Management: Erika Jordan, Laserwords Private Limited
Composition: Laserwords Private Limited
Printer/Binder: Courier/Kendallville
Cover Printer: Lehigh-Phoenix Color/Hagerstown
Text Font: ITC Stone Serif Std

Credits and acknowledgments for content borrowed from other sources and reproduced, with permission, in this textbook appear on appropriate page.

Library of Congress Cataloging-in-Publication Data
Rittenhouse-Olson, Kate.
  Contemporary clinical immunology and serology/Kate Rittenhouse-Olson, Ernesto De Nardin. — 1st ed.
    p. cm.
  ISBN 978-0-13-510424-8 (alk. paper)
  1. Clinical immunology—Textbooks. 2. Serology—Textbooks. I. De Nardin, Ernesto. II. Title.
RC582.R58 2013
616.07′9—dc23
                                                                        2012017853

10 9 8 7 6 5 4 3 2 1

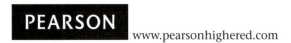
www.pearsonhighered.com

ISBN-13: 978-0-13-510424-8
ISBN-10: 0-13-510424-6

DEDICATION

To the patience and kindness and interest of my students over the last 20 years, I love teaching you—you inspire me with your search for knowledge and your dedication to your future professions. Also to my family, especially to my wonderful husband Jim and my children Jennifer, Anna, and Andrew Diakun, who have watched me type and read into the night. Together, you are the support system that made this book and everything I do possible.

Kate Rittenhouse-Olson

To my family, Ann, Nicole, and Jesse, for putting up with me while I was working on this; to my father, for being the quintessential example of the ultimate free spirit; to my dental, medical, and graduate students, for challenging me all the time; and to my dogs Skippy and Luigi because, well . . . they're really cool dogs.

Ernesto De Nardin

BRIEF CONTENTS

CONTENTS

FOREWORD

Contemporary Clinical Immunology and Serology is part of Pearson's Clinical Laboratory Science series of textbooks, which is designed to balance theory and practical applications in a way that is engaging and useful to students. The authors of and contributors to *Contemporary Clinical Immunology and Serology* present highly detailed technical information and real-life case studies to help learners envision themselves as members of the health care team providing the laboratory services specific to immunology in assisting with patient care. The mixture of theoretical and practical information relating to immunology provided in this text allows learners to analyze and synthesize this information and, ultimately, to answer questions and solve problems and cases. Additional applications and instructional resources are available at www.myhealthprofessionskit.com.

We hope that this book, as well as the entire series, proves to be a valuable educational resource.

Elizabeth A. Zeibig, Ph.D., MLS(ASCP)CM
Clinical Laboratory Science Series Editor
Pearson Health Science

Associate Dean for Graduate Education
Department of Clinical Laboratory Science
Doisy College of Health Sciences
Saint Louis University
St. Louis, Missouri

PREFACE

This first edition of *Contemporary Clinical Immunology and Serology* is written for students that will use, order, or design clinical immunology assays. This includes students in the medical technology/clinical laboratory scientist (MT/CLS) and medical laboratory technician/clinical laboratory technician (MLT/CLT) programs as well as those in biotechnology programs and other science undergraduates and graduates interested in a medically oriented immunology course. Immunology has become an essential part of many scientific careers, and this text and related course is designed to benefit individuals in undergraduate and graduate science courses who want to understand the current state of the art in basic immunology, immunological diseases, and clinical diagnosis using immunological methods. *Contemporary Clinical Immunology and Serology* is also a useful reference for practicing laboratory professionals. Medical residents in allergy, rheumatology, immunology, and internal medicine also will find it useful.

The primary authors, Kate Rittenhouse-Olson and Ernesto De Nardin, have combined over 40 years in teaching immunology to medical technology, biotechnology, dental, medical, and graduate students. They wrote this book with the constant consultation of a team of clinical laboratory scientists at Buffalo, New York, area hospitals, National Reference Laboratories, and colleagues met during interactions with continuing medical laboratory education efforts sponsored by the American Society of Clinical Pathologists (ASCP). *Contemporary Clinical Immunology and Serology* includes the newest techniques used by professionals in the field; this, in turn, ensures that students using this book will be well prepared to work in modern clinical immunology laboratories, understand the data generated by the techniques in these laboratories, and use the conclusions from the results obtained to provide the best patient care.

The material presented in this text has been classroom tested; full-color tables and illustrations have been included to offer the content in the best and most interesting manner. In addition, the inclusion of sample exam questions and cumulative tables help students study the material and gain the knowledge needed to pass the national certification exam.

ORGANIZATION OF *CONTEMPORARY CLINICAL IMMUNOLOGY AND SEROLOGY*

This book is organized in 5 parts: (1) the immune system and its components, (2) the basic principles and methodology of immunological assays, (3) the serology of noninfectious disorders, (4) the serology of infectious disorders, and (5) additional information related to clinical laboratory immunology.

Each section builds on material from the previous sections. Part 1 introduces the innate and acquired immune systems; it begins with an overview of these systems followed by more specific details so that students can apply this information to the subsequent sections. Part 2 addresses the principles and methodologies of different assays, starting with the simpler unlabeled assays followed by the more complex labeled ones. All assays, including the newest techniques such as the multiplex ones, described in this book are currently and routinely performed in modern clinical immunology laboratories. Some older techiques no longer routinely used (eg, complement fixation) are mentioned in passing for historical purposes but are not discussed. Included in Part 2 is a chapter on mathematical calculations and formulas used in various assays from performing serial dilutions to determining the positive predictive value of a particular assay or kit. Understanding the principles and methodology of contemporary clinical immunology techniques is essential for preparing students to work in both a clinical or a research setting.

Parts 3 and 4 build on the material in Parts 1 and 2. Part 3 describes the serology of noninfectious clinical disorders; these include allergy and hypersensitivity, autoimmunity, tumors, hematologic malignancies, transplantation immunology, and primary immunodeficiency diseases. Part 4 discusses the role of the clinical immunology laboratory in the diagnosis of infectious diseases. It begins with a follow-up of immunodeficiency by covering acquired immunodeficiencies including HIV and AIDS and continues with viral diseases, including a chapter on hepatitis and one on the Herpesvirdae family and other viruses. Part 4 then continues with a chapter on bacterial disease, including streptococcal and clostridium infections, syphilis, and Lyme disease. The final chapter in this section covers fungal and parasitic diseases. Part 5 completes the textbook with a chapter on forensic serology, one on basic laboratory safety and regulations, and another on molecular biology techniques.

SUITABLE FOR ALL LEVELS OF LEARNING

Contemporary Clinical Immunology and Serology has been designed for CLT/MLT and CLS/MT students as well as students in biotechnology and those in all health care professions that may use, design, or order these tests. The chapter outlines and detailed objectives provided in the beginning of each chapter allows instructors to select the material and level of content applicable to their specific course. Parts 1 and 2 contain enough background material to prepare the beginning students for subsequent sections and can serve as a review for more advanced students and keep them up-to-date with recent developments in the field.

UNIQUE PEDAGOGICAL FEATURES

Objectives and Detailed Course Outline: Each chapter has its own objectives that were used to generate examination questions for the question bank. Furthermore, the detailed chapter outlines help students find the information specific to the objectives and attempt to help them understand why they are learning the specific material. Each chapter begins with an introduction meant to stimulate interest and ends with a summary to review the key points in the chapter. The many illustrations (with some repetition and redundancy) should help students retain the material in long-term memory.

Key Terms and Glossary: Key terms appear in bold in the chapter text and are defined in the Glossary. Review of these terms allows students to test their knowledge of the material.

Case Studies: Each chapter includes case studies for instructors to use to enrich their lectures. The case study questions are presented in a stepwise manner with information obtained in each leading to subsequent ones so that the case is a summary of the chapter material.

Checkpoints: Checkpoints appear throughout the chapters to help students pause during the reading to determine whether they understand and retain the material that they are reading. The answers to the checkpoints are in the rear of the book.

Summary: To reinforce key points, a summary concludes each chapter and helps students tie the information in it together.

Review Questions: Review questions at the end of each chapter directly relate to the objectives listed at the beginning of the chapter and help students test their understanding of the material. Answers are provided in the rear of the book.

Figures and Tables: Carefully designed figures and tables located throughout the chapters help students visualize and organize the material.

A COMPLETE TEACHING AND LEARNING PACKAGE

Upon adoption of *Contemporary Clinical Immunology and Serology*, a complete teaching and learning package is available. It includes the following:

- Powerpoint lectures and color images contain the material needed to teach each chapter's objectives.

- They are designed to meet each instructor's style and level of teaching, including ready-to-use slides that can be easily adjusted to add or remove content.
- The slides help to ease the transition from previous books to *Contemporary Clinical Immunology and Serology*.
- The test bank of almost 600 questions enables instructors to design exams.
- A fast-paced, game-style review for each chapter section and a cummulative one for the entire text allows competing teams to earn points of varying values for correct answers.
  - Competition is a great way to learn, and this repetitive review helps bring the material from short-term memory to long-term memory.
- A companion website
  - Contains any needed updates to the text material.
    - Clinical laboratory immunology is a rapidly changing field with constant updates in technical elements, diagnostic approaches, and understanding of the complexities of health and disease.
    - These updates keep the text contemporary and pertinent through interactions with clinical laboratories, clinical laboratory publications such as *Advance for Medical Laboratory Professionals*, *LabQ* (American Society of Clinical Pathologists), and *Clinical Diagnostic Laboratory Immunology* (American Society of Microbiology).
- Instructors Resource Manual
  - Contains 11 laboratory exercises that illustrate the course material and can be used as an online laboratory manual.
    - Some of these laboratory exercises also appear in the text, for example, Chapter 6 (immunodiffusion), Chapter 8 (serial dilution), and Chapter 10 (latex agglutination, immunofluorescence),
    - Other laboratory exercises not in the texbook complement the material in it. These include serum protein electrophoresis, immunofixation protein electrophoresis, enzyme immunoassays, venereal disease research laboratory (VDRL) test, rapid plasma reagin (RPR) test, and immunoblot test for Lyme disease.
    - Also included are 100 additional questions that can be used for two laboratory practical examinations.

ACKNOWLEDGMENTS

The labeled immunoassay chapter (Chapter 7) was written after consultation with three area Laboratory Directors, Dr. Daniel Amsterdam (Director, Department of Laboratory Medicine, Erie County Medical Center, Buffalo, New York); James Jarnot (Technical Director of Laboratory Services Catholic Health System, Sisters of Charity Hospital, Buffalo, New York); and Susan F. Howard (Director of Chemistry and Toxicology Laboratory Services, Kaleida Health Systems, Buffalo, New York). They were each kind enough to collect all the immunoassay product inserts so that all the currently utilized assays could be reviewed. We appreciate their help and guidance.

Many thanks to Susan Morey (Figure 8.7(b)) for the serial dilution preparation and for all her help over the last 16 years as my laboratory manager. We would also like to thank Carol Pierce, as she kindly provided the original serial dilution laboratory I adapted for this lab exercise.

Many of the photos of direct and indirect immunofluorescence in Chapter 11 were contributed by Immco Diagnostics, and the authors appreciate the help of Kevin Lawson, Chief Regulatory Officer at Immcodiagnostics.

We appreciate the comprehensive treatment given in Chapter 11 "Organ and Tissue Specific Autoimmunity" which was written by Lucy D. Mastrandrea, M.D., Ph.D. She specializes in pediatric endocrinology and conducts research in diabetes and other endocrine autoimmune disorders. She was an excellent choice as a contributing author for this chapter. We also appreciate the excellent contribution of Kristen Betker, the author of Chapter 21 "Forensic Serology." This chapter is an introduction to the intriguing field of forensic and highlights the importance of immunological techniques for forensic analysis. Kristen is a Forensic Biologist III, and is a supervisor in the DNA section at the Erie County Central Police Services Forensic Laboratory.

The tumor immunology chapter was written after consultation with Beth B. Lynch, Special Chemistry Supervisor, Pathology & Laboratory Medicine, Roswell Park Cancer Institute, Buffalo, NY. The nuclear medicine images were kindly provided by Dr. Dominick Lamonica, Director of Nuclear Medicine, Department of Radiology, Roswell Park Cancer Institute.

The transplantation chapter was written after consultation with Dr. Thomas Shanahan of Immco Diagnostics. He was kind enough to collect all the immunoassay product inserts so that all the currently utilized assays could be reviewed. He also allowed photographs of the equipment and assays in his laboratory and in addition he kindly provided the Figures 14.6 and 14.8.

The fungal and parasite chapter was written with advice from Susan J. Wong, Ph.D., Dipl. A.B.M.L.I. Diagnostic Immunology Laboratory, Wadsworth Center NYSDOH; Eileen M. Burd, Ph.D., DABMM, Director, Clinical Microbiology, Emory University Hospital, Associate Professor, Emory University School of Medicine, 1364 Clifton Rd NE, Atlanta, GA; Susan E. Sharp, Ph.D. DABMM, Director of Microbiology, Kaiser Permanente, Portland, Oregon; Daniel Amsterdam, Ph.D. Professor, Director, Department of Laboratory Medicine, Erie County Medical Center Healthcare Network, Buffalo, NY; and Dr. Fitzroy Orrett, Catholic Health System, Sisters of Charity Hospital.

We would like to thank the late Dr. Mark Wilson for providing the basis for many of the figures in Chapter 9, and Dr. Olga Baker for some of the figures in Chapter 23. Thanks are also extended to Ms. Kshipra Gharpure, Ms. Christine Gaspar and Ms. Nina Thamadilok for modeling for the pictures in Chapter 13 (K.G.) and Chapter 22 (C.G. and N.T.). We would also like to thank Ms. Ginny Gebauer for coming up with the "what's wrong with this picture" concept in Chapter 22.

We would also like to thank Anna Diakun, Julia Abdullah, and Susan Morey for help in proofreading in the later stages of the book.

We understand that it takes a cadre of wonderful collaborators to make the most up-to-date book possible and we thank all the professionals that we have interacted with as we developed this book.

ABOUT THE AUTHORS

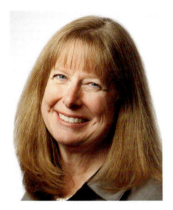

Dr. Kate Rittenhouse-Olson is a Professor of Biotechnology and Clinical Laboratory Sciences, in the School of Medicine and Biomedical Sciences (SMBS) at the University at Buffalo. In 2011, she received the University at Buffalo Faculty Award for Excellence in Mentoring Undergraduates in Research and Creative Activities, and in 2008, she was awarded the SUNY Chancellor's Award for Excellence in Teaching. She has taught the immunology lecture and laboratory course to medical technology and biotechnology students for 20 years. This course is also taken by premed students and other biology majors. She also teaches an immunology course for nuclear medicine students, and teaches immunology lectures for medical, dental and graduate students. She has been editor of the journal, *Immunological Investigations* for 10 years. She has been a section editor for the American Society of Clinical Pathology's teaching case study journal *LabQ* and holds an ASCP certificate as a Specialist in Immunology, ASCP (SI). She is the founding Director of the Biotechnology Program and created the only formal internship program within the SMBS at the University at Buffalo, with ~30 participating companies, and has successfully placed over 200 students in paid internships. She has trained 16 summer high school students (2 Intel semi-finalists, 3 Sidney Farber Cancer Research Awards finalists), 29 undergraduate students since 2000 and has served as major advisor for 42 graduate students. She has ~60 peer reviewed research publications. Her research, funded by the National Institutes of Health, the Department of Defense, the Oishei Foundation, and the Oncologic Foundation of Buffalo, involves studies to improve the immune response to carbohydrate antigens with an emphasis on breast cancer active and passive immunotherapy.

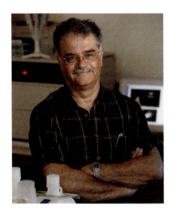

Dr. Ernesto De Nardin is a professor in the Department of Oral Biology and the Department of Microbiology and Immunology in the schools of Medicine and Dentistry at the State University of New York at Buffalo. He teaches immunology and microbiology to first and second year dental and medical students and has acted as a primary mentor for several master students, six Ph.D. students, and five post-doctoral fellows. He is also the director of a Master program and he is actively involved in graduate teaching. He is the associate editor for the journal *Immunological Investigations* and is an editorial board member and reviewer for several peer-reviewed journals. Dr. De Nardin has published over 60 peer-review research articles and book chapters and his research was funded continuously for 21 years by the National Institute of Health. His areas of interest are immunology, inflammation, and the role of genetic polymorphisms in host response. Dr. De Nardin has received numerous awards including the Top 100 Federal Grantees in 2002 and 2005 from the University at Buffalo and a SUNY Chancellor's Award for Excellence in teaching from the State University of New York in 2011.

REVIEWERS

Lisa M Anderson, MHSA, MT (ASCP) SBB
Armstrong Atlantic State University
Savannah, Georgia

Lisa Baker B.S. (ASCP)
Tyler Junior College
Tyler, Texas

Dorothy A. Bergeron, M.S., MLS (ASCP) CM
University of Massachusetts–Dartmouth
North Dartmouth, Massachusetts

Melanie Chapman, M.Ed., MLS (ASCP)
The University of Louisiana at Monroe
Monroe, Louisiana

Janice Costaras, M.S., MT (ASCP) SC
Cuyahoga Community College
Cleveland, Ohio

Daniel P deRegnier, M.S., MT (ASCP)
Ferris State University
Big Rapids, Michigan

Lynne Fantry, MLA, MT (ASCP)
York Technical College
Rock Hill, South Carolina

Dorothy J. Fike, M.S., MLS (ASCP) SBB
Marshall University
Huntington, West Virginia

Amy Lundvall, B.S., MT (ASCP)
Harrisburg Area Community College
Harrisburg, Pennsylvania

Linda E. Miller, Ph.D.
SUNY Upstate Medical University
Syracuse, New York

Valerie Polansky, M. Ed, MT (ASCP)
St. Petersburg College
St. Petersburg, Florida

Diane Schmaus, M.A., MT (ASCP)
McLennan Community College
Waco, Texas

Sherri Sterling B.S., M.B.A., CLS (NCA), MT (ASCP)
University of Massachusetts–Dartmouth
North Dartmouth, Massachusetts

Wendy Sweatt, M.S., CLS
Jefferson State Community College
Birmingham, Alabama

Dick Y. Teshima, MPH, MT (ASCP)
University of Hawai'i at Manoa
Honolulu, Hawaii

Sandra L. Tijerina, M.S., MT (ASCP) SBB, CLSpH (NCA)
University of Texas–Pan American
Edinburg, Texas

M. Lorraine Torres, MT (ASCP), Ed.D.
University of Texas El Paso
El Paso, Texas

Jeffrey Wolz, M.Ed., MT (ASCP)
Arizona State University
Phoenix, Arizona

PART 1
THE SYSTEM AND COMPONENTS

1

Introduction to Immunology

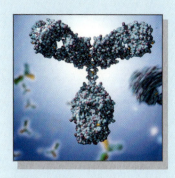

■ OBJECTIVES—LEVEL I

After this chapter, the student should be able to:

1. Define *immunology, immunity, antigen, humoral, serum,* and *plasma.*

2. Give examples of immunity that occurs in simpler species.

3. Compare and contrast the external and internal innate defense systems.

4. Compare and contrast innate immunity and acquired immunity.

5. List factors that affect the innate immune system and describe the resulting effect.

6. Describe the cellular appearance in terms of relative size, nucleus shape, associated CD marker, color when Wright stained, and presence or absence of granules for each of the following cell types: neutrophils, eosinophils, basophils, mast cells, monocytes, macrophages, and dendritic cells.

7. Describe the function(s) of the cell types in (6).

8. Describe the composition of the white blood cells in blood in terms of percentages, and list which cells are found predominately in tissues, not in blood.

9. List the different names for macrophages as they reside in different tissues.

10. Describe phagocytosis and list cells that perform it.

11. Define *phagosome, lysosome, chemotaxin,* and *opsonin.*

12. Describe acute phase proteins and give examples.

13. Describe C-reactive protein, alpha-1 acid glycoprotein, haptoglobin, fibrinogen, and serum amyloid A.

14. Describe cytokines and complement proteins as well as autocrine, paracrine, and endocrine.

15. Describe lymphocytes in terms of amount of cytoplasm, nucleus, product, and antigen specificity.

16. Differentiate between primary and secondary lymphoid organs in terms of functions and organs involved in each.

17. Describe a bursa.

18. Describe the function and architecture of a lymph node, spleen, SALT, and MALT.

19. Diagram lymphatic circulation.

20. Describe the size of a thymus from fetal development to adulthood.

21. Compare and contrast a follicle and a germinal center.

22. Discuss the role of the thymus in T cell maturation.

23. Describe where differentiation and maturation of a B cell occurs from the pre-B cell to a mature B cell and from a B cell to a plasma cell.

24. Explain what a CD marker is, and list CD markers that are on B cells.

25. Identify and discuss the function of the following key antigens on T cells: CD2, CD3, CD4, and CD8.

■ **OBJECTIVES—LEVEL I** (*continued*)

26. Compare and contrast the T-cell receptor on a T cell and the surface immunoglobulin on a B cell.
27. Define *human leukocyte antigen (HLA)* and *major histocompatibility complex (MHC)*.
28. Differentiate T cell subsets on the basis of antigenic structure and function.
29. Explain how natural killer cells differ from cytotoxic T cells.
30. Discuss the principles involved in the analysis of cells by flow cytometry.
31. Analyze data obtained using a flow cytometer.
32. Interpret the use of gating in a particular flow cytometer analysis.
33. Apply the information in this chapter concerning CD markers on particular cell types, and evaluate the significance of flow scattergram data.
34. Define *apoptosis*.

■ **OBJECTIVES—LEVEL II**

After this chapter, the student should be able to:

1. Name seven types of pathogen-associated molecular patterns that trigger the innate immune response.
2. Describe pathogen recognition receptors.
3. Describe Toll-like receptors.
4. Describe antimicrobial peptides, and name two families.

KEY TERMS

acquired immune system
acute phase proteins
acute phase reactants
adaptive immune system
alpha-1 acid glycoprotein
antigen
antigen presentation
antimicrobial peptides
autocrine response
basophil
bone marrow
C-reactive protein (CRP)
cathelicidins
chemotactic factors
complement proteins
complement system
cytokine
defensins
dendritic cells
diapedesis
endocrine response
eosinophil
fibrinogen
flow cytometry
haptoglobin

humoral
immune system
immunity
immunology
inflammation
innate immune system
lectins
macrophages
mast cells
natural immune system
natural killer (NK) cells
neutrophils
opsonin
paracrine response
pathogen-associated molecular patterns (PAMPs)
pattern recognition receptors (PRRs)
phagocytosis
plasma
polymorphonuclear leukocyte
serum
serum amyloid A
T cells
Toll-like receptor (TLR)

▶ INTRODUCTION

When you registered for a course in immunology or decided to read a book about immunology, you may have thought that you would be studying a lot about vaccines. As you opened this book and perused the chapter titles, you probably realized that there is much more to immunology than vaccines, and I can wholeheartedly agree with this conclusion. The immune system is a complicated and wondrous thing to learn about. The knowledge that we have gained about the immune system not only helps us prevent diseases with vaccines, but also helps us diagnose disease and develop drugs to thwart it. New inroads to understanding the immune system continue to help improve health. I hope you enjoy your journey through this book and all your studies of immunology and serology.

Immunology is the study of the reaction when the host encounters a foreign substance. The foreign substance responded to is called an **antigen. Immunity** is the discrimination between self and nonself and the subsequent protection from nonself. The system in an individual that is related to this response is called the **immune system.**

Because every living thing on this planet can be invaded, vertebrates and invertebrates alike needed to develop defense mechanisms. An early evolutionary example of the presence of an immune system includes the fact that some bacteria add a methyl group to their DNA, and if they are invaded by the injection of DNA from a *bacteriophage* (a virus that attacks bacteria), bacterial enzymes will destroy the nonmethylated DNA (Figure 1.1 ■). Another example of a primitive immune system was discovered as a result of an experiment in which a blue sponge and a red sponge were placed in a blender to dissociate them into single cells. These cells were then poured back into an aquarium. If there had been no recognition of the difference between self and nonself, the formation of a purple sponge or a mosaic sponge would have been expected. However, because of self-recognition, the actual result was the formation of a blue sponge and a separate red sponge (Figure 1.2 ■). The self-recognition in the sponges involves surface carbohydrates and lectin interaction. **Lectins** are molecules that specifically bind to carbohydrates. Many

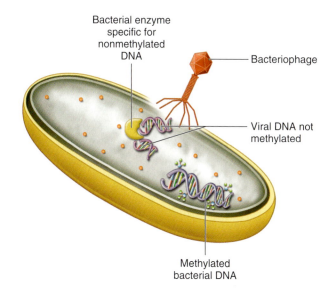

■ **FIGURE 1.1** Bacterial immunity. Bacterial enzymes destroying nonself DNA which entered in an attack by a bacteriophage virus.

other examples of immunity in earlier species exist, and it is important to realize that many of the primitive mechanisms of self-recognition and protection have been maintained in vertebrates where they have been augmented with additional protective mechanisms.

The study of the immune system begins with its separation into the **innate** or **natural immune system** and the **acquired immune system.** The hallmarks of the innate immune system are that it is *available quickly* and is *not specific* for the pathogen in question. Thus, an innate immune response to the measles virus could also work against the influenza virus. The hallmarks of the acquired or **adaptive immune system** are that it is *specific,* has a large *scope,* can *discriminate,* and has a *memory.* The *specificity* engenders a reaction to a particular pathogen without reaction to nonrelated structures. *Scope* involves the fact that the acquired or adaptive immune system is diverse enough that it can react to many different pathogens and molecules, including pathogens that

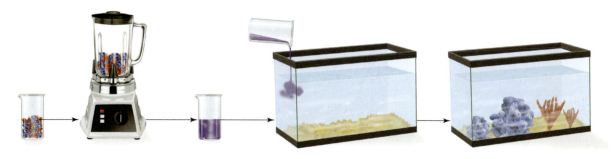

■ **FIGURE 1.2** When a red sponge and a blue sponge are blended together, they reaggregate, not as a purple or mosaic sponge but as a red sponge and a blue sponge because the individual cells recognize self-surface molecules and aggregate.

✪ TABLE 1.1

The Innate and the Acquired Immune Response

Type of Response	Specificity	Molecules Involved in Recognitions	Cells Involved	Time to Response	Memory (enhanced response with next interaction with the same antigen)	Effector Molecules
Innate	Specific to certain patterns recognized in many pathogens called *pathogen-associated molecular patterns (PAMPs)*	*Pattern recognition receptors (PRRs)* can be cell surface or in solution; an important cell surface receptor family is called the *Toll-like receptor* family	Neutrophils, dendritic cells, monocytes, macrophages, mast cells, basophils, eosinophils, and NK cells	Minutes to hours	No	Cytokines Antimicrobial peptides Acute phase proteins Complement Perforins
Acquired	Highly specific; recognizes epitopes with an exact fit	Antibody in solution and on the surface of B cells T-cell receptors on the surface of T cells	Lymphocytes B cells and T cells with antigen presenting cells	Days	Yes	Antibody Cytokines Perforins

have not yet evolved. The concept that the acquired immune system can *discriminate* is based on the fact that the immune system will produce a response only to those molecules that are not present naturally in the individual; that is, there is discrimination between what is self and what is nonself. The acquired immune response improves with subsequent exposure to the pathogen, and this *memory* of the response is the basis of the success of vaccines (1, 2, 3, 4, 5, 6, 7). Table 1.1 ✪ summarizes differences between the innate and the acquired immune response.

Checkpoint! 1.1

A thorn carrying bacteria and a fungus pierces your skin while you are gardening. Cells come and gobble up (phagocytize) the bacteria and the fungus immediately. From what you just learned about the innate and acquired immune system, were these cells from the innate or acquired immune system?

▶ THE INNATE IMMUNE SYSTEM

A piece of meat that you left out on the counter during a hot day would smell of decay by the time you got home. This piece of meat has neither an innate nor an acquired immune system and, thus, would be rapidly invaded. Because you do have these systems, you can be confident that you will not be invaded by bacteria of decay during a normal day. The parts of the innate immune system involved in this protection are those things that separate the inside of the human body from the outside. The innate immune system has components that function at

the interface between the external world and the individual in addition to internal components that protect after entry.

▶ THE INNATE IMMUNE SYSTEM COMPONENTS OF THE EXTERNAL/ INTERNAL INTERFACE

The external components that prevent entry of pathogens include the physical and chemical barriers formed by skin, mucous, and the associated cilia, earwax, lysozyme in tears, and the acidic pH of sweat, stomach acids, urine, and vaginal fluids (Figure 1.3 ■). The normal bacteria of your skin and gastrointestinal tract are also part of the innate immune system. Skin serves as a barrier, and mucous and earwax serve to entrap pathogens prior to entry. Cilia in the respiratory tract push out the invaders, and the reflex that causes coughing and sneezing help push invaders away from the host (Figure 1.4 ■). *Lysozyme* is an enzyme present in tears and saliva that digests the cell wall of gram-positive bacteria. The acidic pH of many fluids inhibits the survival and growth of pathogens. When these innate systems are not intact, an opportunity exists for the entrance of pathogens. It is obvious that there is an increased risk of infection when there is a break in the skin, but what about a pH change? Do you think this pH change would allow for pathogen growth? The answer is yes. For example, previous vaginal douches that were at neutral pH caused a decrease in vaginal acidity, which was thought to increase susceptibility to infection. The next time you are in a store that sells vaginal douches, notice that most brands now say "pH adjusted," "contains

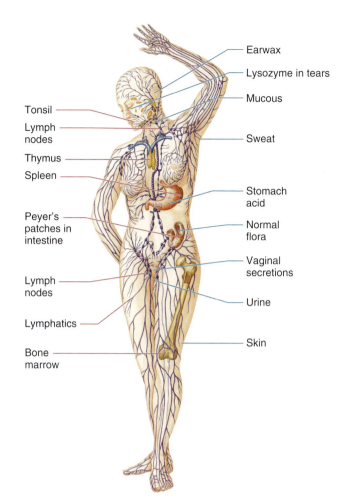

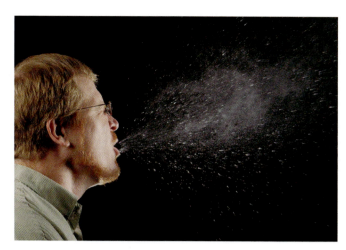

■ **FIGURE 1.3**   (a) Blue arrows (right side): External components of the innate immune system: human body with skin, mucous and the associated cilia, earwax, lysozyme in tears; the acid pH of sweat, stomach acids, urine, and vagina fluids; and the normal bacteria of the skin and gastrointestinal tract labeled. (b) Red arrows (left side): organs of the acquired immune system: tonsil, lymph node, thymus, spleen, Peyer's patches, lymphatics, bone marrow. *Source:* "Human Body image" by Joanna Cameron. DK Human Body Books, reprinted by permission of Dorling Kindersley.

vinegar," or some other expression that indicates that they will not change the protective low pH of the vagina. However, even with this lower pH, vaginal douches still disrupt the mucous layer and the normal flora of the vagina. Perhaps because of this disruption of the innate immune system, vaginal douching has been linked to bacterial vaginosis, pelvic inflammatory disease, cervical cancer, and increased transmission rates of HIV (8).

The normal bacteria that colonize an individual are called their *normal flora*. Alteration of the normal flora through the use of antibiotics can upset the balance in an area and lead to an infection with a pathogen that normally would not be able to grow. An example of this is the gastrointestinal distress that can result after treatment of strep throat or any infection with

an antibiotic. Because antibiotics work systemically, the bacteria in the throat are not the only ones killed, and the removal of the normal gut flora can result in overgrowth of resistant bacteria and the resultant nausea and diarrhea. We will not talk much more about innate defenses, but their importance should not be forgotten.

THE INNATE IMMUNE SYSTEM INTERNAL COMPONENTS

The internal components of the innate immune system include both a cellular and a molecular component that is in the fluid phase of the blood. This fluid phase is called the **humoral** component of the blood, and when blood has been allowed to clot, the fluid phase is called **serum.** If anticoagulants have been added, the fluid phase is different and is called **plasma.** Clotting factors are no longer in the serum because they have joined the clot, but these factors remain in plasma because the blood was not allowed to clot. These internal components of the innate immune system categorized into the cellular components and the humoral components will be discussed separately.

The Cells of the Innate Immune System

The cells of the innate immune system are all white blood cells and include granulocytes (neutrophils, eosinophils, and basophils), monocytes/macrophages, mast cells, dendritic cells, natural killer (NK) cells, and lymphokine-activated killer (LAK) cells. Surface proteins of white blood cells are used along with the cells' microscopic appearance to characterize and differentiate the cells. These surface protein markers were identified using monoclonal antibodies and are numbered beginning with the designation CD for *cluster of differentiation*. An example of the use of CD markers is the commonly used term, the CD4/CD8 ratio, to discuss an AIDs diagnosis (9, 10, 11).

All white blood cells express CD45. Granulocytes, which express CD45 and CD15, have granules in their cytoplasm

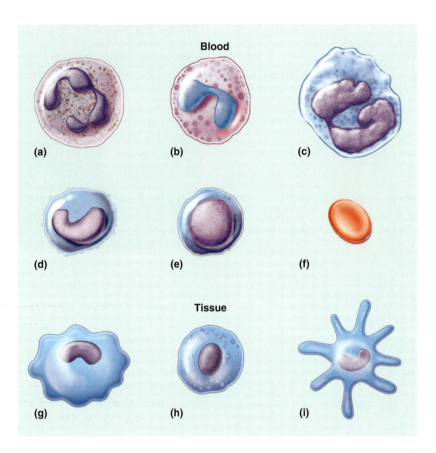

Blood

(a)   (b)   (c)

(d)   (e)   (f)

Tissue

(g)   (h)   (i)

■ **FIGURE 1.5**   The blood cells are shown in (a)–(f) and the tissue white blood cells are shown in (g), (h), and (i). The 3 types of granulocytes: (a) neutrophils, (b) eosinophils, and (c) basophils. As well as a (d) monocyte, (e) lymphocyte, and (f) red blood cell. Next are white blood cells of tissue: (g) macrophage, (h) mast cells, and (i) dendritic cells. *Source:* GOODENOUGH, JUDITH; MCGUIRE, BETTY A., BIOLOGY OF HUMANS: CONCEPTS, APPLICATIONS, AND ISSUES WITH MASTERINGBIOLOGY®, 4th, ©N/A. Printed and Electronically reproduced by permission of Pearson Education, Inc., Upper Saddle River, New Jersey.

(see Figure 1.5 ■ for the three types of granulocytes (neutrophils, eosinophils, and basophils) as well as monocytes, mast cells, and macrophages, which are shown with a lymphocyte and a red blood cell for relative size comparisons). The three types of granulocytes are named for their characteristic staining pattern when using Wright's stain. All granulocytes can be recruited from the blood by chemotaxic factors to enter the tissues that stimulate them to move to the site of an infection. **Neutrophils** are the most abundant type of granulocyte, and they contain neutrally staining granules, that is, their granules do not stain when Wright's stain is utilized. Fifty to 70% of white blood cells in the blood are neutrophils. The nucleus of a neutrophil is irregular in shape with multiple lobes, which gives the neutrophil the alternative name **polymorphonuclear leukocyte** with the shortened names of either *polys* or *PMNs*. Neutrophils are the first cells that enter the site of an acute infection. They reside only about 12 hours in the circulation or one to two days after migration to the tissue. These cells are in the pus of an infected area, and eventually macrophages come into the infected area as well. Neutrophils are very active in **phagocytosis** (engulfment and digestion) of foreign cells and particles. They have recently been found to be involved in the presentation of the antigen to **T cells,** which is one type of cell of the acquired immune system. **Antigen**

presentation, is a process in which a cell of the innate immune system shows or presents the antigen to the cells (lymphocytes) of the acquired immune system. The numbers of neutrophils can increase in an acute infection or inflammation. The **eosinophil** contains red-stained granules after Wright's staining, which indicates that the granules are acidic. These cells are involved in antiparasitic responses and allergic reactions. The numbers of eosinophils can increase during an allergic reaction, parasitic infection, and skin inflammation. In blood, 1 to 3% of the white blood cells are eosinophils. The **basophil,** the rarest of the granulocytes, composes only 0.4 to 1% of white blood cells. The numbers of basophils can be elevated in leukemia, in some allergic responses, in patients with chronic inflammation, and in patients following radiation therapy (9, 10, 11). After Wright's staining, basophils have blue-black-stained granules, indicating that the granules are basic. The function of basophils is not completely defined, but we do know that they play a role in inflammation and allergy.

Mast cells are very similar in appearance to basophils but come from a different lineage. Mast cells have a surface receptor that binds IgE (the antibody molecule involved in allergy) with a high affinity, and this relates to their primary role in allergic and antiparasitic reactions. Mast cells contain granules of histamine and heparin and, when bound to IgE, are responsible for most of the effects in allergic reactions. Mast cells are found in tissues and connective tissues and near mucosal surfaces (9, 10, 11).

Macrophages express CD14 and are the largest white blood cell. They are called *monocytes* while they are in the blood, and when they travel to tissues, they are called *macrophages*. Macrophages are called *Kupfer cells* in the liver, *microglial cells* in neural tissue, *histiocytes* in connective tissue, *osteoclasts* in the bone, *mesangial* cells in the kidney, and either *alveolar macrophages* or *dust cells* when they are in the lungs. When macrophages have accumulated lipids in an arterial wall in a plaque of atherosclerosis in coronary artery disease, they are called *foam cells*. Of the white blood cells in blood, 4 to 6% are monocytes. The number of monocytes in the blood can increase in infection, inflammation, and certain cancers. The life span of a macrophage can be several months. These cells, like neutrophils, are very important in phagocytosis of pathogens. Macrophages are more important in antigen presentation than neutrophils (9, 10, 11).

Dendritic cells, which express CD11c, are found in an immature state in the bloodstream and in a mature state in tissues. The concentration of these cells is very low, but they are very active and efficient in immune processes including phagocytosis and antigen presentation. Dendritic cells are named for the long branching processes that they project (9, 10, 11).

Natural killer (NK) cells are lymphocytes similar to the T and B lymphocytes of the acquired immune system. Unlike B or T cells, however, NK cells do not have the epitope-specific surface receptors of the B cells (immunoglobulin) or T cells (the T-cell receptor), so they are not antigen specific. NK cells are larger and more granular than T or B cells and make up about 10 to 15% of the peripheral blood lymphocytes or about 2 to 3% of the white blood cells of the peripheral blood. NK cells are recognized for their ability to kill tumor cells and virally infected cells but can also respond to bacterial and protozoal infections. NK cells make direct contact with their target and secrete cytotoxic proteins, including perforins and granzymes, which kill the target cell. Perforins function just as their name suggests, by perforating the target cell, causing leakage and lysis. The markers used to differentiate NK cells from other white blood cells are that NK cells are CD3 negative and CD56 and CD16 positive. Because CD16 is a molecule that binds antibody by its Fc region, its presence enables NK cells to bind antibody-coated target cells and kill them by a process called *antibody directed cellular cytotoxicity (ADCC)*. This is one of many places in which the innate immune system works with the adaptive immune system to remove pathogens. A 2009 paper suggests that in addition, NK cells may have memory, thus having some components of the innate immune response and some components of the acquired immune system (12). NK cells also have a surface receptor for a cytokine called *IL-2*, and once they interact with this cytokine, they change and become LAK cells. These cells are much more efficient at killing their target, than NK cells, and partially successful trials have involved the use of LAK cells in cancer therapy. LAK cells also produce cytokines, which increase the immune reaction of other cells. See Table 1.2 for a summary of information about the cells of the innate immune system (9, 10, 11).

✓ **Checkpoint! 1.2**

Which is the largest white blood cell? [Hint: This type of cell has a different name for every tissue it is in.]

⭐ **TABLE 1.2**

The Cells of the Innate Response

Cells of the Innate Immune System	Relative Percent of White Blood Cells in Peripheral Blood	Primary Function	Surface Markers Used to Characterize
Granulocytes neutrophils	50–70%	Phagocytosis—first cell at an infection Antigen presentation	CD15+
Granulocytes eosinophils	1–3%	Allergic and antiparasitic responses	CD15+
Granulocytes basophils	0.4–1%	Not completely defined but have a role in allergy and antiparasitic responses	CD15+
Monocytes Macrophages	4–6% Found in tissues	Phagocytosis Antigen presentation	CD14+
Mast cells	Found in tissues	Primary cell in allergy and antiparasitic responses	Receptor for IgE
Dendritic cells	Found in tissues	Phagocytosis and antigen presentation	CD11c+
Natural killer (NK) cells	2–3% also 10–15% of the lymphocytes	Killing of tumor cells, virally infected cells, some bacteria and protozoan	CD56+ CD16+ CD3−
Lymphokine-activated killer (LAK) cells	Present only when NK cells are activated	Improved killing of tumor cells, virally infected cells, some bacteria and protozoan	CD56+ CD16+ CD3−

The Molecules of the Innate Immune System

Three classes of molecules can be discussed in relation to the innate immune system: (1) recognition molecules, termed pattern recognition receptors, (2) molecules produced in response to an infection, which include cytokines, **antimicrobial peptides,** and **acute phase reactants,** and (3) the **complement proteins** (1, 3, 6, 7, 13, 14).

The innate system is not specific in its reaction to a particular pathogen, so how then can the response be against foreign particles rather than self? The answer to this lies in the pattern recognition molecules that are involved in the innate response. The innate immune system recognizes certain surface molecules that are expressed in groups of microorganisms. The patterns that are recognized are called **pathogen-associated molecular patterns (PAMPs).** Common PAMPs include:

1. Bacterial and viral unmethylated DNA containing increased levels of cytosine with a phosphodiester bound to guanine (CpG dinucleotides) (this is reminiscent of the primitive immunity of some bacteria in the introduction section of this chapter).

2. Surface expression of the terminal sugar (saccharide) mannose that is a common feature on microbial glycolipids and glycoproteins but is not terminal on human structures (this is reminiscent of the self-recognition of sponges in the introduction section).

3. Other fungal-associated saccharides.

4. Lipopolysaccharides (LPS) of the gram-negative cell wall.

5. Peptidoglycans and lipotechoic acids of the gram-positive cell wall.

6. Bacterial flagellin.

7. The amino acid N-formylmethionine found in bacteria but not in mammals.

8. Double-stranded and single-stranded viral RNA.

The molecules of the innate immune system that recognize these PAMPs are called **pattern recognition receptors (PRRs),** PRRs can be either on the cell surface or in solution in the serum. Cell surface PRRs can aid in the phagocytosis of a foreign particle. The cell surface binding of PAMPs to PRRs can also cause the release of effector molecules called **cytokines,** which are secreted by cells and interact with receptors on the surface of cells to create a response. Cytokines can act on the cell that produced them (**autocrine response**), on nearby cells (**paracrine response**), or on distant cells (**endocrine response**) (1, 3, 6, 7, 13, 14). Cytokines will be discussed in more depth in Chapter 4, Cellular Immunity.

An important set of cell surface PRR is called the **Toll-like receptor (TLR)** family of molecules. Each of the 12 different types of Toll-like receptors binds a different PAMP. Binding to any of these molecules causes inflammation, immune cell proliferation, and chemotaxis. The PRRs in solution include

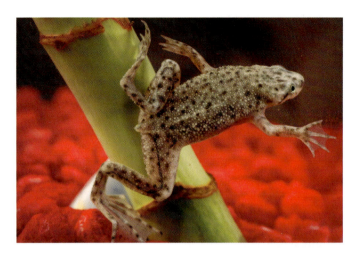

■ **FIGURE 1.6** There is a species specificity to some infections, which involves cell surface molecule recognition. But do not be too complacent, some diseases can be transmitted from other species. This photo is of an aquarium water frog. In 2009, the CDC investigated diarrhea caused by Salmonella associated with contact with water frogs. *Source:* © CDC/Christine Prue.

an acute phase protein called *C-reactive protein.* This protein binds PAMPs and triggers complement binding and phagocytosis of the particle.

Because the ability of a pathogen to infect the host cells is also regulated by recognition of certain surface molecules, a bacterium or a virus has the ability to react with cells bearing certain molecules on their surfaces and will not infect cells that do not express these molecules. The combination of the rapid sequestering of certain pathogens by the innate immune system and the fact that pathogens can infect only cells with certain surface molecules leads to the fact that many infections are species specific, so you will not get the same diseases as your goldfish—no ick (a common goldfish disease) for us. However, do not be too complacent, some diseases can spread from animals to humans. Shown in Figure 1.6 ■ is an aquarium water frog, and such animals have been linked by the CDC to the spread of diarrhea caused by Salmonella (1, 3, 6, 7, 13, 14)!

The antimicrobial peptides produced by the innate immune system in response to infection are usually less than 100 amino acids in length. Similar peptides are found as far back in evolution as prokaryotes. Antimicrobial peptides bind to the cell wall of the microbe and increase the membrane permeability to ultimately cause the pathogen's death. Two major families of antimicrobial peptides in humans are **defensins** and **cathelicidins.** These peptides have very different secondary structures but have a similar function. Both are produced by epithelial cells and phagocytes and provide protection from outside attacks at all epithelial surfaces from the mouth to the anus (1, 3, 6, 7, 13, 14).

The **acute phase proteins** are proteins whose concentrations change with an inflammation, and the levels of these proteins can either be increased or decreased by the inflammation. The elevation of these proteins can cause the increase in

↑ app = ↑ ESR

erythrocyte sedimentation rate (ESR) that is seen with inflammation. The cytokine IL-6 stimulates the production of acute phase proteins, which include C-reactive protein, alpha-1 acid glycoprotein, haptoglobin, fibrinogen, serum amyloid A, and complement proteins (which are discussed separately). An acute phase reactant that is frequently used to assess inflammation is C-reactive protein, the PRR mentioned earlier.

C-reactive protein (CRP) was so named because it reacts with the C-polysaccharide of *Streptococcus pneumonia*. Sensitive assays for increases in this marker have recently been approved to measure risk of cardiovascular disease. CRP is a sensitive indicator of inflammation, rising up to 1000 fold quickly after inflammation and rapidly falling when the inflammation resolves. This marker is involved in the immune system at many levels: It activates complement, is an **opsonin,** and this enhances cell-mediated cytotoxic effects on the pathogen. **Alpha-1 acid glycoprotein** is found to be elevated in some autoimmune disorders. Like many of the acute phase proteins, the liver produces alpha-1 acid glycoprotein. Its primary function may be the inhibition of progesterone and other drugs. It has also been called *orosomucoid*. **Haptoglobin** is an acute phase protein that removes free hemoglobin that has been released through injury and red blood cell lysis. The haptoglobin molecule acts as an antioxidant. **Fibrinogen** is an acute phase protein molecule that is involved in the coagulation pathway. It is converted to fibrin and then fibrin is cross-linked to form a clot. **Serum amyloid A** is an *apolipoprotein,* which is associated with high-density lipoprotein (HDL) in the blood stream. Serum amyloid A is involved with the transport of cholesterol to the liver and in the induction of extracellular matrix degrading enzymes that are involved in repair after infection-induced tissue damage. Additionally, it is a chemoattractant, bringing cells of the innate and acquired immune systems to the site of the infection (1, 3, 6, 7, 13, 14).

The **complement system** contains about 25 proteins; with the origin of some of these proteins found back as far as insects in evolution. Within this system, the roles of the innate and the acquired immune system are truly blended. Three pathways of activation of complement proteins exist: the classical pathway, the alternative pathway and the lectin pathway. These pathways differ in the way that the C3 convertase is formed, and after this step, the pathways are the same with a cascade of proteins each in turn activating other proteins until pathogen lysis occurs. The *classical pathway* functions only with antibody bound to antigen at the onset, so this pathway is linked to the acquired immune system. The *alternative pathway* begins with the spontaneous hydrolysis of some of the C3 that is in the serum, which may bind to surfaces of bacteria, fungi, viruses, or tumor cells and subsequently bind the next molecules of the pathway. The *lectin pathway* begins with the binding of a mannose binding lectin (a PRR) to the mannose on the surface of the pathogen. The mannose-binding lectin is associated with enzymes that bind and cleave the complement component C4. The cleaved C4 subsequently binds to C3 and, thus, complement is activated. Complement will be discussed further in Chapter 4 (1, 3, 6, 7, 13, 14). See Table 1.3 for a summary of the information about the molecules of the innate immune response (1, 3, 6, 7, 13, 14) and Table 1.4 for a summary of the information about acute phase proteins (1, 3, 6, 7, 13, 14).

✓ **Checkpoint! 1.3**

These molecules of the innate immune system can bind to PAMPs.

✪ TABLE 1.3

The Molecules of the Innate Immune Response

Molecules of the Innate Immune System	Targets or Molecules Recognized	Primary Function	Example
Recognition molecules Pattern recognition receptors	Pathogen-associated molecular patterns	Recognition	Toll-like receptors (TLR)
Effector molecules Cytokines	Immune cells	Enhance or decrease immune response	Interleukins Interferons
Effector molecules Antimicrobial peptides	Bacterial cell walls	Protect at epithelial cell surface	Defensins Cathelicidins
Effector molecules Acute phase proteins	Produced in response to infection	Different proteins, different functions Include activating complement to removing free hemoglobin	C-reactive protein Haptoglobin
Effector molecules Complement	3 pathways, recognize (1) surfaces of bacteria, fungi, viruses, tumor cells or (2) mannose (3) antibody bound to antigen	Target cell lysis, improve phagocytosis, increase vascular permeability	Alternative Lectin or classical pathways

☻ TABLE 1.4

Acute Phase Proteins

Acute Phase Reactant	Primary Function
C-reactive protein	Activates complement
	Is an opsonin
	Enhances cell-mediated cytotoxic effects on the pathogen
Alpha-1 acid glycoprotein	Binds drugs and hormones and inhibits their function
Haptoglobin	Clears free hemoglobin
Fibrinogen	Forms clot
Serum amyloid A	Binds cholesterol for clearance
	Recruits enzymes to digest the extracellular matrix
	Chemotactic

The Processes of the Innate Immune System

Inflammation is the result of the responses to harmful stimuli, which can be due to physical (heat, cold, pressure), chemical (acids, bases, other irritants), or microbial factors. Inflammation helps bring the response to the site of the infection, helps eliminate it, repairs the damage, and removes any debris caused by the infection or the response. The hallmarks of inflammation are redness, pain, heat, swelling, and sometimes loss of function. Increased vascular permeability brought about by the cells and soluble substances of the innate response can lead to the heat, redness, and swelling, which in turn can cause pain and sometimes loss of function (Figure 1.7 ■).

To describe inflammation in a particular area, the suffix *-itis* is often added to the name of that area, so *dermatitis, meningitis, tonsillitis,* and *carditis* indicate inflammation of the skin, meninges of the brain, tonsils, and heart, respectively. With inflammation, there is an increased blood supply to the area and migration of first neutrophils and then macrophages to the area. The soluble mediators start and stop the inflammation with factors in the coagulation pathway amplifying the reaction. Neutrophils arrive to the site of the inflammation within 30 to 60 minutes; macrophages arrive between 16 to 18 hours later. The cells come to the site as the result of attraction to chemotactic factors at the site. **Chemotactic factors** include those released by microbes and from the coagulation pathway, the complement pathway, cytokines, and other cellular products. After the neutrophils come to the site, they can phagocytize the microbe (1, 3, 6, 7, 13, 14).

Monocytes, macrophages, and neutrophils can move out of the circulation and into the infected tissues by squeezing through the cells of the intact blood vessel walls by a process called **diapedesis.** Once at the site of infection, phagocytosis is the process by which the leukocyte engulfs and digests the microbe or other particle. The cell first becomes attached to the particle, either by PRRs binding to PAMPS, or through

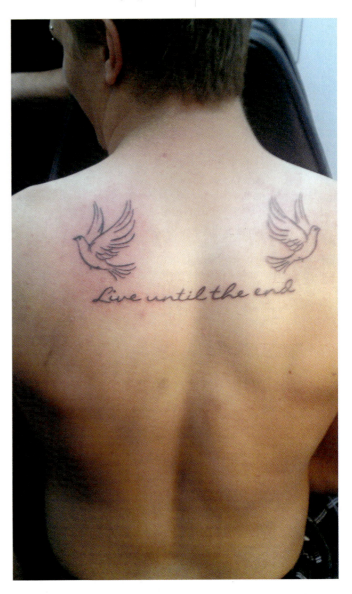

■ **FIGURE 1.7**   Inflammation associated with a new tattoo. Note the redness and swelling. *Source:* Kellee Rogers.

the coating of the particle with opsonins, which are immune factors that enhance phagocytosis. The term *opsonin* is Greek and means *to prepare food for.* These factors, which include breakdown products of complement, C-reactive protein, and antibody molecules, bind to the pathogen and then to receptors on the phagocytic cell in a manner that increases phagocytosis of the particle.

Binding to multiple sites can bring the cell membrane of the phagocytic cell around the particle so that it is completely engulfed. In this way, when the particle is inside the cell, it is surrounded by the cell membrane in a bag called a *phagosome,* which is joined by a second membrane-enclosed bag, this one called a *lysosome,* which is filled with digestive enzymes (Figure 1.8 ■). The new structure formed by the fusion of these two membrane-enclosed bags is called the

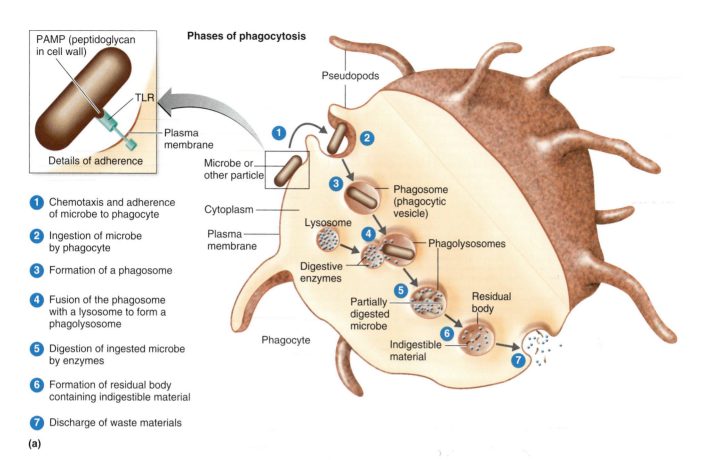

Phases of phagocytosis

PAMP (peptidoglycan in cell wall)

TLR

Plasma membrane

Details of adherence

Pseudopods

Microbe or other particle

Cytoplasm

Plasma membrane

Lysosome

Digestive enzymes

Phagosome (phagocytic vesicle)

Phagolysosomes

Partially digested microbe

Residual body

Indigestible material

Phagocyte

1 Chemotaxis and adherence of microbe to phagocyte

2 Ingestion of microbe by phagocyte

3 Formation of a phagosome

4 Fusion of the phagosome with a lysosome to form a phagolysosome

5 Digestion of ingested microbe by enzymes

6 Formation of residual body containing indigestible material

7 Discharge of waste materials

(a)

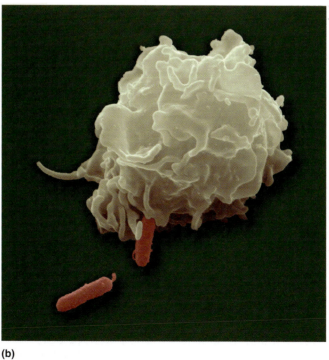

(b)

■ **FIGURE 1.8** (a) The phagocytic process, beginning in the upper left with bacterial attachment and phagocytic cell pseudopod formation, followed by ingestion with the bacteria in a phagosome. The phagosome is joined by a lysosome to create a phagolysosome, the microbe is digested, and waste products are excreted. Some processed peptides from the pathogen may be presented to T cells by this antigen presenting cell. *Source:* TORTORA, GERARD J.; FUNKE, BERDELL R.; CASE, CHRISTINE L., MICROBIOLOGY: AN INTRODUCTION, 10th, ©2010. Printed and Electronically reproduced by permission of Pearson Education, Inc., Upper Saddle River, New Jersey. (b) Scanning electron microscopy showing a phagocytic cell in the process of phagocytizing bacteria. *Source:* © Juergen Berger/Photo Researchers, Inc.

phagolysosome. In this the pathogen is usually killed and broken down by cellular enzymes and the reaction with peroxide anions, hydroxyl radicals, and singlet oxygen produced by a respiratory burst by the phagocytic cell. Some microbes can survive phagocytosis and can actually spread throughout the body while riding in these phagocytic cells (1, 3, 6, 7, 13, 14).

This concludes the discussion of the innate immune system as a separate entity. All further discussions of these cells and molecules will be as they interact with the acquired immune system.

▶ THE ACQUIRED IMMUNE SYSTEM

To begin this section, please remember that the hallmarks of the acquired immune system are that it is *specific,* has a large *scope,* can *discriminate,* and has a *memory.* See Table 1.1 for a summary of the differences between the innate and the acquired immune response.

THE CELLS OF THE ACQUIRED IMMUNE SYSTEM

The key cells involved in the acquired immune response are two types of lymphocytes, the *T lymphocyte* and the *B lymphocyte,* which are also called the *T* and the *B* cells. Lymphocytes are about 20% of the circulating white blood cells and are composed of very little cytoplasm with the resting cell almost full of the nucleus alone. The nucleus can have a slight dent, making it look kidney shaped. These cells get their names from their location of maturation; although they are both derived from the same hematopoietic progenitor, T cells have matured to become T cells in the thymus, while in mammals the B cells have matured to become B cells in the bone marrow and in birds B cells mature in the bursa of Fabricius. This

distinction is important because this easily removable organ in chickens led to the understanding that B cells produce antibody (see Box 1.1 ✪). The acquired immune system is said to have two arms, the humoral and the cellular. The humoral arm is antibody-mediated immunity, and the cellular arm is T-cell-mediated immunity. Both B and T cells recognize antigens through a specific molecule on their surfaces; for the B cell, this is surface immunoglobulin; for T cells, it is called the *T-cell receptor* (2, 4, 5, 6, 7, 8, 10, 15, 16).

ANTIBODY INTRODUCTION—GENERAL STRUCTURE

Antibody molecules are also called *immunoglobulin molecules* and *gamma globulins.* The derivation of the first name is obvious because they have an immune function and are globular proteins, but the second name—*gamma globulin*—takes a little explanation. In serum protein electrophoresis, serum is placed in an electric field in agarose at pH 8.6, and the proteins in the serum, mostly with a negative charge at this pH, are separated into five groups. Albumin is the most anionic protein and thus is the fastest-moving protein toward the anode. Next are the alpha 1 globulins, alpha 2 globulins, then the beta globulins, and finally the gamma globulins (see Figure 1.9 ■). The antibody activity is found in the gamma region, hence, the name *gamma globulins.* The serum protein electrophoresis assay is performed to yield information about certain clinical diseases, such as decreased antibody production (hypogammaglobulinemia) and increased antibody production due to the cancer of antibody-producing cells (myeloma), so this assay will be discussed again later. The 5 types of antibody molecules are IgG, IgM, IgA, IgE, and IgD. There are some similarities between these molecules and some physical differences with the physical differences resulting in biological differences as

✪ BOX 1.1

The Accidental Discovery of the Role of the Bursa in B-Cell Development

The discovery of the role of the bursa for B cell development in birds, was one of the many serendipitous moments in which pivotally important information was discovered accidentally, and not immediately respected. Bruce Glick in 1952 was a scientist in the field of poultry science and was trying to discover the role of the bursa in birds. He had bursectomized several chickens so that he could study the physiologic function of the bursa. A graduate student asked if he could have a few of these chickens to show an undergraduate class that vaccination results in the production of antibodies that can agglutinate Salmonella. A week after this vaccination, much to the hilarity of the undergraduates, when the graduate student mixed the drop of blood with the bacteria nothing happened in the first few samples tried. However, as the graduate student continued, samples from other chickens did agglutinate the bacteria.

The graduate student, Tim Chang, went to talk to Bruce Glick about this and they realized that the animals whose sera did not agglutinate had been bursectomized when they were very young. Further studies showed a link of the bursa to antibody production. Science magazine did not accept this manuscript because they wanted the mechanism explained. This data was subsequently published in the Journal of Poultry Science, and has become a Citation Classic (13).

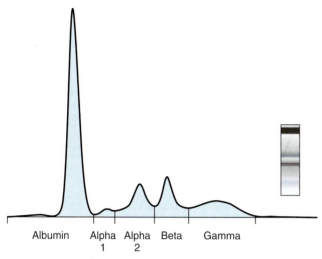

Serum protein electrophoresis

Fractions	%	Reference normal % range	Reference normal concentration range
Albumin	63.0	60.0–71.0	43.00–51.00
Alpha 1	2.1	1.4–2.9	1.00–2.00
Alpha 2	11.2 >	7.0–11.0	5.00–8.00
Beta	11.6	8.0–13.0	6.00–9.00
Gamma	12.1	9.0–16.0	6.00–11.00

■ **FIGURE 1.9** Serum protein electrophoresis is a technique in which serum components separate into 5 different major groups based on their mobility in an electric field. The sample was applied on the right side of the figure. The peak farthest from the origin is albumin, the next contains the alpha 1 globulins, and then the alpha 2, followed by the beta globulins, and finally the gamma globulin peak, which contains the immunoglobulin.

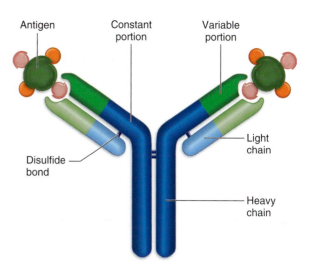

■ **FIGURE 1.10** The basic structure of an antibody molecule. Two heavy chains are joined by two light chains. The antibody contains two binding sites, each of which is formed by a heavy and a light chain. The constant portion of each chain is shown in blue and the variable region in green.

well (Figure 1.10 ■). These will be discussed in Chapter 2. B cells produce antibody in response to the antigen specifically binding to their surface immunoglobulin and can respond to soluble antigen alone. B cells are characterized by this surface immunoglobulin and by the presence of the surface molecules CD19, CD20, and CD21 (2, 4, 5, 6, 7, 8, 10, 15, 16).

 Checkpoint! 1.4

Serum has been taken from a patient and analyzed by serum protein electrophoresis. The patient is immunized with a number of vaccines to prepare for travel and to meet the requirements for college entrance. Blood is drawn 2 weeks later, giving the patient enough time to make antibody. Which peak in the serum protein electrophoresis will be increased?

THE CELLULAR ARM

The cellular arm of the immune response is due to the functions of T cells. T cells respond to antigens that specifically bind to their T-cell receptor (TCR) *and* that are presented by an antigen-presenting cell in either a major histocompatibility

complex (MHC) class I molecule or MHC class II molecule. Additional signals of costimulation through binding of other molecules on the antigen-presenting cells (APCs) and cytokines are also required. The major histocompatibility complex was so named because these antigens were first discovered as a result of their role in the rejection or acceptance (compatibility) of tissue (histo) grafts. These genetically inherited molecules have been found to be important in antigen presentation and in the immune response.

T cells can be divided into helper T cells, cytotoxic T cells, and regulatory T cells. The products of helper T cells are cytokines that can upregulate the immune response; the product of cytotoxic T cells is their direct cytotoxicity (cell killing) of cells bearing the antigen; and the products of regulatory T cells are cytokines that downregulate the immune response when the pathogen is cleared and help prevent autoimmunity. Helper T cells respond to a specific antigen that binds to their TCR in association with the MHC class II molecule, cytotoxic T cells respond to a specific antigen that binds to their TCR in association with the MHC class I molecule, and regulatory T cells bind to their specific antigen through their TCR usually in association with MHC class II molecules but sometimes in association with MHC class I molecules. T cells can be identified by the CD3 marker on their surface, which is part of the T-cell receptor. In addition, helper T cells are CD4+, cytotoxic T cells are CD8+, and regulatory T cells are usually CD4+. CD8+ regulatory cells can also be found with Foxp3+ serving as the marker that characterizes these cells (Figure 1.11 ■) (2, 4, 5, 6, 7, 8, 10, 15, 16). More about these cells and their functions and controls will be described in Chapter 4.

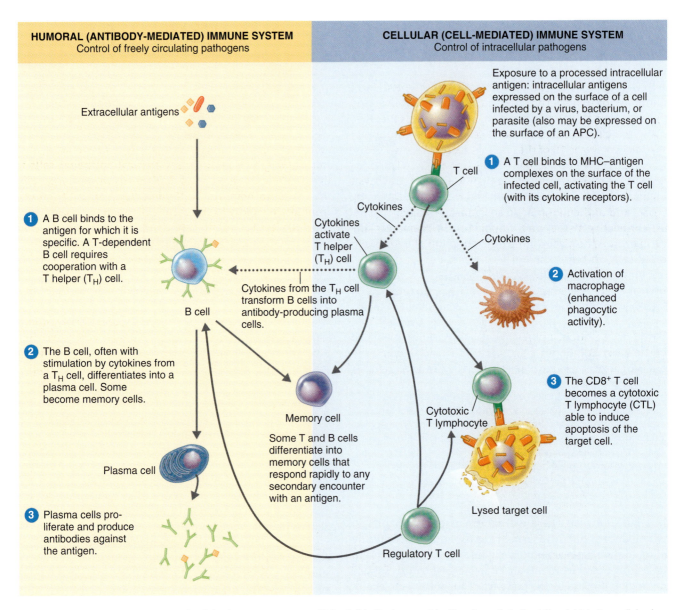

HUMORAL (ANTIBODY-MEDIATED) IMMUNE SYSTEM
Control of freely circulating pathogens

CELLULAR (CELL-MEDIATED) IMMUNE SYSTEM
Control of intracellular pathogens

Extracellular antigens

Exposure to a processed intracellular antigen: intracellular antigens expressed on the surface of a cell infected by a virus, bacterium, or parasite (also may be expressed on the surface of an APC).

T cell

Cytokines

Cytokines activate T helper (T_H) cell

❶ A T cell binds to MHC–antigen complexes on the surface of the infected cell, activating the T cell (with its cytokine receptors).

Cytokines

❶ A B cell binds to the antigen for which it is specific. A T-dependent B cell requires cooperation with a T helper (T_H) cell.

Cytokines from the T_H cell transform B cells into antibody-producing plasma cells.

❷ Activation of macrophage (enhanced phagocytic activity).

B cell

❷ The B cell, often with stimulation by cytokines from a T_H cell, differentiates into a plasma cell. Some become memory cells.

Memory cell

Some T and B cells differentiate into memory cells that respond rapidly to any secondary encounter with an antigen.

Cytotoxic T lymphocyte

❸ The CD8⁺ T cell becomes a cytotoxic T lymphocyte (CTL) able to induce apoptosis of the target cell.

Plasma cell

Lysed target cell

❸ Plasma cells proliferate and produce antibodies against the antigen.

Regulatory T cell

■ **FIGURE 1.11**   The humoral and cellular immune response. At the left is the humoral (or B-cell mediated); at the right is the cellular (or T-cell mediated) immune system. B cells become antibody secreting plasma cells or memory cells with antigen stimulation. T cells are of three general types: (1) helper T cells that secrete cytokines, which upregulate the immune response, (2) cytotoxic T cells that kill target cells after making direct contact with their target, and (3) regulatory T cells, which serve to downregulate the immune response. *Source:* TORTORA, GERARD J.; FUNKE, BERDELL R.; CASE, CHRISTINE L., MICROBIOLOGY: AN INTRODUCTION, 10th, ©2010. Printed and Electronically reproduced by permission of Pearson Education, Inc., Upper Saddle River, New Jersey.

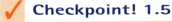 **Checkpoint! 1.5**

Which T cells seem to be on opposite sides of a battle?

▶ THE LYMPHOID ORGANS

The primary lymphoid organs, the bone marrow and the thymus, are where the lymphocytes mature into either T or B cells. Organs in which these white blood cells meet antigens, respond, proliferate, and interact with other lymphocytes are

called *secondary lymphatic organs.* The secondary lymphatic organs include lymph nodes, the spleen, tonsils, mucosal-associated lymphoid tissue (MALT), and skin-associated lymphoid tissue (SALT). MALT includes Peyer's patches in the intestine, tonsils, and the appendix (2, 4, 5, 6, 7, 8, 10, 15, 16).

THE PRIMARY LYMPHATIC ORGANS

The primary lymphoid organs are those in which lymphocytes are generated and the initial differentiation of the lymphoid cells occurs to form mature T cells, B cells, and NK cells. Antigen contact in primary lymphatic organs results in cell death via *apoptosis* (a form of cell suicide), and this process eliminates autoreactive cells (2, 4, 5, 6, 7, 8, 10, 15, 16).

The Bone Marrow

The **bone marrow** is the major site of hematopoiesis after gestation; prior to birth the major sites are the fetal liver and the spleen. Hematopoietic stem cells (HSC) reside in the bone marrow and can become any blood cell type. It is interesting to note that as few as 10 of the HSC can reconstitute all hematopoietic cell types in a lethally irradiated mouse. The bone marrow is the major lymphoid organ, filling the central cavity of all bones. Many cells reside in the bone marrow, including the HSC and all hematopoietic cells, macrophages, stromal cells, connective tissue, and adipocytes. In mammals, the bone marrow is the place for the differentiation of both B cells and NK cells. In birds, the bursa of Fabricius is involved in B cell differentiation. Self-reactive B cells are deleted in the bone marrow by apoptosis (2, 4, 5, 6, 7, 8, 10, 15, 16).

The Thymus

The thymus is a bilobed organ that is below the thyroid and over the heart. It is about 22 grams at birth and increases to about 35 grams at puberty after which it decreases in size. It is largest in proportion to the individual's mass at birth and largest in absolute size at puberty. After puberty, it involutes, and in the adult, the thymus is composed of mostly fat and fibrous tissue. Even though the thymus in the adult appears this way, it still has significant function. Each of the two thymic lobes is broken into lobules. Each lobule has a cortex and a medulla. Lymphoid progenitor cells from the bone marrow enter the thymus at the cortex, and they become immature thymocytes, cortical epithelial cells, and macrophages. Some of these cortical epithelial cells with long extensions have been dubbed the *thymic nurse cells* for their role in helping the thymocytes mature. Thymocytes proliferate rapidly in the cortex. Between the cortex and the medulla are interdigitating dendritic cells, which interact with the thymocytes as they travel toward the medulla. The medulla contains mature and almost mature T cells with medullary epithelial cells, dendritic cells, and macrophages (2, 4, 5, 6, 7, 8, 10, 15, 16). Figure 1.12 ■ shows the structure of the thymus.

Thymocytes begin as CD3−, CD4−, and CD8−, and in the first step in their maturation, T-cell receptors that have either αβ chains or γδ chains develop. The γδ T cells represent a minor population of specialized T cells, which eventually will

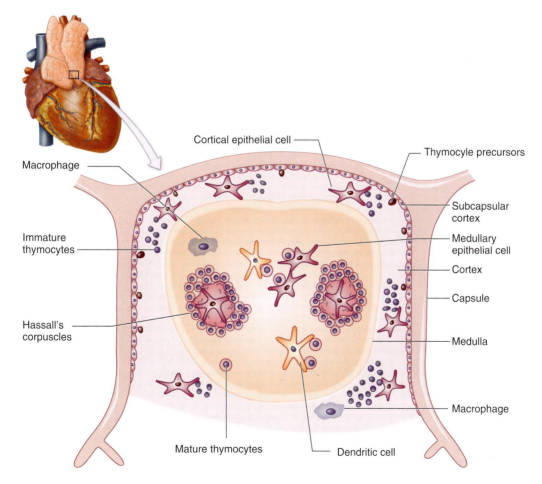

Labels: Macrophage; Cortical epithelial cell; Thymocyte precursors; Immature thymocytes; Subcapsular cortex; Medullary epithelial cell; Cortex; Capsule; Hassall's corpuscles; Medulla; Macrophage; Mature thymocytes; Dendritic cell

■ **FIGURE 1.12**   The thymus, a primary lymphoid organ where T cells mature.

become the T cells of the gut mucosa and the epidermis. They are CD3+, but they are both CD4− and CD8−.

The αβ T cells are first CD3+ and both CD4+ and CD8+ and are called *dual positive.* During maturation, the thymocytes interact in a complex differentiation pathway, which results in the T-cell receptor genetic rearrangement, negative selection of cells that react to self, and positive selection of cells that are able to recognize antigens presented by the class I or class II major histocompatibility molecules. It is thought that only 5% of the entering precursor cells become T cells because of the dual negative and positive selection mechanism after they become CD4+ and CD8+. The T cells further mature and become singly positive for either CD4+ or CD8+. This population is the predominant population of T cells in the body (2, 4, 5, 6, 7, 8, 10, 15, 16).

THE SECONDARY LYMPHATIC ORGANS

In the secondary lymphoid organs, lymphocytes meet trapped antigen and interact with other cells in a manner that can cause them to proliferate. Lymphocytes are antigen specific and direct contact must be made for them to respond to an antigen. Secondary lymphatic are an optimized way of allowing interaction between antigen and the specific lymphocytes. Antigen is brought to the lymph nodes by phagocytic cells and remains trapped there. Lymphocytes circulate through the lymphatic vessels in a fluid called *lymph* that continually recirculates through all of the secondary lymphatic organs. If a relevant encounter occurs, interactions in the secondary lymphatic organs result in B and/or T cell proliferation. The proliferation produces B cells, making the relevant antibody and T cells capable

of a specific cytotoxic or helper response. A maturation of the response through somatic mutation resulting in an increased affinity toward the antigen may also occur (2, 4, 5, 6, 7, 8, 10, 15, 16).

Secondary lymphatic organs include lymph nodes, the spleen, tonsils, MALT (mucosal-associated lymphoid tissue, including Peyer's patches in the intestine, tonsils, and the appendix), and SALT. Lymphatic vessels connect the lymph nodes and help return extracellular fluid from the tissues (2, 4, 5, 6, 7, 8, 10, 15, 16).

The Lymph Nodes

Lymph nodes are located in the areas where lymphatic vessels meet. When you have a sore throat, the lumps in your neck that have increased in size are your cervical lymph nodes and the size increase is brought about by the proliferation of antigen responsive lymphocytes. The lymph nodes are composed of a subcapsular cortex, a paracortex, and an inner medulla. The B and T cells are in different areas in the lymph node with the B cells in the cortex in follicles and germinal centers with macrophages and dendritic cells and with the T cells in paracortical regions with dendritic cells. A follicle becomes a germinal center when the B cells proliferate in response to the antigen. The medullary cords contain macrophages and plasma cells (2, 4, 5, 6, 7, 8, 9, 14, 15, 16). Figure 1.13 ■ shows the structure of a lymph node.

The Spleen

The spleen is located on the upper left side of the body behind the stomach and is about 10 by 5 cm or 2 by 4 inches, increasing in size with infection. Unlike the lymph nodes, which trap

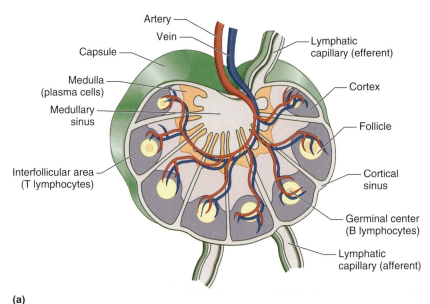

(a)

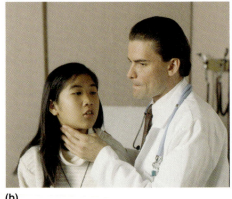

(b)

■ **FIGURE 1.13** (a) Lymph node and (b) the palpation of cervical lymph nodes for enlargement due to infection. *Source:* © Dorling Kindersley.

antigens from the lymphatics, the spleen captures antigens from the blood stream and serves as an area where lymphocytes in the circulatory system can meet antigens. The spleen is surrounded by a thin capsule and is separated into regions of red pulp and white pulp. The red pulp is closest to the capsule and contains red blood cells and macrophages; it functions to remove aged red blood cells. The white pulp forms a coating or sheath (called the *periarteriole sheath*) around the arterioles that enter the spleen. Between the white and the red pulp is an area that contains B-cell-rich follicles and germinal centers (2, 4, 5, 6, 7, 9, 10, 15, 16, 17). See Figure 1.14 ■ for the structure of a spleen.

Mucosa-Associated Lymphoid Tissue

The areas of the body where the inside of the body meets the outside world are often in need of an immune response. These areas are protected by the important MALT (Figure 1.15 ■). MALT includes the respiratory-associated lymphoid tissue (RALT), the gut-associated lymphoid tissue (GALT), and urogenital-associated lymphoid tissue. GALT includes tonsils, the appendix, Peyer's patches, and the lymphocytes, which form the mucosal lining of the gastrointestinal tract. The less common γδ T cells are found in this region. Specialized cells called *M cells* are present in the MALT, which deliver antigens from the lumen by endocytosis to the primary follicles and germinal centers that line the region below the luminal epithelial cells (2, 4, 5, 6, 7, 9, 10, 15, 16).

Skin-Associated Lymphoid Tissue

The skin is an important part of the innate immune system. It contains keratinocytes, which make cytokines, antigen-presenting cells (Langerhans cells, dendritic cells, macrophages, and neutrophils) as well as NK and mast cells. The acquired immune system of the skin is called skin-associated lymphoid tissue (SALT). SALT includes epidermal lymphocytes which contain the less common γδ T cells, and the more usual αβ T cells which can be found in the dermis (2, 4, 5, 6, 7, 9, 10, 15, 16) (see Figure 1.16 ■).

✓ Checkpoint! 1.6

Which two of the following are part of MALT:
SALT, GALT, RALT, ALT?

▶ ASSOCIATED LABORATORY METHOD

The cells of the immune system can be enumerated and differentiated using automated instrumentation in the clinical hematology laboratory. Doing this involves passing the individual cells through a detector and measuring either impedance of conductivity (the ability of cells to block an electric current–yielding cell number, conductivity, and size information) or scattering of light shown through toward the detector (which is blocked to varying extents by cells of different sizes and granularity).

In the clinical immunology laboratory, the analysis of the white blood cells is augmented through the use of fluorescently labeled antibodies to CD markers in flow cytometric analysis using **flow cytometry** (18). This type of analysis is utilized to determine the presence or absence of leukemia, lymphoma, myeloma, HIV, and other immunodeficiency diseases. To perform flow cytometric analysis, heparinized blood is washed, and the cells are pelleted using buffer and heparin and centrifugation. Normal mouse immunoglobulin is added to block nonspecific binding, fluorescently labeled antibodies to the relevant CD markers are added, and the red cells are lysed. The samples are washed and analyzed using a flow cytometer (Figure 1.17 ■).

A flow cytometer analyzes cells through light-scattering and fluorescent emissions after hydrodynamic focusing brings them single file through a laser beam. The amount of forward scatter of the light after it hits the cell is measured and is related to the cell size. The amount of side scatter of the

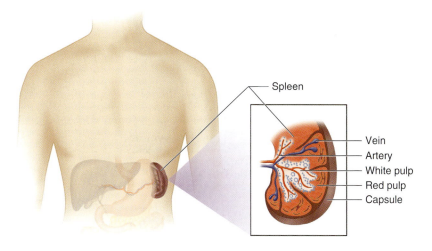

Spleen

Vein
Artery
White pulp
Red pulp
Capsule

■ FIGURE 1.14   The spleen.

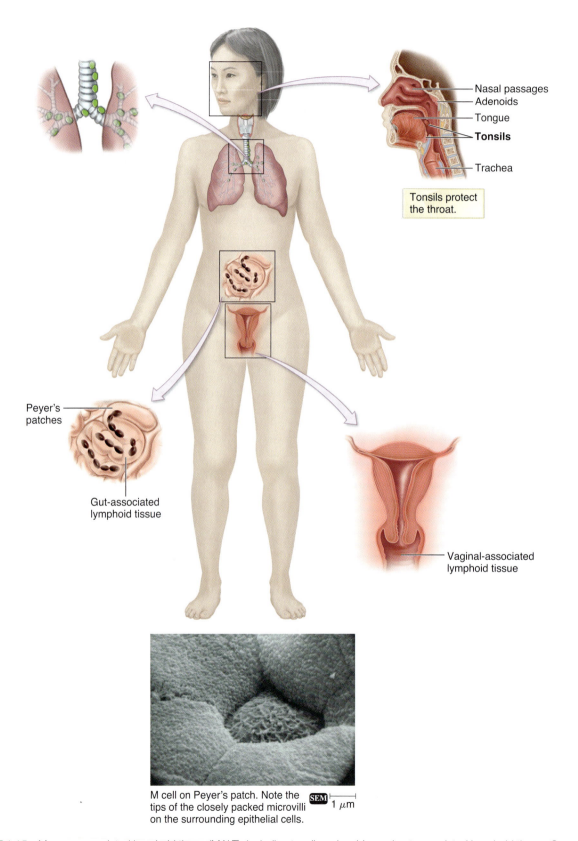

Nasal passages
Adenoids
Tongue
Tonsils
Trachea

Tonsils protect the throat.

Peyer's patches

Gut-associated lymphoid tissue

Vaginal-associated lymphoid tissue

M cell on Peyer's patch. Note the tips of the closely packed microvilli on the surrounding epithelial cells. **SEM** |— 1 μm

■ **FIGURE 1.15** Mucosa-associated lymphoid tissue (MALT), including tonsils, adenoids, and gut-associated lymphoid tissue. *Source:* (a) JOHNSON, MICHAEL D., HUMAN BIOLOGY: CONCEPTS AND CURRENT ISSUES, 5th, ©2010. Printed and Electronically reproduced by permission of Pearson Education, Inc., Upper Saddle River, New Jersey. (b) Kato, T. & Owen, R.L. (2005) in Mucosal Immunology, eds. Mestecky, J., Lamm, M.E., Strober, W., Bienenstock, J. & McGhee, J.R., Mayer, L. (Elsevier Academic Press, San Diego), pp. 131–151.

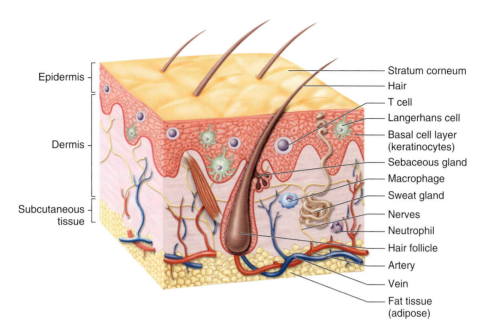

Epidermis

Dermis

Subcutaneous
tissue

Stratum corneum
Hair
T cell
Langerhans cell
Basal cell layer
(keratinocytes)
Sebaceous gland
Macrophage
Sweat gland
Nerves
Neutrophil
Hair follicle
Artery
Vein
Fat tissue
(adipose)

■ **FIGURE 1.16** Skin-associated lymphoid tissue (SALT).

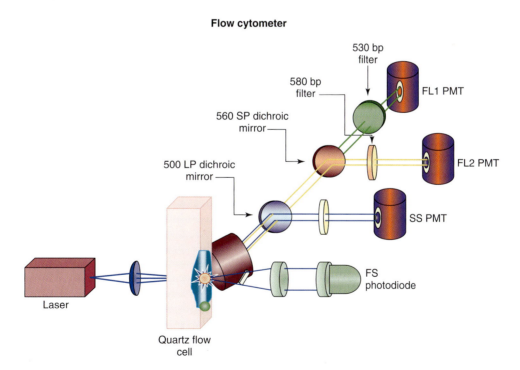

Flow cytometer

530 bp
filter

580 bp
filter

560 SP dichroic
mirror

500 LP dichroic
mirror

FL1 PMT

FL2 PMT

SS PMT

FS
photodiode

Laser

Quartz flow
cell

■ **FIGURE 1.17** Schematic of a flow cytometer. The laser interacts with the cell in the quartz flow cell. Three things happen after the light hits a cell: (1) Some of the light is scattered forward due to the size of the cell and is measured by the forward scatter (FS) photodiode (2) some of the light is scattered due to the granularity of the cell and is measured by the side scatter photomultiplier tube (SS PMT), and (3) the laser light excites the fluorochromes attached to the cell and light emitted from the fluorochrome is measured. The fluorescent light (FL) that is yellowish-orange is measured in the FL2 PMT, and the green light is measured in FL1 PMT.

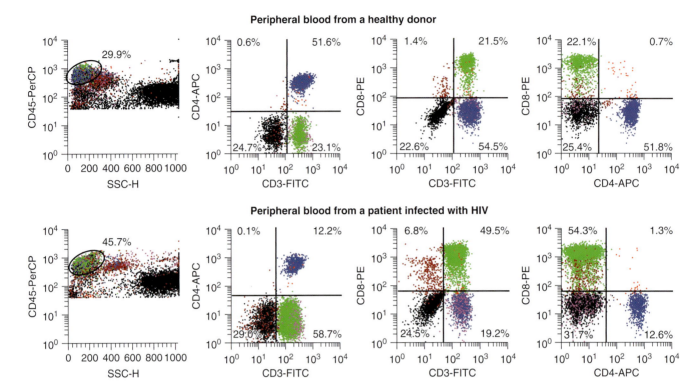

Peripheral blood from a healthy donor

Peripheral blood from a patient infected with HIV

■ **FIGURE 1.18** Flow scattergrams showing results on the top set from a healthy donor and on the bottom set from a patient infected with HIV. The first panel uses CD45, a marker for white blood cells versus side scatter. This panel allows for the gating of white blood cells that have low side scatter—the lymphocytes. All other panels analyze the cells gated in the first panel. The second panel uses CD3, a marker for T cells, and CD4, a marker for helper T cells. The spots in the lower left quadrant represent cells that are negative for both markers. The spots in the upper right quadrant represent cells that are positive for both markers. Those on the upper left are positive for CD4 and negative for CD3. Those on the lower right are positive for CD3 and negative for CD4. Compare the top and bottom set in the second panel and you will see the marked depletion of helper T cells (CD3+ and CD4+) in patients with HIV. The next panel shows the CD3 T cell marker compared with CD8 the cytotoxic T cell marker. In comparing the top and bottom sets, you see that because HIV has caused a depletion of the CD4 cells, the relative number of CD8+ cells in the HIV patient has increased. The last panel shows the lack of CD4 and CD8 dual positive cells. *Source:* Reprinted by permission of Paul Wallace and the Department of Flow Cytometry.

light as it passes through the cell is measured and is related to cell granularity. An example of data that is obtained about white blood cells using a flow cytometer can be seen in Figure 1.18 ■. Two sets of flow scattergrams are shown with the results on the top set from a healthy donor and on the bottom set from a patient infected with HIV. The first panel shows staining with a fluorescent antibody to CD45, which is a marker for white blood cells, and this is plotted versus side scatter. In gating the cells with certain characteristics are selected for further analysis. The gate is the oval around the group that have low side scatter. All other panels analyze the cells gated in the first panel. The second panel uses CD3, a marker for T cells, and CD4, a marker for helper T cells. The dots in the lower left quadrant represent cells that are negative for both markers. The dots in the upper right are quadrant represent cells that are positive for both markers. Upper left are positive for CD4, negative for CD3. Lower right are positive for CD3 and negative for CD4. Compare the second panel in the top versus the one in the bottom and you will see the marked depletion of helper T cells in patients with HIV. The next panel shows the CD3 T cell marker compared with CD8 the cytotoxic T cell marker. Here comparing the top and

bottom panels you see that because HIV has caused a depletion of the CD4 cells the relative numbers of CD8+ cells in the HIV patient has increased. The last panel just shows the lack of CD4 and CD8 dual positive cells (18).

CASE STUDY

On my way home from work, I grabbed the banister on my way up the stairs and got a splinter in my finger. I noticed it but thought that I would take care of it when I got home. When I got home, I made dinner and then worked on some exam questions and forgot about my splinter. The next day the area was red and hot.

1. What was one area of innate immunity that was affected the moment of the entrance of the splinter?

2. What is the red and hot swollen response to the splinter called?

3. I took out the splinter, but I guess I did not clean the area well enough because the next day, pus leaked from the spot. What phagocytic cells of the innate immune response were involved immediately and later?

SUMMARY

Immunology is the study of the host response to a foreign substance. The protection from a foreign substance can be on two levels: (1) the innate or natural response and (2) the acquired immune response. The innate or natural immune response is available quickly, is not specific for the pathogen, and has external components such as the skin and earwax and internal components such as macrophages and acute phase proteins. Pathogen recognition by this system is guided by pathogen-associated molecular patterns that are recognized by pattern recognition receptors. The acquired immune system is characterized by its scope, specificity, memory, and ability to discriminate between similar substances.

The acquired immune system has two arms, the humoral and the cellular. The humoral arm involves antibody molecules that are produced by B lymphocytes. The cellular arm involves the actions of T lymphocytes, helper T cells, cytotoxic T cells, and regulatory T cells. The cells of the acquired immune response differentiate in the primary lymphatics, the bone marrow, and the thymus. In the secondary lymphatics, these cells interact with antigens and further mature and proliferate. Secondary lymphatic organs include the lymph nodes, spleen, the mucosal-associated lymphatic tissue, and the skin-associated lymphatic tissue. The individual cell types can be analyzed utilizing flow cytometry.

REVIEW QUESTIONS

1. Natural or innate immunity is
   a. specific immunity
   b. nonspecific immunity
   c. immunoglobulin
   d. cytotoxic T cells

2. The primary lymphoid organs are the
   a. spleen, lymph node, and tonsil
   b. thymus, bursa of Fabricius, and bone marrow
   c. thoracic duct and vena cava
   d. polymorphonuclear leukocytes

3. Secondary lymphoid organs are the
   a. spleen, lymph node, and tonsil
   b. thymus, bursa of Fabricius, and bone marrow
   c. thoracic duct and vena cava
   d. polymorphonuclear leukocytes

4. MALT relates to the
   a. spleen, lymph node, and tonsil
   b. gastrointestinal and respiratory tract lymphoid tissue
   c. amino terminus of the antibody molecule that contains the paratope
   d. area on an immunoglobulin molecule defined by structure

5. When a phagocytic cell engulfs a bacteria, the bacteria is in the cellular compartment known as
   a. lysosome
   b. chemotaxin
   c. opsonin
   d. phagosome

6. A lymphocyte has
   a. more cytoplasm than nucleus
   b. more nucleus than cytoplasm
   c. equal amounts of cytoplasm and nucleus
   d. segmented nucleus

7. A bursa is where
   a. mammalian B cells develop; a primary lymphoid organ
   b. B cells develop in birds; a primary lymphoid organ
   c. mammalian B cells develop; a secondary lymphoid organ
   d. B cells develop in birds; a secondary lymphoid organ

8. A thymus produces most of its T cells when the person is
   a. in puberty until age 25
   b. in college
   c. elderly
   d. a baby until puberty

9. If I have a bruise on my arm, which acute phase reactant will bind the hemoglobin and bring it to the liver to be cleared?
   a. complement
   b. alpha-1 acid glycoprotein
   c. C-reactive protein
   d. haptoglobin

10. How do some bacteria protect themselves from an invader?
    a. by swimming away
    b. by identifying similar bacteria and staying together
    c. by attacking nonmethylated DNA
    d. by producing antiviral compounds into the surrounding fluid

11. Which cell is a helper cell?
    a. macrophage
    b. B cell
    c. CD4+ T cell
    d. CD8+ T cell

12. A macrophage in the liver is called
    a. microglial cell
    b. alveolar macrophage
    c. histocyte
    d. Kupfer cell

13. A lymphocyte in the innate immune system is called
    a. mast cell
    b. T cell
    c. B cell
    d. NK cell

REVIEW QUESTIONS *(continued)*

14. The patterns that the innate immune system recognizes are called
    a. antigens
    b. epitopes
    c. pathogen-associated molecular patterns
    d. pattern recognition receptors

15. Two families of antimicrobial peptides are
    a. PRRs and PAMPS
    b. defensins and cathelicidins
    c. Toll-like receptors and cytokines
    d. acute phase proteins and complement

16. CD19, CD20, and CD21 are on
    a. NK cells
    b. T cells
    c. macrophages
    d. B cells

REFERENCES

1. Paul WE. The intersection of the innate and the adaptive immune system. In: Paul WE, ed. *Fundamental Immunology*. 6th ed. Philadelphia, PA: Wolters Kluwer/Lippincott Williams & Wilkins; 2008: chap 14.

2. Flajnik MF, Du Pasquier L. Lymphoid tissues and organs. In: Paul, WE, ed. *Fundamental Immunology*. 6th ed. Philadelphia, PA: Wolters Kluwer/Lippincott Williams & Wilkins; 2008: chap 2.

3. Kindt TJ, Goldsby RA, Osborne BA. *Kuby Immunology*. New York, NY: W.H. Freeman and Company; 2006: chap 1.

4. Kindt TJ, Goldsby RA, Osborne BA. *Kuby Immunology*. New York, NY: W.H. Freeman and Company; 2006: chap 2.

5. Kindt TJ, Goldsby RA, Osborne BA. *Kuby Immunology*. New York, NY: W.H. Freeman and Company; 2006: chap 3.

6. Murphy KM, Travers P, Walport M. *Basic Concepts in Immunology in Janeway's Immunobiology*. 7th ed. New York, NY: Garland Science Publishing; 2008: chap 1.

7. Murphy KM, Travers P, Walport M. *Basic Concepts in Immunology in Janeway's Immunobiology*. 7th ed. New York, NY: Garland Science Publishing; 2008: chap 2.

8. Ness RB, Hillier SL, Richter, HE et al. Why women douche and why they may or may not stop. *Sex Transm. Dis.* 2003;30(1):71–74.

9. Williams JL. Hematopoesis. In: McKenzie S and Williams L, eds. *Clinical Laboratory Hematology*. 2nd ed. Boston, MA: Pearson; 2010: chap 3.

10. Laudicina RJ, Simonian Y. The leukocyte. In: McKenzie S and Williams L, eds. *Clinical Laboratory Hematology*. 2nd ed. Boston, MA: Pearson; 2010: chap 7.

11. White blood cell differential count. Lab Tests Online. http://www.labtestsonline.org/understanding/analytes/differential/test.html. Accessed January 16, 2010.

12. Sun JC, Beilke JN, Lanier LL. Adaptive immune features of natural killer cells. *Nature*. 2009. doi: 10.1038/nature07665.

13. Uhlar CM, Whitehead AS. Serum amyloid A, the major vertebrate acute-phase reactant. *Eur. J. Biochem.* 1999;265:501–523.

14. Kiyono H, Kunisawa J, McGhee JR et al. The mucosal immune response. In: Paul WE, ed. *Fundamental Immunology*. 6th ed. Philadelphia, PA: Wolters Kluwer/Lippincott Williams & Wilkins; 2008: chap 31.

15. Akirav E, Liao S, Ruddle NH. Lymphoid tissues and organs. In: Paul WE, ed. *Fundamental Immunology*. 6th ed. Philadelphia, PA: Wolters Kluwer/Lippincott Williams & Wilkins; 2008: section ii, chap 2.

16. Birds, serendipity and red socks make Bruce Glick a poultry legend. *Merial Selections*. 2007;3(2):1–3. http://www.merialselections-digital.com/merialselections/ merialsel2007spring/?pg=2. Accessed February 14, 2011.

17. Hosey RG, Mattacola CG, Kriss V et al. Ultrasound assessment of spleen size in collegiate athletes. *Br. J. Sports Med.* 2006;40:251–254. doi: 10.1136/bjsm.2005.022376.

18. Introduction to flow cytometry. BD Biosciences. http://www.bd.com/videos/bdb/training_ITF/index.html. Accessed January 24, 2009.

PEARSON
myhealthprofessionskit™

Visit www.myhealthprofessionskit.com to access the interactive Companion Website for this textbook. Simply select "Clinical Laboratory Science" from the choice of disciplines. Find this book and log in by using your user name and password to access additional learning tools.

2

Antibody

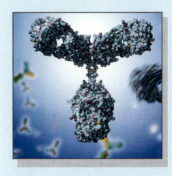

■ OBJECTIVES—LEVEL I

After this chapter, the student should be able to:

1. Draw the basic structure of an immunoglobulin.
2. Define *hinge region*.
3. Draw and label a serum electrophoresis pattern. Explain why the gamma peak is broad.
4. Compare and contrast a polyclonal antiserum with a monoclonal antibody.
5. Describe a myeloma protein and explain how its use aided immunologists.
6. Differentiate between the 5 immunoglobulin types found in humans in terms of chemical, physical, and biological properties.
7. Describe a Bence Jones protein.
8. Compare and contrast the antigenic regions of immunoglobulins, isotype, idiotype, and allotype.
9. Compare and contrast a primary and a secondary immune response.
10. Describe how a monoclonal antibody is produced.

■ OBJECTIVES—LEVEL II

After this chapter, the student should be able to:

1. Draw the result of (1) urea and mercaptoethanol, (2) papain, and (3) pepsin treatment of IgG.
2. Describe how the structure of IgG was elucidated experimentally.
3. Diagram how immunoglobulin diversity occurs within the limits of the amount of DNA utilized, and name the enzymes involved.
4. Solve for the number of antibody-combining sites possible when given the number of V, D, and J heavy chain genes and V and J light chain genes.
5. Compare and contrast antigen-independent diversity and antigen-dependent diversity.
6. Describe how immunoglobulin is purified.

KEY TERMS

affinity	hybridoma cells
allotypic antigen	hypervariable regions
analytical	IgA
ultracentrifugation	IgD
avidity	IgE
complementary determining	IgG
regions (CDRs)	IgM
domain	immunoglobulin
epitope	supergene family
Fab	isotypic determinants
F(ab')₂	light chains
Fc	monoclonal antibody
framework regions	paratope
heavy chains	serology
hinge regions	

▶ INTRODUCTION

Antibody molecules are the products of B cells and are made in response to vaccination and infection. These molecules are key in helping humans fight infection and are vital to many diagnostic tests. Antibodies produced by the patient are used in the clinical laboratory to help diagnose the cause of an infection. Antibodies produced in animals are utilized in laboratory analysis to determine what the infection is by finding the clinically relevant antigen in the patient. **Serology** is the study of the reaction and properties of the serum components of the blood; this science deals mostly with these antibody and antigen reactions *in vitro*. Looking for *antibody* in the patient is important in the diagnosis of infectious disease, allergy, and autoimmune disease. Using antibody to *detect antigen* in the patient's serum, urine, or other body fluids is important in the diagnosis of infectious disease, cancer, pregnancy, illicit drug use, and also in therapeutic drug concentration testing. Antibody molecules are also utilized in research and in the biotechnology industry for many purposes, including determination of the cellular location of antigens, purification of chemicals, and validation of recombinant protein structure. Thus, the antibody molecules that you are about to study are important to many aspects of clinical laboratory analysis, research applications, and biotechnology industrial applications.

▶ GENERAL STRUCTURE

Experiments have been performed to understand the structure and function of immunoglobulin molecules. One of these experiments, serum protein electrophoresis, was described in Chapter 1. In serum protein electrophoresis (SPE), the immunoglobulins, which are the globular proteins with immune function, appear in the gamma, or slowest moving region of

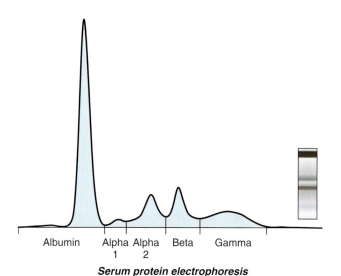

Fractions	%	Reference normal % range	Reference normal concentration range
Albumin	63.0	60.0–71.0	43.00–51.00
Alpha 1	2.1	1.4–2.9	1.00–2.00
Alpha 2	11.2	7.0–11.0	5.00–8.00
Beta	11.6	8.0–13.0	6.00–9.00
Gamma	12.1	9.0–16.0	6.00–11.00

■ **FIGURE 2.1**   Serum protein electrophoresis: Serum placed in an electric field will separate into the 5 regions shown here. The gamma region contains the molecules that bind antigen, the immunoglobulins. A densitometer "reads" the blue gel. When the light goes through the blue area, a peak that corresponds to the density and width of the colored band is seen.

the electrophoretic mobility pattern. In this SPE, the diversity of the immunoglobulin molecules is shown because the gamma peak is broad, rather than narrow as would be seen by a molecule without any diversity. The broadness of the peak is due to the fact that the different binding sites of the immunoglobulin molecules give slightly different electrophoretic mobilities (Figure 2.1 ■).

Analytical ultracentrifugation was utilized to obtain the approximate molecular weight of the various immunoglobulin molecules. A solution containing IgG was placed in a high-speed ultracentrifuge that had optics so that the sedimentation coefficient could be determined. The sedimentation coefficient is related to molecular weight, and the molecular weight was determined before and after treatment with denaturing and dissociating agents. Before treatment with urea, the sedimentation coefficient of IgG was 7S, indicating a molecular weight of 150 000 daltons. The next experiment helped us to understand the structure of the immunoglobulin molecule. When IgG was treated with the enzyme urea to denature it (unfold the molecule) and mercaptoethanol was used to break the disulfide bonds, the molecule changed from a single 7S size sedimentation coefficient in size to 2 different peaks, 1 at 3.5 S and 1 at 2.2 S, corresponding to 50 000 and 22 000 in molecular weight (MW), respectively. Equal amounts of each were produced, and thus it was deduced that the 150 000-dalton molecule was composed of 2 **heavy chains** (50 000 dalton chains) and 2 **light chains** (about 25 000 dalton chains). This work showed that IgG was a 150 000 dalton heterodimer with 2 heavy chains linked to 2 light chains, (H$_2$L$_2$) (1).

The next experiment used 2 different enzymes, papain and pepsin, to study the IgG molecule. IgG treated with papain was broken into 2 different pieces, which were about 50 000 daltons. When these were analyzed, it was found that there was 1 piece that could crystallize (called **Fc** for Fragment crystallizable) that did not bind to the antigen and twice as much of the second piece that could bind antigen (called **Fab** for *Fragment antigen binding*). Thus, areas of different functions were separated with 2 antigen-binding regions for each crystallizable piece. The ability to crystallize involves the homogeneity of this region, and the lack of ability to crystallize showed that IgG molecules purified from serum contain variability in the part of the molecule that bound antigen.

IgG was also treated with pepsin, and the result was (1) a dimeric **F(ab')$_2$** that could cross-link 2 antigens and was slightly more than twice the molecular weight of the Fab and (2) small fragments of the Fc area. The last piece of data needed to determine the structure of the IgG antibody molecule utilized antibody raised in animals against the fragments of the human IgG to deduce the structure. Antibody to the Fab region was found to react with the heavy and light chain, and antibody against the Fc region was found to react against the heavy chain only. Putting all this information together, the structure could be deduced (Figure 2.2 ■), and what was happening during each of these processes could also be deduced (see Figure 2.3(a) ■ IgG after urea and mercaptoethanol, 2.3(b)

IgG after Papain, and 2.3(c) IgG after Pepsin) (1). Knowledge of how these enzymes break apart the immunoglobin molecule is still important because sometimes fragments rather than whole immunoglobulin are used in certain studies and assays.

✓ **Checkpoint! 2.1**

The enzyme with the e in it eats up the Fc region to little bits. Name the enzyme.

The antigen-binding site is at the N-terminal end of both the heavy chain and the light chain. The antigen-binding site is called the **paratope,** and the part of the antigen that it binds is called the **epitope.** The paratope and the epitope are related in a lock-and-key fit. The binding of the epitope to the paratope is by *noncovalent* bonds, which include van der Waals bonds, hydrogen bonds, electrostatic or ionic bonds, and hydrophobic and hydrophilic interactions. The **affinity** of the reaction is the sum of the attractive interactions between the paratope and the epitope. The **avidity** of the reaction is the sum of the binding of all paratopes of the antibody molecule and the epitopes. In the case of IgG, the avidity is twice the affinity because 2 paratopes can bind to epitopes (1, 2, 3, 4, 5, 6, 7, 8).

Further analysis of both the heavy and light chains showed that both contain **domains** of about 110 amino acids with intrachain disulfide bonds that form loops causing a globular

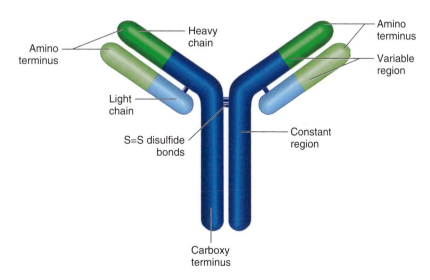

■ **FIGURE 2.2** Schematic of an IgG molecule: Two heavy and 2 light chains are linked together by disulfide bonds. The number and position of the disulfide bonds varies according to the subclass.

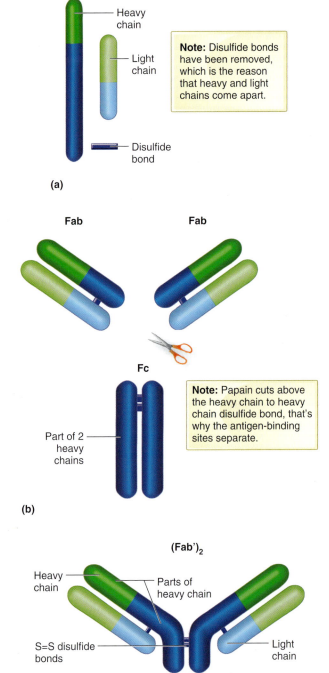

Note: Disulfide bonds have been removed, which is the reason that heavy and light chains come apart.

Note: Papain cuts above the heavy chain to heavy chain disulfide bond, that's why the antigen-binding sites separate.

Note: The enzyme cuts below the disulfide bond, which is the reason that the two antigen-binding sites stay together.

■ **FIGURE 2.3** (a) IgG after treatment with urea plus mercaptoethanol. (b) IgG after treatment with papain. (c) IgG after treatment with pepsin.

area to form. The light chain has 1 domain near the amino terminal end that is called V_L for variable light chain domain and 1 domain at the carboxy terminus end that is called C_L for constant domain of the light chain. The heavy chain has 1 variable domain V_H and 3 or 4 constant domains called C_H1, C_H2, C_H3, and C_H4 with the numbering beginning next to the variable region. The variable regions of different heavy and light chains have different binding abilities due to several **hypervariable regions.** There are 3 hypervariable regions in the V_L and 3 hypervariable regions in the V_H. Stretches in the variable domains between the hypervariable regions are called **framework regions.** The shape of the paratope must be a complement of the shape of the epitope for a good fit for the epitope, so these hypervariable regions are also the **complementary determining regions (CDRs)** (1, 2, 3, 4, 5, 6, 7, 8).

Some of the structural studies of immunoglobulin were facilitated by the discovery of myeloma proteins, which are identical immunoglobulin molecules produced by a clone of tumor cells (myeloma cells) that are plasma cells. These immunoglobulin molecules are identical, containing identical Fab as well as Fc regions. They are a natural type of monoclonal antibody.

▶ CLASSES, SUBCLASSES, AND LIGHT CHAINS

The 5 main classes of immunoglobulin molecules are IgG, IgM, IgA, IgD, and IgE. These classes are based on the different heavy chains of the molecules. The heavy chains are γ, μ, α, δ, and ε, respectively. These immunoglobulin classes all have structural similarities in that they are composed of one or more units of the 2 heavy chains and 2 light chains held together by disulfide bonds as in the structure that was just described for IgG (Figure 2.1; Table 2.1 ✪). These structures are part of the **immunoglobulin supergene family,** which is a group of glycoproteins that share a common ancestral gene. This ancestral gene coded for about 110 amino acids and was duplicated and underwent divergence. Members of this family are involved in antigen recognition and cellular interactions and include immunoglobulin, the T-cell receptor (TCR), major histocompatibility complex (MHC) class I and class II molecules, and CD markers including CD4, CD8, and CD19 among others (1, 2, 3, 4, 5, 6, 7, 8).

The different immunoglobulin classes share the same basic structure, but differences in their heavy chains lead to their classification as either IgG, IgM, IgA, IgD, or IgE. These differences in the heavy chains also lead to their different biologic functions. The Fc region, as can be seen in the antibody structure, is made up of only parts of the heavy chain whereas the Fab region is composed of the heavy and the light chains combined. Thus, the difference in the biological activity of the immunoglobulin classes is based on their heavy chain

✪ TABLE 2.1

Immunoglobulin Class (3–11)

Class	Structure	Subclasses	Function	Molecular Weight	Complement Binding	Opsonic	Agglutination/ Precipitation
IgG		IgG$_1$ IgG$_2$ IgG$_3$ IgG$_4$	Predominant immunoglobulin in serum Passes from mom to baby through placenta	150 000	Yes	Yes	Yes
IgA		IgA$_1$ IgA$_2$	Protection at mucosal surfaces Dimers held together by J chain Secretory chain wrapped around Fc regions, makes IgA less susceptible to proteolytic cleavage	445 000 dimer 160 000 monomer	No—classical pathway Yes—alternative pathway	Yes	Yes
IgM		IgM	First antibody produced Low affinity, but multiple binding sites allow for higher avidity	900 000 serum pentamer 180 000 B cell surface monomer	Yes	Yes	Yes
IgD		IgD	B cell Maturation marker	175 000	No	No	No
IgE		IgE	Antiparasitic response Allergy	190 000	No	No	No

differences in the Fc region. IgG, IgA, and IgD have a **hinge region** between the C_H1 and C_H2 domains that allows flexibility. This region is not globular because it has a stretch of prolines, which gives this region flexibility, and it allows the paratopes on the antibody molecule to have some flexibility in the distance from each other so that they can reach and bind two epitopes. IgM and IgE do not have a hinge region but have the extra constant region C_H4 instead. Glycosylation (little bit of sugar molecules added to the amino acids of the immunoglobulin) occurs at the C_H2 of IgG, IgA, and IgD and at the C_H3 of IgM and IgE (refer to Figure 2.4 ■, which shows how the hinge can bend and where the glycosylation, domains, and CDRs are) (1, 2, 3, 4, 5, 6, 7, 8).

IgG is the immunoglobulin that is in highest concentration in the serum, about 80% of the immunoglobulin in the serum is IgG. The heavy chains in this molecule are called the *gamma* (γ) *heavy chains*. IgG has a high diffusion coefficient, so it travels from the blood vessels to the extravascular space to protect there as well. Humans have 4 slight variations of this molecule called *subclasses,* which are called IgG$_1$, IgG$_2$, IgG$_3$, and IgG$_4$ (Table 2.2 ✪). These subclasses are numbered according to their concentration in serum; IgG$_1$ has the highest concentration and IgG$_4$ the lowest. Subclasses are much more similar to each other in terms of amino acid sequence and function than immunoglobulins of different classes (3, 4, 5, 6, 7, 8).

IgG functions in the serum to help fight infection through (1) opsonization (preparing the foreign particle for phagocytosis), (2) complement activation (with lytic and opsonic effects), (3) neutralization of toxins and viruses

Immunoglobulin G (IgG)

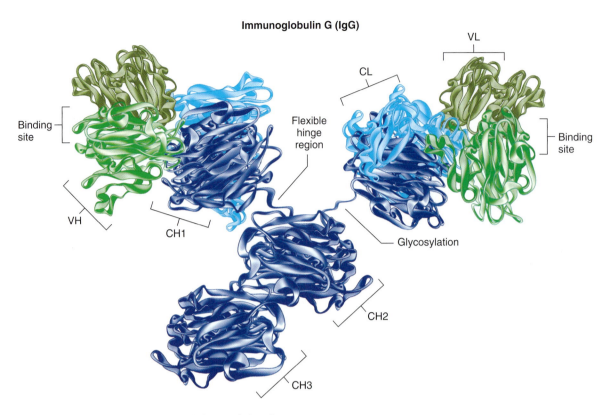

■ **FIGURE 2.4**   IgG: hinge, glycosylation, and domains.

⭐ **TABLE 2.2**				
IgG Subclasses (3–11)				
Subclass	Placental Transfer	Complement Activation	Opsonic	Half-Life
IgG$_1$	+	+	++	23
IgG$_2$	+/−	+/−	+/−	23
IgG$_3$	+	+	++	8
IgG$_4$	+	−	+	23

(usually by blocking binding), and (4) enhancing clearance by causing agglutination and precipitation reactions by cross-linking the particulate (agglutination) or soluble antigen (precipitation). (See Figure 2.5 ■ depicting all the functions of IgG.) IgG$_1$ and IgG$_3$ are best at opsonization; IgG$_3$ is best at complement activation; IgG$_1$ activates complement; IgG$_2$ has minimal ability to activate complement; and IgG$_4$ does not activate complement (Table 2.2). IgG$_1$, IgG$_3$, and IgG$_4$ can pass through the placenta and protect the fetus. The half-lives of IgG$_1$, IgG$_2$, and IgG$_4$ are the longest of the immunoglobulins at 23 days. The half-life of IgG$_3$ is 8 days (3, 4, 5, 6, 7, 8).

Because of the long half-life of the IgG molecules and the fact that they are transferred to the fetus by the mother, maternal IgG is an effective part of a baby's defenses for the first few months of life. This can be important knowledge clinically. For example, a baby who seems fine at birth but between 2 and 6 months of life starts showing signs of sinopulmonary disease and skin infections might have an immunodeficiency disease, the inability to make immunoglobulin. The reason the infant was fine the first few months was due to the passively transferred maternal immunoglobulin, which stayed protective for a few of its biological half-lives. In addition, the facts that the IgG in the newborn is from mom and that any IgM present has been produced by the infant is very important diagnostically. IgG to rubella in the newborn would indicate that a vaccinated mom's immunoglobulin had been passively transferred to the infant through the placenta. IgM to rubella in the newborn is a much more serious indicator, suggesting that the infant's immune system has made antibody to rubella as the result of infection (3, 4, 5, 6, 7, 8).

IgA is the next highest in serum concentration but has little function in serum where it is present as a monomer with a molecular weight of about 160 000 daltons. IgA is the primary functional immunoglobulin in secretions and is present there in dimers, where it serves as a primary defense to prevent entrance of invaders. IgA dimers are aligned with the Fc regions, together and the Fab regions facing out. The 2 chains are held together by a 15 000 dalton J (joining) chain. IgA in secretions also contains an extra chain called

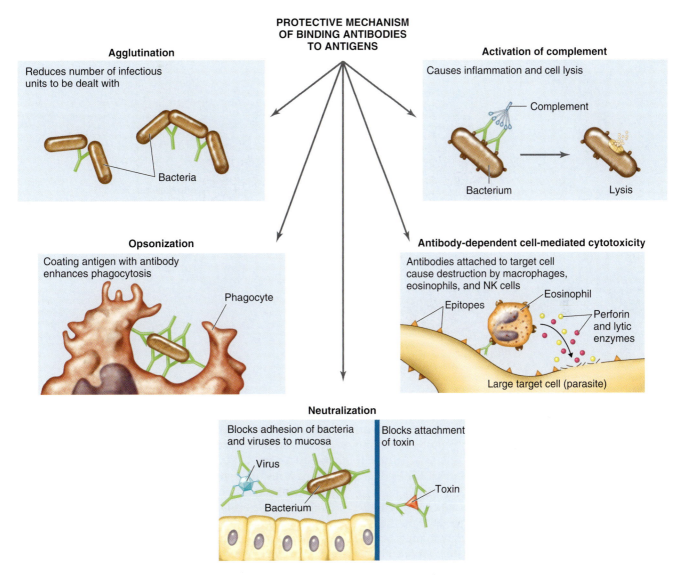

**PROTECTIVE MECHANISM
OF BINDING ANTIBODIES
TO ANTIGENS**

Agglutination

Reduces number of infectious
units to be dealt with

Bacteria

Activation of complement

Causes inflammation and cell lysis

Complement

Bacterium   Lysis

Opsonization

Coating antigen with antibody
enhances phagocytosis

Phagocyte

Antibody-dependent cell-mediated cytotoxicity

Antibodies attached to target cell
cause destruction by macrophages,
eosinophils, and NK cells

Epitopes   Eosinophil

Perforin
and lytic
enzymes

Large target cell (parasite)

Neutralization

Blocks adhesion of bacteria
and viruses to mucosa

Blocks attachment
of toxin

Virus

Bacterium

Toxin

■ **FIGURE 2.5** Depiction of all immunoglobulin functions. *Source:* TORTORA, GERARD J.; FUNKE, BERDELL R.; CASE, CHRISTINE L., MICROBIOLOGY: AN INTRODUCTION, 10th, ©2010. Printed and Electronically reproduced by permission of Pearson Education, Inc., Upper Saddle River, New Jersey.

the secretory piece that is synthesized by an epithelial cell. The synthesis of IgA is interesting because IgA dimers that are joined with the J chain bind to an epithelial cell via a receptor that is a precursor of the secretory piece (100 000 daltons). The IgA is brought into the epithelial cell attached to this secretory piece and transverses the epithelial cell. At the opposite side of the cell at the secretory lumen, part of the secretory piece is cleaved, and the IgA dimer attached to the remaining secretory piece (70 000 daltons) is secreted—Figure 2.6(a) ■ and (b). This final secreted IgA_2 is about 445 000 daltons and was made by 4 genes (heavy chain, light chain, secretory piece, J chain, not including the genes required for the enzymes of glycosylation) and 2 different cells (3, 4, 5, 6, 7, 8)!

There are 2 different subclasses of IgA, IgA_1, and IgA_2. IgA_1 is the main component of serum IgA whereas IgA_2 is the main

component of secreted IgA. IgA_2 has a smaller hinge (nonglobular) region and thus is less susceptible to proteolytic cleavage (9, 10, 11).

Secretory IgA functions by preventing the entrance of pathogens. It does this by cross-linking multiple epitopes to cause aggregates that are easily removed by the ciliated cells of the mucous membranes and by gut peristalsis. It also functions by blocking antigens that are involved in adhesion of the bacteria, virus, or toxin. IgA does not bind complement by the classical pathway but may activate the alternative pathway in some cases. Neutrophils, macrophage, and monocytes have Fcα binding receptors on their surfaces, so IgA is opsonic in facilitating phagocytosis by these cell types (9, 10, 11).

IgA is not transferred through the placenta to the fetus but is transferred through breast milk to the newborn. Breast

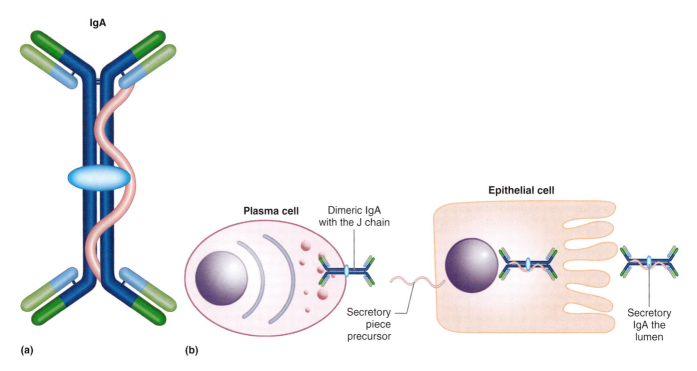

IgA

Plasma cell

Dimeric IgA with the J chain

Epithelial cell

Secretory piece precursor

Secretory IgA the lumen

(a)   (b)

■ **FIGURE 2.6**   (a) IgA. (b) IgA production.

milk contains numerous proteins, oligosaccharides, and fatty acids that help augment the infant's innate immune system. IgA is one of the most important breast milk proteins because of its ability to augment a *specific* response to a particular pathogen. Human breast colostrum contains 17.35 g/L IgA, and human breast milk contains 1 g/L IgA. Nearly 90% of the immunoglobulins in either colostrum or milk are of the IgA class. Colostrum is the early form of milk produced in the first days after delivery. It looks more like serum than milk and is a very concentrated form of nutrition, containing more protein but less fat than later milk does. Protection of the newborn from enteric pathogens is an important role of human secretory immunoglobulins (9, 10, 11).

About 5 to 10% of the immunoglobulin in serum is **IgM,** which is a pentamer that is composed of 5 of the 2 heavy chain and 2 light chain units. It has a starfishlike shape with the Fc regions in the center and the Fab arms extended out (Figure 2.7 ■). Serum IgM is the largest of the immunoglobulins with a molecular weight of 900 000 daltons (Table 2.1). IgM is called a *macroglobulin* because of its large molecular weight. A tumor in which tumor plasma cells make IgM is called a *macroglobulinemia* because of this. Each of the five 2 heavy and 2 light chain units is a little heavier than those in an IgG molecule because of the extra C_H domain, C_H4, and the molecular weight of each of these units is 180 000. The 5 units are held together by a J (joining) chain. This chain has several cysteine residues, which form disulfide bonds with the carboxy terminal area of the Fc regions to hold the units together. The J chain is 15 000 daltons. Each monomer has 2 binding sites, so potentially the 10 paratopes of the IgM molecule could bind 10 epitopes. This

is the case if the antigens are quite small and there is no steric hindrance; however, some steric interactions usually occur, and functionally, only about 5 paratopes bind to epitopes at 1 time (3, 4, 5, 6, 7, 8).

The arms of the different monomers of the IgM molecule can bind to epitopes either spatially within the same plane as the IgM molecule or above or below the plane. This flexibility in binding allows IgM to bridge particulate or cellular

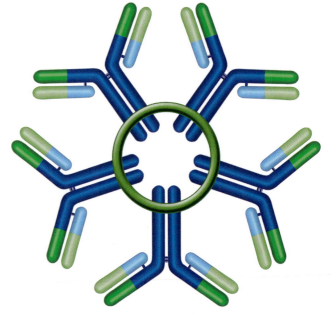

■ **FIGURE 2.7**   IgM.

antigens together to cause agglutination. The "reach" of the different paratopes allows IgM to bring together cells that are slightly charged because the repulsion due to the charge is diminished over this great binding distance (see Figure 2.8 ■ for the bridging ability of IgM). Because of the number of binding sites and the length of the reach between paratopes on the opposite sides of the molecule, IgM is the best immunoglobulin at agglutination (bridging together particulate antigens) and precipitation (bridging together soluble antigens). IgM is also best at fixing complement by the classical pathway. It also is opsonic and neutralizes toxins and viruses very well (3, 4, 5, 6, 7, 8).

IgM is the first immunoglobulin produced in response to an antigen and this immunoglobulin is produced without

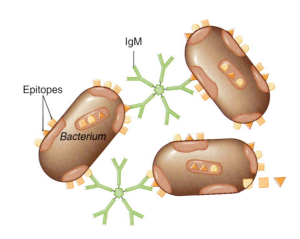

(c)

■ **FIGURE 2.8** *(continued)* (c) IgM agglutination of bacteria. *Source:* TORTORA, GERARD J.; FUNKE, BERDELL R.; CASE, CHRISTINE L., MICROBIOLOGY: AN INTRODUCTION, 10th, ©2010. Printed and Electronically reproduced by permission of Pearson Education, Inc., Upper Saddle River, New Jersey.

the somatic mutation events that result in higher affinity binding sites of the other immunoglobulin classes. While the affinity of each epitope to paratope reaction of IgM with the antigen is low because of this lack of affinity maturation, the avidity of the interaction is the sum of all the paratopes and epitopes that are interacting, so the avidity can be high. IgM is the first immunoglobulin produced in a newborn, and elevations in it after birth indicate an infection. The half-life of IgM is 10 days. It does not cross the placenta from the mother to the baby nor does it enter extravascular spaces because it is too large to diffuse through the blood vessels. The J chain on the IgM molecule, like the J chain on the IgA molecule, can bind to receptors on secretory cells and thus IgM can enter external secretions. IgA is the predominant immunoglobulin in secretions, but IgM can also play a role in secretions (3, 4, 5, 6, 7, 8, 9, 10, 11, 12).

IgM also is present on the surface of B cells as a surface receptor for antigen. Surface IgM is monomeric rather than pentameric and contains a slightly different Fc region because membrane IgM contains transmembrane and cytoplasmic regions that are removed by RNA splicing when the cell is producing the secreted form of IgM. The expression of IgM on the surface of an immature B cell is an important part of the cell's maturation process. IgM can be expressed on the surface of immature and mature B cells, plasma cells, and memory B cells. Most of the surface IgM, which is a surface receptor for specific antigen, is found on the immature and mature B cells, and this IgM is a surface receptor for specific antigen. When the antigen binds to the surface IgM, signals are sent into the B cell, resulting in cellular activation and proliferation to become plasma cells and memory cells. Until recently, all memory cells were thought to have undergone a class switch from IgM to IgG or another class, and IgM positive memory B cells were not thought to exist; however, they

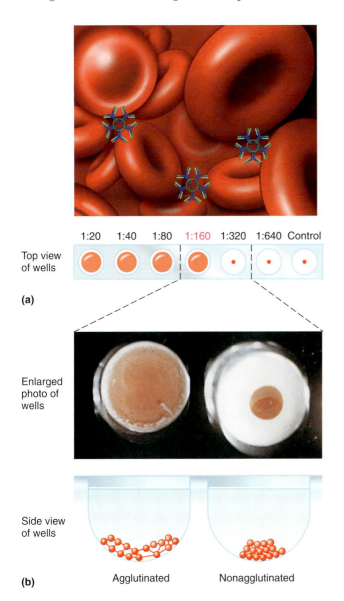

1:20 1:40 1:80 1:160 1:320 1:640 Control

Top view of wells

(a)

Enlarged photo of wells

Side view of wells

Agglutinated   Nonagglutinated

(b)

■ **FIGURE 2.8** The bridging ability of IgM: (a) Pictorial view of IgM bridging of red cells. (b) Macroscopic view of IgM bridging of red cells used in blood typing. Agglutinated cells show a spread appearance in the tube while nonagglutinated cells form a button.

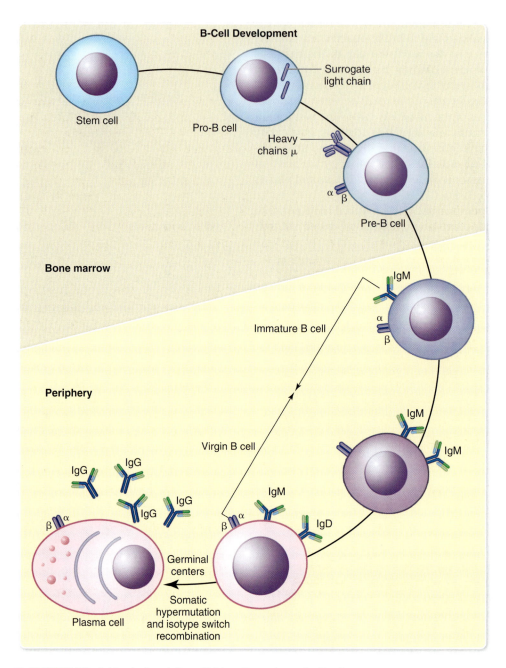

■ FIGURE 2.9   IgM only, then IgD and IgM on the surface of a B cell.

have been isolated, and they represent a specialized population of memory B cells (3, 4, 5, 6, 7, 8).

IgD is about 0.2% of the total serum immunoglobulin; it is present in such low concentrations in human serum that its biologic function in serum has not been characterized. It has a molecular weight of 180 000. IgD is on the surface of mature B cells and functions as a specific antigen receptor, a molecule that facilitates antigen specific B-cell activation, and a maturation marker for the B cell. IgM appears on the surface of B cells first; the addition of the IgD receptors appears to

help the B cell respond to signals from T cells and to switch to synthesis of IgG, IgA, or IgE—see Figure 2.9 ■ (a) IgM and (b) IgD and IgM on the surface of a B cell. IgD does not bind complement, is not opsonic, and is not transferred to the fetus through the placenta (3, 4, 5, 6, 7, 8).

IgE is present in serum in the lowest concentration of any of the immunoglobulins, only about 0.02% or less of all of the serum immunoglobulins. Although only very low concentrations are present in serum, this immunoglobulin can cause dramatic effects because it is the immunoglobulin responsible for the type of allergy called *immediate type hypersensitivity*. It is approximately 190 000 MW, containing an extra C_H domain. The C_H3 domain binds to mast cells, basophils, eosinophils, and Langerhans cells with very high affinity. Plasma cells that make IgE are located along the respiratory tract; the skin, alimentary tract, and mast cells that bind the IgE are located nearby (Figure 2.10 ■). After the IgE is bound to the mast cells, binding of the antigen causes mast cell degranulation, which releases histamine, heparin, and chemotactic factors. These substances cause the classic symptoms of allergy, hay fever, asthma, vomiting, diarrhea, hives, shock, and even anaphylactic death. These negative aspects of IgE would not indicate a reason for its production to have been maintained in our genome. IgE has an important protective role less thought of in the United States because it has a protective role for pathogens that have penetrated the IgA response at the mucosa, such as parasites. IgE triggers an inflammatory response that brings eosinophils and neutrophils to the area. Eosinophils can destroy parasitic worms, so IgE is an important part of the antiparasitic response. IgE does not pass through the placenta, bind complement, or enhance phagocytosis (3, 4, 5, 6, 7, 8).

 Checkpoint! 2.2

Which immunoglobulin molecules have a J chain?

The classes just described are based on the heavy chains of the molecules, but there are also 2 types of light chains, kappa (κ) and lambda (λ). There are no functional differences between these light chain types, and they are present in roughly a 2:1 ratio. Light chains have been found in the urine of patients with a type of tumor called *myeloma* in which plasma cells have become tumor cells. These light chains were one of the first diagnostic markers of a tumor found in an easily assayable fluid. These proteins are called Bence Jones proteins (3, 4, 5, 6, 7, 8).

 Checkpoint! 2.3

Bence Jones proteins were found after a scientist heated urine of myeloma patients and found that a protein precipitated out of solution upon heating and as the urine got hotter, the protein went back into solution. Don't you wonder how a scientist knew to stare at urine as it was being heated? What are the Bence Jones proteins?

Vaccination of an animal with human immunoglobulin will result in the production of antibodies to different regions of the human immunoglobulin. The regions that are specific for the heavy chain type of the immunoglobulin molecule are called its **isotypic determinants** or the *isotype,* these

First exposure

Step 1: The invader (allergen) enters the body.
 Allergen

Step 2: Plasma cells produce large amounts of class IgE antibodies against the allergen.
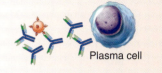 Plasma cell

Step 3: IgE antibodies attach to mast cells, which are found in body tissues.
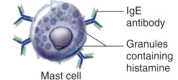
IgE antibody

Granules containing histamine

(a)   Mast cell

Subsequent (secondary) response

Step 4: More of the same allergen invades the body.
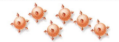

Step 5: The allergen combines with IgE attached to mast cells. Histamine and other chemicals are released from mast cell granules.
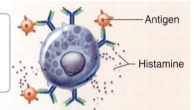
Antigen

Histamine

Step 6: Histamine causes blood vessels to widen and become leaky. Fluid enters the tissue, causing swelling.
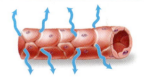

• Histamine stimulates release of large amounts of mucus.
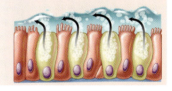

• Histamine causes smooth muscle in walls of air tubules in lungs to contract.

(b)

■ **FIGURE 2.10** (a) IgE binding to a mast cell. (b) IgE bound to a mast cell and cross-linked by antigen-causing mast cell degranulation. *Source:* GOODENOUGH, JUDITH; MCGUIRE, BETTY A., BIOLOGY OF HUMANS: CONCEPTS, APPLICATIONS, AND ISSUES WITH MASTERINGBIOLOGY®, 4th, ©N/A. Printed and Electronically reproduced by permission of Pearson Education, Inc., Upper Saddle River, New Jersey.

determinants are involved in the class (G, A, M, D, E) of the molecule. To determine whether an immune reaction in an infant is due to the infant's own IgM or maternal IgG reacting with the antigen, it is important to have an antibody that is specific for the IgM isotype (or class). Antibody to human immunoglobulin can also react with allotypic determinants on the immunoglobulin molecule. **Allotypic antigens** are different on different members of the same species and are inherited as the result of simple mendelian genetics. So, a child would inherit the allotypic markers of the immunoglobulin molecules from his or her mother and father. Also present on the immunoglobulin molecule is the epitope formed as the result of the paratope's unique structure. The paratope is unique in its reaction with the epitope and as such has a unique combination of amino acids that can be antigenic. This antigen in the paratope is called the *idiotype of the molecule*. The idiotype of an immunoglobulin as an antigen is more important than it sounds because a paratope must have a good fit with an epitope, and an antibody that binds to a paratope could look like the original epitope and thus could stimulate or regulate an immune response to the original antigen. The study of anti-idiotypic antibodies remains of interest to those searching for new ways to develop vaccines as well as for those searching for new ways to downregulate an immune response

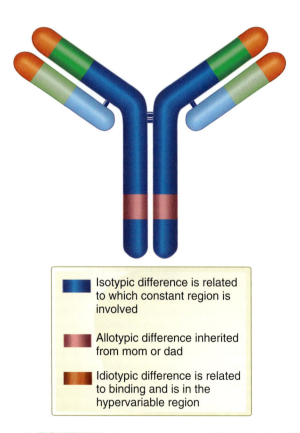

Isotypic difference is related to which constant region is involved

Allotypic difference inherited from mom or dad

Idiotypic difference is related to binding and is in the hypervariable region

■ **FIGURE 2.11**   Isotype, allotype, and idiotype.

(3, 4, 5, 6, 7, 8). See Figure 2.11 ■ for diagrammatic explanation of allotypic, isotypic, and idiotypic antigens.

▶ DIVERSITY

The hallmarks of the acquired immune system are that it is *specific*, has a large scope, can discriminate, and has a memory. The question at this time is how immunoglobulin helps accomplish these hallmarks. Just for fun, let's look at some numbers. The molecular weight of the IgG is 150 000 with about 214 amino acids in each light chain and about 448 in each heavy chain for a total of about 1324 amino acids. With 3 nucleotides required for each amino acid, almost 4000 nucleotides would be required to produce 1 antibody molecule. The estimated number of different antibody specificities that are produced is around 10^8, so if each antibody molecule were produced by a different full-length gene, an enormous amount of DNA (approximately $4 * 10^{11}$ nucleotides) would be required. The human genome project has reported that there are $2.85 * 10^9$ nucleotides in the human genome, so if the immunoglobulin molecules were made in the conventional way, just the diversity of the immunoglobulin would use more than all of the DNA in a human, and that is without even calculating the diversity of the T-cell receptors (3, 4, 5, 6, 7, 8)!

Jerne and Burnet coined the *clonal selection theory*, which proposes how the diverse immunoglobulin repertoire could exist. The key idea behind this theory is the existence of lymphocytes that can react with only 1 antigen before any encounter with antigen has occurred. When these lymphocytes interact with an antigen, they proliferate and make a clone of cells that respond to that antigen only. So, a lymphocyte inside of a human body that is ready and waiting to react to the flu virus will not be able to help at all when a person is infected with a different virus because each lymphocyte has its own epitope to which it can respond. The reaction with the antigen is by a surface receptor; on B cells, the reaction is via surface immunoglobulin (IgM or IgD); and on T cells, the surface receptor is the T-cell receptor. This still leaves a dilemma as to how all these immunoglobulins and T-cell receptors are made in a way that conserves use of DNA. Several events guide the development of the antibody repertoire: (1) *antigen-independent* random recombinational events of DNA gene segments during B-cell maturation, (2) *antigen-dependent* clonal deletion of self-reactive B cells, and (3) *antigen-dependent* somatic mutation and affinity maturation (3, 4, 5, 6, 7, 8).

✓ **Checkpoint! 2.4**

One property of the adaptive or acquired immune system that is key to the success of vaccines, I am sure that you remember, is _____.

ANTIGEN-INDEPENDENT DIVERSITY

During antigen-independent, random recombinational events of DNA gene segments during B-cell maturation, the mechanism that is used begins with the fact that the variable regions and the constant regions are formed by different gene segments. The heavy chain variable region is encoded by 3 gene segments—the V, D, and J—and after recombination, in which the 3 are joined to each other, the 3 are joined to the heavy chain constant region. The light chain variable region is encoded by 2 gene segments—the V and J—that are joined to the light chain constant region after a recombinational event. Tonegawa discovered that genes from chromosome 14 make human immunoglobulin heavy chains, genes from chromosome 2 make kappa light chains, and genes from chromosome 22 make human immunoglobulin lambda light chains (3, 4, 5, 6, 7, 8).

The multiple binding sites in the variable region produced prior to interaction with the antigen is the result of random recombination of (1) the heavy chain of the over 50 different V_H gene segments, with 27 functional D gene segments and 6 J gene segments and either (2) for the kappa light chain, about 40 Vκ gene segments and 5 Jκ gene segments or for the lambda light chain (3) 30 Vλ gene segments, and 4 Jλ gene segments (Figure 2.12 ■). The number of different heavy chains that can be made is $50 * 27 * 6 = 8100$, and the number of different kappa light chains that can be produced is $40 * 5 = 200$. The number of antibody-combining sites that can be made with heavy chains plus the kappa light chain is $8100 * 200 = 1.6$ million. The number of antibody-combining sites using the lambda light chain is an additional $8100 * 120 = 0.96$ million. Now we can account for 2.6 million different antibody specificities (3, 4, 5, 6, 7, 8).

Genetic rearrangement must occur for functional immunoglobulin to be made. Think of these genetic regions as beads on a string with the V region beads colored light blue, the D region beads colored green, the J region beads colored dark blue, and the constant region beads colored orange. The V region contains 50 different segments (50 different beads colored light blue in our visualization), and one of these 50 light blue bead segments must be brought next to 1 of the 27 green bead segments of the D region, 1 of the 6 dark blue bead segments of the J region, and 1 of the orange bead segments of the constant regions. The constant regions are further downstream and are in the following order for the heavy chain class type: μ, δ, γ3, γ1, α1, γ2, γ4, α2, and ϵ. Initially, each B cell that produces immunoglobulin rearranges the VDJ with the μ constant region for the initial production of IgM (3, 4, 5, 6, 7, 8).

To get the V, D, and J segments together, an interesting bit of DNA manipulation occurs. On either side of these segments are nonamers or heptamers with a matching complementary heptamer or nonamer downstream. Here *complementary* is meant in the genetic sense, so if the nonamer on the 5' side

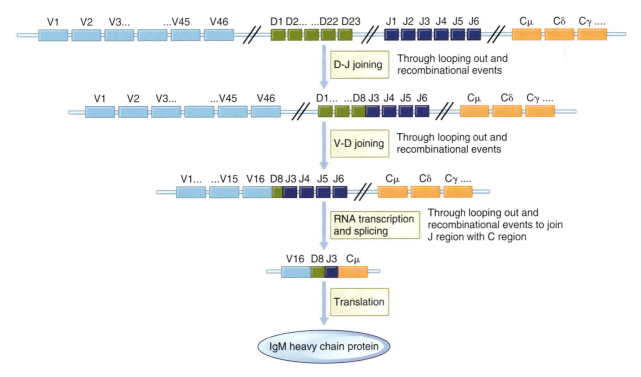

■ **FIGURE 2.12**   The occurrence diversity of the immunoglobulin binding site. Nonamer binding loops together sections for the splice out and recombination, which results in bringing together VDJ regions to form the specificity of the antibody.

of the coding region was GGTTTTTGT, the complementary nonamer on the 3' side would be CCAAAAACC; if brought together in the random movement of the DNA, the complementary regions would bind to each other GG to CC and AAAAA to TTTTT, and so on bind, causing a loop to be made by these recombination signal sequences (RSS). This loop is cut out and the pieces are annealed together through the use of 3 enzymes, the recombinase activating genes 1 and 2 (RAG1, RAG2), and terminal deoxynucleotidyl transferase (TdT). The joining process itself has some built-in variability with slight changes in where the junction occurs and an addition or deletion of nucleotides that can result in a different binding site. These changes can also result in a reading frame shift which may cause a nonproductive rearrangement and utilization of the other chromosome for rearrangement to form the immunoglobulin. The changes in the way the regions are combined during the recombinational event affect the CDR3 because this complementary determining region involves amino acids that would be encoded by inserted nucleotides. Combining all these things, antigen-independent diversity can encode for tens of millions of different specificities (3, 4, 5, 6, 7, 8).

Antigen-Dependent Clonal Deletion

The next process, *antigen-dependent clonal deletion* of self-reactive B cells, decreases diversity in a mechanism that helps maintain the self-non-self-recognition system of the acquired immune response. If a maturing B cell meets and binds with its antigen prior to maturation, a maturational arrest occurs, preventing the B cell from becoming mature. In addition, interaction of the maturing B cell with membrane-bound antigen can result in apoptosis, a process by which the B cell, after receiving certain signals, produces enzymes that degrade its own DNA in effect committing cellular suicide (3, 4, 5, 6, 7, 8).

ANTIGEN-DEPENDENT SOMATIC MUTATION AND AFFINITY MATURATION

The final process in the development of the antibody repertoire is antigen-dependent somatic mutation and affinity maturation. When a B-cell receptor (surface immunoglobulin) or a T-cell receptor binds antigen, rapid proliferation of the cell occurs, resulting in each offspring cell being identical in B-cell receptor or T-cell receptor to the original parental cell unless mutation occurs during this rapid proliferation. Mutation frequently occurs during this rapid proliferation because the hypervariable regions in these genes mutate at a rate 100 000 times the mutation rate of other regions of the genome. Most of these mutations are substitutions, not deletions or additions, so the reading frame is not affected. This process affects each of the antibody's CDRs. This somatic mutation can result in the production of a higher-affinity B-cell receptor, and as the amount of antigen wanes, the cells with the higher-affinity receptors' preferential take up antigen and are preferentially selected to continue proliferating. Thus, the affinity of the immunoglobulin improves in this process,

Checkpoint! 2.5

An individual's immunoglobulin diversity develops through 3 processes: _____, _____, and _____.

which is called *antigen-dependent affinity maturation* (3, 4, 5, 6, 7, 8).

The final detail in the production of immunoglobulin is the heavy chain class switching. The first immunoglobulin made by the B cell is IgM, and downstream of the μ gene segment are gene segments for all other heavy chain types. T-cell help guides the class switching through the secretion of cytokines that cause the B cell to excise the μ gene segment and combine the VDJ region with a different heavy chain class. It is still within the 1 cell-1 specificity rule because although the immunoglobulin that is produced has a different heavy chain type, its binding site remains the same. A B cell can complete more than 1 class switch, but the subsequent classes can be selected only from downstream gene segments because the intervening segments have been spliced out (Figure 2.12b) (3, 4, 5, 6, 7, 8).

When stimulated by its antigen, a mature B cell can become either a plasma cell that dies in a relatively short period of time (weeks) after producing antibody or a memory B cell that survives for years. The production of memory B cells that have undergone class switching and affinity maturation is the reason that a secondary response (the second time the pathogen is seen) is an improvement over the primary response (Figure 2.13 ■). The primary response has a longer lag time

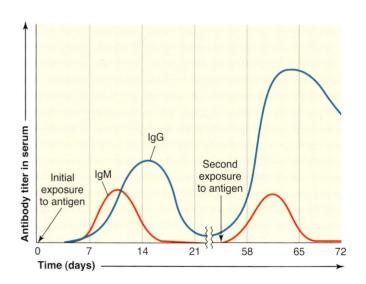

■ **FIGURE 2.13** The primary and secondary adaptive responses. *Source:* TORTORA, GERARD J.; FUNKE, BERDELL R.; CASE, CHRISTINE L., MICROBIOLOGY: AN INTRODUCTION, 10th, ©2010. Printed and Electronically reproduced by permission of Pearson Education, Inc., Upper Saddle River, New Jersey.

before any measurable antibody is produced because only a small number of B cells are initially reactive with the antigen and these are clonally expanded to produce the higher number of memory cells that await secondary interaction with the antigen. The secondary response is also greater in magnitude; for this same reason, a larger set of reactive cells at the beginning makes a much larger set of plasma cells, which have a higher affinity due to the somatic mutation that occurred in the primary response (3, 4, 5, 6, 7, 8).

▶ MONOCLONAL ANTIBODIES

The discovery of myeloma proteins facilitated studies on immunoglobulin. These proteins are produced when the patient has a myeloma tumor that originated as 1 plasma cell. These plasma cell tumors proliferate, forming a clone of identical cells. The clones produce antibody molecules, which are identical and these are a type of natural monoclonal antibody. This antibody, however, is not usually of a known specificity and was not produced in response to an antigen. Now **monoclonal antibodies** are routinely prepared intentionally; the most frequently used type is the mouse monoclonal antibody.

Monoclonal antibodies are important because they are a consistent source of antibody of a defined specificity and sensitivity that can be utilized in clinical assays to identify antigens and can also be used for a variety of research purposes. Polyclonal antibody for clinical use was routinely prepared by vaccinating large animals to create a pool of antiserum to be utilized for clinical studies, but when the pool was depleted, the development of a similar pool was time consuming and validation was difficult. Antiserum contains antibody to multiple epitopes on the molecule with which the animal was vaccinated, and antiserum contains other antibodies that the animal produced for its own immune response. The polyclonality of the antiserum utilized increases the likelihood that cross-reactivities that decrease the specificity of the assay will occur. Kohler and Milstein received a Nobel Prize in 1984 for the development of a technique for producing monoclonal antibodies of a desired specificity. Development of a monoclonal antibody source allows the continuous use of an antibody of defined specificity to 1 epitope that can be more easily replenished. Monoclonal antibodies are produced by a clone of cells called **hybridoma cells.** The word *hybridoma* refers to the fact that these cells are hybrids formed through the combination of 2 cell types, a spleen cell, and a myeloma cell. The myeloma cell is a tumor cell with a plasma cell origin. This cell, like all tumor cells, can reproduce indefinitely. The spleen cell from an immunized animal is a plasma cell–producing antibody of the specificity that is desired (3, 4, 5, 6, 7, 8) (Figure 2.14 ■).

The animal is immunized until it is making a high titer of antibody of the desired specificity; then it is sacrificed, and its spleen cells are harvested. A single cell suspension is made

of the spleen cells, which are mixed with the myeloma cells in a tube. The tube is centrifuged and the cells are pelleted. Then an agent, such as polyethylene glycol, is added to cause the cells to fuse. Polyethylene glycol addition changes the cell membranes so that when the cells are in contact, the membranes can then intercalate, and the 2 cells become one (3, 4, 5, 6, 7, 8).

This fusion process is random, so spleen cells can fuse with spleen cells, myeloma cells with myeloma cells, spleen cells with myeloma cells and the cells can remain separate. The next part of the process is selecting the desired cells. Spleen cells and spleen cell–spleen cell hybrids will not survive long in culture, so the spleen cell–myeloma cell hybrids need to be selected from the myeloma cell–myeloma cell hybrids and the myeloma cells alone. This selection process actually begins with the selection of the myeloma cells as the fusion partner. The myeloma cells chosen have 2 properties that make them useful for this technique; 1 property is that they do not make any immunoglobulin of their own (ie, they are nonsecretors), and the other important property is a defect in one of the pathways used to make DNA. In a cell, DNA can be made either by the De Novo pathway or the salvage pathway. The myeloma cells have a defect in an enzyme, so they cannot make DNA through the salvage pathway. After the fusion, the cells are placed in a media that contains 3 things: aminopterin, which blocks the De Novo pathway of DNA synthesis; thymidine; and hypoxanthine, which provide the precursors needed for the salvage pathway. This media is called HAT (hypoxanthine, aminopterin, and thymidine). The only cells of our possibilities that can survive in this media are the spleen cell–myeloma cell hybrids (3, 4, 5, 6, 7, 8).

The next selection that needs to be made is for the hybridoma cell which makes the desired antibody. The fused cells are grown in 96 well plates diluted so that each well will contain only a clone derived from 1 cell. After sufficient time for cell growth and antibody production (about 2 weeks), the supernatants of these wells are tested for reactivity with the desired antigen and as a control, are tested for reactivity with antigens that may have an undesired cross-reactivity. The wells with the desired specificity are grown, subcloned, and frozen for use for years (3, 4, 5, 6, 7, 8).

✓ Checkpoint! 2.6

One reason that monoclonal antibodies are especially useful is because after an assay using a monoclonal antibody has been developed, the monoclonal antibody can be used in the assay for many years because the cells producing them are stable. This long-lived property of the cell that produces the monoclonal antibody comes from one of the cells used to make the hybridoma. This cell is the _____.

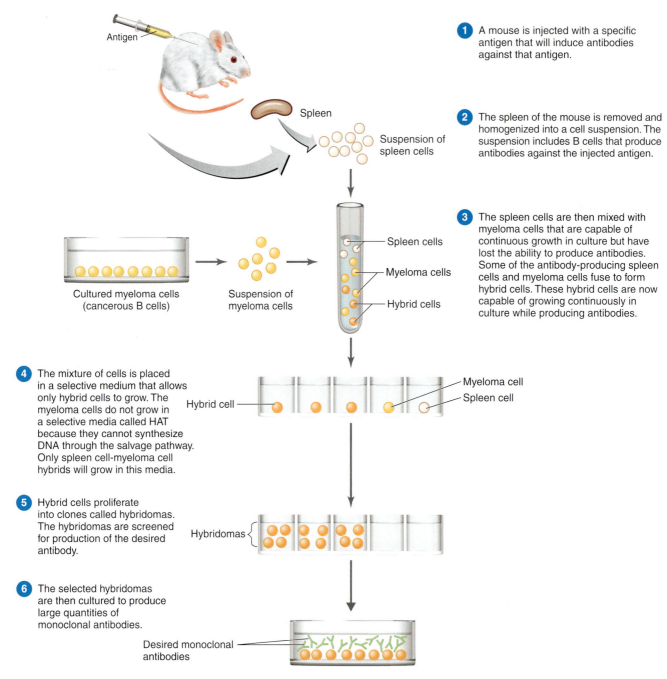

Antigen

Spleen

Suspension of spleen cells

Cultured myeloma cells (cancerous B cells)

Suspension of myeloma cells

Spleen cells

Myeloma cells

Hybrid cells

Hybrid cell

Myeloma cell

Spleen cell

Hybridomas

Desired monoclonal antibodies

1 A mouse is injected with a specific antigen that will induce antibodies against that antigen.

2 The spleen of the mouse is removed and homogenized into a cell suspension. The suspension includes B cells that produce antibodies against the injected antigen.

3 The spleen cells are then mixed with myeloma cells that are capable of continuous growth in culture but have lost the ability to produce antibodies. Some of the antibody-producing spleen cells and myeloma cells fuse to form hybrid cells. These hybrid cells are now capable of growing continuously in culture while producing antibodies.

4 The mixture of cells is placed in a selective medium that allows only hybrid cells to grow. The myeloma cells do not grow in a selective media called HAT because they cannot synthesize DNA through the salvage pathway. Only spleen cell-myeloma cell hybrids will grow in this media.

5 Hybrid cells proliferate into clones called hybridomas. The hybridomas are screened for production of the desired antibody.

6 The selected hybridomas are then cultured to produce large quantities of monoclonal antibodies.

■ **FIGURE 2.14**   The myeloma cells do not grow in a selective media called HAT because they cannot synthesize DNA through the salvage pathway. Spleen cell–myeloma cell hybrids will grow in this media. *Source:* TORTORA, GERARD J.; FUNKE, BERDELL R.; CASE, CHRISTINE L., MICROBIOLOGY: AN INTRODUCTION, 10th, ©2010. Printed and Electronically reproduced by permission of Pearson Education, Inc., Upper Saddle River, New Jersey.

► ANTIBODY PURIFICATION

To purify an antibody or any protein, solubility characteristics, molecular weight, and binding affinities can be utilized. Commonly used methods of purifying antibody include ammonium sulfate precipitation and affinity purification. *Affinity purification* of antibody can utilize specific antigen column chromatography or Fc binding column chromatography. Fc-binding affinity columns include proteins A, G, and L, which are available commercially. Protein A is purified from *Staphylococcus aureus* and binds human IgG1 and IgG2 as well as a variety of other animal immunoglobulins but does not bind IgG3. Protein G is prepared from either group C or group B streptococcal bacteria and reacts with human IgG1, IgG2, IgG3, and IgG4 as well as a variety of other animal immunoglobulins. Protein L is purified from Peptostreptococcus and binds to kappa light chains. The choice of affinity column depends on the species type and the isotype of the immunoglobulin that is being purified. These proteins are all virulence factors for the bacteria because they hold the Ab by the Fc region in an orientation that prevents its biologic activity (3, 4, 5, 6).

CASE STUDY

Emma is a baby girl who was born healthy and weighed 8 lb, 12 oz at birth. Soon after birth, she developed an infection.

1. What was the type of immunoglobulin that Emma was born with because it was passively transferred from her mom through the placenta?

2. Emma also has IgM antibody to a respiratory virus called *respiratory syncytial virus*. What does this mean?

3. While Emma is fighting the infection, she makes an immunoglobulin that mainly works in secretions. What is it?

4. Emma recovers from her infection but develops a rash after being fed cow's milk at 6 months. What immunoglobulin will we look for when we look for an immune response in Emma to the cow's milk?

SUMMARY

Experimental evidence using an ultracentrifuge showed that the molecular weight of IgG was 150 000. Urea and mercaptoethanol treatment coupled with the ultracentrifuge analysis showed that IgG was made of 2 different things, a heavy chain and a light chain. The heavy chain is twice the molecular weight of the light chain, and 2 of each chain were present in the molecule. Use of the enzyme papain, which broke the antibody into 2 Fab regions (fragments antigen binding) and 1 Fc region (fragment crystallizable), showed that there were separate areas on the molecule, one that bound antigen and contained some variability and one that was the same on each immunoglobulin molecule. Use of the enzyme pepsin showed that these antigen-binding regions could be isolated while linked to each other as (Fab')$_2$. The use of antibody to IgG showed that the Fab region was made of the light chain and the heavy chain and that the Fc region was made just of heavy chain (1). Thus, the basic structure of immunoglobulin shown in Figure 2.2 was deduced.

The IgG structure was shown to contain domains: a variable domain on each of the heavy and light chains, 1 constant-region domain on the light chain, and 3 constant-region domains on the heavy chain. The variable region was found to contain 3 hypervariable regions, which form the paratope, or antigen-binding region of the antibody molecule. These areas are also called *complementary determining regions*. The binding of the antibody to the antigen is by a paratope binding an epitope noncovalently. The forces that hold an antigen to antibody include van der Waals bonds, hydrogen bonding, electrostatic or ionic bonds, and hydrophobic and hydrophilic interactions (3, 4, 5, 6, 7, 8).

Based on the heavy chain type, there are 5 main classes of immunoglobulin molecules, IgG, IgM, IgA, IgD, and IgE. These molecules have different biological functions. IgG is the highest in serum levels and has multiple biologic functions including (1) opsonization, (2) complement activation,(3) neutralization of toxins and viruses, (4) agglutination and precipitation reactions, and (5) transfer through the placenta to protect the fetus and newborn. The 4 IgG subclasses have slightly different biological activities. IgA is the major immunoglobulin in secretions and performs blocking functions to prevent pathogen entrance. It is present in secretions as a dimer with a secretory piece and a J chain. IgA is transferred to the newborn with breast milk. IgM is a 900 000 dalton pentamer, which is the first antibody formed in an immune response. The presence of IgM indicates an acute infection. IgM and IgD are surface molecules on B cells that can bind antigen, which causes B-cell activation. IgD is a differentiation marker for B cells. IgE is important in the immune response to parasites and is the immunoglobulin that is responsible for the type of allergy called *immediate-type hypersensitivity* (3, 4, 5, 6, 7, 8).

The number of different antibody molecules and T-cell receptors is enormous, and their synthesis occurs in a unique way. The events that guide the development of the antibody repertoire include (1) antigen-independent random recombinational events of DNA gene segments during B-cell maturation, (2) antigen-dependent clonal deletion of self-reactive B cells, and (3) antigen-dependent somatic mutation and affinity maturation. T-cell help activates the B cell to undergo heavy chain class switching. T-cell receptors also undergo antigen-independent random recombinational events of DNA gene segments during B-cell maturation and antigen-dependent clonal deletion of self-reactive B cells (3, 4, 5, 6, 7, 8).

Monoclonal antibody production involves the hybridization of an antibody-producing cell and a myeloma cell. The antibody-producing cell, usually a spleen cell from a mouse, supplies the desired antibody production, and the myeloma cells confer immortality. Also involved are methods to select the hybridoma cells that produced the desired antibody. The myeloma cells have a defect in DNA synthesis by the salvage pathway and will not survive in the HAT media unless fused to the spleen cell, which can supply the necessary enzyme. The cells are plated at low dilution in individual wells so that individual clones of cells are obtained. The clone that produces the desired specificity is selected using enzyme immunoassays of the supernatants. Antibody purification methods commonly used include ammonium sulfate precipitation and affinity purification using materials that bind the Fc region of the molecule (3, 4, 5, 6, 7, 8).

REVIEW QUESTIONS

1. Mature B cells have
   a. IgD and IgM on their surface
   b. IgM as the only Ab on their surface
   c. VDJ rearrangement of the heavy chain of IgA
   d. expression of TCR

2. Which molecule is best at defense before entry?
   a. IgA
   b. IgE
   c. IgM
   d. IgG

3. If there were 200 V regions, 5 D regions, and 10 J regions, how many different heavy chains could be made?
   a. 215
   b. 2050
   c. 1000
   d. 10 000

4. Pepsin cleaves an antibody molecule
   a. to its heavy and light chains
   b. to 2 Fab + 1 Fc
   c. to (Fab')$_2$ + fragments
   d. to J chain

5. Which molecule has 4 antigen-binding sites?
   a. IgA
   b. IgE
   c. IgM
   d. IgG

6. Which hardly moves in an electric field?
   a. albumin
   b. α_1 globulins
   c. α_2 globulins
   d. γ_2 globulins

7. The amino terminus of the antibody molecule contains
   a. the Fc region
   b. the mast cell-binding site
   c. the paratope
   d. the CH3 region

8. A paratope is
   a. part of an antibody molecule that binds to an epitope
   b. part of an antigen that binds to an epitope
   c. part of the epitope that is highly charged
   d. 2 binding molecules

9. Which of the following is *not* involved in the antibody and antigen interactions?
   a. van der Waals forces
   b. hydrogen bonding
   c. hydrophobic–hydrophillic interactions
   d. convalent bonds

10. Characteristics of IgG include that it is
    a. 900 000 daltons, first one secreted in an immune response, 10 binding sites
    b. 165 000 dalton monomer but usually present as dimer in secretions, protects at surfaces
    c. least in terms of concentration but has most effects in allergy and parasitic infections
    d. largest concentration of all antibodies in serum, MW 150 000 daltons, placental transfer
    e. a differentiation marker on B cells

11. Characteristics of IgM include that it is
    a. 900 000 daltons, first one secreted in an immune response, 10 binding sites
    b. 165 000 dalton monomer but usually present as dimer in secretions
    c. least in terms of concentration, has most effects in allergy and parasitic infections
    d. largest concentration of all antibodies in serum, lymph fluids, cerebrospinal fluid peritoneal fluid, MW 150 000 daltons, placental transfer
    e. differentiation marker on B cells

REVIEW QUESTIONS *(continued)*

12. An isotype is
    a. an area on an immunoglobulin molecule defined by codominant mendelian traits
    b. an area on an immunoglobulin defined as a *unique structure* that binds to the antigen
    c. an area on an immunoglobulin that is involved in the class of the immunoglobulin
    d. none of the above

13. An idiotype is
    a. an area on an immunoglobulin molecule defined by codominant mendelian traits
    b. an area on an immunoglobulin defined as a *unique structure* that binds to the antigen
    c. an area on an immunoglobulin that is involved in the class of the immunoglobulin
    d. none of the above

14. Characteristics of IgA include
    a. 900 000 daltons, first one secreted in an immune response
    b. usually present as dimer in secretions, protects at outside-inside interfaces
    c. *reaginic antibody,* is least in terms of concentration, has most effects in allergy and parasitic infections
    d. largest concentration of all antibodies in serum, lymph fluids cerebrospinal fluid peritoneal fluid, MW 150 000 daltons
    e. differentiation marker on B cells

15. Characteristics of IgE include
    a. 900 000 daltons, first one secreted in an immune response
    b. usually present as dimer in secretions, protects at outside-inside interfaces
    c. least in terms of concentration, has most effects in allergy and parasitic infections
    d. largest concentration of all antibodies in serum, lymph fluids cerebrospinal fluid peritoneal fluid, MW 150 000 daltons
    e. differentiation marker on B cells

16. Which molecule is the best at agglutination and at complement fixation?
    a. IgA
    b. IgE
    c. IgM
    d. IgG

17. An IgG molecule has
    a. 1 antigenic-binding site
    b. 2 identical antigenic-binding sites
    c. 2 different antigenic-binding sites
    d. 10 different antigenic-binding sites

18. Papain cleaves an antibody molecule to
    a. its heavy and light chains
    b. 2 Fab + 1 Fc
    c. 2(Fab')$_2$ + fragments
    d. J chains

19. In monoclonal antibody production, the myeloma cells are used
    a. to grant immortality to the fused cell
    b. to confer the proper Ab-producing quality on the fused cell and to allow the cell to grow in HAT media
    c. to confer the proper Ab production and to confer immortality
    d. none of the above

REFERENCES

1. Silverstein AM. *A History of Immunology.* 2nd ed. New York, NY: Elsevier; 2009: chap 3.
2. Silverstein AM. *A History of Immunology.* 2nd ed. New York, NY: Elsevier; 2009: chap 4.
3. Kindt TJ, Goldsby RA, Osborne BA. *Kuby Immunology.* New York, NY: W.H. Freeman and Company; 2006: chap 4.
4. Kolar GR. The immunoglobulins: Structure and function. In: Paul WE, ed. *Fundamental Immunology.* 6th ed. Philadelphia, PA: Wolters Kluwer/Lippincott Williams & Wilkins; 2008: chap 3.
5. Murphy KM, Travers P, Walport M. *Janeway's Immunobiology.* 7th ed. New York, NY: Garland Science Publishing; 2008: part I, chap 1.
6. Murphy KM, Travers P, Walport M. *Janeway's Immunobiology.* 7th ed. New York, NY: Garland Science Publishing; 2008: chap. 2.
7. Turgeon ML. Antigens and antibodies. In: Turgeon, ML. *Immunology and Serology in Laboratory Medicine.* 4th ed. St. Louis, MO: Mosby; 2009: chap 2.
8. Stevens CD. *Clinical Immunology and Serology: A Laboratory Perspective.* 3rd ed. Philadelphia, PA: F.A. Davis; 2009.

9. Kiyono H, Kunisawa J, McGhee JR et al. The mucosal immune response. In: Paul WE, ed. *Fundamental Immunology*. 6th ed. Philadelphia, PA: Wolters Kluwer/Lippincott Williams & Wilkins; 2008: chap 31.

10. Palmeira P, Costa-Carvalho BT, Arsalanian C, et al. Transfer of antibodies across the placenta and in the breast milk from mothers on intravenous immunoglobulin. *Pediatr Allergy Immunol*. 2009;20:528–535.

11. Wheeler TT, Hodgkinson AJ, Prosser CG, et al. Immune components of colostrum and milk—A historical perspective. *J. Mammary Gland Biol Neoplasia*. 2007;12:237–247.

12. Van der Perre, P. Transfer of antibody via mother's milk. *Vaccine*. 2003;21:3374–3376.

PEARSON

myhealthprofessionskit™

Visit www.myhealthprofessionskit.com to access the interactive Companion Website for this textbook. Simply select "Clinical Laboratory Science" from the choice of disciplines. Find this book and log in using your user name and password to access additional learning tools.

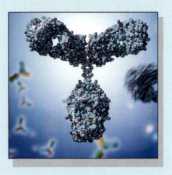

3

Antigens, Epitopes, and Immunogenicity

■ OBJECTIVES—LEVEL I

After this chapter, the student should be able to:

1. Define and describe the basic requirements for immunogenicity.
2. Define and describe *antigen, immunogen,* and *antigenic determinant* or *epitope.*
3. Describe the major role of MHC components in an immune response and the specific roles that MHC class I and MHC class II molecules play in the response.
4. Explain what a haplotype is in regard to inheritance of major histocompatibility complex (MHC) antigens.
5. Compare and contrast a linear versus a conformational epitope.
6. Describe what a hapten is and how it helped define the specificity of the immune system.
7. Describe what a carrier is.
8. Rank the immunogenicity of carbohydrates, lipids, nucleic acids, and proteins.
9. Describe adjuvant and list examples.
10. Define *cross-reactivity* and its effect on assays and responses.

■ OBJECTIVES—LEVEL II

After this chapter, the student should be able to:

1. Compare the terms *autoantigen, alloantigen, heteroantigen,* and *heterophile antigen.*
2. Describe the structural differences between class I and class II MHC molecules.
3. Describe the structure of the T-cell receptor and its associated components.
4. Describe the major steps in antigen processing and presentation by an antigen-presenting cell.

KEY TERMS

adjuvant
alloantigens
antigenic determinants
antigen-presenting cell
antigen processing
autoantigens
conformational epitopes
cross-reactivity
endogenous antigen
epitopes
exogenous antigen

foreignness
haptens
heteroantigens
immunogen
immunological cross-reactivity
invariant chain (Ii)
linear epitopes
major histocompatibility complex (MHC)
phylogenetic
T-cell receptor (TCR)

▶ INTRODUCTION

In a highly organized military defense system, what makes an enemy an "enemy"? No single characteristic feature, not a uniform, not a flag, not a nationality, nor a particular weapon used can categorically and automatically classify any entity as an enemy. Rather, an enemy is a complex set of features that, when interpreted according to one's own environment, may render an entity "foreign" and thus a potentially harmful agent. In this chapter, we describe the concept of immunological foreignness, antigenicity, and immunogenicity and how the immune system goes about "recognizing" antigenic traits. It is important to understand that the immune system cannot distinguish a "good" from a "bad" antigen; indeed, in many situations, the immune system reacts to a harmless antigen and in doing so causes more damage to the host than the antigen itself. We discuss examples of these situations with hypersensitivity and autoimmunity. The immune system can recognize only what is "self" versus "nonself," which, in turn, is dictated by various complex mechanisms that function during the development of the immune system itself. Recognition of antigens in the immune system is achieved by various sets of molecules, including secreted as well as membrane-bound immunoglobulins, T-cell receptors, and products of the genes belonging to the major histocompatibility complex. This chapter will discuss these molecules and their role in antigen recognition.

▶ REQUIREMENTS FOR IMMUNOGENICITY

A compound's composition and size can determine whether that compound can elicit an immune response and can influence the strength of that response. The basic characteristics that determine immunogenicity are (1) foreignness, (2) molecular size, (3) chemical complexity, (4) susceptibility to recognition, uptake, and degradation by antigen-presenting cells, (5) indirectly, the method of introduction of the antigen, and (6) the presence of certain chemicals that can act as immune adjuvants.

FOREIGNNESS

The concept of **foreignness** refers to the **phylogenetic** relationship between the host and the antigen. In general, the farther apart they are in this relationship, the better is the response to the antigen. So, for example, a compound from a plant can stimulate a better immune response in a human than a component from a very close species, such as another primate. This is not to say that members of the same species cannot generate immune responses against each other; however, in general, the more phylogenetically distant the antigen from the host, the better the response (1). Such "distance" can

be described within 3 different sets of antigens: **Autoantigens** are self-antigens (ie, antigens that are part of the host). As expected, these antigens are not immunogenic to the host, at least under normal conditions. Antigens that are from other members of the same species as the host are termed **alloantigens,** which can elicit an immune response in the host. **Heteroantigens** are antigens from a species different from the host, for example, a different animal, a plant, or a microorganism. Interestingly, some heteroantigens, although may share similarities and have epitopes that can cross-react. These are called *heterophile antigens;* their clinical relevance is that this **cross-reactivity** may affect procedures such as blood transfusions because these antigens are relevant when dealing with blood groups.

 Checkpoint! 3.1

What is a protein from your own body called?

Is this protein more or less immunogenic than a protein from a bacterium?

SIZE AND COMPLEXITY

The size of the antigen is also a major factor in immunogenicity: In general, the larger its size, the stronger its immunogenicity. In general, antigens of less than 1000 daltons are nonimmunogenic, 1000 to 6000 are sometimes immunogenic, and molecules of more than 6000 daltons, if foreign, are generally immunogenic. **Haptens** are small compounds that cannot stimulate an immune response unless they are linked to a much larger immunogenic molecule. The larger molecule to which a hapten is linked is called the *carrier molecule.* There are exceptions to the immunogenicity and size rule: Many small compounds such as glucagon (3400 daltons) can be immunogenic, and large homopolymers (ie, components made of numerous repeating units of simple compounds) do not elicit an immune response. But, in general, size is usually related to chemical complexity, and both affect the immunogenicity of an antigen. Chemical complexity also implies more numerous and diverse antigenic determinants, which are the critical recognition factors for the immune system. Larger, more complex antigens have a better chance to have epitopes recognized by helper T cells; they may also be better recognized and therefore be more susceptible to phagocytosis by antigen-presenting cells (1).

NATURE

Proteins, with their overall large size and chemical complexity, make strong immunogens; their secondary, tertiary, and quaternary structures contribute to this immunogenicity by displaying

TABLE 3.1

Immunogenicity of Different Types of Antigens

Antigen	Immunogenicity
Proteins	+++
Carbohydrates	++
Lipids	+/−
Nucleic acids	−

both linear as well as conformational epitopes. Proteins are usually thymic-dependent antigens (ie, after being processed by antigen-presenting cells, a relevant epitope is presented to a T cell and stimulates it, which, in turn, secretes cytokines that increase and mature the immune response). Carbohydrates, usually made of repeating units from a limited number of sugars, are immunogenic but less so than proteins, and the response to these saccharides is usually T-cell independent. Anticarbohydrate responses are important in the responses to blood groups, bacteria, and tumor-associated antigens. At the end of the list come lipids and nucleic acids, which are usually not immunogenic unless covalently linked to an immunogenic carrier (Table 3.1 ❂). Although they occur rarely, antibodies that react to DNA are very important clinically, however, because they are present in some individuals with systemic lupus erythematosus (SLE) and can indicate a more severe form of the disease. These antibodies may be causative for some of the kidney damage seen in SLE.

✓ Checkpoint! 3.2

At first glance, if a pathogen has both a protein antigen and a carbohydrate antigen that do not cross-react with human antigens, which would you use to make the most effective vaccine?

STATE AND SITE

Immunization protocols can also influence the immunogenicity of an **immunogen.** For example, particulate antigens (such as a whole microorganism or segments of tissue) often elicit responses after inoculation by intracutaneous or intravenous routes at a broad range of doses. Soluble antigens, on the other hand, may require more fastidious and critical schedules/doses of immunizations (eg, repeated immunizations) (1).

ADDITION OF IMMUNE-ENHANCING AGENTS

The use of an **adjuvant** can also increase the response to an immunogen. Adjuvants are chemicals that, when mixed with immunogen, enhance the immune response to

that immunogen. However, the immunogen itself must be immunogenic per se (ie, adjuvants cannot make a nonimmunogenic compound immunogenic or act as immunogenic carriers). Adjuvants tend to be chemicals that can stimulate a localized inflammatory reaction at the site of their injection by recruiting to the site phagocytic and inflammatory cells, which facilitate better uptake of the antigen. In addition, adjuvants are thought to increase the size of the immunogen and to physically maintain the antigen within the area of inflammation by causing a slower antigen release so that more immune cells arriving at the site participate in the response to that antigen. Adjuvants vary in composition from aluminum salts to mineral oil and often contain bacteria or bacterial products. Examples are alum, Freund's adjuvant (a mineral oil and water mixture either free from or containing bacterial products), lipopolysaccharide (LPS), and muramyl dipeptide.

▶ ANTIGENIC DETERMINANTS (EPITOPES)

If we look at the recognition of a person as an analogy, recognizing a person's face involves the prior recognition of several different features of that face. This may include color of eyes, color of hair, characteristic facial features, and a limited number of other small but essential factors that are critical components of that face. The recognition of these components as a specific individual is based on their nature as well as their specific arrangement in space in relationship to each other and precedes the subsequent recognition of the face as a whole. Such a process then leads to a conceptual conclusion that ultimately results in the total recognition of that person's face. Likewise, the immune system recognizes an antigen by distinguishing a limited number of immunogenic components of that antigen. These components, called **antigenic determinants** or **epitopes,** are restricted portions of a molecule that are involved in the actual binding with the combining site of a particular antibody. The number of distinct antigenic determinants on an antigen molecule varies in size and chemical complexity. The nature and the special arrangement of these antigenic determinants plays a crucial role in the ability of the immune system in recognizing the antigen (1, 2). Epitopes can be linear or conformational. **Linear epitopes** are usually related to the amino acid sequence of a particular antigen; they are not affected by the 3-dimensional structure of the antigen in space; on the other hand, **conformational epitopes** depend on the antigen's 3-dimensional structure and, in turn, depend on the antigen's secondary and tertiary conformation. So, the unfolding of a protein antigen, as in denaturation, will affect the recognition of conformational epitopes but not of linear epitopes (1, 2). A diagram of linear epitopes is shown in Figure 3.1 ■.

Each epitope will be recognized by and stick to the binding site of a particular immunoglobulin or T-cell receptor (1, 3),

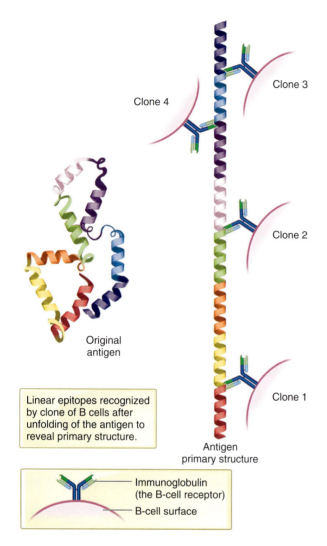

Linear epitopes recognized by clone of B cells after unfolding of the antigen to reveal primary structure.

Immunoglobulin (the B-cell receptor)

B-cell surface

FIGURE 3.1 Schematic diagram showing polyclonal response by B cells against linear epitopes.

and a particular antibody-producing cell synthesizes immunoglobulins that recognize a particular epitope of a particular antigen. Therefore, an individual's normal antibody response to an antigen involves the production of different immunoglobulins, each recognizing different epitopes of the same antigen (Figure 3.2 ■) (1). The size of an epitope can vary, depending on the immune molecule with which it reacts. So, for example, epitopes recognized by surface immunoglobulins on B cells can vary between 6 and 15 amino acid or 2–7 sugars; class I MHC molecules can recognize peptides of 8–10 amino acids, and class II can accommodate peptides of 13–18 amino acids (4, 5).

CROSS-REACTIVITY

Because nature is often made of repeating patterns, antigenic determinants—or epitopes—may be shared by different antigens; the fact that epitopes can be shared in nature can lead

to **immunological cross-reactivity.** *Cross-reactivity* is the reaction of an antibody with an antigen other than the one that induced its formation. Occasionally something cross-reacts because it contains the same epitope but in different areas elsewhere on the molecule; at other times, something can cross-react because it contains an area very similar to the epitope. Sometimes cross-reactivity is useful, but we must be careful that cross-reactivity does not cause us to misdiagnose a patient. An example of cross-reactivity proving useful is with tetanus toxin and tetanus toxoid. The toxin (native and harmful) and the toxoid (modified and nontoxic) are different biologically and chemically but cross-react immunologically. This allows for the development of an antitoxin vaccine while avoiding the use of the toxin as the immunizing agent.

> ### ✓ Checkpoint! 3.3
>
> *The fact that bacteria that causes Strep throat have an epitope that cross-reacts with the heart tissue components can cause a disease called rheumatic heart disease, where antibodies produced to the bacteria react with and injure the heart. This is due to a phenomena called* ~~immunologreat cross-reactivity~~

Sometimes cross-reactivity requires extra steps in an assay to prevent misdiagnosis, and this is the case with the shared epitopes of the molecules of luteinizing hormone, follicle-stimulating hormone, and human chorionic gonadotropin. A pregnancy test must contain antibodies that are very specific to human chorionic gonadotropin but that do not cross-react with the others; otherwise, a pregnancy test would be positive when a woman is ovulating. The clinical significance of immunological cross-reactivity spans from the development of vaccines, to hypersensitivity, to autoimmunity; some of these issues are covered in different chapters.

▶ MAJOR HISTOCOMPATIBILITY COMPLEX

The **major histocompatibility complex (MHC)** is a region formed by genetic loci discovered during the study of rejection of foreign tissue, thus the term *histo* (tissue) *compatibility*. However, it has since been found that this genetic region plays a central role in both humoral and cell-mediated immunity. The region is composed of a family of a large number of genes on chromosome 6. The MHC genes are found in most vertebrates and participate in immune responses to both foreign as well as self-antigens. The 3 classes of MHC gene products are I, II, and III. Classes I and II represent distinct structural entities exhibiting similar overall structures; class III contains a diverse collection of different genes, including some encoding for complement components as well as some that encode for cytokines and

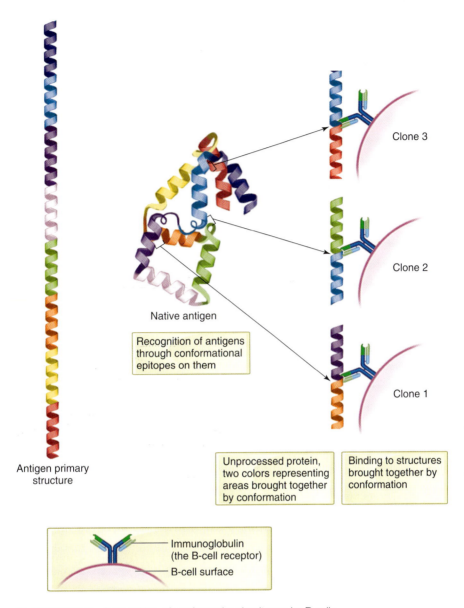

Native antigen

Recognition of antigens
through conformational
epitopes on them

Antigen primary
structure

Clone 3

Clone 2

Clone 1

Unprocessed protein,
two colors representing
areas brought together
by conformation

Binding to structures
brought together by
conformation

Immunoglobulin
(the B-cell receptor)

B-cell surface

■ **FIGURE 3.2**   Recognition of conformational epitopes by B cells.

some other soluble proteins (1). A diagram of the different MHC genes is shown in Figure 3.3 ■.

Only a portion of the genes in the MHC plays a direct role in immune responses; these include the genes that are assigned to the human leukocyte antigen (HLA) group, which, in turn, encode for proteins that participate in antigen presentation from an antigen-presenting cell to a T cell. Often the terms *MHC* and *HLA* are interchangeably used; however, *HLA* refers to the gene products (proteins) that are involved in antigen presentation, while *MHC* refers to the area of the genome that encodes for these products as well as others not directly involved in antigen presentation. As we will see when we discuss antigen presentation to T cells, the diversity of the MHC is a critical requirement for the diversity of an immune response in humans, and MHC restricts antigen recognition by T cells (6, 7).

MHC haplotypes are highly polymorphic (ie, the genes have many alternate forms). These alleles are inherited, one set of alleles from each parent, and each set of alleles is codominantly expressed, that is, the products of both sets of genes are expressed on cell surfaces. MHC classes I and II belong to the immunoglobulin superfamily, sharing some structural similarities with immunoglobulins. However, unlike the genes for immunoglobulins and T-cell receptors, MHC genes are not rearranged; therefore, the repertoire of a person's MHC is limited by the haplotypes inherited from each parent. These genes are inherited as linked sets like beads in a string; a particular HLA, ABC, DR, DP, and DQ set is inherited as a unit from each parent, so 4 different sets can be inherited. After HLA typing of the parents and one sibling, the segregation of the sets as well as the 4 possible inheritance patterns can be

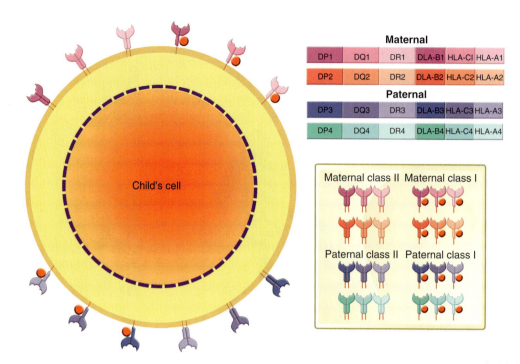

Maternal

DP1	DQ1	DR1	DLA-B1	HLA-CI	HLA-A1
DP2	DQ2	DR2	DLA-B2	HLA-C2	HLA-A2

Paternal

DP3	DQ3	DR3	DLA-B3	HLA-C3	HLA-A3
DP4	DQ4	DR4	DLA-B4	HLA-C4	HLA-A4

■ **FIGURE 3.3**   MHC genes and expression.

determined. Because of the inherited MHC, different individuals may respond differently to a particular antigen. The MHC genes are the most polymorphic genes in the human genome; each locus may have a very large number of different alleles, and the theoretical diversity in the MHC is estimated to be more than 1 trillion. An example of MHC genetic control of the immune response is an inherited tendency called a *hole in the repertoire,* which occurs when an individual fails to respond to a certain antigen. The most graphic example of this that comes to mind is that some individuals do not respond to poison ivy, an antigen that causes the rest of us to have an unwanted response. This lack of responsiveness is an inherited tendency.

Class I molecules are involved in antigen presentation of **endogenous antigens** (ie, a foreign entity that appears from within the cell, such as fragments from a foreign protein after the cell has been infected by an organism that replicates intracellularly such as a virus or some bacteria). Because all nucleated cells have the potential to be infected by a virus or an intracellular microorganism, class I molecules are found on *all* nucleated cells. Class I molecules are encoded by 3 different regions of the MHC: A, B, and C. These molecules are composed of a single polypeptide chain of approximately 45 kilodalton (kDa), associated noncovalently with a smaller component of approximately 12 kDa called *β2 microglobulin,* which plays a role in maintaining the proper 3-dimensional structure of the α chain. A

hydrophobic region of the α chain anchors the molecule to the membrane; the peptide-binding site of the α chain (ie, where the antigen fragment binds) is divided into the most polymorphic regions of the molecule, specifically α1 and α2. Another region, α3, functions as a binding site for the CD8 molecule on cytotoxic T cells (1, 6, 7).

Unlike class I molecules, which are found on all nucleated cells, class II molecules are found only on certain immune cells, specifically antigen-presenting cells such as those of the monocyte–macrophage lineage, B cells, and dendritic cells. They are structurally different than class I molecules because class II molecules are composed of 2 polypeptide chains, the α chain (approximately 33kDa in size), and the β chain (approximately 28 kDa), which are associated noncovalently and anchored to the cell membrane by a hydrophobic region of each of the chains (Figure 3.4 ■). As with the class I molecules, class II molecules are also encoded by different regions of the MHC, specifically, the DR, DP, and DQ regions. Each chain is further divided into 2 domains: α1 and α2, and β1 and β2. The association of the 2 chains on the cell membrane creates a peptide-binding cleft composed of the α1 and β1 domains; it is in this cleft that a fragment of degraded antigen can bind for antigen presentation. Like the class I molecules, the peptide-binding cleft is where the majority of the polymorphism is found. The major functional difference between class I MHC and class II MHC is in the nature of the antigen they recognize. Class I molecules are associated with

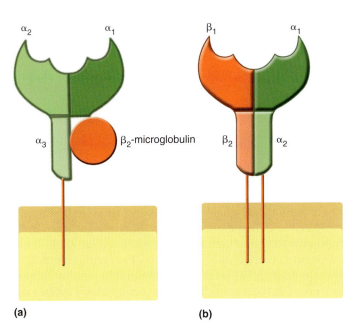

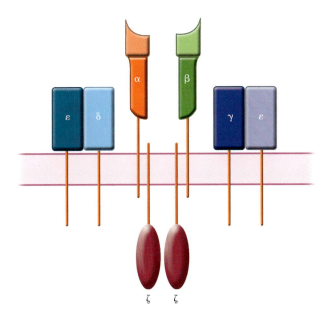

(a)   **(b)**

■ **FIGURE 3.4** (a) Schematic representation of MHC class I molecule, consisting of 3 α-domains and 1 β$_2$-microglobulin molecule, the peptide-binding groove is situated between domains α$_1$ and α$_2$. (b) Schematic representation of MHC class II molecule, consisting of 2 α-domains and 2 β-domains, the peptide-binding groove is situated between domains α$_1$ and β$_1$.

■ **FIGURE 3.5** Diagram of the α-β T-cell receptor complex including associated CD3 proteins.

recognition of endogenous antigens, and class II molecules are involved in the recognition of **exogenous antigens** (ie, antigens that are present extracellularly—an infectious microorganism or a foreign protein—and that have been engulfed by an antigen-presenting cell). The different roles that MHC class I and MHC class II molecules play in an immune response will be clear when we discuss antigen processing and presentation. See Figure 3.4 for diagrams of MHC classes I and II molecules.

▶ T-CELL RECEPTORS

T cells, like B cells, are capable of recognizing a large number of different antigens. This recognition is achieved through surface molecules called **T-cell receptors (TCR),** (1) which also belong to the immunoglobulin superfamily of proteins and share some structural features with immunoglobulins. They are composed of 2 heterodimers (either α, β or γ, δ) covalently linked by a single disulfide bond and have a variable region, a single "immunoglobulin-like" constant region, a membrane-spanning region, and a connecting peptide or hinge-like region; some (α, β heterodimers) exhibit a cytoplasmic tail (Figure 3.5 ■). The variable regions of the heterodimers form the binding site for antigen peptides; their diversity is randomly created by rearranging variable region genes just like immunoglobulins, and such rearrangement follows similar mechanisms and nomenclature as for immunoglobulins (ie, VJ and VDJ recombinations) (1, 8). However, there are

also differences between T-cell receptors and immunoglobulins: T-cell receptors exist only on the cell surface and are not secreted like immunoglobulins. Also, somatic mutations do not appear to contribute to the random repertoire of T-cell receptor specificities as they do for immunoglobulins, and there is no rearrangement of the constant region genes such as the ones that achieve isotype switch in immunoglobulins. In addition, the V-J junctional diversity is much higher in T-cell receptors than in immunoglobulins. This may be due to the small fragments of degraded antigen that T cells recognize. The T-cell receptor heterodimers in the cell membrane are associated with a group of membrane proteins called the *CD3 complex,* which includes CD3γ, δ, and ε as well as the ζ chains. The CD3 complex does not determine antigen specificity as the T-cell receptor heterodimers do; on the other hand, the CD3 complex is involved in transmembrane signaling transmission and subsequent cell activation (1).

▶ ANTIGEN PROCESSING

To discuss antigen processing and presentation, let's first review some facts. Antigens that are taken up by **antigen-presenting cells** such as macrophages or dendritic cells tend to be strong immunogens; antigens that remain in solution, however, are usually weak ones. T cells from a person immune to a microorganism will not bind directly to that organism, but they will bind either to antigen-presenting cells that have ingested that organism (class II presentation) or that have been infected by that organism (class I presentation). This suggests that although T cells are essential for an immune response to a particular antigen, their role in recognizing the antigen differs from the role of cells that encounter the antigen in the first place. This, in turn, leads to **antigen processing** and presentation, a mechanism that comprises a series of essential cellular and biochemical events that activate CD4+ and CD8+ T cells after an accessory or antigen-presenting cell binds a particular antigen, internalizes it, processes it biochemically, and then presents it to the T cell (1, 6, 7).

An antibody response to a protein antigen is usually directed to its conformational determinants, which are displayed on the protein in its natural state, and may be based on the folded form of the protein itself. B cells, which produce antibodies to the original form of the antigen, must recognize an antigen in its natural state; therefore, B-cell clones reactive to a particular antigen must interact with it before its chemical processing. In contrast, T cells recognize denatured or native protein molecules that the host has biochemically processed. These differences make it necessary for antigen-presenting cells to "break down and alter" the antigen so that T-cell recognition and activation can occur. The recognition of an antigen by an antigen-presenting cell differs according to the nature of the antigen-presenting cell itself as was described in Chapter 1. For example, macrophages may recognize an antigen by having receptors for certain carbohydrate moieties, or receptors for complement components, or receptors for the Fc portion of immunoglobulin molecules. During opsonization, an antigen may be covered by the C3 complement component or by immunoglobulin, thus becoming more "visible" to a macrophage that has receptors for these components. B cells, in turn, recognize the antigen via their surface immunoglobulin whereas dendritic cells, the most common antigen-presenting cells, take up antigens by recognizing patterns and features that are common to microbial surfaces or by a process called *pinocytosis,* which involves ingesting large amounts of surrounding material and fluids (1).

Once an antigen is internalized, it goes through a process that breaks it down into components, which, after further processing, ultimately can bind to components encoded by the genes of the MHC. This is a critical step because a direct relationship exists between the immunogenicity of an antigen and the binding strength of its processed peptides with MHC molecules. In other words, strong immunogens bind better to MHC than weak immunogens. Therefore, the T-cell response to a particular immunogen depends on whether the immunogen contains components capable of interacting with MHC molecules (1, 6, 7).

When an endogenous antigen is involved, antigen peptides are processed so they can bind to class I MHC molecules; in the case of an exogenous antigen, however, such peptides bind to MHC class II molecules. The first step in this process is the uptake of an antigen by the antigen-presenting cell and its internalization into specific intracellular vesicles. Within these vesicles, antigens are processed by various cytoplasmic proteases, and the resulting products are then transported to the rough endoplasmic reticulum (RER). This transport is carried out by a group of proteins called *ABC proteins,* a family of proteins that transport various molecules (including antigen peptides) across membranes. Peptides are transported by certain ABC proteins called *transporters* associated with antigen processing (specifically TAP-1 and TAP-2) into the RER where class I and class II (among other molecules) are synthesized and assembled (9). The specificity of the MHC molecules for different antigens is somewhat promiscuous; MHC molecules have a binding site that can only partially discriminate between antigens, and many different antigens (peptides) can bind to the same MHC-binding site. This is so because the binding site of the MHC molecules tends to recognize common chemical motifs rather than highly specific sequences or structural features. The binding site of MHC molecules is a complex 3-dimensional structure with a variety of pockets, protrusions, ridges, invaginations, and depressions, so the binding of an antigen peptide here depends on the nature of the side chains of that peptide and their complementarity with the MHC molecule's binding groove (4, 5).

Although MHC class I and class II molecules follow similar mechanisms throughout antigen processing and presentation, the interaction of peptides with MHC class I and class II occurs at different sites in the cell (Table 3.2 ✪). Following synthesis

✪ TABLE 3.2

MHC Class I and Class II Molecules

Type of MHC Molecule	T Cell Type That It Reacts With	Type of Antigen	On Which Cells	Antigen Size	Antigen Added to the MHC in the
Class I	CD8+ cytotoxic T cell	Endogenous (from inside the cell as in an infected cell)	All nucleated cells in body	Peptides 8–10 amino acids long	Golgi
Class II	CD4+ helper T cell	Exogenous (picked up from the environment)	Antigen-presenting cells such as cells of the monocyte–macrophage lineage, B cells, and dendritic cells	Peptides 13–18 amino acids long	Endosomal compartment after invariant chain removal

in the RER, both classes I and II molecules are transported to the Golgi compartment. In the Golgi, classes I and II segregate: Class I molecules interact with the antigen peptides; peptides which fulfill the requirements for fitting into the binding groove, will combine with MHC molecules, and the MHC-peptide complex goes directly to the cell surface for antigen presentation.

On the other hand, class II molecules in the RER are complexed to an additional component called the **invariant chain (Ii)** whose function is to prevent class II molecules from binding peptides derived from endogenous antigens. The class II-invariant chain complex is transported to an acidic endosomal or lysosomal compartment where the invariant chain is dissociated from the class II molecule and swapped with the antigen peptide; the class II-peptide complex is then transported to the cell surface for antigen presentation. Incidentally, as much as MHC components play a critical role in immune responses, their regulation can also modulate the response in which they are involved. The quantity of MHC class II on monocytes and macrophages varies; interferon-γ released by activated T cells during antigen presentation binds to receptors on young phagocytes. This causes, among other changes, an increase of MHC class II molecules (1, 6, 7). Refer to Figure 3.6 ■ for differences in the antigen-processing pathways between MHC molecules class I and class II.

► DIFFERENT ROLES FOR MHC CLASSES I AND II MOLECULES IN AN IMMUNE RESPONSE

As we have seen, class I and class II MHC molecules follow similar mechanisms in antigen presentation to T cells. However, they have a different role in an immune response. In addition, the size of the epitope they recognize varies; class I MHC molecules can recognize peptides of 8 to 10 amino acids, whereas class II can accommodate peptides of 13 to 18 amino acids. MHC class I molecules bind antigenic peptides in the endoplasmic reticulum. These peptides tend to be fragments of self-proteins or foreign components that come from within the cell, such as a viral component or a fragment of an intracellular organism or even tumor components. Fragments are also derived from proteins that have been newly synthesized but may not be formed or folded correctly. Overall, a large number of *intracellular proteins* (including host proteins) are processed that way and presented in association with class I molecules. Most do not activate T cells, however, because T cells expressing self-reactive T-cell receptors are eliminated during the thymic processes involved in T-cell maturation. Peptides that are derived from foreign host proteins inside an infected cell, on the other hand, are recognized by T cells, specifically the cytotoxic T cells. After processing of antigen and association with class I components, the MHC–peptide complex is brought to the surface and recognized by a CD8+ T cell (cytotoxic T cell). This recognition is achieved because the CD8 molecule on the cytotoxic T cell acts as a receptor for the class I molecule and the specificity of antigen recognition is achieved by the T-cell receptor on the cytotoxic T cell recognizing the antigen peptide that is associated with the class I molecule. What follows is the activation of the CD8+ T cell, which ultimately results in killing the infected antigen-presenting cell. Thus, MHC class I molecules are involved in the elimination of "altered" self-cells such as a virally infected cell.

In contrast, class II molecules must travel from the endoplasmic reticulum to an endosomal compartment before they can interact with antigenic peptides where the invariant chain is removed and antigen peptides are then allowed to interact with the class II molecule. These compartments usually contain antigenic peptides that derived from phagocytosed exogenous antigens such as an ingested extracellular microorganism. The MHC class II-peptide complex is then transported to the surface where a CD4+ (helper) T cell recognizes it as the CD4 molecule acts as a receptor for the MHC class II molecule. Antigen specificity, once again, is dictated by the antigen peptide interacting with the T-cell receptor on the CD4+ cell (1, 6, 7). T-cell activation follows, and the mechanisms following this activation will be described in Chapter 4.

> ✓ **Checkpoint! 3.4**
>
> *Because every cell in your body can become infected, every cell may need to present the antigens from this internal infection to CD8+ T cells that can kill them to get rid of the infection. What molecule is involved in this presentation?*

► THE EXQUISITE SPECIFICITY OF THE IMMUNE SYSTEM

Haptens are low molecular weight compounds that are not immunogenic (ie, they cannot elicit an immune response by themselves) but can become antigenic if conjugated to an immunogenic carrier (eg, protein) by acting as novel antigenic determinants of the carrier. The immune response generated by the hapten-carrier conjugate elicits antibodies to not only the carrier itself but also antibodies specific for the hapten. Haptens can be artificially made or can occur in nature; natural haptens can become linked to self-proteins and provoke an immune response to that self-protein. For example, certain antibiotics such as penicillin can create hapten self-protein conjugates that create hypersensitivity reactions, some of which can be fatal. Another example is poison ivy; the plant contains certain small compounds that can act as haptens, link to self-proteins during exposure, and cause self-reactive responses, which are reflected in the rash typical of the reaction to poison ivy. Because they are very carefully prepared and chemically well defined, artificially created haptens, on

Pathway of class I MHC-associated antigen presentation

1	2	3	4	5
Proteins or other endogenous antigens in cytosol	Proteins are processed and degraded	Peptides from degradation are transported to the ER	Antigen peptides are associated with MHC class I molecules	Antigen peptide-MHC class I complex is expressed on cell surface

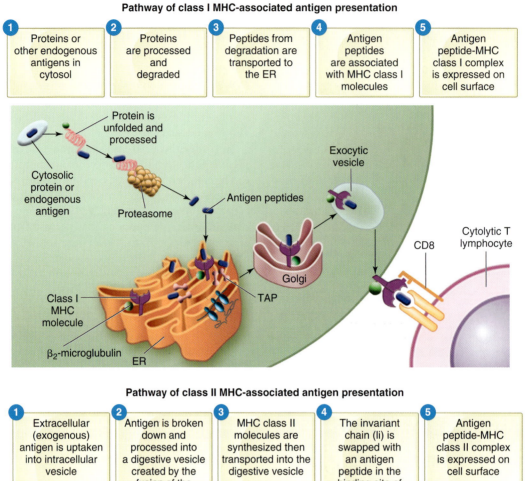

Pathway of class II MHC-associated antigen presentation

1	2	3	4	5
Extracellular (exogenous) antigen is uptaken into intracellular vesicle	Antigen is broken down and processed into a digestive vesicle created by the fusion of the endosome and the lysosome	MHC class II molecules are synthesized then transported into the digestive vesicle	The invariant chain (Ii) is swapped with an antigen peptide in the binding site of the MHC class II molecule	Antigen peptide-MHC class II complex is expressed on cell surface

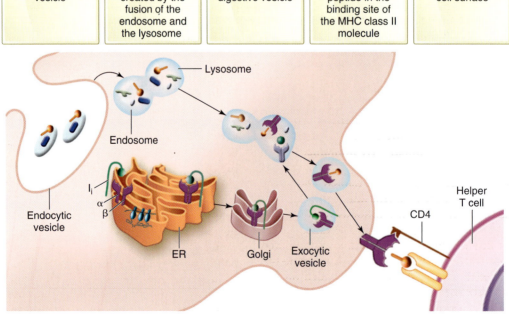

■ **FIGURE 3.6** Differences in the antigen-processing pathways between MHC molecules class I and class II.

Hapten	Antisera to:			
	Aminobenzene	o-Aminobenzoic acid	m-Aminobenzoic acid	p-Aminobenzoic acid
Aminobenzene	+++	–	–	–
o-Aminobenzoic acid	–	+++	–	–
m-Aminobenzoic acid	–	–	+++	–
p-Aminobenzoic acid	–	–	–	+++

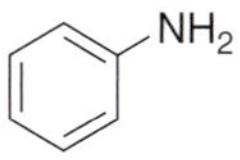

Aminobenzene

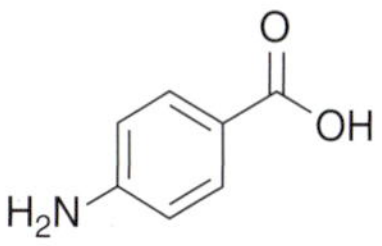

p-aminobenzoic acid

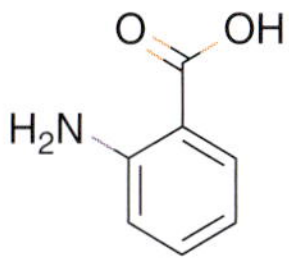

o-aminobenzoic acid

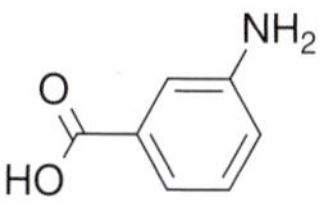

m-aminobenzoic acid

■ **FIGURE 3.7** Landsteiner's experiment demonstrating the exquisite specificity of the immune system.

the other hand, have been used to study the specificity of antigen–antibody reactions.

Using haptens, Karl Landsteiner (10) demonstrated the exquisite specificity of the immune system in a classical experiment. In it, laboratory animals were immunized using hapten-carrier conjugates. The animal's antibody response was then tested against the carrier, against the hapten, and, more importantly, with closely related haptens linked to a different immunogenic carrier. In this way, the antibody response specific to a particular hapten independent of the carrier could be measured. The immunizing hapten and the closely related haptens were all derivatives of aminobenzene. The antibody's level of reactivity with a specific hapten depended on the overall configuration of the hapten itself. Refer to Figure 3.7 ■ for the results of the experiment. When using aminobenzene with a carboxyl group at the para position (para-aminobenzoic

acid), antibodies from the immunized animal reacted with the original immunizing hapten configuration (ie, with the carboxyl group in the para position) but did not cross-react with aminobenzene if the carboxyl groups were at the meta or ortho position. The same was true if the original immunizing configuration had the hydroxyl groups in the meta position: Antibodies would react with meta-aminobenzoic acid but not with para- or ortho-benzoic acid. On the other hand, when using aminobenzene with different side groups but in the same para position, different levels of antibody reactivity were seen. It must be emphasized that these differences in hapten structure (ie, a change in position of a conjugate on an aromatic ring) are infinitely minuscule compared to the enormity of the molecular size of a protein and that from these experiments came the realization that the diversity of specificity of an immune response can be immense.

CASE STUDY

A company is trying to develop a vaccine for a certain infectious disease. After studying the microorganism causing the disease, researchers identify one of its components as highly immunogenic, so they decide to undergo a clinical trial and use such component as a vaccine. The study participants respond well to the vaccination and develop a strong antibody response to both the component and the whole organism. However, after a while, some of the study participants start developing autoimmune hemolytic anemia.

The same company changes its protocol and now looks for a safer component for the vaccine. After much biochemical manipulation of different components of the microorganism, researchers find a peptide that is unique to the organisms by boiling and then solubilizing one of the components of the microorganism in detergent. They test this linear peptide and find it to be immunogenic in laboratory animals (ie, the animals mount a strong antibody response to the peptide). However, when they test the antibody response to the whole organism, they get none.

The company is also trying to develop a diagnostic kit to identify the organism using antibodies raised against a small (molecular weight of approximately 150 daltons) yet highly specific (ie, unique to that organism) aromatic compound found only on the surface of that organism. Injecting the small compound in laboratory animals does not generate an immune response to it, so the company decides to mix the compound with complete Freund's adjuvant (a powerful immunologic adjuvant) before administering to the animals. Yet even with the use of such powerful adjuvant, no antibody response to the compound is obtained.

1. What do you think is a possible reason for some of the study participants starting to develop autoimmune hemolytic anemia?

2. With the new protocol, why do you think the company got no antibody response to the whole organism?

3. For the diagnostic kit, the company decided to mix the compound with complete Freund's adjuvant but still got no antibody response. What do you think the reason is?

4. What would you suggest as an alternate approach to make an antibody preparation against the small compound?

SUMMARY

The immunogenicity of an antigen depends on several factors including foreignness; molecular size; chemical complexity; susceptibility to recognition, uptake, and degradation by antigen-presenting cells; the method of the antigen's introduction; and the presence of immune adjuvants. *Foreignness* refers to the phylogenetic relationship between the host and the antigen: In general, the farther apart they are in this relationship, the better the response to the antigen. When size is concerned, in general, the larger the size of the antigen, the stronger is its immunogenicity:

Size is usually related to chemical complexity and both affect the immunogenicity of an antigen. Chemical complexity, in turn, implies more numerous and diverse antigenic determinants, which are the critical recognition factors for the immune system. Immunogenicity depends on the nature of a particular antigen; proteins are usually strong immunogens. Carbohydrates are immunogenic, but less so than proteins. Lipids and nucleic acids are usually not immunogenic unless covalently linked to an immunogenic carrier. Immunogenicity can also be affected by immunization protocols and route of entry as well as mixing the immunogen with an immunologic adjuvant. The basis of immune recognition relies on the concept of epitopes, or antigenic determinants, that are restricted portions of a molecule involved in the actual binding with the combining site of a particular antibody, T-cell receptor, or MHC molecule. Epitopes can be shared among different entities, and such sharing can result in cross-reactivity, which is the reaction of an antibody with an antigen other than the one that induced its formation.

The major histocompatibility complex (MHC) plays an essential role in antigen recognition because antigen recognition by T cell is restricted to the repertoires of the MHC. Of the different MHC components, class I and class II MHC molecules are involved in antigen recognition. Class I molecules are involved in antigen presentation of endogenous antigens (ie, a foreign entity that appears from within the cell, such as fragments from a foreign protein) after the cell has been infected by an organism such as a virus or some bacteria that replicates intracellularly. On the other hand, class II molecules are involved in the recognition of exogenous antigens (ie, antigens that are present extracellularly—an infectious microorganism or a foreign protein and that have been engulfed by an antigen-presenting cell). The involvement of MHC molecules in antigen recognition is demonstrated in antigen processing, a mechanism that comprises a series of essential cellular and biochemical events that activate CD4+ and CD8+ T cells after an accessory or antigen-presenting cell binds a particular antigen, internalizes it, processes it biochemically, and then presents it to the T cell. During this mechanism, antigen peptides derived from antigen processing are combined with either class I or class II MHC molecules, depending on whether the antigen is endogenous or exogenous. In this regard, antigen processing by class I and class II molecules follows slightly different cellular pathways. Unlike the genes for immunoglobulins and T-cell receptors, MHC genes are not rearranged and therefore the repertoire of a person's MHC is limited by the haplotypes inherited from each parent. At the end of these pathways, an antigenic peptide with an MHC molecule is presented to a T cell, which recognizes the peptide via a molecule called *T-cell receptor*. T-cell receptors belong to the immunoglobulin superfamily of proteins and share some structural features with immunoglobulins; the T cell uses them to recognize antigen peptides. Overall, these mechanisms allow for an immunological recognition that is exquisitely specific (ie, the immune system can distinguish very small chemical and structural differences between otherwise similar antigens), thus providing a large repertoire of possible recognition specificities to the host.

REVIEW QUESTIONS

1. Which is *not* true of antigenic determinants (or epitopes)?
   a. They are restricted portions of a molecule that are involved in the actual binding with the combining site of a particular immunoglobulin molecule.
   b. The number of distinct antigenic determinants on an antigen molecule varies with its size and chemical complexity.
   c. An antigen must have a minimum number of antigenic determinants before it can become immunogenic.
   d. A polyclonal antibody response involves the production of different immunoglobulins, each recognizing different epitopes of the same antigen.

2. The sharing of 1 or more identical antigenic determinants between 2 different antigens is defined as
   a. chemotaxis
   b. receptor cross-linking
   c. immune complexes
   d. immunological cross-reactivity

3. During antigen processing, transportation of antigen peptides to the RER is thought to be mediated by
   a. ABC proteins
   b. MHC class II molecules
   c. MHC class I molecules
   d. B-cell receptors

4. Which is *correct* about MHC class II molecules?
   a. Every nucleated cell expresses them.
   b. They are involved in the presentation of endogenous antigens.
   c. They are involved in the presentation of antigen peptides to CD8+ T cells.
   d. None of the above.

5. During antigen processing, antigen–peptide interaction with MHC class II molecules probably occurs
   a. in the nucleus of the antigen-presenting cell
   b. at the surface of the antigen-presenting cell
   c. in the mitochondria of the antigen-presenting cell
   d. in an endosomal or lysosomal compartment

6. In general, which of the following makes the best immunogen?
   a. a very large homopolymer
   b. a very large protein
   c. a polysaccharide
   d. a very long nucleic acid

7. A MHC class I molecule
   a. can bind most peptides that are 9 amino acids long
   b. can bind only whole proteins
   c. can bind a specific antigen only, which is determined by an event that occurs during maturation in the absence of antigen
   d. can bind a specific antigen only, which is determined by an event that occurs during maturation in the presence of antigen

8. Helper T cells interact with
   a. CD4+ molecules
   b. CD8+ molecules
   c. class I molecules
   d. class II molecules

9. Class II molecules
   a. must be transported from RER to an endosomal compartment before binding peptides
   b. bind to antigen in the RER
   c. bind to a blocking protein called ABC protein
   d. can only bind peptides smaller than 8 amino acids

10. Which of these is least immunogenic?
    a. protein
    b. polysaccharides
    c. self-proteins
    d. all of the above are immunogenic

11. Class II molecules
    a. are on every nucleated cell in the body
    b. have identical alleles in individuals of the same species
    c. are on B cells and macrophages but not on every nucleated cell
    d. are on T cells only

12. To be immunogenic, which of the following is *not* important?
    a. charge
    b. foreignness
    c. chemical complexity
    d. molecular weight

13. Which of the following does *not* act as an adjuvant?
    a. Freund's
    b. water
    c. LPS
    d. alum

14. CD4 on T cells binds to
    a. CD4
    b. MHC class I molecules
    c. MHC class II molecules
    d. CD8

15. Which of the following is important in the induction of the immune response?
    a. amount of antigen
    b. timing of the injections
    c. route of the injections
    d. all of the above are important

REFERENCES

1. Janeway CA, Travers P, Walport M, et al. *Immunobiology*. 5th ed. New York, NY: Garland Publishing; 2001.

2. Davis DR, Cohen GH. Interactions of protein antigens with antibodies. *PNAS USA*. 1996;93:7.

3. Davis MM, Boniface JJ, Reich Z, et al. Ligand recognition by alpha beta T cell receptors. *Annu. Rev. Immunol.* 1998;16:523.

4. Freemont DH, Matsumura M, Stura EA, et al. Crystal structure of 2 viral peptides in complex with murine MHC class I H-2Kb. *Science*.1992;357:91.

5. Freemont DH, Hendrickson WA, Marrack P, et al. Structures of an MHC class II molecule with covalently bound single peptides. *Science*.1996;272:1001.

6. Cresswell P, Ackerman AL, Giodini A, et al. Mechanism of MHC class I-restricted antigen processing and cross-presentation. *Immunol. Rev.* 2005;207:147.

7. Pieters J. MHC class II-restricted antigen processing and presentation. *Adv. Immunol.* 2000;75:159.

8. Garcia KC, Degano M, Stanfield RL, et al. An αβ T cell receptor structure at 2.5 A and its orientation in the TCR-MHC complex. *Science*. 1996;274:209.

9. Li P, Gregg JL, Wang N, et al. Compartmentalization of class II antigen presentation: Contribution of cytoplasmic and endosomal processing. *Immunol. Rev.* 2005;207:206.

10. Landsteiner K. *The specificity of serological reactions* (rev. ed.). New York, NY: Dover Press; 1962.

PEARSON
myhealthprofessionskit™

Visit www.myhealthprofessionskit.com to access the interactive Companion Website for this textbook. Simply select "Clinical Laboratory Science" from the choice of disciplines. Find this book and log in using your user name and password to access additional learning tools.

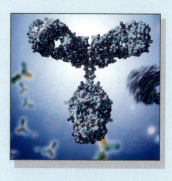

4

Cellular Immunity

■ OBJECTIVES—LEVEL I

After this chapter, the student should be able to:

1. List and describe the general features of cytokines.
2. Compare and contrast the role of helper T cells and cytotoxic T cells after antigen presentation.
3. Compare and contrast the function of helper T cell subsets (ie, Th1 and Th2).
4. Describe the function of IL-2 as a cytokine prototype.
5. Describe laboratory assays to measure T-cell function.
6. Describe assays for cytokines.
7. Differentiate among and define the terms *autocrine effect, paracrine effect,* and *endocrine effect.*

■ OBJECTIVES—LEVEL II

After this chapter, the student should be able to:

1. Describe and compare the different classes of cytokines based on their function.
2. Describe the function of cytokines involved in innate immunity.
3. Describe the function of cytokines involved in adaptive immunity.
4. Describe the molecular mechanisms behind SCID and as example of aberrations of cytokine function.

KEY TERMS

acute phase response
adhesins
autocrine effect
chemokines
cytokines
cytotoxic T cells
double negative thymocytes
double positive thymocytes
endocrine effect
haplotype
helper T cells
immunoglobulin superfamily
immunological tolerance
integrins
MHC restriction
negative selection
paracrine effect
pleiotropic
positive selection
redundant
regulatory T cells
synergistic

INTRODUCTION

In Chapter 3, we used the analogy of a highly organized military defense system to describe the immune system. As in any such complex system, its efficient function depends on the coordinated and successful interaction among the different components of the system. So, for example, a successful military action of defense relies on the communication and collaboration of different officers, soldiers, specialized forces, laboratory scientists, support personnel, and others that ultimately coordinate the successful completion of such defensive response. An immune response likewise relies on the coordinated interaction among different cells and molecules of the immune system and the careful regulation of such interactions. In this chapter, we will describe the nature and mechanisms of many of these interactions and the functions that result from them. In particular, we will discuss the activation of T cells, the subsequent responses that result from this activation, and the molecules that are critical players in these responses.

CELLULAR INTERACTIONS

Interactions among immune cells are essential to a strong and successful immune response; they result in a wide variety of events from activation to maintenance to inhibition of a particular response, and they are the very basis of an "immune network." Early experiments showed that the collaboration between antigen-presenting cells (such as B cells or macrophages) and T cells was essential for an immune response to a particular antigen to occur. In the first experiment, mice were lethally irradiated to "wipe out" their immune cells; they were then injected with bone marrow from other mice of the same strain (a source of B cells), thoracic duct lymphocytes from other mice of the same strain (a source of T cells), or a mixture of both. The ability of the mice receiving the different combinations of injections to mount an immune response to a particular antigen was then tested. Only the mice injected with a combination of both B and T cells were able to mount an immune response to the antigen. The results of the experiment are shown in Table 4.1 ✪. This demonstrated that at least the presence of both types of cells was necessary for the

immune response to take place. Later experiments demonstrated that the interaction between antigen-presenting cells and T cells also depended on T cells recognizing the MHC **haplotype** of the antigen-presenting cell. In other words, the antigen-presenting cell and the T cell had to share the same MHC haplotype for the interaction to be successful. In these experiments, macrophages from guinea pigs of a particular strain (strain 2) were allowed to react with an antigen so that the animals would process it and present it on their surface. These antigen-sensitized macrophages were then mixed with T cells from the same strain (strain 2) with T cells from a different strain (strain 13) or with T cells from offspring of a 2x13 strain combination (2x13F$_1$). The levels of activation of the T cells from the different strains were then evaluated. The results of this experiment showed that T cells could be activated only when they were mixed with macrophages from their same or similar strain (ie, T cells from strain 2 could be activated only by macrophages from strain 2 or 2x13F$_1$, not from macrophages from strain 13). Likewise, T cells from strain 13 could be activated only by macrophages from strain 13 or 2x13F$_1$, not from macrophages from strain 2 (Table 4.2 ✪). The results of this experiment demonstrated that only antigen-presenting cells that bear the same MHC haplotype could activate T cells (2). Thus, the response of a T cell to a processed antigen is said to be **MHC restricted.**

ANTIGEN-PRESENTING CELLS

A variety of cells can act as antigen-presenting cells including B cells, macrophages, dendritic cells, fibroblasts, thymic epithelial cells, vascular endothelial cells, and others (1). However, as we have discussed in Chapter 3, the major antigen-presenting cells are dendritic cells, macrophages, and B cells. These are usually classified as *professional antigen-presenting cells.* Dendritic cells are the most efficient of the antigen-presenting cells (3); they express high levels of MHC class II molecules and can activate naïve helper T cells. Macrophages also express MHC class II molecules, but their expression usually follows phagocytosis of an antigen such as a microorganism. The method of antigen detection by these cells also varies

✪ TABLE 4.1

Dependence of an Immune Response (+ + +) on the Presence of Both B and T Cells in Irradiated and Reconstituted Mouse Hosts

Cells Injected	Immune Response
B cells	−
T cells	−
Both	+++

✪ TABLE 4.2

MHC Restriction of Immune Responses. Cell Activation (+ + +) Could Occur Only After the Interaction of MHC Matched-T Cells and Macrophages

Source of T Cells	Antigen-Primed Macrophages		
	Strain 2	Strain 13	2x13F$_1$
Strain 2	+++	−	+++
Strain 13	−	+++	+++
2x13F$_1$	+++	+++	+++

with the cell type: Macrophages recognize an antigen by having receptors for certain carbohydrate moieties, complement components, or receptors for the Fc portion of immunoglobulin molecules. B cells recognize the antigen via their surface immunoglobulin whereas dendritic cells take up antigens by recognizing patterns and features that are common to microbial surfaces or by pinocytosis.

► SUBSETS OF T CELLS

If we go back to the analogy of the military defense system, T cells can be considered as the major officers of the immune army. As such, they regulate, direct, modulate, and participate in the immune response, and different subsets of T cells play different roles in such response. As indicated in Chapter 1, there are 3 major subsets of T cells: **helper T cells, cytotoxic T cells,** and **regulatory T cells.** Each subset is characterized by different functions as well as different surface markers. Helper T cells express the CD4 marker and are thus described as CD4+ T cells. Cytotoxic T cells, bearing the CD8 marker, are CD8+ whereas regulatory T cells, usually CD4+, also bear unique distinctive markers such as CD25. Functions for the different subsets also differ; helper T cells recognize processed antigens that have been presented in conjunction with MHC class II molecules; their usual role is to upregulate an immune response (1).

Two major subsets of helper T cells have been described: Th1 and Th2. Th1 helper T cells stimulate a response more dependent on cell-mediated immune functions such as cytotoxic T cells, activation of macrophages, and phagocytosis. On the other hand, Th2 helper T cells tend to stimulate both an immune response that is directed more toward an antibody response and B cells to make such antibodies against a particular antigen (1, 4). A more recently described subset of helper T cells, Th17, has been implicated in the pathogenesis of autoimmunity. Th1 or Th2 populations, however, dominate most immune reactions.

Cytotoxic T cells recognize processed endogenous antigens that are presented in conjunction with MHC class I antigens, and their role is to kill the cell that is presenting the particular antigen. The main role of regulatory T cells is to act as chaperones of the immune system by downregulating immune responses. The action of each subset is usually mediated by a wide variety of both cell surface and secreted molecules that are described later. See Table 4.3 ✪ for a summary of the function of the different subsets of T cells.

► T-CELL DEVELOPMENT IN THE THYMUS

Considering their cardinal importance in an immune response, it is surprising to note that the great majority (> 95%) of thymocytes, which are precursors of T cells, die before

✪ TABLE 4.3

Different Subsets of T Cells and Their Function

Cells	Cell Function
Th1 helper T cells	Modulate and coordinate an immune response and steer it toward a cell-mediated response
Th2 helper T cells	Modulate and coordinate an immune response and steer it toward an antibody-mediated response
Cytotoxic T cells	Kill target cells (eg, cells that have been infected by an endogenous antigen such as a virus)
Regulatory T cells	Act as regulator of the immune response; play an important role in immunological tolerance

becoming mature T cells. This high selection involves several subsequent steps and occurs during the journey of thymocytes from the bone marrow into the thymus (1, 5). As the precursors enter the thymic cortex, they do not express either CD4 or CD8 molecules. These cells are usually referred to as **double negative thymocytes** (ie, they express neither marker). Double negative cells spend several days in the cortex where they proliferate and undergo T-cell receptor gene rearrangement; the β chain of the T-cell receptor is the first to be rearranged followed by the combining of the β chains with the precursor of the α T-cell receptor chain called $pT\alpha$. This combination is a precursor of the final T-cell receptor and is complexed with the CD3 component described in Chapter 3. This process allows the further proliferation of the thymocyte, stops any further rearrangement of the β chain genes, and allows the thymocyte to express both CD4 and CD8 molecules. Cells that do not make a successful rearrangement of the β chain genes usually do not continue proliferating and die. The cells expressing both CD4 and CD8 molecules are called **double positive thymocytes.** Once they have become double positive, thymocytes begin rearranging their α chains; only thymocytes that are double positive and have a fully assembled T-cell receptor/CD3 complex on their surface are allowed to continue to proliferate.

► IMMUNOLOGICAL TOLERANCE

Immunological tolerance refers to a state of unresponsiveness specific for a particular antigen. Tolerance is induced by prior exposure to that antigen, and although it can be induced to non-self antigens, most importantly, it prevents the body from attacking itself (self-tolerance). As we discussed when dealing with the specificity of immunoglobulin and T-cell receptor epitope-binding sites, such specificity is achieved through random rearrangement of both immunoglobulin and T-cell-receptor variable region genes (ie, the VJ and VDJ rearrangements discussed in Chapters 1 and 3). This happens because the immune system relies on the concept that because everything in nature is made of repeating patterns, generating a very large repertoire of different randomly selected patterns ensures that such antigen receptor molecules have that particular specificity to recognize a particular antigen at a particular point in time. This, however, creates a problem: because the repertoire of specificities is made randomly, an immunoglobulin or a T-cell receptor molecule may, by chance, express a random specificity that can recognize self-epitopes. This, in turn, would lead to an autoimmune reaction; so, cells bearing these self-reactive receptors must be eliminated. Therefore, the prevention of self-reactivity is not genetically programmed; rather, processes that occur in the thymus during the development of T cells from precursors prevent self-reactivity (1). Two screening processes that achieve MHC restriction as well as prevent the maturation of self-reactive T cells are **positive selection** and **negative selection**. In positive selection, double positive thymocytes with functional T-cell receptors within the thymus are presented MHC molecules of either class I or II. Only the thymocytes that are capable of recognizing self-MHC molecules are allowed to survive; any thymocyte that does not recognize self-MHC dies within the thymus. It appears that the binding with MHC somehow stimulates cellular processes that are necessary for the further proliferation of the thymocyte. This process of elimination ensures the MHC restriction of the T-cell repertoire. The recognition of either MHC class I or MHC class II molecules may also determine what T-cell subset a thymocyte will become (ie, either CD4+ or CD8+). CD4+ T cells interact with MHC class II molecules, whereas CD8+ T cells interact with MHC class I molecules. Therefore, positive selection may also determine whether a particular thymocyte will become a helper T cell or a cytotoxic T cell.

Thymocytes undergo another selection process, namely **negative selection.** In this process, developing thymocytes are presented self-peptides; the reaction of these cells with self-peptides, in turn, results in either killing the self-peptide-recognizing cell or receiving a strong signal that results in the cell's apoptosis or programmed cell death. Presentation of self-antigens is carried out by professional antigen-presenting cells, most notably bone marrow-derived dendritic cells and macrophages (although specialized thymocytes and thymic epithelial cells also have the ability to delete self-reactive cells). This ensures that the repertoire of mature T cells does not contain autoimmune or self-reacting T cells. The processes of positive and negative selection are not perfect, and not all self-reactive T cells are eliminated. For example, negative selection depends on many factors such as the accessibility of developing T cells to self-antigens, the combined avidity of the T-cell receptor (TCR) and CD4/CD8 molecules for MHC and self-antigens, and the identity of the cells presenting self-antigens. Because of this, regulatory T cells play a major role in the downregulation of any potentially reactive T cell that

may have escaped negative selection. See Figure 4.1 ■ for a summary of the selection of T cells from precursors in the thymus. Only mature T cells enter the circulation; the presence of dual positive T cells or any other T-cell precursor in the blood stream indicates that a leukemia or lymphoma may be present.

 Checkpoint! 4.1

Why is it that the bulk of central tolerance is achieved by mechanisms that affect T cells (ie, positive and negative selection) even though B cells can also be self-reactive?

► ANTIGEN PRESENTATION TO T CELLS

As we saw in Chapter 3, antigen presentation to the different T-cell types follows similar yet somewhat different pathway mechanisms; and presentation to different subsets of T cells leads to the response to substantially different types of antigens (1, 6, 7). Antigen presentation to CD8+ T cells (cytotoxic T cells) follows the recognition of an endogenous antigen, such as an intracellular microorganism, and the activation of CD8+ T cells result in the cytotoxic T cell's killing of the antigen-presenting cell. This prevents multiplication of the pathogen within the infected cell, and subsequent infection of other cells. On the other hand, presentation of antigen to CD4+ T cells (helper T cells) results in the augmentation of the immune response to that antigen. In this case, the function of helper T cells is to "help" other immune cells respond to infections from extracellular pathogens. In addition, the subsequent response to the pathogen can differ mechanistically, depending on the subsets of helper T cells that are stimulated (ie, Th1 or Th2) (4). See Figure 4.2 ■ for a diagram of an antigen-presenting cell interacting with a T cell.

ANTIGEN PRESENTATION TO CD4+ T CELLS

Following antigen processing, an antigen-presenting cell expresses antigen peptides on its surface associated with MHC class II molecules (this was described in Chapter 3). It also migrates to the lymph nodes or other secondary lymphoid organ where antigen presentation to T cells occurs. Naïve T cells enter the lymphoid tissues via specialized vessels called *high endothelial venules.* They continuously go back and forth between the bloodstream and the lymphoid tissues and constantly interact with a very high number of antigen-presenting cells. These interactions result in two events; (1) they reinforce the screening of positive selection by presenting self-MHC molecules and (2) they ensure the expansion of the

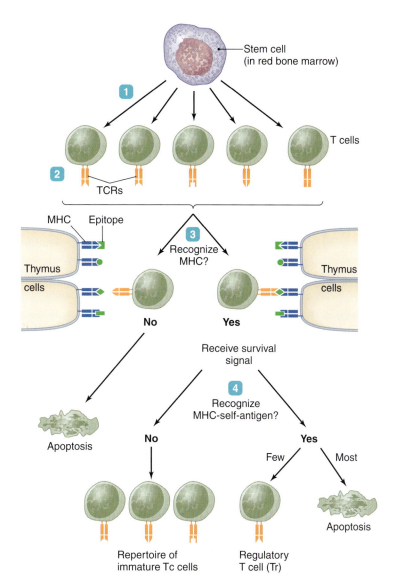

■ **FIGURE 4.1** Positive and negative selection during T-cell development. *Source:* BAUMAN, ROBERT W., MICROBIOLOGY WITH DISEASES BY BODY SYSTEM, 3rd, ©2012. Printed and Electronically reproduced by permission of Pearson Education, Inc., Upper Saddle River, New Jersey.

T-cell clones that have T-cell receptor specificities for presented foreign peptides. The TCR on a helper T cell then recognizes peptides lodged in the binding groove of MHC molecules. This dictates the antigen specificity of the response because a particular peptide and a particular MHC haplotype form a unique structure to be recognized by the TCR (1, 8). However, antigen recognition and interactions between the antigen-presenting cell and the T cell do not depend exclusively on TCR and MHC.

Other relevant molecules are involved in cell-to-cell interactions in an immune response. These can be either surface molecules or secreted molecules, such as cytokines, which will be discussed later. Surface molecules play two major roles: they promote and maintain cell-to-cell adhesion, and they participate in transmembrane-signaling transmission. Two surface molecules we have already discussed are CD4, which

acts as a ligand for MHC class II molecules, and CD8, which acts as a ligand for MHC class I molecules. Other molecules involved in the antigen-presenting cell-T cell interactions are adhesive molecules such as **adhesins** belonging to the **immunoglobulin superfamily** and **integrins.** These molecules play a critical role in cell-to-cell interactions; they also act as co-stimulatory signals for T cell activation (9).

Examples of co-stimulatory signal molecules are the B7 molecules on the surface of the antigen-presenting cell; these bind another member of the immunoglobulin superfamily, CD28, and this binding, in turn, is required for the clonal expansion of naïve T cells (10, 11). Once this binding has occurred and the naïve T cell has been activated, the T cell expresses other surface molecules including CD154 (also called *CD40 ligand*), which binds a CD40 molecule on antigen-presenting cells. The ligation of CD40 further activates the T cell, which

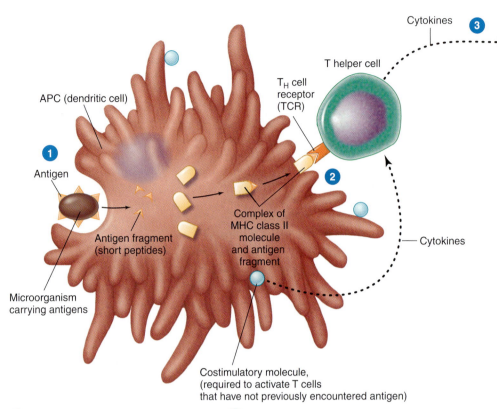

Cytokines

③ A T cell recognizes an antigen presented by a dendritic cell; the dendritic cell produces co-stimulatory molecules; the T cell becomes activated allowing proliferation and development of effector functions

T helper cell

T_H cell receptor (TCR)

APC (dendritic cell)

①

Antigen

②

Complex of MHC class II molecule and antigen fragment

Antigen fragment (short peptides)

Cytokines

Microorganism carrying antigens

Costimulatory molecule, (required to activate T cells that have not previously encountered antigen)

① An APC encounters and ingests a microorganism. The antigen is enzymatically processed into short peptides, which combine with MHC class II molecules and are displayed on the surface of the APC.

② A receptor (TCR) on the surface of the CD4+ T helper cell (T_H cell) binds to the MHC–antigen complex. If this includes a Toll-like receptor, the APC is stimulated to secrete a costimulatory molecule. These two signals activate the T_H cell, which produces cytokines.

③ The cytokines cause the T_H cell to proliferate and to develop its effector functions.

■ **FIGURE 4.2**   Antigen presentation to a T cell. *Source:* TORTORA, GERARD J.; FUNKE, BERDELL R.; CASE, CHRISTINE L., MICRO-BIOLOGY: AN INTRODUCTION, 10th, ©2010. Printed and Electronically reproduced by permission of Pearson Education, Inc., Upper Saddle River, New Jersey.

proliferates more. It appears that this complex back-and-forth system of stimulatory signals prevents the activation of T cells to self-antigens. This is because antigen-presenting cells express B7 molecules by detecting the presence of infections through detection mechanisms of the innate immune system, so only antigen-activated, antigen-presenting cells can activate naïve T cells. In addition, the recognition of an antigen without these co-stimulatory mechanisms actually leads to the inactivation of peripheral T cells. Refer to Figure 4.3 ■ for a depiction of the molecular interaction between an antigen-presenting cell and a helper T cell.

ANTIGEN PRESENTATION TO CD8+ T CELLS

The main role of cytotoxic T cells is to kill the cell that is presenting the particular antigen. In general, this antigen is part of an intracellular organism such as an intracellular bacterium or a virus that has infected the cell.

The ultimate goal of the action of a cytotoxic T cell is to eliminate this source of pathogen so that other cells do not become infected. Because of this, the actions of a cytotoxic T cell can be very powerful and very profound, so, in general, activation of a CD8+ T cell requires stronger secondary signals than those required by the activation of a CD4+ T cell. There is some evidence that the activation of CD8+ T cells may actually require the coparticipation of CD4+ cells recognizing the same endogenous antigen on the antigen-presenting cell. In this case, the CD4+ cell sends signals that increase the co-stimulatory activity of the pathogen-infected antigen-presenting cell. The interaction of the cytotoxic T cell with its target cell involves tight cell-to-cell binding modulated by a variety of surface molecules called *cell-adhesion molecules*. The cell surface adhesion molecule interaction results in focusing effector molecules from the cytotoxic T cell and their concentrated release onto the target cell from intracellular granules within the cytotoxic T cell (12). These effector molecules include perforin, which

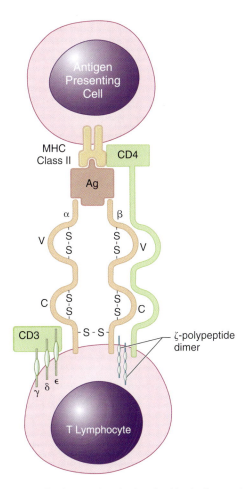

■ FIGURE 4.3 Surface molecules involved in the interaction between an antigen-presenting cell and a CD4+ T cell.

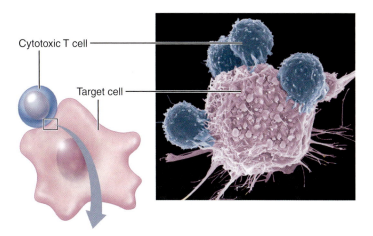

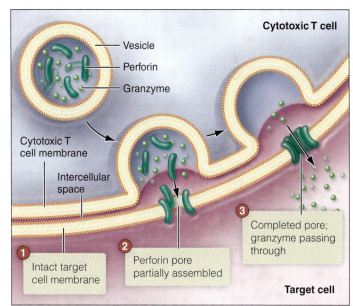

■ FIGURE 4.4 Interaction between a CD8+ T cell and its target. *Source:* JOHNSON, MICHAEL D., HUMAN BIOLOGY: CONCEPTS AND CURRENT ISSUES, 6th, ©2012. Printed and Electronically reproduced by permission of Pearson Education, Inc., Upper Saddle River, New Jersey.

can puncture the target cell membrane, as well as various enzymes or cytokines, which can trigger target cell death (Figure 4.4 ■).

 Checkpoint! 4.2

Antigen-presenting cells express MHC class II molecules, which are presented to a helper T cell after an antigen peptide from a processed exogenous antigen has been associated with them. The helper T cell then recognizes the MHC class II/antigen complex presented by the antigen-presenting cell. Why then do these antigen-presenting cells also express MHC class I molecules?

 Checkpoint! 4.3

To help remember which molecule presents to which cell, the answer is 8. That is MHC class II present to CD4 cells, 2 times 4 is 8, and MHC class I molecules present to CD8 cells, so 1 times 8 is also 8.

▶ ACTIVATION OF T CELLS

What does a T cell do after becoming activated? It proliferates and various mechanisms come into action. Various genes such as cellular proto-oncogenes (which regulate cell growth and differentiation), cytokine genes, and cytokine receptor genes are activated followed by secretion of cytokines, expression of cytokine receptors, and mitotic activity (1). Activated T cells produce the cytokine interleukin-2 (IL-2). They also start expressing receptors for IL-2. This process also requires the co-stimulatory signals described previously. Naïve T cells usually express low-affinity receptors for IL-2; upon stimulation, activated T cells start expressing high-affinity receptors for IL-2, and the binding of IL-2 to this receptor further drives the clonal expansion of the activated T cell (11, 13).

Activated T cells can divide many times and produce a very large number of activated antigen-specific daughter cells, thus expanding the immune response to that antigen. This is a critical step in both T-cell activation and the immune response to an antigen in general. At this point, the activated T cells can attain different functions by differentiating into either Th1 or Th2 cells; this, in turn, dictates whether a response will be more an antibody-mediated or a cell-mediated one (1, 4). The secretion of different cytokines results in different functions in an immune response, as we discuss next.

▶ CYTOKINES

If the coordinated and successful interaction among the different components of a system is required for that system to function, the communication mechanisms used by those components are just as crucial for that system's efficient functioning. **Cytokines** are the chemical "radio communications" among cells of the immune system; their functions are essential for most mechanisms involved in a successful immune response. There are many types of cytokines, usually characterized by their function, and new ones are being discovered all the time. Cytokines are peptide mediators that allow cell-to-cell communication; they function beyond the immune system and are involved in many other functions including bone metabolism, central nervous system function, and tissue development (1, 14).

Cytokines are also used clinically; for example, the interferon families of cytokines are used in cases of hairy cell leukemia, multiple sclerosis, and hepatitis. Interleukin-2 is used to treat cancer of the kidneys and melanoma, whereas granulocyte-macrophage colony-stimulating factor (GM-CSF) is used in neutropenia. In addition, antibody to the cytokine tumor necrosis factor (TN) alpha is used to downregulate the immune response for the treatment of a variety of autoimmune diseases. We discuss their general actions as they relate to an immune response and present a few selected examples.

GENERAL PROPERTIES OF CYTOKINES

The terminology to describe cytokines in the literature has varied throughout the years; terms such as *lymphokines, monokines, interleukins,* and *chemokines* have been and/or are used to describe cytokines, the different terms based on either a particular function, the cell that secretes it, or that it acts upon. Cytokines carry their function by binding to specific receptors on the surface of the cell they act upon and although their actions differ, they have several properties in common. Cytokines are **pleiotropic,** which means that one cytokine can act on multiple cells and have multiple functions. For example, IL-4 from an activated helper T cell can induce a B cell to undergo an isotype switch to produce IgE, but this cytokine can also inhibit the action of macrophages. IL-4 can also induce Th2 differentiation. Cytokines can also be

redundant (ie, two or more can have the same function). For example, IL-2, IL-4, and IL-5 can induce B-cell proliferation. Their action can be **synergistic** (ie, their combined action is greater than the sum of the actions of a single cytokine). Interferon gamma (INFγ) and TNF in combination can greatly increase the expression of MHC class I molecules on different cell types. On the other hand, their action can also be antagonistic, the action of one cytokine having the opposite effect of the action of another cytokine. For example, INFγ can induce the activation of macrophages whereas IL-4 inhibits it. This process creates a network of cytokines that can fine-tune a particular response (1, 14, 15, 16).

Cytokine secretion is a brief, self-limited event; it is usually associated with the new transcription of cytokine genes, which results in a transient production of the cytokine. Cytokine mRNAs are unstable as are many cytokine proteins, and cytokines are usually internalized after binding to target cells. Because of this, cytokines in general act locally, and their actions are carried out during a short period of time. However, some cytokines can act systemically, carrying their action at distal sites. A cytokine can have an **autocrine effect** by acting on the cell that secretes it, a **paracrine effect** by acting on a nearby cell, and in some cases, can have an **endocrine effect,** which involves entering the circulation and acting on a distal target cell. Cytokines frequently regulate synthesis of other cytokines and/or cytokine receptors, resulting in a cascade or networks; for example, IL-17 triggers production of IL-6 and IL-8 and synergizes with IL-1 and TNF. This results in sequential responsiveness, such as IL-5 inducing the IL-2 receptor in B cells (1, 14, 15, 16).

 Checkpoint! 4.4

Why are so many different cytokines needed, considering that many of them have the same effect on a particular cell or tissue?

FUNCTIONS OF CYTOKINES

The functions of cytokines are numerous and varied; most cytokines are involved in cell proliferation; some, such as IL-7, IL-4, and IFNγ, are also involved in cell differentiation; others (TNF family, IL-2) may result in cell apoptosis. Others, such as the interferons, have antiviral properties. Cytokines can be divided into 3 different functional categories: those that regulate innate immunity, those that regulate adaptive immunity, and those that regulate hematopoiesis (1, 14).

Cytokines That Regulate Innate Immunity

Cytokines that regulate innate immunity are usually produced by mononuclear phagocytes and stimulate early responses to microbes. Classical cytokines involved in innate immunity are IL-1, IL-6, tumor necrosis factor alpha (TNFα), and interferon alpha and beta (INFα, INFβ). Initially described as a factor that could induce fever, IL-1 is a major proinflammatory cytokine; it is a key regulator of host responses to microbial infection and a major modulator of extracellular matrix catabolism and bone resorption. Major sources of IL-1 include monocytes and activated macrophages as well as fibroblasts and dendritic cells. The systemic effects of IL-1 are mostly due to IL-1β; it is one of the earliest cytokines to be produced after an infection, and it can initiate a cascade of events called the **acute phase response.** IL-1 can induce the production of various other cytokines, including IL-6 and various chemokines, and can upregulate adhesion molecules, which are components used for cell migration so that cells can arrive at sites of infection. IL-1 also plays a role in hematopoiesis.

IL-6 is produced mainly in response to IL-1 and plays a major role in the acute phase response. Its actions range from participating in B-cell and T-cell activation and differentiation, to fever induction, to regulation of antibody synthesis. Interestingly, IL-6 can act as an inflammatory cytokine and as an anti-inflammatory one by modulating various T-cell functions. TNFα is a principal mediator of host response against gram-negative bacteria; its major source is the LPS (endotoxin)-activated macrophage, and it is produced by activated T cells, NK cells, and mast cells. TNFα was named this way because it was originally isolated from tumor cells; its actions include the modulation of T-cell activation, the regulation of adhesion molecules, and the modulation of expression of MHC class II molecules. The actions of TNFα are different and depend on TNFα concentrations; if secreted in large amounts, such as in the chronic exposure to gram-negative bacterial infections, TNFα can have harmful systemic effects such as septic shock. As a potent inflammatory cytokine, TNFα can also be involved in autoimmune disease tissue damage as we will discuss in a different chapter.

Two kinds of interferon are produced as part of the innate immune response: α-interferons, produced by virally infected blood leukocytes, and β-interferons, produced by tissue cells and fibroblasts. They are produced in response to bacterial and viral infections, invasion by parasites, and the presence of tumor cells. They were so named because they "interfered" with the replication of certain viruses. The main functions of INFα and INFβ are antiviral and antitumor. Their antiviral functions interfere with the molecular mechanisms that allow a virus to replicate intracellularly, including reducing intracellular protein synthesis, degrading RNA, and inducing virus-infected cell apoptosis, thereby limiting the infection from spreading (1, 17).

CYTOKINES THAT REGULATE ADAPTIVE IMMUNITY

T cells (especially helper T cells) produce cytokines that regulate adaptive immunity during specific immune response. They regulate the activation and the differentiation of cells involved in T-dependent immune responses. Classical examples are IL-2, IL-4, IL-5, IL-10, and gamma interferon (INFγ). IL-4 plays a major role in B cell activation, isotype switch to IgE, and suppression of Th1 cell functions. Secretion of IL-4 induces the differentiation of Th0 cells into Th2 cells, thus steering the immune response into an antibody-mediated one. IL-4 can also stimulate B cells to produce IgE and thus is a major player in type I hypersensitivity (see Chapter 9). In addition, while promoting the differentiation of Th2 cells, it can also inhibit the production of Th1 cells, further propagating an antibody-mediated response. Similar actions are also characteristic of IL-5, which can also promote B cell differentiation and increase antibody secretion. IL-5 can also modulate the action of allergy-related cells such as eosinophils and thus has been implicated in allergic reactions such as allergic rhinitis and asthma (1, 4).

INFγ can stimulate an immune response in a variety of different ways and thus plays a major role in both innate and acquired immunity. Its functions are numerous and can range from increasing antigen presentation by antigen-presenting cells, to increasing the expression of both class I and class II MHC molecules, to upregulating the differentiation of Th1 cells while downregulating the activity of Th2 cells, to promoting the activity of NK cells. INFγ can also modulate isotype switching and regulate the function of various adhesion molecules, thus regulating cell migration (18).

IL-10, on the other hand, is a downregulator of immune responses; it is an anti-inflammatory cytokine produced by mononuclear cells. As such, it inhibits the synthesis of cytokines such as IL-2, IL-3, TNFα, and INFγ. It also downregulates the expression of class II MHC molecules and various co-stimulatory molecules on antigen-presenting cells.

Cytokines That Regulate Hematopoiesis

Cytokines that regulate hematopoiesis are produced by the bone marrow and thymic stroma and stimulate the development of specific lineages of immune cells. For example, IL-7 stimulates the development of T and B cells, IL-15 of NK cells, IL-3 of myeloid cells, and G-CSF of neutrophils.

Th1 and Th2 Cytokines

Cytokines can influence the subsets of helper T cells that are derived from T-cell activation (ie, Th1 or Th2), which, as described, exert different overall effects on the immune system. For example, Th1 cells develop when the activated T cell is exposed to IL-12 (usually from the antigen-presenting cell, especially dendritic cells). On the other hand, Th2 cells develop when the activated T cell is exposed to IL-4 (usually from extracellular sources). The Th1 and Th2 subsets, in turn, can also release different cytokines: Th1 cells, in response to microbes that infect or activate macrophages and NK cells, produce IFNγ. In contrast, Th2 cells produce IL-4, IL-5, and IL-10 in response to helminthes and allergens, generating an antibody-mediated response (1, 4).

Checkpoint! 4.5

Give some examples of how cytokines can affect the function of other cytokines.

Cytokine Receptors

Because the action of cytokines depends on specific receptors on the surface of the cell they act upon, there are also multiple families of cytokine receptors, which, although different, share structural features. There are common structural features shared by different types of cytokine receptors, which are usually dimers or higher-order multimers. Various cytokines share similar receptor subunits. Cytokine signaling usually involves cross-linking receptor subunits (ie, binding the cytokine to its receptor) and brings the receptor subunits together. This, in turn, activates a series of enzymes (especially kinases) associated with the subunits, resulting in the recruitment of cellular molecules such as transcription factors to activate the cell to make the response to the cytokine.

Chemokines

Cells of the immune system can move from one site to another by a process called *chemotaxis,* which is the directed movement of cells along a concentration gradient of chemoattractants, which may be derived from the tissue or an infecting organism. **Chemokines** are chemoattractant cytokines that regulate the recruitment and movement of a variety of different cells (1, 19, 20).

Interleukin-2 (IL-2) and Its Receptor—A Model Cytokine System

IL-2 was one of the first cytokines to be discovered and described; it was first found to be a growth factor for T cells, thus providing a crucial step in allowing their study (21). IL-2 plays a central role in T-cell expansion and maintenance of T-cell homeostasis. It induces the proliferation of *newly activated* T cells as well as the proliferation and differentiation of NK cells; it also plays a role in the proliferation and antibody production of B cells. IL-2 is also critical in preventing autoimmunity and maintaining peripheral tolerance by modulating the development of T-regulatory cells (thus, IL-2 can also downregulate an immune response). Activated T cells produce IL-2, which is also responsible for clonal expansion of those T cells.

The receptor for IL-2 (Figure 4.5 ■) consists of different subunits: IL-2Rα, which is not required for signaling but acts as an affinity modulator, and IL-2Rβ/γc, which is necessary and sufficient for signaling. Initially, T cells that recognize antigen are preferentially stimulated by low concentrations of IL-2. Cell stimulation, in turn, results in the production of a higher-affinity IL-2 receptor.

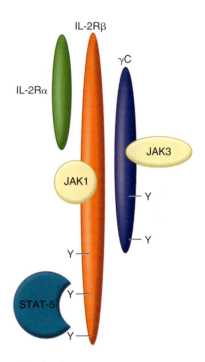

■ **FIGURE 4.5**   The basic structure of the IL-2 receptor.

► ASSAYS FOR MEASURING T-CELL FUNCTION

Measurements of T-cell function can be carried out at various levels of T-cell activation from the activation of early signal transduction mechanisms, to the expression of various molecules, to full-blown proliferation. Suni, Maino, and Maecker (22) published an excellent review on measurements of T-cell functions. Classical assays for measuring T-cell functions have concentrated on T-cell proliferation. Three of these assays are the tritiated thymidine uptake assay, the mixed lymphocyte reaction, and the Cr^{51} release cytotoxicity assay. In general, uptake of tritiated (ie, radioactive) thymidine has been used to demonstrate cell proliferation by the cell taking up thymidine while making new DNA. The radioactive label of the tritiated thymidine allows for precise measurement of the uptake; thus, it is a reflection of cell proliferation.

The mixed lymphocyte reaction has been used in transplantation to evaluate the histocompatibility of lymphocytes between a donor and a recipient. Lymphocytes from 2 subjects are mixed together in vitro and allowed to incubate together in culture for a few days. Lymphocytes, which are not histocompatible, will stimulate each other and, in doing so, will proliferate. This proliferation can be measured by the uptake of tritiated thymidine. If the lymphocytes from the different subjects are compatible, no proliferation will occur, and no uptake of tritiated thymidine will be observed. The mixed lymphocyte reaction can also be carried out as a 1-way test in which 1 set of lymphocytes (ie, from one of the subjects) is inactivated using radiation or substances such as mitomycin before mixing it with the other set. In this case, the proliferation can be measured on only one of the lymphocytes sets; the proliferation of the other set is turned off by radiation or drug treatment before the assay.

The Chromium^{51} (radioactive Chromium Cr^{51}) released cytotoxicity assay, on the other hand, has been used to measure the killing by CD8+ cytotoxic T cells. This assay is based on the fact that CD8+ cells bind to target cells that are then killed. The target cells are incubated with Cr^{51}; the cells spontaneously take in the Cr^{51} in their cytosol. The CD8+ cells are then allowed to incubate with the target cells after excess Cr^{51} has been washed off. Spontaneous release of Cr^{51} is measured in the absence of CD8+ cells, and total release of Cr^{51} can be measured by lysing the target cell with a specific detergent. The release of Cr^{51} as the result of the action of the CD8+ cells on the target cells can then be calculated by using the following formula:

(Specific Release − Spontaneous Release)
÷ (Maximum Release − Spontaneous Release)

The percentage of specific cytotoxicity thus obtained is a reflection of the specific activity of the CD8+ cells on the target cells.

T-cell function can also be determined by measuring the production of T-cell–associated cytokines such as IL-2 or IL-4.

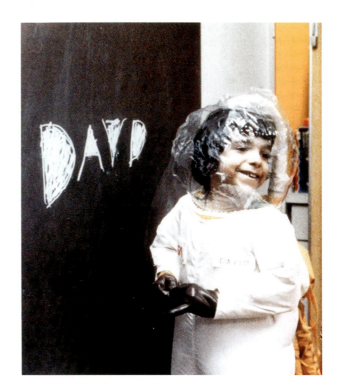

■ **FIGURE 4.6** David Vetter, the "bubble boy." *Source: Science Source / Photo Researchers, Inc.*

The Importance of Cytokines in Immune Responses

X-linked severe combined immunodeficiency (X-SCID) is a condition that affects lymphocytes and is characterized by a very low number of both T and B lymphocytes, severe susceptibility to numerous different infections, and profound immunodeficiency. This condition was made popular by a PBS documentary on the "bubble boy," David Vetter (Figure 4.6 ■) who, because of this condition, was forced to live in a completely sterile environment (the bubble) until his death at age 12 and by a film starring John Travolta, also featuring a bubble boy. In 1993, it was discovered that X-SCID was due to mutations in the γc subunit of the IL-2 receptor; it was thus assumed that this condition was caused by a defective IL-2 receptor, which would result in defective IL-2 function. However, animal studies had shown that IL-2 knockout animals (ie, animals that could not produce IL-2) did not exhibit such a severe immunodeficiency. The answer to this mystery came with studies of other cytokine receptors; these studies demonstrated that the γc subunit of the receptor for IL-2 is actually shared by the receptors of several other cytokines, including receptors for Il-2, IL-4, IL-7, IL-9, IL-13, and IL-15. Thus, aberrations of the function of this γc subunit would affect not only the IL-2 function but also the function of numerous other cytokines, resulting in multiple functional aberrations in the immune system. This highlights the critical role that cytokines play in an immune response.

SUMMARY

Cell-to-cell interactions in the immune system are the basis for an immune response and are essential for a well-coordinated and efficient immune response to an antigen. Many of these interactions occur at different phases of the immune response and involve a variety of different cells and different molecules, both surface and secreted. A critical interaction in antigen recognition and response is the interaction between an antigen-presenting cell and a T cell. Although different cells can act as antigen-presenting cells, the professional antigen-presenting cells are dendritic cells, macrophages, and B cells. There are also different subsets of T cells, specifically, helper T cells, cytotoxic T cells, and regulatory T cells; each has different functions. Helper T cells modulate and coordinate an immune response; cytotoxic T cells kill target cells (eg, cells that have been infected by an endogenous antigen such as a virus) whereas regulatory T cells act as regulators of the immune response and play an important role in immunological tolerance. Furthermore, helper T cells are subdivided into two major groups: Th1 and Th2. Th1 cells tend to promote a cell-mediated immune response whereas Th2 cells promote an antibody-mediated immune response. A third subset of helper T cells, Th17, has been implicated in the pathogenesis of autoimmunity. Th1 or Th2 populations, however, dominate most immune reactions.

T cells are produced in the bone marrow but develop in the thymus where more than 95% of them die off before becoming mature T cells. The selection of T cells involves a process called *immunological tolerance,* which, in turn, involves two major steps: positive selection and negative selection. In positive selection, only thymocytes that are capable of recognizing self-MHC molecules are allowed to survive; this ensures the MHC restriction of the T-cell repertoire. In negative selection, MHC-restricted thymocytes are presented self-peptides; the reaction of these cells with self-peptides, in turn, results in either the killing of the self-peptide-recognizing cell, or in the production of a strong signal that results in the apoptosis or programmed cell death of the self-peptide-recognizing cell. Negative selection ensures that the repertoire of mature T cells does not contain self-reacting T cells. Antigen presentation to T cells involves different pathways, depending on whether the antigen is endogenous or exogenous. Antigen presentation to CD8+ T cells (cytotoxic T cells) follows the recognition of an endogenous antigen, such as an intracellular microorganism, and the activation of CD8+ T cells result in the cytotoxic T cell's killing the antigen-presenting cell. On the other hand, presentation of antigen to CD4+ T cells (helper T cells) results in the augmentation of the immune response to that antigen. Antigen presentation depends on critical molecules such as MHC molecules, T-cell receptors, and antigen peptides; however, several other molecules also play a role in both cell-to-cell adhesion and cell activation. Examples include adhesion molecules, which play a role in cell-to-cell attachment and transmembrane signal transmission, as well as various cytokines. A summary of the activity of the different T cell subsets appears in Table 4.4 ✪.

Cytokines are peptide mediators that allow for communication among cells; they are the critical communication networks of the immune system. There are many different cytokines, and more are discovered on a regular basis; they are usually classified according to their functions. They share common properties: They are pleiotropic, which means that 1 cytokine can act on multiple cells and have multiple functions; they are redundant (ie, 2 or more cytokines can have same function) they can be synergistic (ie, their combined action is greater than the sum of the actions of a single cytokine); as well as antagonistic (ie, the action of one cytokine having the opposite effect of the action of another cytokine).

Cytokines usually have localized effects, but in some cases, they can have systemic effects by acting on distal sites. Cytokine effects can vary from cell proliferation to cell differentiation, to apoptosis, to hematopoiesis, to antiviral properties. Cytokines of the innate immune system include IL-1, IL-6, tumor necrosis factor alpha (TNFα), and interferon alpha and beta (INFα and INFβ). Examples of cytokines that regulate the adaptive immune system are IL-2, IL-4, IL-5, IL-10, and INFγ. Cytokines can also steer an immune response toward a cell-mediated or antibody-mediated response, depending on which subset of helper T cells—Th1 or Th2—they stimulate. All cytokines act on cells by binding to specific receptors on the cell surface; these receptors have many common components and are classified according to their structure. *Chemokines* are cytokines that modulate cell movement and chemotaxis; the common 7 transmembrane domains characterize their receptors. Refer to Table 4.5 ✪ for a summary of the activity of various cytokines.

T-cell function is generally measured using its activation; classical assays for measuring T-cell proliferation are the tritiated thymidine uptake assay, the mixed lymphocyte reaction, the Cr^{51} release cytotoxicity assay, and cytokine production.

✪ TABLE 4.4

Summary of T-Cell Types

Cells	Function	Markers	Effector Molecules
Th1 helper T cells	Modulate and coordinate an immune response Steer toward a cell-mediated response	CD4	INF-γ, TNF-β,
Th2 helper T cells	Modulate and coordinate an immune response Steer toward an antibody-mediated response	CD4	IL-4, IL-5, IL-6, IL-10, TGF-β
Cytotoxic T cells	Kill target cells that have been infected by an endogenous antigen such as a virus	CD8	Perforin, various degradative enzymes, INF-γ, TNF-α,
Regulatory T cells	Act as downregulators of the immune response Play an important role in immunological tolerance	Usually CD4, CD25	IL-10, TGF-β

⭐ **TABLE 4.5**

Summary of Cytokine Activity

Immune Branch	Cytokine	Produced by	Main Function

Innate immunity	IL-1	Monocytes
		Activated macrophages
		Fibroblasts
		Dendritic cells
			Induces
			  acute phase response
			  production of various other cytokines and chemokines including IL-6
			Upregulates adhesion molecules

	IL-6	Activated macrophages
		T cells
			Induces
			  acute phase response
			  fever
			Regulates antibody synthesis
			Participates in B-cell and T-cell activation and differentiation

	TNFα	Activated macrophages
		Activated T cells
		NK cells
		Mast cells
			Modulates
			  T-cell activation
			  expression of MHC class II molecules
			Regulates adhesion molecules expression

Adaptive immunity	IL-2	Activated T cells	Induces proliferation of
			  newly activated T cells
			  NK cells
			  antibody production of B cells
			Modulates development of T-regulatory cells

	IL-4	Th2 cells
		Mast cells
			Induces
			  B-cell activation
			  isotype switch to IgE
			  suppression of Th1 cell functions, differentiation of Th0 cells into Th2 cells

	IL-5	Th2 cells
		Mast cells
			Promotes
			  B-cell differentiation and increase antibody secretion
			Modulates
			  action of allergy-related cells such as eosinophils

	IL-10	Mononuclear cells	Downregulates
			  immune response
			  synthesis of cytokines such as IL-2, IL-3, TNFα, and INFγ
			  expression of class II MHC molecules and various co-stimulatory molecules on antigen-presenting cells.
			Has anti-inflammatory effects

Innate and adaptive immunity	INFγ	NK cells
		Cytotoxic T cells
		Th1 cells
			Increases
			  antigen presentation
			  expression of both class I and class II MHC molecules
			  differentiation of Th1 cells' activity of NK cells
			Downregulates
			  activity of Th2 cells

REVIEW QUESTIONS

1. David (the bubble boy's) SCID was due to defects in genes encoding for
   a. the IL-2 receptor alpha
   b. the IL-2 receptor gamma
   c. the CD4 molecule
   d. the CD8 molecule

2. In T-cell tolerance, positive selection is associated with
   a. presentation of self-antigens to the T cell
   b. production of a large number of B cells
   c. deletion of self-reactive T cells
   d. MHC restriction of the T cell repertoire

3. In T-cell tolerance, negative selection involves
   a. presentation of self-antigens to a T cell
   b. MHC restriction of the T cell
   c. deletion of self-reactive antigen-presenting cells
   d. elimination of T-independent antigens

4. T cells mature in the
   a. thymus
   b. spleen
   c. pancreas
   d. lymphatics

5. Which of the following cytokine receptor subunits possesses no signaling capacity but acts as an affinity modulator?
   a. IL-2Rγc (IL-2 receptor gamma chain)
   b. IL-2Rα (IL-2 receptor alpha chain)
   c. IL-17RA (IL-17 receptor A)
   d. IL-2Rβ (IL-2 receptor beta chain)

6. IL-2 is made by T cells and can trigger T cells.
   a. true
   b. false

7. A T cell that is positive for CD4 and CD8 is
   a. a helper and a killer T cell
   b. a double negative thymocyte
   c. an immature or a tumor cell
   d. a T-suppressor cell

8. Antigen presentation to T cells is performed by
   a. monocytes
   b. macrophages
   c. B cells
   d. any of the above
   e. A and B only

9. When a cell makes a cytokine that affects a distant cell, the response is called
   a. paracrine
   b. endocrine
   c. autocrine
   d. allocrine

10. CD8+ cells require interaction with
   a. class I molecules
   b. class II molecules
   c. both class I and class II molecules
   d. gamma delta cells

11. IL-6 is made by
   a. mast cells
   b. B cells
   c. T cells
   d. macrophages

REFERENCES

1. Murphy K. *Janeway's Immunobiology.* 8th ed. New York, NY: Garland Publishing; 2012.

2. Rosenthal AS, Shevac EM. Function of macrophages in antigen recognition by guinea pig T lymphocytes. I. Requirement for histocompatible macrophages and lymphocytes. *J. Exp. Med.* 1973;138:1194.

3. Schlienger K, Craighead N, Lee KP, et al. Efficient priming of protein antigen-specific CD4+ T cells by monocyte-derived dendritic cells. *Blood.* 2000;96:3490.

4. O'Garra A, Arai N. The molecular basis of T helper 1 and T helper 2 cell differentiation. *Trend Cell Biol.* 2000;10:542.

5. Bradley LM, Harbertson J, Freschi GC, et al. Regulation of development and function of memory CD4 subsets. *Immunol. Res.* 2000; 21:149.

6. Cresswell, P, Ackerman, AL, Giodini, A, et al. Mechanism of MHC class I-restricted antigen processing and cross-presentation. *Immunol. Rev.* 2005;207:147.

7. Pieters, J. MHC class II-restricted antigen processing and presentation. *Adv. Immunol.* 2000;75:159.

8. Davis MM, Boniface JJ, Reich Z, et al. Ligand recognition by alpha beta T cell receptors. *Annu. Rev. Immunol.* 1998;16:523.

9. Madri JA, Graesser D. Cell migration in the immune system: The evolving interrelated roles of adhesion molecules and proteinases. *Dev. Immunol.* 2000;7:103.

10. Bour-Jordan H, Blueston JA. CD28 function: A balance of costimulatory and regulatory signals. *J. Clin. Immunol.* 2002;22:1–7.

11. Cerdan C, Martin Y, Courcoul M, et al. CD28 costimulation regulates long-term expression of the three genes (alpha, beta, gamma) encoding the high affinity IL-2 receptor. *Res. Immunol.* 1995;146:164.

12. Edwards KM, Davis JE, Browne KA, at al. Antiviral strategies of cytotoxic T lymphocytes are manifested through a variety of granule-bound pathways of apoptosis induction. *Immunol. Cell Biol.* 1999;77:76.

13. Minami Y, Kono T, Miyazaki T, et al. The IL-2 receptor complex: Its structure, function and target genes. *Anu. Rev. Immunol.* 1993;11:245.

14. Gilman A, Goodman LS, Hardman JG, et al. *Goodman & Gilman's the pharmacological basis of therapeutics.* New York, NY: McGraw-Hill; 2001.

15. Carpenter LR, Moy JN, Roebuck KA. Respiratory syncytial virus and TNF alpha induction of chemokine gene expression involves differential activation of Rel A and NF-kappa B1. *BMC infectious diseases.* 2002;2:5.

16. Tian B, Nowak DE, Brasier AR. A TNF-induced gene expression program under oscillatory NF-kappaB control. *BMC genomics.* 2005;6:137.

17. Guidotti LG, and Chisari FV. Cytokine-mediated control of viral infections. *Virology.* 2000;273:221.

18. Liu YJ. IPC: Professional type 1 interferon-producing cells and plasmacytoid dendritic cell precursors. *Annu Rev Immunol.* 2005;23:275–306.

19. Balkhill F. The molecular and cellular biology of the chemokines. *J. Viral Hepat.* 1998;5:1.

20. Bravo J, Heat JK. Receptor recognition by gp130 cytokines. *EMBO J.* 2000;19:2399.

21. Gordon J, Maclean LD. A Lymphocyte-stimulating factor produced in vitro. *Nature.* 1965;208:795–796.

22. Suni MA, Maino VC, and Maecker HT. *Ex-vivo* analysis of T cell function. *Current Opinion in Immunol.* 2005;17:434–440.

PEARSON myhealthprofessionskit™

Visit www.myhealthprofessionskit.com to access the interactive Companion Website for this textbook. Simply select "Clinical Laboratory Science" from the choice of disciplines. Find this book and log in using your user name and password to access additional learning tools.

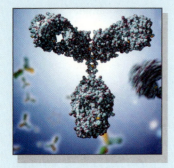

CHAPTER OUTLINE

5

Complement

■ OBJECTIVES—LEVEL I

After this chapter, the student should be able to:

1. Describe the classical pathway of complement activation in terms of C1 and its subunits; C4 and its subunits; C2 and its subunits; and C3 and its subunits, C5, C6, C7, C8, and C9.

2. Describe for all elements in Objective I what is required for activation of each particular piece (what initiates this system, what previous components are needed for each step, whether Ca++ and Mg++ are needed). The student also should be able to describe the biologic activities of each subunit.

3. For the alternative complement pathway, list the activating substances for initiation of this system and describe the role of C3b, factor B, factor D, properdin, factor H, and factor I in this pathway.

4. Describe the 3 different functions—recognition, activation, and membrane attack—of each of the 3 pathways.

5. Describe the central role of C3 for all pathways.

6. Describe regulators of the complement system, both fluid phase and membrane bound.

7. Name and describe the functions of the subunits that are anaphylatoxins and chemotaxins as well as those that are involved in immune adherence and in opsonization.

8. Interpret case histories with emphasis on the nature of the disease, the effect of the disease on complement levels, and the role of the clinical laboratory tests in the diagnosis and evaluation of the disease for hereditary angioedema, paroxysmal nocturnal hemoglobinuria, and other diseases with complement deficiency.

9. Compare the effect of complement on fragile cell types such as red blood cells, white blood cells, thrombocytes, and gram-negative bacteria versus the effect of complement on yeasts, molds, plants, most mammalian cells, and gram-positive bacteria.

10. Describe the laboratory method and the controls for the following assays involving complement: complement immunoassays, complement activity measurements, CH50, and AH50. In addition, describe why serum is used rather than plasma for complement assays.

11. Interpret the results of the assays named in Objective 10, determine when they show alterations in complement levels, whether they indicate genetic disorders and whether they are secondary to other diseases: (1) acute inflammatory conditions and (2) chronic conditions.

12. Describe the method and purpose of heat inactivation of serum.

■ OBJECTIVES—LEVEL II

After this chapter, the student should be able to:

1. Name and describe the functions of the subunits that are involved in (1) the production of inflammatory mediators, (2) B-cell activation, and (3) memory.

2. Name and describe the functions of the subunits that are involved in (1) immune adherence and (2) opsonization.

KEY TERMS

AH50 assay	classical pathway
alternative pathway	factor XIIa
anaphylatoxin	lectin pathway
apoptosis	membrane attack
CH50 assay	complex (MAC)
chemotaxis	regulators of complement

▶ INTRODUCTION

We have seen that antibodies and T cells have specific receptors so that they can specifically identify invaders, but what weapons do they have to kill the invaders? In this analogy, the complement proteins are one of the weapons used by the antibody to destroy the invaders. You will soon see that complement is a very powerful weapon indeed. The complement system includes about 35 different proteins that are synthesized by the liver, monocytes, macrophages, and epithelial cells. The synthesis of these proteins increases in acute inflammation when the levels of complement components can rise, whereas in chronic inflammation or in liver disease, the levels can decrease. These proteins received their name because they were found to complement (or help) the antibody in the lysis of bacteria. A series of experiments showed that serum from an immunized animal could lyse the bacteria of the strain that was used to immunize it. When this serum was heated to 56°C for 30 minutes, it no longer lysed the bacteria; however, the serum could still confer protection when transferred to an unimmunized animal. These experiments showed that a heat-labile substance complemented the activity of the antibody in the lysis of bacteria. It is important to note that complement-mediated lysis occurs only to relatively fragile cell types, such as gram-negative bacteria and red blood cells. Although lysis of gram-positive cells does not occur, interaction of complement with the antibody on the surface of these cells does help in the clearance of the gram-positive bacteria because it facilitates phagocytosis (1, 2, 3, 4, 5).

▶ FUNCTIONS OF COMPLEMENT

Although lysis of bacteria is an important function of complement, complement proteins play additional important roles in immunity. Complement has roles in (1) the host defense against infection (lysis of bacteria, opsonization, and chemotaxis and leukocyte activation), (2) clearance of immune complexes from the circulation and tissues, and in clearance of apoptotic cells, (3) interactions with the coagulation pathway, (4) joining the forces of the innate immune system with the acquired immune system, and (5) the enhancement of immunological memory through interactions with B cells and follicular dendritic cells. **Chemotaxis** is when a chemical causes movement of cells to a site, and **apoptosis** is programmed cell death, a process by which cells after the receipt of certain signals commit suicide (Figure 5.1 ■) (1, 2, 3, 4, 5, 6, 7).

Three different pathways of complement activation lead to cell lysis: the classical pathway, the alternative pathway, and the lectin pathway. These pathways all lead to the activation of C3, and after its activation, all pathways converge and activate the components C5 through C9 in succession. These different pathways are individually described later. By convention, complement components are numbered, and each component is activated by one or more of the activated components before it. An activated complex is denoted by a bar over the top of its name (as in $\overline{C4bC2a}$). Some of the components are cleaved upon activation; in these cases, the larger cleavage product lands on the cell that initiated the activation, and the smaller piece floats away. When a particular component is broken into 2 pieces, the pieces are called *a* and *b*, for example C3a and C3b. Additional breakdown during degradation causes the formation of other pieces such as C3d. Usually the piece that floats away and has its biological activities in solution is the *a* component. The exception to this is the complement component C2; in this case, the piece labeled C2a lands on the surface of the cell and C2b floats away. A component that has enzyme activity and affects the next piece is called a *convertase;* for example, in the case of $\overline{C4bC2a}$, it is called C3 convertase (1, 2, 3, 4, 5).

▶ THE FORMATION OF C3 CONVERTASE BY EACH PATHWAY

CLASSICAL PATHWAY

The **classical pathway** is so named because it was the first pathway to be discovered. It is initiated by an antibody bound to an antigen. The classes of antibody that activate the classical pathway include IgM and IgG and subclasses IgG3, IgG1, and IgG2 (listed here in order of their efficiency of complement activation). After these antibody types bind to the antigen, a conformational change occurs, revealing a site on the antibody molecule that binds the C1q molecule. C1q is part of the Ca^{+2} ion-dependent C1 molecular complex of C1q, C1r, and C1s. The fact that the C1q binding site on these antibody molecules is revealed only upon antigen binding by the antibody molecule is one of the many important controls of the complement cascade. This control prevents the activation of complement by free-circulating immunoglobulin. C1q can also be activated by C-reactive protein, some gram-negative bacteria including E. coli, several viruses, some protozoa, and mycoplasmas. **Factor XIIa** of the coagulation pathway can also activate C1q; in fact, this is only one of the places where interactions occur between these 2 pathways (6). Most direct activation of complement by pathogenic organisms occurs through the **alternative pathway** or the **lectin pathway** (1, 2, 3, 4, 5, 6, 7, 8, 9, 10).

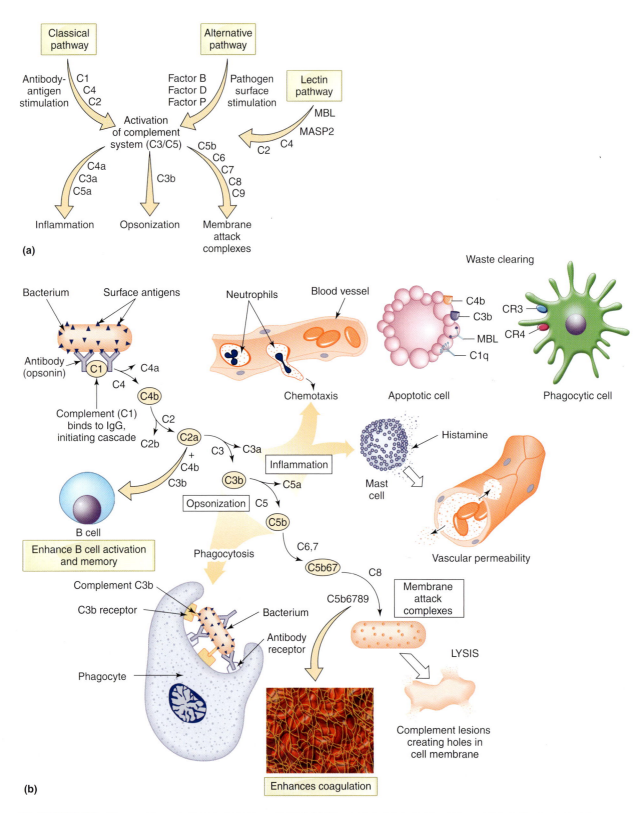

■ **FIGURE 5.1**   Three pathways of complement combined. (a) Figure shows a summary of how each pathway proceeds. (b) The biological effects of complement activation.

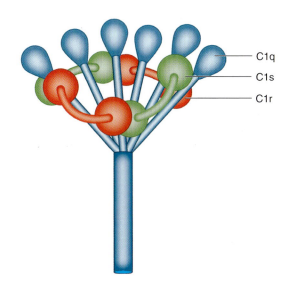

■ **FIGURE 5.2** C1qrs. A schematic of C1 showing structure and C1q, r, and s.

C1q is an interesting molecule with 6 arms with globular heads joined at their base (Figure 5.2 ■). The C1r and C1s molecules are wrapped around the C1q. When 2 of the globular heads of the C1q molecule are bound to antibody molecules (which, in turn, are bound to an antigen), a mechanical shift of the C1q activates C1r and then C1r activates C1s. C1q must bind 2 of its globular heads to 2 sites to initiate this activation; this can occur by binding to 2 Fc units of 1 IgM molecule or to 2 Fc units of 2 different IgG molecules. Because the arms of C1q have only a limited reach, the epitopes that are bound by the IgM or the IgG molecules must be close to each other. An example of this concept can be seen in the hemolytic disease of the newborn in which an Rh-negative mother can produce IgG antibodies to an Rh-positive fetus's red blood cells (see Chapter 9). The Rh antigens tend to be far apart, so when anti-Rh antibodies cross the placenta, they bind to the baby's red blood cells but are unable to initiate complement activation. Thus, the baby's red blood cells are not lysed; instead, they are aggregated by the antibody, which on their surfaces binds the Fc receptors on phagocytic cells for cellular destruction by the phagocytic cells (8).

Next, C1s cleaves C4 into C4a and C4b (Figure 5.3 ■). C4a is released into the fluid phase (and has anaphylatoxin activity), and C4b lands on the cell surface. C4 is the only component that acts out of its numerical sequence; it was given the name C4 because it was the fourth component to be discovered. This is an amplification step; every molecule of C1 cleaves about 30 molecules of C4. C4b has a very short half-life unless it lands on a cell surface. On the cell surface, C4b forms a Mg^{+2} ion-dependent complex with C2; C2 is then cleaved by C1s, forming C2a (the larger piece), which lands on the surface, and C2b (the smaller piece), which floats away and has prokinin activity and causes edema. This step also

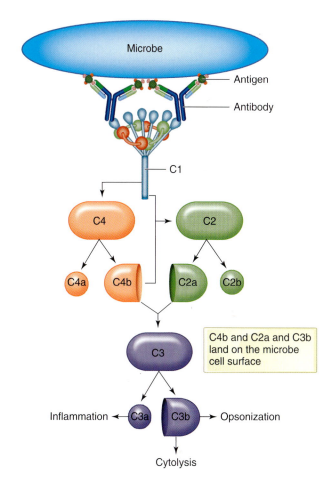

■ **FIGURE 5.3** Classical complement activations. IgM and IgG3, IgG1, and IgG2 activate the classical pathway of complement after a conformational change caused by antigen binding. C1q binds to the bound antibody and is part of the Ca^{+2} ion-dependent C1 molecular complex of C1q, C1r, and C1s. When 2 of the globular heads of the C1q molecule are bound C1q activates C1r and then C1r activates C1s. Next C1s cleaves C4 into C4a and C4b. C4a is released into the fluid phase and C4b lands on the cell surface. On the cell surface, C4b forms a Mg^{+2} ion-dependent complex with C2; C2 is then cleaved by C1s, forming C2a (the larger piece), which lands on the surface, and C2b (the smaller piece), which floats away. This brings us to the C3 convertase of the classical pathway C4b2a.

has some amplification effects with about four C2 cleaved for every C1. This brings us to the C3 convertase of the classical pathway C4b2a. The classical pathway is a combination of the acquired and the innate immune systems, usually beginning with antibodies of the acquired immune system and joining with the complement proteins of the innate immune system to destroy bacteria. Refer to Table 5.1 ✪ for a summary of the characteristics of the components of the classical pathway (1, 2, 3, 4, 5, 6, 7, 8, 9, 10).

✪ TABLE 5.1

Classical Complement

Component	Pathway and Stage	Activity	Split to a and b	Additional Important Information
C1 made of C1q, C1r, and C1s	Classical: Recognition	C1q binds antibody C1q bound to Ab at 2 sites activates C1r, which activates C1s, which activates C4	No	Requires Ca^{+2} to stay together
C4	Classical: Activation	C4a released into the fluid phase C4b attaches to the surface	Yes	C4a, a weak anaphylatoxin An amplification step (~30x)
C2	Classical: Activation	C2b released into the fluid phase C2a lands on the surface	Yes	C2a forms a complex with C4b which is Mg^{++} dependent An amplification step (~4x)
C3	All pathways: Activation	C3a released into the fluid phase C3b lands on the surface	Yes	C3a, an anaphylatoxin and a chemotaxin C3b, an opsinogen
C5	All pathways: Membrane attack	C5a released into the fluid phase C5b lands on the surface	Yes	C5a, the most potent anaphylatoxin and a chemotaxin
C6, C7, C8, C9	All pathways: Membrane attack	C6 binds C5b, C7 binds, and then C8 binds, 1 C9 binds and then additional C 9 binds, polymerizes	No	C9 inserts into the membrane, and several C9 molecules bind, forming a polymer tube through the membrane

ALTERNATIVE PATHWAY

In the alternative pathway, microorganisms and certain structures called *activator surfaces* can directly interact with the complement proteins and initiate the complement cascade. Lipopolysaccharide-containing bacterial cell walls, fungi, viruses, some parasites including trypanosomes, endotoxins, and aggregated IgG2, IgA, and IgE (Figure 5.4 ■) are all activator surfaces. The proteins involved in the activation of C3 instead of C1, C4, or C2 of the classical pathway are C3w and C3b, factors B and D, and properdin. A small amount of C3w is produced by hydrolysis of C3 by water in a process called *tick-over*. C3w is also called *C3(H20)* or *tick-over-formed C3b*. When bound by an activator surface, C3w binds factor B, and after action by factor D, $\overline{C3wBb}$, which is a C3 convertase forms. Thus more C3b is made, and more factor B binds and is cleaved to form Ba which floats away and Bb which binds to the activator surface. Addition of properdin stabilizes this compound. The association of multiple C3b, Bb units, and properdin forms a potent C5 convertase, and thus the membrane attack complex begins. The alternative pathway can also begin with C3b made by the classical pathway or the lectin pathway. It is a powerful amplifier of those pathways. See Table 5.2 ✪ for a summary of the characteristics of the components of the alternative pathway (1, 2, 3, 4, 5, 6, 7, 8, 9, 10).

LECTIN PATHWAY

In the lectin pathway, either mannose-binding lectin (MBL) or serum ficolin bind to surface terminal carbohydrates (either mannose or N-acetylgalactosamine) on the pathogen.

These sugars are internal structures in human glycoproteins and glycolipids but are terminal structures on pathogens, so they are accessible to MBL and ficolin binding only on pathogens. MBL-associated serine protease-2 (MASP-2) binds to the MBL and cleaves C2 and C4, creating the same C3 convertase that was in the classical pathway. MASP-1 can become associated with MBL but cleaves C2 only and thus may enhance the pathway but does not work independently. See the summary of the characteristics of the components of the lectin pathway in Table 5.3 ✪ (1, 2, 3, 4, 5, 9, 10, 11). See Figure 5.5 ■ for the lectin pathway and Figure 5.6 ■ for the mannose-binding lectin.

✓ **Checkpoint! 5.1**

If EDTA is used in a tube and chelates calcium and other metal ions, which complement pathway do you think would be most affected?

 C5-9

After C3 convertase is generated by one of the three pathways just discussed, C3 is converted to C3a and C3b. This is an amplification step with several hundred C3 converted for each step via the classical or lectin pathway and amplification in the alternative pathway. C3b lands in many places on the pathogen and is opsonic. The C3b that lands next to the C3 convertase forms a C5 convertase. C5 splits into C5a and C5b.

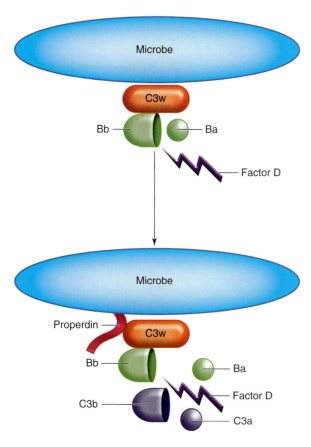

■ **FIGURE 5.4** Alternative pathway recognition and activation. C3w is on the surface of the microbe; factor B binds next to it; factor D interacts but does not land; factor B is split to Bb, which lands; properdin lands and stabilizes the complex; and C3 is converted to C3a and C3b, C3b binds to the surface. Ba and C3a float away.

C5a floats away, and C5b lands on the cell surface. C6 binds C5b, then sequentially C7 binds, C8 binds, and then one C9 binds followed by additional C9 binding. C9 polymerizes and forms a donut shaped hole in the membrane. The C5-9 complex is also called the **membrane attack complex (MAC)** (Figure 5.7) (1, 2, 3, 4, 5, 6, 7, 8, 9, 10).

> ✓ **Checkpoint! 5.2**
>
> *All of the pathways share certain components. What are these shared components?*

▶ **BIOLOGICAL EFFECTS OF FRAGMENTS**

The fragments that float away during complement activation have important and powerful effects. C5a, C3a, and C4a are all anaphylatoxins, and C5a is more powerful than C3a, which is more effective than C4a. An **anaphylatoxin** is a small peptide that causes histamine release from mast cells, smooth muscle contraction, and increases in vascular permeability. These 3 fragments also cause chemotaxis, generation of oxygen radicals, and potentiate inflammation (1, 2, 3, 4, 5).

> ✓ **Checkpoint! 5.3**
>
> *The classical pathway makes 1 more anaphylatoxin than the lectin pathway or the alternative pathway. What is it?*

⚙ **TABLE 5.2**

Alternative Pathway

Component	Pathway and Sage	Activity	Split to a and b	Additional Important Information
Called C3w or C3(H20) or Tick-over formed C3b	Alternative pathway: Recognition	Upon landing on an activator surface, has affinity for factor B		
Factor B	Alternative pathway: Recognition	Binds to C3w when on an activator surface	Yes	Ba unknown activity / Bb lands on surface
Factor D	Alternative pathway: Activation	Cleaves factor B when bound to surface-bound C3w	No	Does not become part of the complex
Properdin	Alternative pathway: Activation	Stabilizes C3wBb	No	
C3wBb	C3 convertase	Cleaves more C3 to C3a+b		
C3wBbC3b	C5 convertase	Cleaves C5 to C5a+C5b		

⊘ TABLE 5.3

Lectin Pathway

Component	Pathway and Stage	Activity	Split to a and b	Additional Important Information
Mannose-binding lectin (MBL) Ficolin	Lectin: Recognition; binds mannose Lectin: Recognition; binds N-acetylglucosamine	Recognizes mannose and N-acetylglucosamine in a Ca^{2+} dependent manner Pattern recognition receptor	No	MBL is an opsonin Both have multiple carbohydrate recognition domains (CRD); multiple CRDs need to bind, repetitive carbohydrates on fungi, viruses, bacteria, and parasites to initiate reaction
MBL-associated serine protease MASP-1	Lectin: Activation	Cleaves C2 to C2a + C2b		
MBL-associated serine protease MASP-2	Lectin: Activation (key)	Cleaves C4 and C2 Creates same C3 convertase as seen in the classical pathway C4bC2a		Ca^{+2} dependent

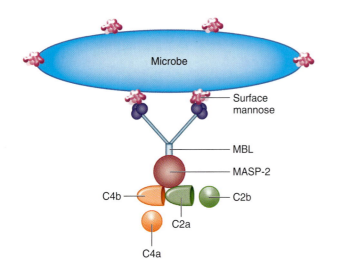

■ FIGURE 5.5 The lectin pathway of recognition and activation. Either MBL or serum ficolin bind to surface terminal carbohydrates that have either mannose or N-acetylgalactosamine as a nonreducing terminus on the pathogen. These sugars are internal structures in human glycoproteins and glycolipids but are terminal structures on pathogens, so they are accessible only on pathogens. Mannose-binding lectin-associated serine protease-2 (MASP-2) binds to the MBL and cleaves C2 and C4, creating C2a and C2b and C4a and C4b. C2b and C4a diffuse away and C2aC4b forms the same C3 convertase that was in the classical pathway. MASP-1 can become associated but cleaves C2 only and thus may enhance the pathway but does not work independently.

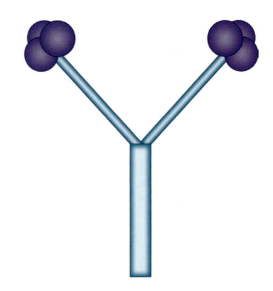

■ FIGURE 5.6 Mannose-binding lectin. Note the similarity in structure to C1q. MBL can have 2 to 6 globular carbohydrate-binding regions, 2 are shown.

present on red blood cells and other cells. Red blood cells bound to these complexes are brought to the spleen and liver where the immune complexes are transferred to phagocytic cells for processing (1, 2, 3, 4, 5, 10).

 Checkpoint! 5.4

What is the classical pathway opsonic molecule that is not shared with the other pathways?

C3b, C4b, iC3b (a breakdown product of C3b), and C1q are all opsonic molecules. They bind cellular receptors on phagocytic cells and increase phagocytosis. C1q, C3b, C4b, and iC3b are also involved in immune complex clearance through binding to the complement receptor 1, which is

C3dg, C3d, and iC3b, all breakdown products of C3b, are involved in B-cell activation through their interaction with CR2. Sublytic amounts of C5-9 can increase coagulation and inflammation (1, 2, 3, 4, 5, 10).

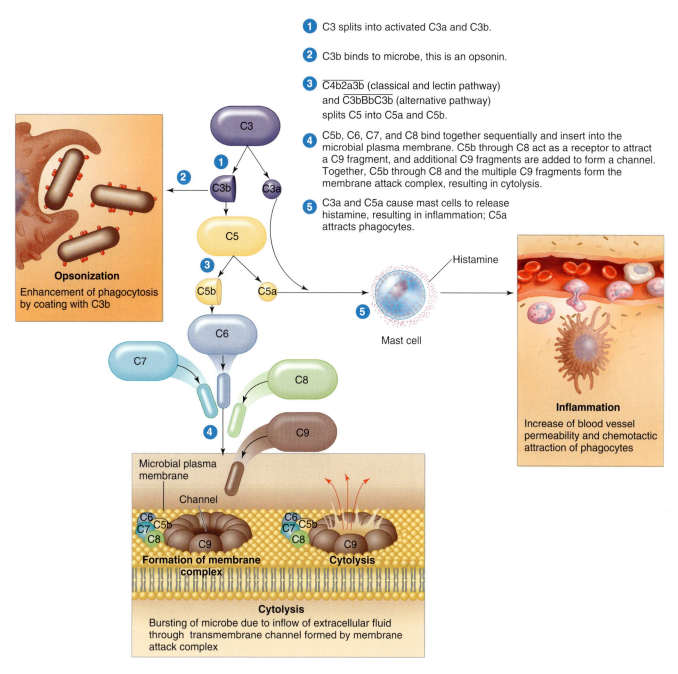

1 C3 splits into activated C3a and C3b.

2 C3b binds to microbe, this is an opsonin.

3 $\overline{C4b2a3b}$ (classical and lectin pathway) and $\overline{C3bBbC3b}$ (alternative pathway) splits C5 into C5a and C5b.

4 C5b, C6, C7, and C8 bind together sequentially and insert into the microbial plasma membrane. C5b through C8 act as a receptor to attract a C9 fragment, and additional C9 fragments are added to form a channel. Together, C5b through C8 and the multiple C9 fragments form the membrane attack complex, resulting in cytolysis.

5 C3a and C5a cause mast cells to release histamine, resulting in inflammation; C5a attracts phagocytes.

Opsonization
Enhancement of phagocytosis by coating with C3b

Inflammation
Increase of blood vessel permeability and chemotactic attraction of phagocytes

Histamine

Mast cell

Microbial plasma membrane

Channel

Formation of membrane complex

Cytolysis

Cytolysis
Bursting of microbe due to inflow of extracellular fluid through transmembrane channel formed by membrane attack complex

■ **FIGURE 5.7** Formation of membrane attack stage of complement. C3b containing structures (see above) on the pathogen surface splits C5 to C5a and C5b. C5b, C6, C7, and C8 sequentially bind to the pathogen surface and attract multiple C9 molecules. The C9 molecules form a channel and cell lysis can occur. It takes multiple C9 pores to cause cell lysis. The fragments that diffuse away have biologic activity. C3a, C5a, and C4a have anaphylatoxin activity and chemotactic activity. C3b is a potent opsonin. *Source:* TORTORA, GERARD J.; FUNKE, BERDELL R.; CASE, CHRISTINE L., MICROBIOLOGY: AN INTRODUCTION, 10th, ©2010. Printed and Electronically reproduced by permission of Pearson Education, Inc., Upper Saddle River, New Jersey.

▶ REGULATORS OF COMPLEMENT

The complement system is a powerful tool used by the immune system to lyse cells, clear bacteria, viruses, and immune complexes, increase inflammation, and interact with the coagulation system. If left unchecked, such a powerful system could cause severe collateral damage to cells and tissues,

so controls must be present in both the fluid phase and on the cell surfaces.

Several proteins control the classical pathway. First, C1 inhibitor (C1INH) inactivates C1 by causing C1r and C1s to dissociate from C1q. C4b-binding protein (C4BP), decay-accelerating factor (DAF), membrane cofactor protein, and complement receptor 1(CR1) are additional factors that interact with C3b and C4b so that they can be inactivated by factor I (11).

CR1 has an additional important function: It plays a role in immune adherence in which the CR1 on platelets and red blood cells binds to C3b-coated immune complexes. The red blood cells and platelets bring the complexes to the liver and spleen where the immune complexes are stripped off and the red blood cells and platelets returned to circulation. DAF, which is on most cells, keeps them from being damaged when complement products produced in a nearby inflammatory response land on them. The normal cell damage that would be caused by these complement products is called bystander lysis (11).

 Checkpoint! 5.5

How does complement help clear immune complexes?

The alternative pathway is controlled by factor H, which blocks the binding of factor B. In the fluid phase, the binding affinity of factor H to C3w is higher than factor B, so an activator surface is needed for this pathway to activate complement. Factor H bound to C3b interacts with factor I, and factor I breaks down C3b to C3f and then to iC3b, which can be broken down to C3c and C3dg. DAF also can dissociate the alternative pathway C3 convertase. The lectin pathway is inhibited by C1INH because C1INH also inhibits binding of MBL-MASP-2.

The terminal components are controlled by S protein, which also is called *vitronectin*. If some $\overline{C5b67}$ enters the fluid phase, S protein binds and prevents bystander cell damage by these membrane-active components. A membrane inhibitor called *CD59* or *membrane inhibitor of reactive lysis* of these terminal components, is present on the cell surfaces of all blood cells, endothelial cells, and epithelial cells and blocks C9 insertion into the membrane. Refer to Table 5.4 ✪ for a summary of the characteristics of the soluble **regulators of complement.**

 Checkpoint! 5.6

Hereditary angioedema can cause severe and rapid swelling in an area on the person's body. This is caused by a complement deficiency in an inhibitor that has roles in the classical pathway and the lectin pathway, although its name sounds as if it has an effect only on the classical pathway. What is this inhibitor?

▶ ADDITIONAL FUNCTIONS

CR2 (CD21), a complement receptor on B cells and follicular dendritic cells, binds various breakdown products of C3. It is involved in B-cell activation and in immunoglobulin class switching. CR3 and CR4 bind particles with iC3b on their surface and are receptors involved in the increased phagocytosis of particles coated with complement. Collectin receptors are specific receptors for C1q and increase phagocytosis. In addition, the collectin receptors enhance the binding of C1q to Fc receptors. See Table 5.5 ✪ for a summary of the characteristics of the cell surface regulators of complement.

✪ **TABLE 5.4**

Soluble Regulators of Complement

Regulator	Compound It Affects	How It Occurs
C1INH	C1	Dissociates C1 complex
	MBL-MASP-2	Inhibits MBL-MASP-2 binding
		Inhibits clotting and kinin pathways
C4BP	C3b, C4b	Interacts with C3b, C4b, allows for inactivation by factor I
DAF	C3b, C4b	Interacts with C3b, C4b, allows for inactivation by factor I
		Protects cells from bystander lysis
		Can dissociate alternative pathway C3 convertase
sCR1	C3b, C4b	Interacts with C3b, C4b, allows for inactivation by factor I
		Is also present on cell surfaces, see Table 5.5
Factor H	Factor B	Blocks binding of factor B to C3w
Factor I	C3	Breaks down C3
S-protein	$\overline{C5b67}$	Binds fluid phase $\overline{C5b67}$ and prevents bystander lysis
CD59	C9	Blocks insertion of C9 into the membrane

✪ **TABLE 5.5**

Cell Surface Regulators

Receptor	Function
CR1	Immune adherence
CR2	B-cell activation
CR3	Phagocytosis
CR4	Phagocytosis
Collectin receptors	Phagocytosis

► MEASUREMENT OF COMPONENTS

Two types of assays exist for complement proteins: (1) functional assays that measure the lytic function of the components and (2) antigenic assays that measure the amount of each protein using traditional serologic assays.

FUNCTIONAL ASSAYS

Two types of functional assays are used; the first is the **CH50 assay,** which measures the function of complement initiated through the classical pathway. The second is the **AH50 assay,** which measures the function of complement initiated through the alternative pathway.

The CH50 assay begins with antibody-coated sheep red blood cells and tests the ability of the patient's serum to lyse the red blood cells. Hemoglobin released from these cells is used as a measure of lysis. Newer tests rely on neoantigens formed with the formation of the membrane attack complex (12).

The AH50 relies on the fact that rabbit red blood cells can directly activate the alternative pathway of complement. In this test, rabbit red blood cells are mixed with the serum to be tested, and the amount of hemoglobin released by the cells is proportional to the amount of alternative pathway activity (12).

Both the CH50 and the AH50 require the complement components C3 and C5-9. The CH50 also requires C1, C2, C4, and C1INH, and the AH50 requires factor B, factor D, properdin, and factors H and I (12).

ANTIGENIC ASSAYS

Serologic tests are also important; for example, measurement of C4a indicates activation of complement through the classical or lectin pathway, and Bb can be measured as a marker for the activation of the alternative pathway. Terminal pathway activation can be determined by measuring C3a, C5a, and SC5b-9. Measurements of individual complement components can be performed by radial immunodiffusion (12).

> ✔ **Checkpoint! 5.7**
>
> *If I had a defect in a complement component that caused an amino acid change so that there was a point mutation and the component did not work anymore, which type of complement assay would be best to see this defect?*

Acute inflammation can raise complement levels. Conversely, genetic deficiencies and deficiencies as the result of chronic activation can lower levels of complement. However, the most common cause for measurements of low complement levels is incorrectly processed serum samples. The samples must be obtained in a red top tube. Serum samples but not plasma samples can be used in complement assays because in plasma collection the chelation that occurs using EDTA or heparin will decrease calcium and magnesium. Calcium is needed to keep C1q, r, and s together and magnesium is needed for C2 activation by the classical pathway and for factor B activation in the alternative pathway. The serum should be separated from the clot and should be frozen and stored at −70° C until analysis (12).

► COMPLEMENT DEFICIENCIES

Deficiencies in the C1, C4, and C2 recognition and activation parts of the classical pathway are linked to autoimmune connective tissue diseases such as systemic lupus erythematosus (SLE) and recurrent infections with staphylococci and streptococci. Deficiencies in the lectin pathway are associated with bacterial infections in infants. Deficiencies in C1INH, which is involved in inhibiting both the classical and lectin pathways because of the interactions of the coagulation and complement pathways and vascular permeability, can cause hereditary angioedema, a rare disease, which, as its name indicates, runs in families (see Chapter 15). People with this disease experience rapid swelling of an effected site. The swelling can constrict airways and can be life threatening (13).

Because of its role as a central hub, deficiencies in C3 are profound, affecting all pathways, phagocytosis, immune complex clearance, and class switching from IgM to IgG. Alternative pathway deficiencies are related to increased and severe pus-forming infections. People who are deficient in the terminal components (the membrane attack complex components) have increased and severe *Neisseria meningitides* infections and SLE. Deficiencies of DAF and CD59 are related to paroxysmal nocturnal hemoglobinuria, an anemia due to complement-mediated red blood cell destruction because patients with these deficiencies do not have membrane inhibitors of complement (13).

 CASE STUDY

I was in college working in an immunology laboratory. I was new to the lab and after training I started my experiment, which involved trying to cause lysis of lymphoma cells using antibody to the lymphoma cells and human complement. The human complement was from my own serum. Everyone in the laboratory performed this same experiment using her or his own complement. Everyone else's worked, but my experiment did not: The lymphoma cells in my experiment were still alive. We repeated this every day and still my results did not improve. I overheard the professor say that if I could not get it right, I would have to leave! On Friday, I asked one of the other

CASE STUDY *(continued)*

students if he would switch serum with me. He did, and on this day, my experiment worked but his did not.

1. What do you think happened?
2. Which complement system is involved in antibody-mediated lysis?
3. How would I test to see whether I have a defect in the classical pathway?
4. How could I check my activity in the alternative pathway?
5. The AH50 was normal, so with this result and an abnormal CH50, what complement components may be involved in my defect?
6. What antigenic assay could I do to measure these components?

SUMMARY

Originally discovered due to its ability to complement antibody in the lysis of bacteria, the additional roles of complement in immune complex clearance, opsonization, chemotaxis, inflammation, and B-cell activation and memory cell formation have become apparent.

The 3 pathways of complement activation activate C3 and form the C5-9 membrane attack complex. The differences between these pathways are the ways that the C3 is activated. In the classical pathway, C1q binds antibody, activating C1r and C1s. C4 is split into C4a and C4b. C4b on the cell surface reacts with C2 causing the split of C2a and C2b. C2a lands near C4b and forms the C3 convertase. In the alternative pathway, C3w, which had been produced by hydrolysis of C3 by water in a tick-over process, binds to an activator surface such as lipopolysaccharide containing bacterial cell walls, fungi, viruses, and some parasites, endotoxins, and aggregated IgG2, IgA, and IgE. There it interacts with factor B and with the action of factor D, forms $\overline{C3wBb}$ that, stabilized by properdin, is a C3 convertase (1, 2, 3, 4, 5, 6, 7, 8, 9, 10). The lectin pathway begins with the mannose-binding lectin binding mannose on the pathogen and then binding MASP-2. This cleaves C2 and C4, forming the same C3 convertase as the classical pathway does (10).

C5a, C3a, and C4a are all anaphylatoxins, which cause histamine release from mast cells, smooth muscle contraction, and increases in vascular permeability. These 3 fragments also cause chemotaxis, generation of oxygen radicals, and potentiate inflammation. C3b, C4b, iC3b (a breakdown product of C3b), and C1q are all opsonic molecules. C1q, C3b, C4b, and iC3b are involved in immune complex clearance by binding to CR1 and clearance in the spleen and liver by phagocytic cells. C3dg, C3d, and iC3b, which are all breakdown products of C3b, are involved in B-cell activation through their interaction with CR2. Sublytic amounts of the membrane attack complex C5-9 can increase coagulation and inflammation (1, 2, 3, 4, 5, 6, 7, 8, 9, 10).

C1INH inactivates C1 and MBL-MASP-2. C4b-binding protein (C4BP), decay-accelerating factor (DAF), membrane cofactor protein and complement receptor 1 (CR1) are factors that interact with C3b and C4b so that they can be inactivated by factor I. CR1 is involved in immune adherence in clearance of immune complexes. DAF is on most cells and keeps them from being hurt by bystander lysis (1, 2, 3, 4, 5, 6, 7, 8, 9, 10).

The alternative pathway is controlled by factor H, which blocks the binding of factor B and interacts with factor I so that factor I can break down C3b. DAF also can dissociate the alternative pathway C3 convertase. The terminal components are controlled by S protein, also called *vitronectin,* and by CD59, an inhibitor of the terminal component-driven lysis that is present on cell surfaces (1, 2, 3, 4, 5, 6, 7, 8, 9, 10).

CR2 (CD21) is a complement receptor on B cells and follicular dendritic cells is involved in B-cell activation. CR3 and CR4 bind particles with iC3b on their surface and increase phagocytosis of particles coated with complement. Collectin receptors are specific receptors for C1q and increase phagocytosis (11).

Functional assays for complement include the CH50 for the classical pathway and the AH50 for the alternative pathway. Antigenic assays are used for individual components and measurements of C4a, Bb are done for the different pathways, and C3a, C5a, and SC5b-9 are used to measure terminal pathway activation (12).

Deficiencies in complement are related to increased pus-forming infections and staphylococcal, streptococcal, or *Neisseria meningitides* infections depending on the component. They are also related to increases in the incidence of SLE or SLE-like syndromes (13).

REVIEW QUESTIONS

1. The correct order for the classical complement pathway is
   a. C1, C2, C3, C4, C5, C6, C7, C8, C9
   b. C1, C4, C3, C4, C5, C6, C7, C8, C9
   c. C1, C4, C2, C3, C5, C6, C7, C8, C9
   d. C1, C2, C3, C5, C4, C6, C7, C8, C9

2. Which of the following is the worst clinical deficiency to have?
   a. C1
   b. C2
   c. C3
   d. C4

3. Which of the following is *not* a functional assay for complement?
   a. CH50
   b. radial immunodiffusion
   c. AH50
   d. none of the above

4. Which of the following is *not* associated with elevated complement levels?
   a. acute inflammatory conditions
   b. acute myocardial infarction
   c. acute streptococcal bacteremia
   d. systemic lupus erythematosus

5. What sample can be directly used for complement measurements?
   a. EDTA plasma
   b. heparin plasma
   c. serum
   d. chelated blood

6. A patient who is admitted to the hospital and is found to have an acute infection would have
   a. elevated CH50
   b. lowered CH50
   c. lowered level of C2
   d. lowered level of C3

7. C5a can cause
   a. smooth muscle contraction and vasodilation
   b. immune adherence
   c. opsonization
   d. all of the above

8. Which of the following can activate the alternate pathway of complement?
   a. barbitol buffer
   b. gram-positive bacteria
   c. lipopolysaccharide from gram-negative bacteria
   d. sheep red blood cells

9. C1q can interact with
   a. IgM
   b. IgD
   c. low density of IgG
   d. A and B

10. Which of the following is (are) involved in regulation of complement activity?
    a. C1 esterase inhibitor
    b. factor H
    c. C4b-binding protein
    d. all of the above

11. Complement components can lyse
    a. gram-negative bacteria
    b. gram-positive bacteria
    c. plant cells
    d. yeasts

12. What is the order in which the alternative pathway of complement is used?
    a. C1, C2, C3, C4, C5, C6, C7, C8, C9
    b. C3w, factor B, factor D, $\overline{C3bBb}$, properdin stabilization
    c. C3w, factor D, factor A, $\overline{C3bBb}$, factor H
    d. C3w, factor B, factor D, $\overline{C3bC4b}$, properdin stabilization

13. Which complement component(s) is (are) cleaved?
    a. C3
    b. C7
    c. C8
    d. C9
    e. A and D

14. Which is the weakest anaphylatoxin of the following?
    a. C5a
    b. C3a
    c. C4a
    d. all of the above are equivalent in terms of their anaphylatoxin activity

15. A complement deficiency involving an inadequacy in the decay-accelerating factor can cause which of the following?
    a. damage to the host's cells due to bystander lysis
    b. angioedema of the skin
    c. increased susceptibility to systemic Neisseria infections
    d. SLE

16. Complement components are synthesized by
    a. the spleen
    b. macrophages
    c. the liver
    d. all of the above

17. A patient is admitted to the hospital and is found to have high levels of circulating immune complexes from a chronic systemic lupus erythematosis. Which of the following would the patient have?
    a. an elevated CH50
    b. a lowered CH50
    c. elevated levels of C2
    d. elevated levels of C3

REVIEW QUESTIONS (continued)

18. The alternative pathway for activation needs which of the following?
    a. C1-9 and factor B, properdin, factor I, and factor H
    b. C3, properdin, factor B, an activator surface
    c. lipids
    d. all of the above

19. C5a can cause
    a. smooth muscle contraction
    b. vasodilation
    c. chemotaxis
    d. all of the above

20. Which complement component requires Ca++ ions to stay together?
    a. C1
    b. C3
    c. C2
    d. C4

21. Which of the following is an opsoninogen?
    a. C3a
    b. C3b
    c. C5a
    d. C5b

22. Which are molecules that inhibit the alternative pathway?
    a. C1INH
    b. factor B and D
    c. factor D and C 2 inhibitor
    d. factor H and I

23. Interaction of complement and coagulation can occur with
    a. C4-causing clot formation
    b. sublytic amounts of C5-9 causing coagulation
    c. C3b-causing clotting
    d. none of the above

REFERENCES

1. Mayer G. Complement. *Immunology,* chap 2. http://pathmicro.med.sc.edu/ghaffar/complement.htm. Accessed September 19, 2010.

2. Ricklin D, Hajishengallis G, Yang K, et al. Complement: A key system for immune surveillance and homeostasis. *Nature Immunology.* 2010;11:785–797.

3. Volanakis JE. Overview of the complement system. In: Volankis KJ, Frank M, eds. *The Human Complement System in Health and Disease.* New York, NY: Marcel Dekker; 1998, chap 2.

4. Speth C, Prodinger WM, Wurzner R, et al. Complement. In: Paul WE, ed. *Fundamental Immunology.* 6th ed. Philadelphia, PA: Wolters Kluwer/Lippincott Williams & Wilkins; 2008.

5. Stevens CD. *Clinical Immunology and Serology: A Laboratory Perspective.* 3rd ed. Philadelphia, PA: F.A. Davis; 2009: chap 6.

6. Amara U, Rittirsch D, Flierl M, et al. Interaction between the coagulation and complement system. *Adv Exp Med Biol.* 2008;632:71–79.

7. Hess C, Schifferli JA. Immune adherence revisited: Novel players in an old game. *News Physiol Sci.* 2003;18:104–108.

8. Lu JH, Teh BK, Wang L, et al. The classical and regulatory functions of C1q in immunity and autoimmunity. *Cell Mol Immunol.* 2008;5(1):9–21.

9. Phillips AE, Toth J, Dodds AW, et al. Analogous interactions in initiating complexes of the classical and lectin pathways of complement *J. Immunol.* 2009;182:7708–7717.

10. Wallis R. Interactions between mannose-binding lectin and MASPs during complement activation by the lectin pathway. *Immunobiology.* 2007;212(4–5):289–299.

11. Tas SW, Klickstein L, Barbashov, SF, et al. C1q and C4b bind simultaneously to CR1 and additively support erythrocyte adhesion *J. Immunol.* 1999;163:5056–5063. http://www.jimmunol.org/cgi/content/full/163/9/5056. Accessed May 26,2012.

12. Giclas PC. How to distinguish between acquired and inherited complement deficiency. *Lab Q Clinical Laboratory Volume No. CL-15 Section Emerging Technologies* p.113–120. 2006.

13. Sjöholm AG, Jönsson G, Braconier JH, et al. Review: Complement deficiency and disease: An update. *Molecular Immunology.* 2006; 43(1–2):78–85.

PEARSON myhealthprofessionskit™

Visit www.myhealthprofessionskit.com to access the interactive Companion Website for this textbook. Simply select "Clinical Laboratory Science" from the choice of disciplines. Find this book and log in by using your user name and password to access additional learning tools.

PART 2
THE ASSAYS

6

Agglutination and Precipitation Reactions: The Unlabeled Immunoassays

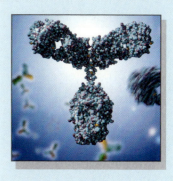

■ **OBJECTIVES—LEVEL I**

After this chapter, the student should be able to:

1. Define *precipitation.*
2. Discuss affinity and avidity and their influence on antigen-antibody reactions.
3. Explain how the prozone, postzone, and equivalence affect the amount of lattice cross-linked precipitates.
4. Compare and contrast the 2 optical-enhanced techniques: turbidity and nephelometry.
5. Interpret Ouchterlony immunodiffusion patterns.
6. Compare and contrast agglutination and precipitation.
7. Using what they have learned about agglutination and precipitation reactions, determine the effect of a hapten on a precipitation or an agglutination reaction.
8. Describe the physiologic conditions that can be altered to enhance agglutination.
9. Compare and contrast direct agglutination, passive agglutination, reverse passive agglutination, and agglutination inhibition.
10. Describe the direct antiglobulin test and evaluate situations to determine when it should be utilized.
11. Describe the indirect antiglobulin test and evaluate situations to determine when it should be utilized.
12. Describe the following instrument enhanced agglutination techniques: PETINA, PACIA, and QUELS.
13. Discuss conditions that must be met for optimal results in agglutination testing (equivalence, zeta potential).

■ **OBJECTIVES—LEVEL II**

After this chapter, the student should be able to:

1. Compare and contrast single diffusion and double diffusion.
2. Describe the principle of the kinetic (Fahey) and the endpoint method (Mancini) of radial immunodiffusion.
3. Define *zeta potential* and describe the effect of decreasing it on agglutination.

CHAPTER OUTLINE

KEY TERMS

affinity
agglutination
avidity
direct agglutination
direct antiglobulin
  test (DAT)
double diffusion gel
  precipitation
equivalence
Fahey method
identity
indirect antiglobulin
  test (IAT)
lattice
Mancini method
nephelometry
nonidentity

partial identity
particle-counting
  immunoassay (PACIA)
particle-enhanced
  turbidimetric inhibition
  assay (PETINA)
passive agglutination
postzone
precipitation
prozone
quasi-elastic light scattering
  method (QUELS)
radial immunodiffusion (RID)
reverse passive
  agglutination
turbidometry
zeta potential

► INTRODUCTION

In the unlabeled immunoassays, you can actually see part of what we have been discussing in previous chapters: the antibody molecules that have bound to antigen! The precipitation and agglutination reactions were the first immunoassays developed and rely on the fact that antibodies and most antigens have multiple binding sites. The multiple binding sites of the antibodies and antigens result in the formation of large complexes when antigens and antibody meet at appropriate concentrations (Figure 6.1 ■). Two types of reactions can result from the cross-linked structures that form: precipitation and agglutination reactions. **Precipitation** is the cross-linking of a soluble antigen to create an insoluble precipitate that is visible. **Agglutination** is the cross-linking of particulate antigens (bacteria, cells, or latex particles) to form larger complexes that are also visible. These assays are not very sensitive because a positive reaction of antibody and antigen is actually seen unamplified by the human eye. Using optics to register the differences between uncomplexed and complexed antigen and antibody results in some improvement of the sensitivity of agglutination and precipitation reactions. Two such optical techniques are turbidometry and nephelometry (1, 2, 3, 4).

All serologic reactions, whether unlabeled or labeled, rely on the affinity, avidity, and specificity of the antibody to bind to the antigen.

AFFINITY AND AVIDITY

Affinity is a measure of the strength of the binding of 1 Fab region with its corresponding epitope on the antigen. The affinity constant Ka is defined as follows:

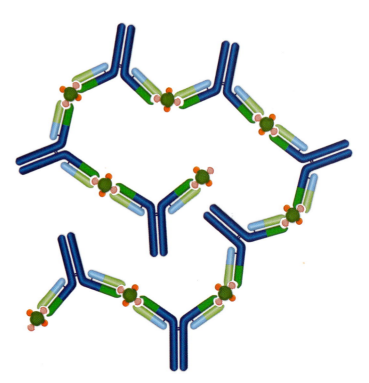

■ **FIGURE 6.1** Antigen (dark green and orange) and antibody (blue and green) binding forming a complex.

$$Ka = \frac{[AbAg]}{[Ab][Ag]}$$

Where [AbAg] is the concentration of the complexed antibody and antigen, and [Ab] is the concentration of the free antibody, and [Ag] is the concentration of the free antigen.

From the preceding equation, we can see that the higher the affinity, the more of the antibody and antigen that is complexed in comparison to the amount that is free. Thus, the higher the affinity, the more sensitive is the reaction because more of the antigen and antibody will be in the complexed form, and this form will be visualized. **Avidity** is the number of binding sites times the affinity. So, IgG with its 2 binding sites has an avidity of 2 times the affinity, and IgM with its 10 binding sites has a theoretical avidity of 10 times its affinity constant. This increase due to the number of binding sites is particularly important for IgM reactions because IgM has, on average, a weaker affinity than IgG because IgG is usually produced after the somatic mutational events (see Chapter 2) that improve affinity. One must also remember that steric hindrance can affect the binding of all binding sites and thus lower avidity. Steric hindrance affects the binding when the antigens bound are big enough to block binding by the other binding site(s) of the immunoglobulin molecule (1, 2, 3, 4, 5, 6).

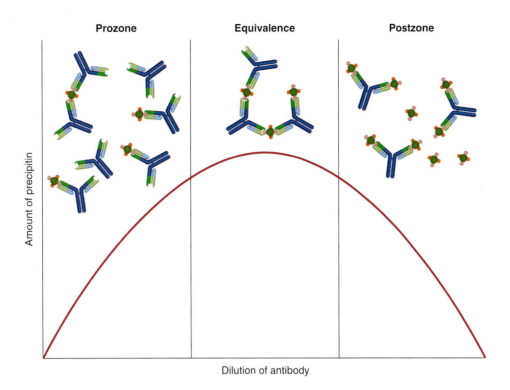

■ **FIGURE 6.2**   A depiction of the amount of precipitin that would form with different ratios of antigen and antibody. The prozone has antibody excess, and only small complexes with 2 antibody molecules and 1 antigen form. At equivalence, the number of paratopes roughly equals the number of epitopes, and the largest complexes form. The postzone has excess antigen, and the small complexes are formed of 2 antigens per antibody molecule.

EQUIVALENCE, PROZONE, AND POSTZONE

In the formation of antigen and antibody complexes, large complexes are formed when the antigen and antibody meet at a concentration in which the number of paratopes (antibody binding sites) approximately equals the number of epitopes; this part of the precipitation curve is called **equivalence** (Figure 6.2 ■). When there is too much antibody, 2 antibodies are bound to every bivalent antigen and there is no need for bridging of 2 antigen molecules by an antibody molecule. In this situation, little or no precipitate would form, which makes it appear that the patient does not have an antibody to the antigen when, in fact, he or she has too much antibody for the multiple bridging required for precipitation or agglutination reaction to occur. This part of the precipitation or agglutination curve is called the **prozone.** Most of the precipitation occurs when the ratio of antibody to antigen is just right (ie, the number of paratopes approximately equals the number of epitopes). When the amount of patient antibody is low so that each IgG antibody is bound by 2 antigen molecules, there is no bridging of 2 antibody molecules by the antigen, so little or no precipitation occurs. This situation is called the **postzone.** In both the prozone and the postzone situations, the patient would appear negative for antibody to the tested antigen. In a prozone situation, the patient's serum can be diluted and tested again to reach equivalence. In the case of a postzone reaction, the patient's blood can be drawn again in 1 or 2 weeks to allow the patient to form more antibodies (an increase in titer) to bring the reaction to the zone of equivalence (1, 2, 3, 4, 5, 6).

 Checkpoint! 6.1

The patient really looks sick with an autoimmune disease that is caused by antibody; however, the agglutination reaction is negative. What should you do?

▶ IMMUNODIFFUSION TECHNIQUES

Proof that an antibody is reacting with an antigen is at its simplest when you can actually see the precipitate that forms when the 2 interact, forming the lattice structure.

Precipitation, as a method of detecting antigen-antibody interactions, is a very easy technique; it usually involves just placing the antigens and the antibody in different wells in an agar plate, allowing the diffusion to occur, and analyzing the pattern of precipitation that results. However, this is the least sensitive serological technique because it requires the visualization of 2 substances in solution as they come out of solution. It is not amplified by the antigen being on a particle, nor is it amplified by any methods to link this reaction to another more visible reaction. The measuring limit of precipitation is approximately 20 microgram/ml of antibody and antigen. However, it is still a clinically important assay for fungal antigens and for some research purposes because it can give information concerning the relatedness of antigens and the minimum number of antigen and antibody pairs, which is difficult to garner in any other way. Two examples of immunodiffusion gel precipitation methods are **double diffusion gel precipitation** reactions, which are also called *Ouchterlony reactions* or *immunodiffusion (ID) reactions*, and single diffusion precipitation, which is also called **radial immunodiffusion (RID)** (1, 2, 3, 4, 5, 6).

OUCHTERLONY

In double diffusion gel precipitation, also known as Ouchterlony analysis, both the antibody and the antigen diffuse through agar or agarose. As they diffuse radially, their concentration diminishes (Figure 6.3 ■); at the point in the diffusion where the relative concentrations of antibody and antigen reach equivalence, a precipitin line appears, which is formed by the **lattice** (cross-linked) structure formed by the complexes. Double immunodiffusion gel precipitation analyses are unique in that they allow for determination of antigenic relatedness of an unknown test material with a known antigen. Specifically, double diffusion gel precipitation allows the determination of whether the unknown is identical, partially

identical, or nonidentical with the known antigen. Double diffusion gel precipitation is a *qualitative* procedure and is utilized clinically in the diagnosis of some fungal infections including coccidiomycosis and is used in research to determine relatedness. The qualitative procedure has also been used to analyze serum from patients with autoimmune disorders and to determine the specificity of antibodies found in antinuclear antibody testing. However, in the case of autoimmunity, immunodiffusion has largely been replaced by enzyme immunoassays.

To compare antigenic relatedness, 2 different antigen preparations are placed in different wells, and the antiserum is placed in a third well. The antigens and antibodies diffuse in a circle out of the well, and only some of the antibody and antigen will actually be in the reaction because much of it diffuses in the wrong direction. When the antibody and the antigen meet at equivalence, they form a precipitin line (Figure 6.4 ■). One of 3 patterns can occur when the precipitin line forms: lines of **identity, nonidentity,** or **partial identity.**

1. When the 2 different antigen preparations contain the same antigen, a line of identity will form (Figure 6.4(b)). The arc shape of this line is the result of the intersection of the circular shapes of the diffusion from each well so that the reagents react at equilibrium in an arc.

2. When the antigens are completely different (Figure 6.4(c)), 2 different lines of precipitation form, one made of 1 antibody and its antigen, and the other made of the second antibody and its antigen. In the figure, observe that the red antibody to "pink and purple" antigen can go through the wall formed by the blue antibody and "dark green and orange" antigen lattice. This happens because precipitin walls are permeable to everything except to the reagents of which they are composed. An additional blue antibody would not get through this wall because it would bind to the orange epitopes and make the wall thicker. Similarly,

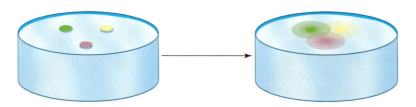

■ **FIGURE 6.3** To illustrate how antibody and antigen diffuse from the wells, we depict colored dye diffusing from the wells. In diffusion of color from each well, the dye is most concentrated as it leaves the well, and as it goes farther, the concentration and the amount of color decreases. Where 2 colors meet a mixed color forms. In an antibody and antigen reaction where the two reactants met at appropriate concentrations the lattice precipitin product forms.

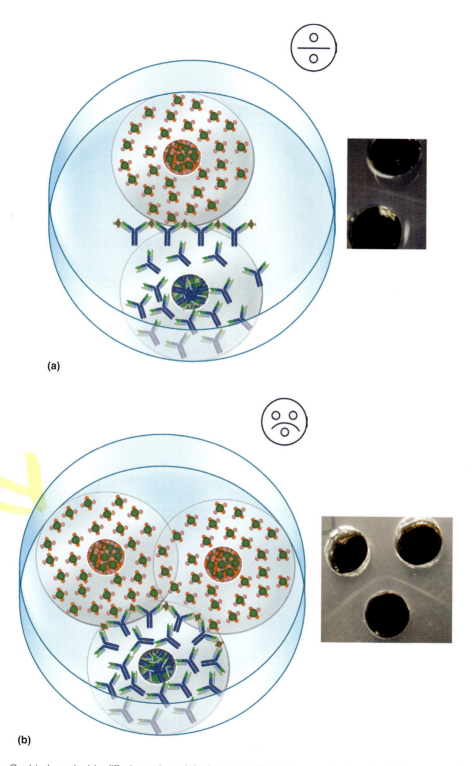

■ **FIGURE 6.4** (a) An Ouchterlony double diffusion gel precipitation assay. The antigen and antibody solutions are most concentrated at the wells. When the Ag and Ab meet at equivalence, they form the lattice precipitin structure. (b) Two wells are filled with the same antigen, and when they diffuse to the antibody, they make a line of identity.

(continued)

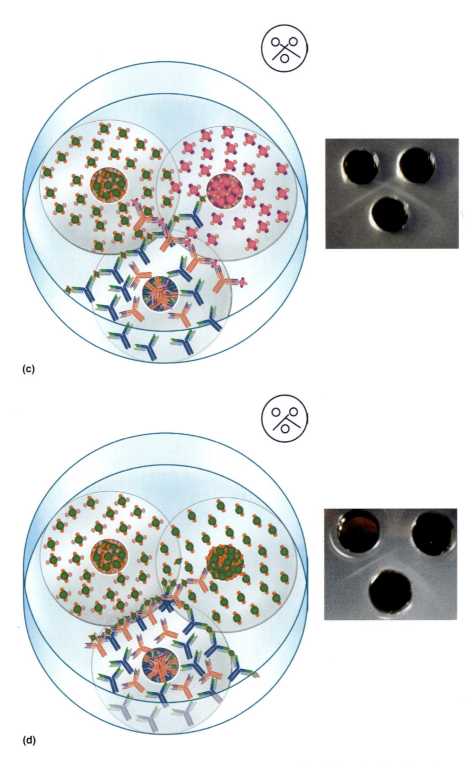

(c)

(d)

■ **FIGURE 6.4** *(continued)* (c) Two wells are filled with different antigens and when they diffuse, they form lines that cross which is called a line of nonidentity. (d) Two wells are filled with related or partially identical antigens. The well on the left contains an antigen with an additional epitope when compared with the antigen in the well on the right. The precipitin line on the left is formed by the reaction of an antibody to the shared epiotpe, and this line continues on the right, as in a line of identity. Also in the line on the left is the reaction of an antibody to the unique epitope and the antigen with the unique epitope. This reaction line continues beyond the line of identity because the antibody to the unique epitope is not stopped as it comes to the line formed by the antigen without this epitope and antibody to the shared epitope. For simplicity, the antigen has been drawn with 2 to 4 epitopes, but proteins usually have more than this number of epitopes.

the orange and green antigen would not get through this wall but would bind to blue antibody and make the wall thicker.

3. When the antigens in the 2 wells are similar (Figure 6.4(d)) but the antigen in the well on the left contains an additional epitope (the pink piece), the antibody to the shared epitopes forms a line similar to a line of identity, but on the left, the antibody to the additional piece can also react. This antibody can also go through the wall made of the antigen without the pink epitope and its antibody, thus making a "spur" on the well on the left. The spur is made of antibody to the extra epitope and the antigen that contains the extra epitope. This line is called a *line of partial identity*. The spur always points to the simpler antigen.

Although the double diffusion gel precipitation reaction is qualitative rather than quantitative, it can be set up so that relative concentrations of the antigens can be determined. When the antigen and antibodies are diffusing from their respective wells, their concentration decreases as they move farther from the well, so when the antibody concentration in 2 wells is the same, the 2 wells containing the antigen opposite the 2 antibody wells would form precipitin lines in different places if their antigen concentrations are different. The antigen with the higher concentration would form a precipitin line closer to the antibody well because it would diffuse further before its concentration decreased to the level needed for equivalence (Figure 6.5 ■) (1, 2, 3, 4, 5, 6, 7).

RADIAL IMMUNODIFFUSION

Radial immunodiffusion utilizes an adaptation of the diffusion principle involving decreasing concentrations as one moves away from the source well to develop a quantitative immunoprecipitation technique. In radial immunodiffusion, single diffusion of the antigen takes place into a gel that already contains the antibody evenly distributed throughout (ie, the gel is poured with the antibody already mixed with it). Thus, as in Figure 6.5, the antibody concentration is held at a constant, and different concentrations of the antigen diffuse into it. Because the antigen is diffusing out of a circular well into the gel, the precipitation will be in a circle with its diameter reflecting the concentration of the antigen and with a more concentrated antigen traveling farther to become dilute enough for the precipitation to occur at equivalence (Figure 6.6 ■). A standard curve is prepared by using 3 different concentrations of the antigen in 3 different wells; the patient's results (ie, the diameter of the precipitation line from the patient's sample) are then compared to this standard curve, and an approximate concentration of antigen in the patient's sample is then obtained.

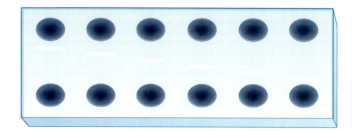

■ **FIGURE 6.5** Concentration affects where the precipitin line forms. When 1 reactant is held at a constant concentration and the other reactant is varied in concentration, the place where the precipitin line forms changes in relation to the concentration.

Two slightly different methods are utilized for quantitating the results of radial immunodiffusion. The **Fahey method** allows the diffusion to proceed for 18 hours and the diameter is proportional to the log of the concentration. It is plotted using semilog paper with the diameter

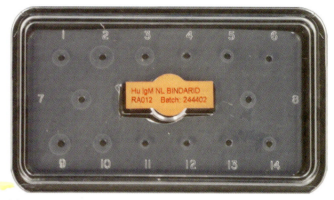

(a)

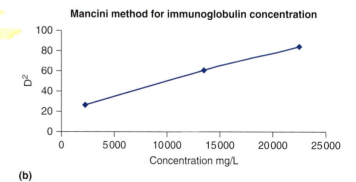

(b)

■ **FIGURE 6.6** (a) A photograph of a radial immunodiffusion reaction for measurement of patient IgA concentrations. In this example the Ag concentration in well 2 is greater than that in well 3, or, well 5. (b) A plot of the Mancini method of determining immunoglobulin concentration.

of the precipitin line on the arithmetic axis and concentration on the y-axis. The Fahey method is also called the kinetic method. Conversely, in the **Mancini method** or end-point method, the reactants are allowed to come to equilibrium (in 48 to 72 hours), and the square of the diameter is directly proportional to the concentration (Figure 6.6(b)). Radial immunodiffusion is used to measure IgG, IgM, and IgA levels. Serum concentrations of IgE and IgD are not high enough to be read by this relatively insensitive method. These immunoglobulins are being measured as antigens, not as antibodies. The antibody in these commercial kits is anti-human immunoglobulin that is Fc specific. Concentrations of complement components are also determined this way.

 Checkpoint! 6.2

Should you use the Fahey method for RID or the Mancini method to get the patient's result faster?

Another method that utilizes immunoprecipitation is immunofixation electrophoresis. In this method a patient's serum proteins are separated as in serum protein electrophoresis 6 times in 6 different lanes (Chapters 1 and 2). After the electrophoretic separation, each individual lane is overlaid with a different monospecific antisera, anti-IgG in 1 lane, and then anti-IgM, anti-IgA, anti-kappa, and anti-lambda in each subsequent lane. The sixth lane is treated with a protein fixative. After washing, the precipitated proteins are stained for improved visualization using Commassie blue (1, 2, 3, 4, 5, 6, 7). This method is used for identification of which immunoglobulin class is elevated in myeloma. It is discussed in detail in Chapter 13.

Other methods that utilize diffusion and electrophoresis were developed to speed up the reaction and improve sensitivity. These methods include immunoelectrophoresis, counter-current immunoelectrophoresis, and rocket immunoelectrophoresis. *Immunoelectrophoresis* is serum protein electrophoresis followed by double diffusion gel precipitation. *Counter-current electrophoresis* is the Ouchterlony technique enhanced and made quicker by using an electric current to bring the antigen and antibody together. *Rocket electrophoresis* is radial immunodiffusion using an electric current to bring the antigen into the antibody-containing gel. The shape of the precipitin line is the shape of a rocket. The height is proportional to the concentration of the antigen. None of these is used clinically any longer (1, 2, 3, 4, 5, 6, 7).

INSTRUMENTAL METHODS TO ENHANCE SENSITIVITY

Nephelometry and **turbidometry** use optical analysis methods to acquire and analyze antibody and antigen lattice formation. When antibodies and antigens are mixed in solution, the lattice structures begin to form and an initial cloudiness of the solution is followed by the lattice structures precipitating out of solution. In turbidometry, the initial cloudiness is measured by passing a light through the solution and determining the amount of light that comes directly across the solution into the detector. This is a measure of the amount of light that is lost due to scatter by the lattice structures. The amount of scatter is proportional to the concentration of the molecules in the lattice structures. Nephelometry is similar to turbidometry but does not measure the light directly across from the light source but at a 10° to 90° (70° typically used) angle from the light source. Both instrumental methods are much more sensitive than detecting precipitation with the naked eye and have been made more sensitive with the use of laser light as the light source. Nephelometry is more sensitive than turbidometry (Figure 6.7 ■). Immunoglobulin concentrations for IgG, IgM, and IgA as well as kappa and lambda light chains, complement proteins, and acute phase reactants are measured this way (7, 8, 9, 10).

 Checkpoint! 6.3

You were just hired, and the lab supervisor tells you to run an assay using the nephelometer. You have never seen one before and there are 2 instruments in the lab: One is a nephelometer and one is a turbidometer. You see that one of the instruments says that the light is detected at a 70° angle. A note on this instrument also gives the sensitivity range; it is more sensitive than the other instrument. Is this the correct instrument to use?

▶ AGGLUTINATION TECHNIQUES

HISTORY

The fact that serum from a patient could specifically agglutinate bacteria that caused an infection was discovered just before the 20th century. This discovery contributed evidence to the idea that the humoral (serum) part of the blood provided defense against infection. Soon after its discovery, bacterial agglutination was used to diagnose typhoid fever. Agglutination, the drawing together of particles that contain antigen to form a visible lattice or clump, is not very sensitive

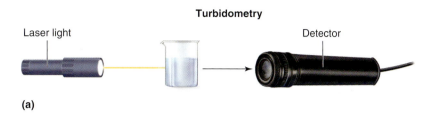

Turbidometry

Laser light   Detector

(a)

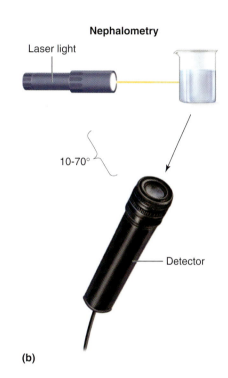

Nephalometry

Laser light

10-70°

Detector

(b)

■ **FIGURE 6.7**   (a) A turbidometry detector measures laser light directly across from the light source. The sample, the light source, and the detector are shown. (b) A nephelometry detector measures light at a 10° to 70° angle from the light source. The sample, the light source, and the detector are shown.

because nothing amplifies the actual antibody-antigen reaction. However, agglutination is more sensitive than precipitation because the larger antigen particles enhance visualization. Agglutination of particles that naturally have the antigen on their surface is called **direct agglutination.** The increased sensitivity of agglutination over precipitation was the reason for the development of **passive agglutination,** agglutination of particles that have been covalently coated with antigens (Figure 6.8(a) ■). Latex beads are the most commonly used particles for passive agglutination, although red blood cells that have been treated with tannic acid so that antigens will stick to them have also been used. Both direct and passive agglutination assays test for antibody that holds the antigen-coated particles together (1, 2, 3, 4, 5, 6, 7).

To test for antigen, different agglutination assays were developed. One of these is an inhibition agglutination assay. In this type of assay, agglutination is seen after mixing the antigen-coated particles from the kit and antibody supplied with the commercial kit. To determine if antigen is present in the patient's serum, the patient's serum is mixed with the kit antibody and if antigen is present in the serum it will bind to the kit antibody. Subsequent addition of the antigen-coated particles will not result in agglutination. So, in this inhibition assay, absence of agglutination is a positive result for antigen in the patient's serum (Figure 6.8(b)). Another type of agglutination assay that measures antigen is called **reverse passive agglutination.** In reverse passive agglutination, the particles have been coated with antibody (with the Fc regions down against the particle and with the Fab regions facing out), and antigen binding to antibody on 2 different particles holds the particles together. This can be used to detect bacterial or other antigens in solution; see Figure 6.8(c).

Refer to Figure 6.8(d) for an example of a clinically used agglutination reaction. This is a latex agglutination reaction for rheumatoid factor, an IgM antibody to the Fc region of IgG that is produced in patients with rheumatoid arthritis. In this assay for rheumatoid factor, the latex beads are coated with human IgG with the Fc region facing out. This human IgG is the antigen. If the patient has the rheumatoid factor antibody, the beads will be held together and agglutinated. Agglutination is seen in the figure in wells 1, 3, and 4. No agglutination is seen in well 2. When the milky white particles are not agglutinated, the suspension looks like milk, while

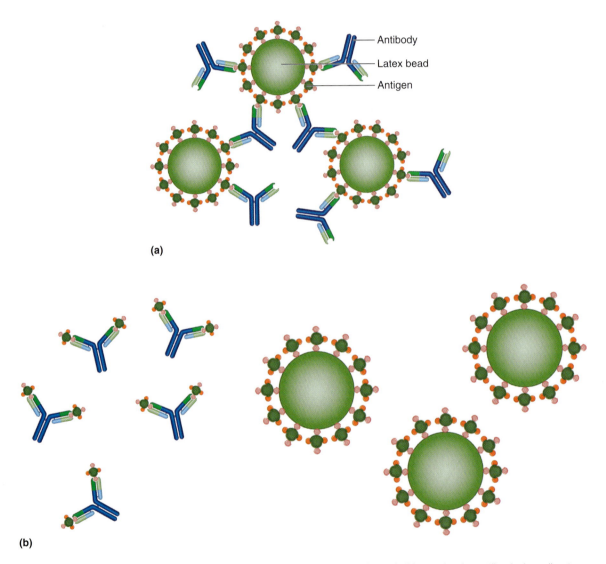

(a)

(b)

■ **FIGURE 6.8**   (a) An agglutination reaction. Antigen-coated latex beads are held together by antibody. In a direct agglutination reaction, the antigen is naturally part of the particle, but in passive agglutination, the antigen is attached to the particle. (b) An agglutination inhibition reaction. Commercial kit materials would create an agglutination reaction as seen in (a). If the patient's serum has antigen in it, mixing the patient's serum with the antibody first and then adding the antigen-coated beads would result in the reaction seen here. The antibody is bound by soluble antigen and no longer causes agglutination of the particles.

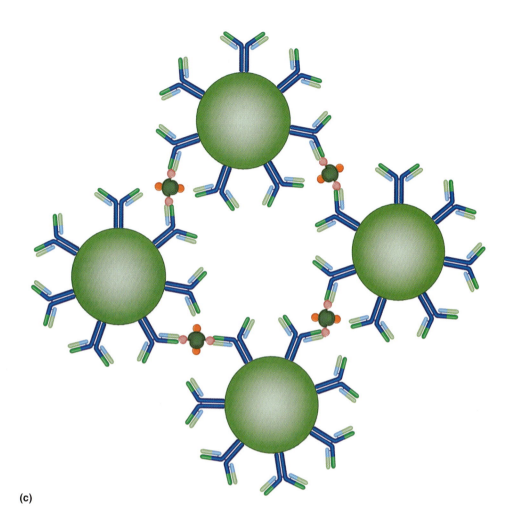

(c)

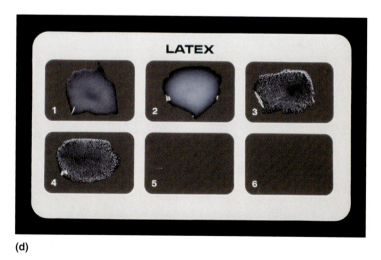

(d)

■ **FIGURE 6.8** *(continued)* (c) A reverse passive agglutination reaction. The antibody is bound to the particles, and antigen in the patient serum or urine causes the particles to become agglutinated. (d) A latex agglutination reaction. This is an analysis for rheumatoid factor. Immunoglobulin is bound to the latex particles with the Fc facing out. For this disease, the Fc of immunoglobulin is the antigen that the patient makes antibody to. The patient's IgM to the Fc of IgG binds the particles together. A weak positive is seen in well 1, a negative control in well 2, and strong positives in wells 3 and 4.

agglutination looks gritty with a clearing of the background (1, 2, 3, 4, 5, 6, 7).

Checkpoint! 6.4

Which of the following measures antibody?
A. *direct agglutination*
B. *reverse passive agglutination*
C. *agglutination inhibition*
D. *passive agglutination*

EFFECT OF A CHARGE ON THE PARTICLE

When agglutination is performed using charged particles such as bacteria or red blood cells, the antibodies pull together 2 particles that would naturally repel each other like 2 north poles of a magnet pushing each other apart. If you have ever held 2 north poles of a magnet together, you will remember that the closer you brought them together, the harder they pushed apart. Agglutination is similar in that with agglutination of charged particles, the closer the particles are brought together, the more they repel. This property results in the fact that IgM works much better for agglutination of charged particles than IgG because of the increased reach between the antigen-binding sites of IgM. IgM is also very good at agglutination because it has so many binding sites. Where the particle has a charge, the pH of the reaction is important because it affects the charge. The charge on the particle is called the **zeta potential** of the particle. If the charge or zeta potential increases, the apparent titer would decrease because it would take more immunoglobulin to hold these charged particles together. Methods have been adapted to improve binding of charged particles: using low ionic strength (LISS) media to decrease charge, using increased viscosity media to decrease the water of hydration, altering the temperature to improve antibody binding, treating the red cells with enzymes to decrease surface charge, and agitation or centrifugation to increase interaction. IgM antibodies agglutinate best between 4°C and 27°C, and IgG antibodies agglutinate best at 37°C. See Figure 6.9(a) ■ for IgM hemagglutination (agglutination of red blood cells) (1, 2, 3, 4, 5, 6, 7).

Because of the repulsive effect of charge, sometimes IgG antibodies do not cause agglutination of the particles; in this case, an anti-human immunoglobulin can be added to cross-link the Fc regions of the IgG molecules that are bound to the particle. The addition of the anti-human immunoglobulin increases the distance between the particles and allows agglutination to occur (1, 2, 3, 4, 5, 6). Figure 6.9(b) ■ shows IgG and anti-human immunoglobulin-mediated hemagglutination.

There are 2 types of agglutination with red blood cells (hemagglutination), the direct antiglobulin test and the indirect antiglobulin test. Both tests involve IgG and anti-human immunoglobulin-mediated hemagglutination (see Figure 6.9(b)). Anti-human immunoglobulin is antibody that is made in another species and binds to the Fc region of human immunoglobulin. It is used to detect human antibody in a number of reactions in the serology lab. The **direct antiglobulin test (DAT)** measures whether antibody is present on an individual's red blood cells. For example, this test can determine whether an infant's red blood cells

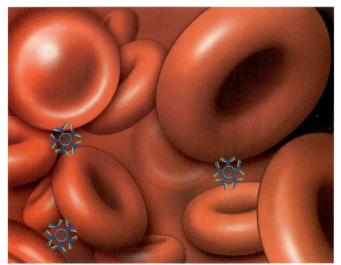

(a)

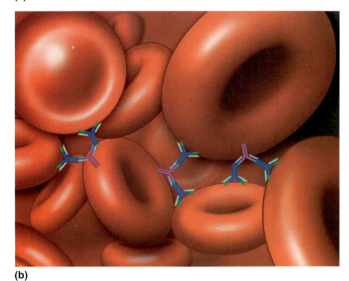

(b)

■ FIGURE 6.9 (a) Hemagglutination with IgM antibody. (b) Hemagglutination with IgG binding to the rbcs and an anti-human immunoglobulin added to bridge the IgG antibodies.

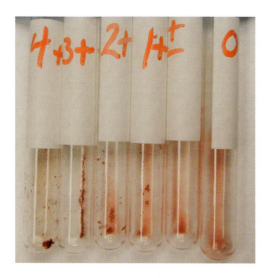

(c)

■ **FIGURE 6.9** *(continued)* (c) A photograph of a hemagglutination reaction. In the tube labeled 0, there is no agglutination, in the tube labeled +/−, a small amount of agglutination is seen and as the numbers increase, there is progressively more agglutination. In the tube labeled 4+, you can see that the red blood cells are in 1 large clump.

have their mother's anti-Rh on their surface and whether a patient has an autoimmune hemolytic anemia, a transfusion reaction, or antibody to drug-sensitized red blood cells. Anti-human immunoglobulin is added directly to red cells from the patient which are then observed for agglutination. Using an **indirect antiglobulin test (IAT),** the clinical laboratory looks for the presence of patient antibody to red blood cells. Compared with the previous example, this test would be used to see whether a mother has anti-Rh antibodies. It can also be used to test for transfusion compatibility. The patient's serum is added to the red blood cells and after incubation and washing, anti-human immunoglobulin is added. The cells are centrifuged and observed for agglutination. Figure 6.9(c) shows different degrees of hemagglutination from no agglutination to a 4+ agglutination reaction in which the cell button comes off the bottom of the tube in 1 clump (1, 2, 3, 4, 5, 6, 7).

INSTRUMENTAL METHODS TO ENHANCE AGGLUTINATION SENSITIVITY

Similar to the way the sensitivity of precipitation assays are enhanced using the optical-enhanced methods of nephelometry and turbidometry, agglutination assays are also enhanced with optical detection methods, including the **particle-enhanced turbidimetric inhibition assay (PETINA),** the **particle-counting immunoassay (PACIA),** and the **quasi-elastic light scattering method (QUELS).**

PETINA is used to determine the serum concentration achieved with administration of a therapeutic drug. The need for this monitoring of therapeutic drug concentration occurs because different individuals metabolize drugs differently and certain concentrations of the drug must be maintained but not exceeded for efficacy without toxicity. This *therapeutic drug monitoring* is particularly important with the anti-clotting drug Coumadin, but is important for many other drugs as well. In a PETINA for therapeutic drug concentration, the commercial kit comes with a specific drug linked to particles and an antibody to the drug. Mixing antibody with these particles will cause increased turbidity of the solution because it agglutinates the particles. When the patient's serum containing that particular drug is added to this mixture, it will bind the antibody, so no antibody is left to bind the particles. This drug in the patient's serum *inhibits* the cross-linking of the particles by the antibody because the antibody-binding sites are bound to the drug in the patient's serum and are not free to cross-link the particles. Therefore, no agglutination indicates the presence of the drug in the patient's sample. This is diagramed in Figure 6.8(b), the agglutination (or lack thereof) is detected using turbidometry and has enhanced sensitivity for measuring drug concentrations over nonoptically enhanced methods (7, 8, 9, 10).

In PACIA, an agglutination reaction occurs, but this reaction is observed by counting the residual nonagglutinating particles. They are measured by an optical cell counter calibrated to count single particles and to exclude aggregated particles according to size. The particles are brought through a detector and measured either by the change in conductance as the particles go through the detection path or they are measured as they go through a detector by light scattering. This assay is more sensitive than nephelometry because dimers are easily gated as agglutinated particles whereas most other techniques need agglutination of higher order before it is detected. These assays are much more sensitive than noninstrumental agglutination techniques, reaching down to 10^{-10} molar (9).

QUELS, or quasi-elastic dynamic light scattering method, measures changes that are related to diffusion coefficients. Diffusion coefficients, in turn, are related to particle size, shape, flexibility, and particle-to-particle interactions. Fluctuations in light intensity are measured after a laser light is shined on the sample. The amplitude of the scattered wave of light is proportional to particle size. For QUELS to be an accurate representation of aggregation of the particles, the sample must be dust free because dust will register as aggregated particles. This method works best when the light is scattered by a single particle, not by the light hitting multiple particles, so this method works best at low concentrations (10).

Checkpoint! 6.5

Match the items 1 through 3 to the proper letter A through C.

1. *PACIA*
2. *PETINA*
3. *QUELS*

A. *uses inhibition*
B. *counts nonagglutinating particles*
C. *uses the fact that little particles and big particles scatter light differently*

 CASE STUDY

You are working at a biotechnology company. Your supervisor asked you to improve the sensitivity of a latex agglutination assay. This assay has been especially designed to need no instrumentation because it will be used in third-world countries in laboratories. Currently, 20% of the patients with this disease do not test positive until they have already developed significant illness due to the infection. If they tested positive earlier, they would have received antibiotics and would not have become so ill.

1. To improve the sensitivity, a smaller amount of patient's immunoglobulin should agglutinate the particles. Latex particles are not charged. How can you design the agglutination assay to be more sensitive?

2. If the assay had been done with red blood cells (negatively charged particles), how could you increase the sensitivity of the assay in relation to charge?

SUMMARY

In precipitation and agglutination reactions, the complexes of molecules of antibody and antigen are visible with the naked eye. In these reactions, the key to the development of lattice (cross-linked) structures that we can visualize is the fact that antibodies always have more than 1 binding site and most antigens also have more than one binding site. To form these lattice structures, antibody and antigen must be at or near equivalence; too much antibody causes a false negative (prozone) and too much antigen causes a false negative (postzone) as well. The most commonly performed precipitin techniques are immunodiffusion plates also called *double diffusion gel precipitation reactions* or *Ouchterlony reactions*. Antibody and antigen detection for fungal infections are still sometimes performed with this technique. The pattern of the precipitin line allows one to determine whether antigens are identical, partially identical, or nonidentical. See Table 6.1 ✪ for a summary of precipitin reactions. Agglutination reactions are more sensitive than precipitation reactions because fewer of these larger particles are needed to form a visible reaction. Agglutination reactions can be direct assays, which are performed on an antigen that is naturally a part of the particle or they can be passive agglutination when the antigen is covalently attached to a carrier such as a latex bead. Direct and passive agglutination reactions are used to measure antibody, and reverse passive and agglutination inhibition assays are used to measure antigen. In testing to see whether a baby has received placentally transferred anti-RH antibodies from his or her mother, an agglutination assay is done with the baby's red blood cells. This assay measures whether antibody is bound to these red blood cells. Anti-human immunoglobulin is added to the red cells, and if this causes agglutination, the baby has this anti-RH antibody on his or her red blood cells. This is a direct antiglobulin test (DAT). To test whether a woman has anti-RH in her serum, it is mixed with RH+ red blood

✪ **TABLE 6.1**

Summary of Precipitation Reactions

Assay	Double Diffusion Gel Precipitation	RID	Nephelometry	Turbidometry
Step 1	Place antiserum in 1 well	Place antigen in well	Add antibody and antigen together, place in instrument	Add antibody and antigen together, place in instrument
Step 2	Place antigens in wells across from antiserum	Allow diffusion to occur	Visualize light that is scattered at a 10–90° (usually 70°) angle	Visualize light that is directly across from the light source
Step 3	Allow diffusion to occur	Visualize and interpret reaction	Create a standard curve	Create a standard curve
Step 4	Visualize and interpret reaction Document as number of lines present and pattern of identity, nonidentity, or partial identity	Draw standard curve using D^2 versus concentration for Mancini or Fahey on semilog paper with D versus concentration on the y-axis		

cells and then anti-human immunoglobulin is added. This is an indirect antiglobulin test (IAT). Charged particles repel, so more antibody is needed to hold charged particles together. To increase the sensitivity of an agglutination assay with charged particles, the ionic strength of the media is reduced to lower particle charge. Refer to Table 6.2 ✪ for a summary of agglutination reactions.

Media viscosity can also be increased to decrease charge, clinical laboratories do this by adding 22% bovine serum albumin to the reaction. Instrumental methods can be employed to increase the sensitivity of precipitation (nephelometry and turbidometry) and agglutination reactions (PETINA, PACIA, and QUELS) (1, 2, 3, 4, 5, 6, 7, 8, 9, 10).

✪ TABLE 6.2

Summary of Agglutination Reactions

Assay	Direct Agglutination	Passive Agglutination	Inhibition Agglutination	Reverse Passive Agglutination	Direct Antiglobulin Test	Indirect Antiglobulin Test
Step 1	Add patient's serum to red blood cells or bacteria	Add patient's serum to antigen-coated particles	Add patient's serum or urine to kit-supplied antibody	Add patient's serum or urine to antibody-coated particles	Draw red blood cells from newborn	Prepare RH+ red blood cells
Step 2	Mix	Mix	Add antigen-coated particles from the kit	Mix	Add anti-human immunoglobulin	Add patient's serum
Step 3	Visualize presence or absence of agglutination	Visualize presence or absence of agglutination	Mix	Visualize presence or absence of agglutination	Visualize presence or absence of agglutination	Add anti-human immunoglobulin
Step 4			Visualize presence or absence of agglutination			Visualize presence or absence of agglutination
Detects	Antibody	Antibody	Antigen	Antigen	Anti-RH on infant's red blood cells	Anti-RH in patient's serum

LABORATORY EXERCISE

INSTRUCTIONAL OBJECTIVES

At the conclusion of this lab, the student will be able to:

COGNITIVE DOMAIN

1. Define *precipitation.*
2. Discuss the principle of radial immunodiffusion (RID).
3. Compare and contrast the overnight (Fahey) and the endpoint (Mancini) methods of interpreting results.
4. Discuss several sources of error in quantifying immunoglobulins by RID.
5. Define *prozone.*
6. Describe the requirement for multiple epitopes and for a certain minimal molecular size for the antigen for a precipitation reaction to occur.
7. Discuss how initial concentration in the well of an RID or Ouchterlony plate affects where the precipitin line forms and equivalence occurs.

PSYCHOMOTOR DOMAIN

1. Identify and interpret the reactions of identity, partial identity, and nonidentity in an Ouchterlony double diffusion plate.
2. Perform and interpret the results of an IgG RID procedure.

LABORATORY EXERCISE *(continued)*

3. Define *lattice formation* and be able to draw a molecular depiction to explain lattice formation in a precipitation reaction. Also define *prozone* and *postzone* and draw the effect of excess Ab or Ag on lattice formation.

4. Define *equivalence* in terms of the answer to Objective 3. In addition, draw the way that the concentration of the Ag and the Ab changes as the distance from the well of origin increases.

DOUBLE IMMUNODIFFUSION (OUCHTERLONY): LABORATORY PART 1

Double immunodiffusion allows the determination of antigenic relatedness of an unknown test material with a known antigen. This technique allows for determining whether the unknown is identical, partially identical, or nonidentical with the known. Double immunodiffusion is a *qualitative* procedure, largely a research tool, and used in the laboratory for analysis of serum from patients with autoimmune disorders.

You and a partner will prepare an Ouchterlony system, set up as follows:

1. Fill a Petri dish with 1% agarose in phosphate-buffered saline (PBS) with azide to a depth of 3 mm. Allow to cool.

2. Cut 3- to 4-mm holes in the agarose. Remove the plugs by suction.

3. Prepare an Ouchterlony reaction (one person should do the identity plate, and one the nonidentity) as follows:
   a. Label under the wells carefully with a sharpie. Do not get ink between the wells.
   b. Add 40 microliters of antibody of bovine serum to A wells.
   c. Add 40 microliters of albumin to wells labeled C (1–10 mg/ml).
   d. Add 40 microliters of bovine IgG (1–10 mg/ml) to the well labeled D on only one of the plates.
   e. Incubate overnight on a flat surface.
   f. Observe, draw, and interpret patterns.*

*The exact concentration of antigen required depends on the particular antiserum that you are using. Run a test immunodiffusion prior to using these concentrations in class.

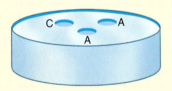

Plate 1 Nonidentity

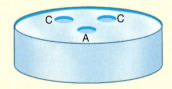

Plate 2 Identity

4. Interpret the following:

   a. Fusion: Identity of antigens

   b. Crossing over: Nonidentity

c. Spur formation: Partial identity

Variables in the double diffusion method include size of the antigen wells relative to the antibody well, concentration of antiserum, and time.

RADIAL IMMUNODIFFUSION: LABORATORY PART 2

MATERIALS

1. Bindarid™ RID plate from The Binding Site Ltd. Birmingham, UK (RN004.3, RN010.3, RN012.3, or RK002)
2. Serum samples for testing

PROCEDURE

1. Remove the RID plate from the foil pouch, remove the lid, and allow condensation to evaporate for 10 to 15 minutes.
2. Mix calibrators gently before using.
3. Fill wells with 5 microliters of the samples and calibrators. Do not leave the plate open for an extensive period of time.
4. Incubate the RID plate at room temperature (20° to 24° C) for 18 hours for the Fahey method or 48 hours for the Mancini method (72 hours for IgM; the larger molecular weight molecule takes a longer time to diffuse).
5. Measure the diameter of each precipitin ring from the back of the plate using the jeweler's eyepiece or the RID ruler. Measure the diameter to the nearest 0.1 mm and then square it.
6. Draw a standard curve on linear graph paper for the Mancini method (concentration on the x-axis; d^2 on the y-axis). This will give a straight line. Determine the immunoglobulin concentration of the sample by squaring the diameter, plotting it on the y-axis, and reading the concentration from the standard curve on the x-axis.
7. Plot the Fahey method as above, but the line will be curved. For a straight line for the Fahey method, use semilog paper with the diameter on the arithmetic axis and concentration on the y-axis.

REVIEW QUESTIONS

1. In an Ouchterlony plate, a precipitin line of identity forms between 2 Ags and an Ab, the 2 lines
   a. cross
   b. merge
   c. cross on 1 side only
   d. form 2 separate lines

2. A prozone effect
   a. occurs in agglutination and precipitin reactions when there is antigen excess
   b. occurs in agglutination and precipitin reactions when there is antibody excess
   c. occurs in agglutination but not in precipitation reactions
   d. occurs in enzyme immunoassay and fluorescent immunoassays when there is antigen excess

3. Which of the following describes agglutination?
   a. soluble Ag + soluble Ab
   b. particulate Ag + soluble Ab
   c. reaction that requires instrumentation to read
   d. reaction that requires covalent binding to the Ab molecule

4. Which of the following enhances agglutination of charged particles?
   a. increasing the ionic strength
   b. removing albumin from the reaction buffer
   c. decreasing viscosity
   d. decreasing ionic strength

REVIEW QUESTIONS (continued)

5. A direct agglutination reaction involves an
   a. antigen that is already part of the particle
   b. antigen that has been covalently attached to the particle
   c. antigen that has been attached with van der Waals forces to the particle
   d. antibody that has been covalently attached to the particle

6. Agglutination reactions involve all of the following except
   a. van der Waals, hydrophobic and hydrophilic interactions, electrostatic interactions, hydrogen bonding
   b. covalent attachment of something to an antibody molecule
   c. Ab and Ag reaction
   d. zones of equivalence

7. In radial immunodiffusion by the Mancini method, the
   a. concentration of the antigen is directly proportional to the ring diameter
   b. concentration of the antigen is inversely proportional to the ring diameter
   c. concentration of the antigen is directly proportional to the ring diameter squared
   d. time required is less than that for the Fahey method

8. A direct antiglobulin test
   a. measures the amount of antibody in the RH− mom that reacts with the RH+ fetal red blood cells
   b. determines whether anti-RH is already present on the newborn's red blood cells
   c. measures the amount of antibody produced by the fetus to the mother's red blood cells
   d. uses cross-linking antibodies of the IgD type

9. When a light shines directly through a solution and the amount of light that goes through the sample (directly across) is measured as the amount of complex formation, this is called
   a. nephelometry
   b. turbidometry
   c. spectrophotometry
   d. fluorescence

10. If a patient shows the signs and symptoms of severe rheumatoid arthritis but the 1:40 dilution of her sera did not show an agglutination reaction,
    a. we should use an enzyme immunoassay instead, because we need a more sensitive assay
    b. we should test for other forms of arthritis
    c. we should serially dilute the serum and run the test again
    d. we should report to the physician that she is negative for rheumatoid factor

11. A physician came into your laboratory and wants a stat result on the immunoglobulin level in a patient's sera. You have an RID commercial kit for immunoglobulin levels. How soon can you give the physician the results, remembering that the physician wants a stat, or fast, result?
    a. 18 hours by the Mancini method
    b. 18 hours by the Fahey method
    c. 48 hours by the Mancini method
    d. 48 hours by the Fahey method

12. If an Ouchterlony were repeated using twice as much total antigen concentration in the well as used originally, the precipitin line would be
    a. closer to the antibody well
    b. closer to the antigen well
    c. in the same place
    d. not enough information is available to decide between the above answers

REFERENCES

1. Bailey G. Ouchterlony double immunodiffusion. *The Protein Protocols Handbook*. 1996;part VII:749–752. doi: 10.1007/978-1-60327-259-9_135.
2. Saubolle MA. Laboratory aspects in the diagnosis of coccidioidomycosis. *Ann N Y Acad Sci*. 2007;1111(1).
3. Silverstein AM. Cellular versus humoral immunity. In: Silverstein AM, ed. *A History of Immunology*. 2nd ed. Elsevier, NY: 2009: chap 2.
4. Stevens CD. *Clinical Immunology and Serology: A Laboratory Perspective*. 3rd ed. Philadelphia, PA: F.A. Davis Co; 2009; chap 8.
5. Stevens CD. *Clinical Immunology and Serology: A Laboratory Perspective*. 3rd ed. Philadelphia, PA: F.A. Davis Co; 2009: chap 9.
6. Berzofsky JA, Berkower IJ, Epstein SL. Antigen-antibody interactions and monoclonal antibodies. In: Paul WE, ed. *Fundamental Immunology*. 6th ed. Philadelphia, PA: Wolters Kluwer/Lippincott Williams & Wilkins; 2008.
7. Kaplan LA, Pescoe A, Kazmierczak SC. Clinical chemistry: Theory, analysis, correlation. *Laboratory Techniques*. 4th ed. chap 12.

8. Bangs Laboratories, Inc. Tech Note 304 Light-Scattering Assays. April 2008. http://www.bangslabs.com/sites/default/files/bangs/docs/pdf/304.pdf

9. Beckman Coulter, Inc. The Chemistry Information Sheet Theophylline Kit. https://www.beckmancoulter.com/wsrportal/techdocs?docname=/cis/A18559/AG/EN_THE.pdf

10. Lomakin A, Teplow DB, Benedek GB. Quasielastic light scattering for protein assembly study. In: Sigurdsson EM, ed. *Methods in Molecular Biology*. Totowa, NJ: Humana Press; 2005:153–174. http://web.mit.edu/physics/benedek/ArticlesMore/Lomakin2005.pdf

PEARSON
myhealthprofessionskit™

Visit www.myhealthprofessionskit.com to access the interactive Companion Website for this textbook. Simply select "Clinical Laboratory Science" from the choice of disciplines. Find this book and log in by using your user name and password to access additional learning tools.

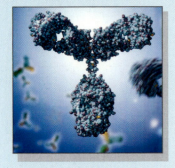

7

Labeled Immunoassays

■ OBJECTIVES—LEVEL I

After this chapter, the student should be able to:

1. Describe the creation of the first labeled immunoassay.
2. Describe the typical constituents of a labeled assay.
3. Identify standards that an antibody must meet to be used for immunoassay.
4. Distinguish between heterogeneous and homogeneous enzyme immunoassays.
5. Describe applications for homogeneous enzyme immunoassays.
6. Explain the principle of direct immunoassays.
7. Explain the priniciple of indirect immunoassays.
8. Explain the principle of sandwich or capture immunoassays.
9. Explain the principle of competitive immunoassays.
10. Compare and contrast enzyme immunoassay and radioimmunoassay as to ease of performance, shelf life, sensitivity, and clinical application.
11. Compare and contrast direct and indirect techniques.
12. Explain the principle of a Western blot assay.
13. Explain why it is sometimes important to perform a Western blot assay rather than an enzyme immunoassay to determine whether a patient has an antibody to a particular disease.
14. Relate the principle of fluorescence polarization immunoassay.
15. Discuss advantages and disadvantages of each type of immunoassay.
16. Compare and contrast the immunoassays in terms of sensitivity

■ OBJECTIVES—LEVEL II

After this chapter, the student should be able to:

1. Describe how a multiplex assay allows for the analysis of multiple antibody and antigen reactions at one time.
2. Describe assay-specific factors that may affect a particular immunoassay (substrate or enzyme effects).
3. Describe patient-specific factors that may affect an immunoassay.

KEY TERMS

anti-human immunoglobulin	immunochromatographic sandwich assay
chemiluminescence	indirect immunoassay
colloid particles	multiplexed fluorescent microbead assays
competitive immunoassay	optical immunoassays
direct immunoassay	recombinant immunoblot assay (RIBA)
fluorescence	
fluorescence polarization immunoassay	rheumatoid factor
heterogeneous assays	sandwich assay
homogeneous assays	spectrophotometer
human anti-mouse antibody (HAMA)	steric hindrance
	Western blot

▶ HISTORY AND INTRODUCTION

The unlabeled immunoassays discussed in Chapter 6 have the advantage of ease of use and are still utilized when the concentrations of the reactants are high enough to visualize. However, relying on actually seeing the antibody and antigen reaction requires a large amount of the immune complex to be formed and is inherently insensitive. With the use of nephelometry and turbidometry, instrumentation improves the ability to visualize the reaction, but the sensitivity is still limited. The vast potential for earlier disease detection and for research applications inspired scientists to look for ways to increase the sensitivity of visualization of antibody and antigen reactions. As in the unlabeled immunoassays, the affinity and the specificity of the antibody utilized in the assay is a key component in any immunoassay. The first assay in which a marker or label was covalently attached to the antibody or antigen to increase the sensitivity of detection was the radioimmunoassay (RIA) developed in 1959 by Rosalyn Yalow who won the Nobel prize for this discovery (1). In this competitive RIA, antigen from the patient competed with radiolabeled antigen for binding to a fixed amount of antibody. Reactants were measured at concentrations that were not visible to the human eye. Yalow's assay, which was developed to help study the clearance of insulin, became the predecessor of many sensitive assays in which a detectable marker or label is attached to either an antibody or antigen. In these assays, the reaction of antibody and antigen complex formation is detected with a thousandsfold increase in sensitivity. Yalow compared the change brought about by this technique to viewing the sky with a powerful telescope compared to viewing it by eye alone (1).

 Checkpoint! 7.1

Who invented the labeled immunoassay?

 Checkpoint! 7.2

What was the first label used in a labeled immunoassay?

This enhanced view of immune reactions is not only brought about by radiolabels; antibody or antigen can alternatively be labeled with enzymes (enzyme immunoassays (EIA) or enzyme-linked immunosorbant assays (ELISA)), fluorescent compounds (fluorescent immunoassay (FIA)), chemiluminescent labels, and colloid particles. In the 1970s, Engvall and Perlman developed an enzyme label for the antibody-antigen reaction to use instead of a radioactive tag (2). In these immunoassay reactions, it is essential to be able to measure the amount of the label that is bound to the antigen-antibody interaction and to separate this bound label from the amount of label that is on unbound antigen or antibody. This is done most often by using a solid phase for the reaction and washing away unbound reactant. This type of assay, requiring separation of bound from free is called a **heterogeneous assay. Homogeneous assays** do not require a separation or washing step to separate the bound antigen and antibody molecules from the free ones. Homogeneous assays can be accomplished because the binding of an antigen to an antibody affects the activity of the label in such a way as to cause a measureable change.

 Checkpoint! 7.3

A patient's urine was applied to a chromatographic membrane and the reactants traveled up the membrane to the point where the Ag + Ab complexes bound to a spot on the membrane and the free Ab and Ag kept traveling. Is the reaction homogeneous or heterogeneous?

Radiolabels are detected by either gamma counters or liquid scintillation counters. Enzyme labels are detected by the addition of a substrate, which the enzyme changes to produce either (1) a color change that can be measured in a **spectrophotometer,** (2) **fluorescence** that can be measured fluorometrically, (3) a flash of light (**chemiluminescence**) that can be measured with a luminometer, or (4) a change in optical reflection in optical immunoassays (OIA). Fluorescent labels are detected in a spectrofluorimeter by detecting the amount of fluorescence at the emission wavelength after application of the excitation wavelength of light. The chemiluminescent assay is based on (1) labeling either an antigen or antibody with a chemiluminescent compound, (2) separating the bound from the free label, (3) activating the chemiluminescent compound with a "trigger" followed by (4) the subsequent measurement of the light in a luminometer or on employing a photomultiplier tube for maximal sensitivity.

In colloid immunoassays, colloid particles are detected by eye after separation in a process called *immunochromatography.* These large colored **colloid particles** must be attached to the antibody or antigen in a way that does not cause **steric hindrance.** The optical immunoassay is based on the changes in the reflection of light after antigen and antibody binding to a surface. The optical immunoassay is also visualized by eye. Because they do not require instrumentation, the colloid and the optical immunoassays are useful for point-of-care testing. The colloid immunoassay is frequently utilized in over-the-counter home diagnostic kits such as pregnancy tests. In colloid immunoassays, these tiny colloid particles allow visualization of the reaction.

▶ TYPES OF HETEROGENEOUS ASSAYS

Many permutations of heterogeneous assays are utilized in the clinical laboratory. Variations can include whether (1) the antigen or the antibody is labeled, (2) the antigen antibody complex is detected directly or, (3) a second anti-immunoglobulin antibody that is labeled is utilized, (4) the antigen or antibody is captured by a capture molecule to a solid phase and detected by a second molecule, and (5) if an inhibition step is performed in which labeled and unlabeled reactants compete. Most of these heterogeneous assays are performed using solid-phase attachment of one of the reactants to a microtiter plate, a slide, or a bead. The use of the solid phase allows the rapid separation of the bound molecules from the free ones by washing steps to remove free labeled reagent so that only the bound label is measured (2).

DIRECT IMMUNOASSAY

A **direct immunoassay** utilizes a labeled antibody binding to an antigen or a labeled antigen binding to an antibody. The direct immunoassay is typically used to detect an antigen in a cell preparation or biopsy sample. An example of the use of a direct assay is a direct fluorescent immunoassay in which antibody to anthrax is labeled with a fluorescent compound and the antigen source is a suspect skin lesion biopsy. The biopsy sample, which has been prepared, sectioned, and placed on a microscope slide, is incubated with a purchased fluorescently labeled antibody to anthrax. After a suitable incubation period, the slide is washed and observed under a fluorescent microscope. The wash step removes the fluorescently labeled antibody that has not bound to the anthrax antigen. This type of assay is used to find antigen in infected tissues and in cultured cells. See Figure 7.1 ■ for direct assays with an enzyme, a fluorescent, and a radiolabeled tag. Please note that the only differences between a direct enzyme immunoassay, a direct immunofluorescent assay, a direct radioimmunoassay and a direct chemiluminescent assay are the label that is conjugated and the method of detection used (Table 7.1 ✪).

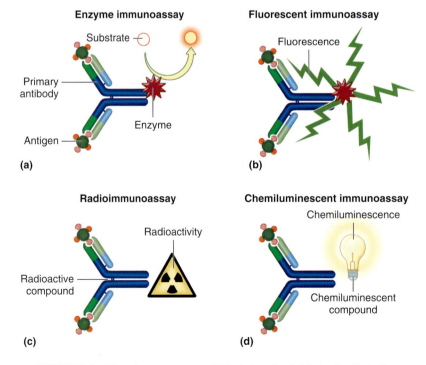

Enzyme immunoassay

Substrate

Primary antibody

Enzyme

Antigen

(a)

Fluorescent immunoassay

Fluorescence

(b)

Radioimmunoassay

Radioactivity

Radioactive compound

(c)

Chemiluminescent immunoassay

Chemiluminescence

Chemiluminescent compound

(d)

■ **FIGURE 7.1**   Direct immunoassays. A labeled antibody binds directly to the antigen. The label on the antibody can be (a) an enzyme, (b) a fluorochrome, (c) a radioisotope, or (d) a chemiluminescent compound.

⊗ TABLE 7.1				
Direct Immunoassays				
Assay	A. Enzyme Immunoassay	B. Fluorescent Immunoassay	C. Radioimmunoassay	D. Chemiluminescent
Label	Enzyme	Fluorochrome	Radioactive molecule	Chemiluminescent compound
Detection method	Spectrophotometer/ Fluorimeter/ Luminometer	Fluorimeter	Gamma or scintillation counting	Luminometer

INDIRECT IMMUNOASSAY

An **indirect immunoassay** utilizes an unlabeled antigen, an unlabeled antibody, and a labeled antiglobulin to detect the reaction of the initial antibody and antigen complex. This immunoassay is generally used to measure a patient's antibody titer to a known antigen. An example of this type of assay is the use of an indirect enzyme immunoassay to measure a patient's titer or level of antibody to rubella (Figure 7.2 ■). A kit in which the rubella antigen is coated on wells in a microtiter plate is purchased, and the patient's sera is diluted and added to a well.

After an incubation period, the nonbinding antibody is washed off and then a second antibody, an anti-human immunoglobulin that is enzyme labeled, is added. After a suitable incubation and another wash step to remove the secondary antibody that has not bound, a substrate for the enzyme is

added and incubated. Depending on the substrate, the enzyme reaction is subsequently read using a spectrophotometer, fluorimeter, or luminometer. This use of a labeled anti-human immunoglobulin was developed because it would not be practical nor would it create a very sensitive assay if each patient's immunoglobulin had to be purified and labeled before each assay for disease. The **anti-human immunoglobulin** step can be performed to detect either all immunoglobulins, IgM only (using a heavy chain-specific anti-human IgM), IgG only (using a heavy chain-specific anti-human IgG), or IgE only (using anti-human IgE). Because IgM is present in acute infections, this ability to detect a specific isotype can help determine whether the antibody that is present is due to a past or current infection. The use of IgG-specific immune conjugates can help determine immune status, and IgE-specific immune conjugates can help diagnose allergy. Any of the other labels could be used in an indirect immunoassay as well as the indirect enzyme immunoassay depicted here. An indirect fluorescent immunoassay, indirect radioimmunoassay, indirect chemiluminescent assay, indirect immunocolloid assay, and indirect optical immunoassay could all be performed. Once again, the only difference would be the label utilized and the method of detection. The ability to use any label type is consistent with all methods that will be discussed.

In a variation of an indirect assay, labeled protein A is used instead of a labeled anti-human IgG antibody. Protein A is isolated from *Staphylococcus aureus* and, like the anti-human immunoglobulin, binds immunoglobulin at the Fc region.

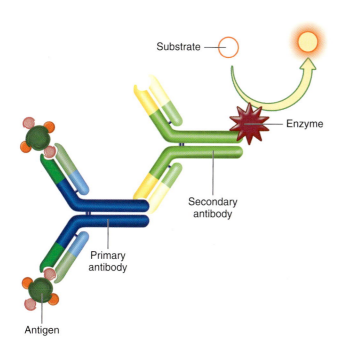

Substrate

Enzyme

Secondary antibody

Primary antibody

Antigen

■ **FIGURE 7.2**   Indirect enzyme immunoassay. A patient's antibody reacts with the antigen, which is detected with the addition of an anti-human immunoglobulin labeled with an enzyme. The enzyme reacts with a colorless substrate, which changes to a colored product.

> ✓ **Checkpoint! 7.4**
>
> *Do you think it would be a better idea just to label the patient's antibody instead of using the indirect immunoassay in which a labeled anti-human immunoglobulin is used to detect the patient's immunoglobulin?*

SANDWICH OR CAPTURE IMMUNOASSAY

A **sandwich assay** usually captures antigen between 2 molecules of antibody, one of which captures the antigen to a solid phase while the other is labeled and used to visualize the reaction (Figure 7.3(a) ■). These assays are commonly performed on disposable membrane cassettes. An

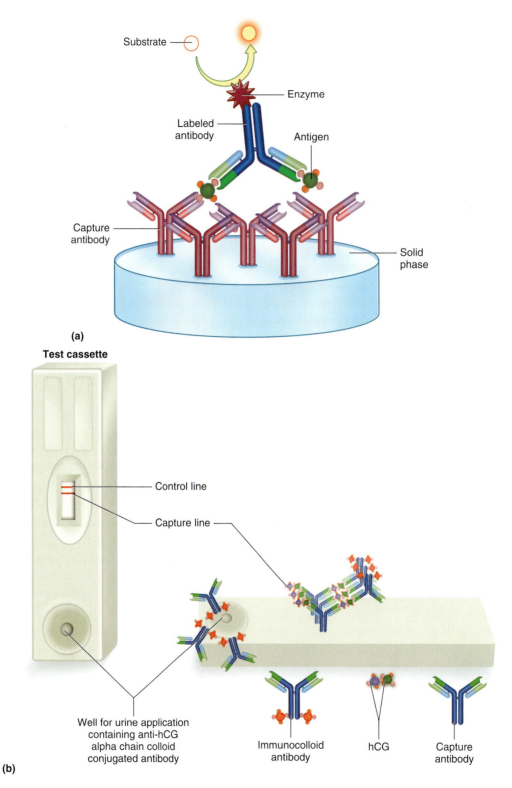

Substrate

Enzyme

Labeled
antibody

Antigen

Capture
antibody

Solid
phase

(a)

Test cassette

Control line

Capture line

Well for urine application
containing anti-hCG
alpha chain colloid
conjugated antibody

Immunocolloid
antibody

hCG

Capture
antibody

(b)

■ **FIGURE 7.3**   (a) Sandwich or capture enzyme immunoassay. The first antibody captures antigen from a body fluid (or from any sample), this is followed by the addition of the second labeled antibody, which also reacts with the antigen. The enzyme on the detecting antibody converts the substrate to a colored product. (b) Colloid-labeled immunochromatographic sandwich assay. The separating properties of chromatography facilitate a capture or sandwich assay. The detecting antibody reacts with the antigen and travels along the chromatographic membrane until it is captured by the capture antibody along the positive line of the test strip.

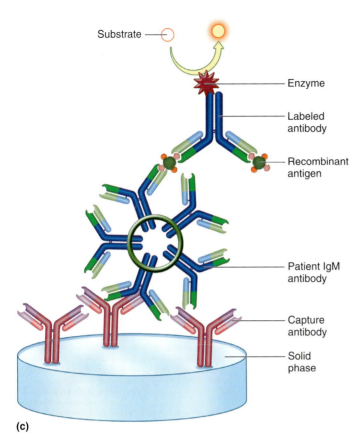

Substrate

Enzyme

Labeled antibody

Recombinant antigen

Patient IgM antibody

Capture antibody

Solid phase

(c)

■ **FIGURE 7.3** *(continued)* (c) Sandwich or capture enzyme immunoassay for patient IgM (double capture: IgM capture, Ag capture).

example of a sandwich assay is a pregnancy colloid labeled **immunochromatographic sandwich assay;** see Figure 7.3(b). In this assay, the 2 antibodies react with the 2 different subunits of human chorionic gonadotropin (hCG), a hormone produced by trophoblastic tissue and excreted in the urine. This capture assay allows for the detection and isolation of hCG, which is present at very low concentrations in the urine. The use of a capture assay increases the specificity of the reaction. The alpha subunit of hCG is nearly identical for luteinizing hormone, follicle-stimulating hormone, thyroid-stimulating hormone, and human chorionic gonadotropin, whereas the beta subunit has hCG-specific epitopes. hCG in the patient's urine is complexed with antibody to the α region of hCG attached to a red colloid. A second antibody, which is directed against an antigenic determinant on the β subunit, is immobilized on the membrane window. This second antibody will also attach to the urine hCG, forming a sandwich. Color capture on this line indicates a positive test. The capture antibody can also be attached to the membrane so that it forms a plus sign if the urine contains hCG (3). The control line is a second antibody capture line after the HCG capture line. This line shows that the reagents are working and that the applied sample is sufficient. See Figure 7.3(b). It is important to note

that the antigen must have more than 1 epitope to utilize a sandwich assay.

A capture assay can also be used to detect immunoglobulin by sandwiching immunoglobulin between a solid-phase antigen and a labeled antigen; an example of this is an assay for the IgM antibody. The antigen is coated on the solid phase, the patient's sera is added, and then after washing, a labeled antigen is added. Bound IgM will have ample binding sites left for reaction with the labeled antigen.

Adaptations have been developed to ensure that an assay for antibody is IgM specific. In many diseases, it is imperative for a prognosis to determine whether the infection responsible for the current illness is caused by a particular pathogen. IgG positivity may indicate only a past infection, so to determine whether the serologic positivity is related to the current illness, paired antibody titers early and late in the infection are compared. For quicker results, the presence or absence of IgM to the pathogen can be determined. IgM is usually present only in the first weeks of an infection and thus indicates an acute infection with this pathogen. However, IgM determinations can be negatively affected by the presence of IgG to the pathogen. When the patient's serum is diluted and incubated with antigen, the presence of IgG to the test antigen will block the binding of IgM to it. This is true even if IgG is present in lesser amounts because it usually has a higher affinity of binding to the antigen and thus would preferentially bind, causing a false negative reaction for the presence of IgM to the antigen (4).

A false positive reaction for IgM to the antigen can occur if the patient has IgG to the pathogen and has IgM rheumatoid factor. **Rheumatoid factor,** which is present in most patients with rheumatoid arthritis, is defined as antibody to the Fc region of the IgG immunoglobulin. It is usually, but not always, of the IgM class. The reason that the rheumatoid factor can cause a false positive is that it can bind to the Fc region of any antibody in the assay, including the capture antibody and the detecting antibody. An adaptation of the capture assay has been developed to detect pathogen-specific IgM without interference with serum IgG to the pathogen; in this example, the pathogen is West Nile virus (WNV). The solid phase is coated with anti-human IgM, the patient's serum is added, and the patient's IgM is attached to the solid phase. Next the antigen, a recombinant WNV Ag, is added. If the patient has IgM specific for this virus, the antigen will be captured. Then an enzyme-labeled mouse monoclonal antibody to the WNV antigen is added. After washing, a substrate is added. The amount of the patient's IgM to WNV will be proportional to the amount of color conversion; see Figure 7.3(c). In this adaptation, the anti-human IgM captures the IgM, and the antigen is captured between the IgM and the enzyme-labeled antibody to the antigen. Another adaptation that measures IgM specifically is the removal of the patient's IgG prior to the performing assay. To do this, the patient's sera is treated with anti-human IgG at precipitating concentrations to remove the IgG prior to incubation with the plated antigen (4).

COMPETITIVE ASSAYS

When an antigen is small and has either only one epitope or if binding to multiple epitopes would create steric hindrance, a capture immunoassay would not work, so a competitive assay would be utilized. *Steric hindrance* refers to a reaction that is inhibited because the bulk of the molecule is in the way of the reaction. In a **competitive immunoassay,** a test kit analyte competes for limited reagent with the analyte in the patient's sample. Antigen can compete for reaction with the antibody, or the antibody can compete for the antigen. An example of a competitive immunoassay for antigen used clinically is the measurement of total homocysteine, which is a risk factor for cardiovascular disease and can assist in the diagnosis of patients with hyperhomocysteinemia or homocystinuria. Homocysteine, at a molecular weight of approximately 138

daltons, is too small to be utilized in a capture assay. In the competitive enzyme immunoassay for patient plasma homocysteine levels, beads are coated with S-adenosyl-L-homocysteine antigen (Figure 7.4(a) ■). The patient serum sample is incubated with an enzyme to cause the formation of S-adenosyl-L-homocysteine from homocysteine present in the serum. The prepared patient sample and an alkaline phosphatase labeled mouse monoclonal antibody to S-adenosyl-L-homocysteine are added to the beads coated with S-adenosyl-L-homocysteine. The patient S-adenosyl-L-homocysteine and the tube S-adenosyl-L-homocysteine compete for binding with the antibody so that the more antigen the patient has, the fewer alkaline phosphatase-labeled antibodies will bind to the beads. The reduction in alkaline phosphatase-labeled antibody will result in a lower formation of the colored product following the addition of the substrate. A standard curve is

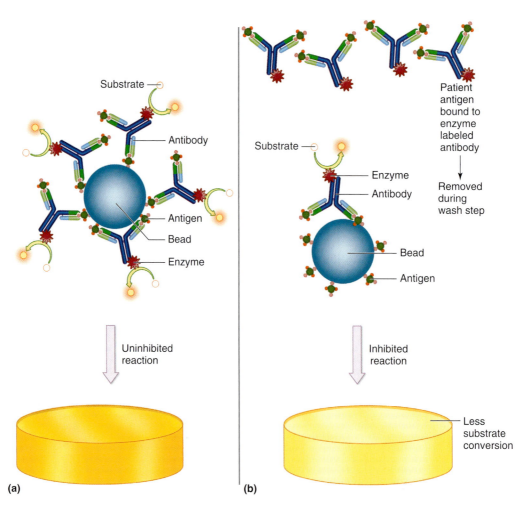

(a)   (b)

■ **FIGURE 7.4** Competitive enzyme immunoassay. (a) Shows the uninhibited reaction and (b) shows the inhibited reaction, in which the binding of the labeled antibody to the patient's antigen in solution blocks the binding of the antibody to the well and results in a decrease in substrate conversion.

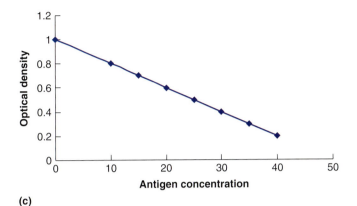

(c)

■ **FIGURE 7.4** *(continued)* (c) The relationship of substrate conversion (as measured by optical density) to the amount of patient antigen in a competitive assay showing the inverse relationship of antigen concentration to color formed in a competitive assay.

utilized to relate the amount of enzymatic substrate conversion to the amount of homocysteine present in the sample; refer to Figure 7.4(b) (5). The pretreatment step for the conversion of homocysteine to S-adenosyl-L-homocysteine was utilized because of the difficulty in forming an antibody to an unmodified amino acid.

An example of a competitive assay for antibody is a microparticle enzyme immunoassay for antibody to hepatitis A antigens. In this assay, microparticles that have been coated with hepatitis A virus (HAV) antigens are incubated with the patient's sera, and then the microparticles are incubated with an enzyme-conjugated antibody to the HAV antigens. In this case, only

the antigenic sites that have not been bound with the patient antibody will be available to this enzyme-labeled antibody. The microparticles are washed and then incubated with the enzyme substrate. For this analysis, a standard curve is created with the amount of patient antibody inversely related to the amount of substrate conversion. (Table 7.2 ✪) (6).

WESTERN BLOT

A **Western blot** is an adaptation of an enzyme immunoassay. It is a technique that begins with the electrophoretic separation of proteins utilizing a sodium dodecyl sulfate polyacrylamide gel electrophoresis (SDS-PAGE) that separates proteins by their molecular weight. The next step utilizes a transfer of these proteins to nitrocellulose, which is a suitable solid phase for the final step of a direct or an indirect enzyme immunoassay. This more expensive and labor-intensive assay is performed when the diagnosis is either difficult or the appropriate diagnosis is critical, or both. An example of a clinically used Western blotting technique for diagnosis is the Western blot for HIV. In this assay, instead of using a solid phase coated with HIV antigens, the proteins from HIV-infected cells are electrophoretically separated using SDS-polyacrylamide gel electrophoresis. The proteins are transferred to nitrocellulose, then non-fat dried milk is added, to block the remaining nonspecific binding sites on the nitrocellulose. The nitrocellulose is cut into strips from top to bottom and each strip is used to test one patient's serum. These strips are sold in diagnostic test kits already prepared with the electrophoretically separated HIV antigens on them. In the clinical

✪ TABLE 7.2

Steps of the Heterogeneous Immunoassays

Assay	Direct	Indirect	Competitive Direct Immunoassay	Sandwich—Solid Phase Ab-Ag-Ab	Sandwich Ag-Ab-Ag	Western Blot
Step 1	Solid-phase Ag incubated with labeled Ab	Solid-phase Ag incubated with Ab	Labeled Ab mixed with patient antigen	Ab (capture Ab), incubated with Ag	Solid-phase Ag (capture Ag), incubated with patient Ab	Polyacrylamide gel electrophoresis of virus or bacterial proteins
Step 2	Wash	Wash	Add mixture to solid-phase antigen	Wash	Wash	Transfer to nitrocellulose
Step 3	Visualize	Add labeled Ab	Wash	Add labeled Ab	Add labeled Ag	Block nonspecific binding sites
Step 4		Wash	Visualize inverse relationship	Wash	Wash	Add patient Ab
Step 5		Visualize		Vsualize	Visualize	Wash
Step 6						Add labeled antihuman immunoglobulin
Step 7						Wash
Step 8						Visualize

laboratory, an indirect enzyme immunoassay is performed on the nitrocellulose strip. The patient's serum is added, incubated, and washed, and then an enzyme-conjugated anti-human immunoglobulin is added. After incubation and washing, the appropriate substrate is added. Diagnosis occurs by comparing the patient's nitrocellulose strip with a positive control strip. For HIV diagnosis, there must be an antibody to two of the major antigens, which include p24, p31, gp41, and gp120/160 (Figures 7.5 ■ and 7.6 ■) (7). This creates a high specificity for the assay, which gives no false positives because

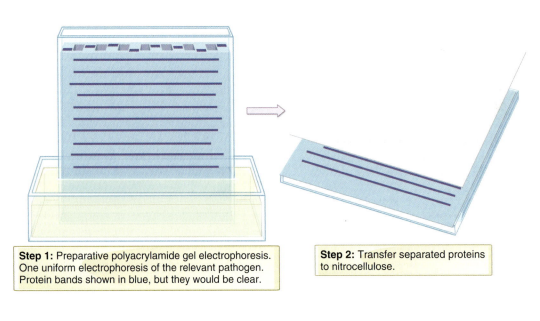

Step 1: Preparative polyacrylamide gel electrophoresis. One uniform electrophoresis of the relevant pathogen. Protein bands shown in blue, but they would be clear.

Step 2: Transfer separated proteins to nitrocellulose.

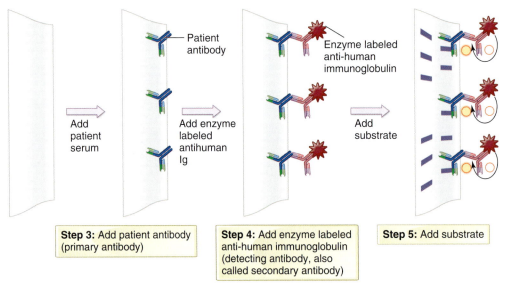

Step 3: Add patient antibody (primary antibody)

Step 4: Add enzyme labeled anti-human immunoglobulin (detecting antibody, also called secondary antibody)

Step 5: Add substrate

Nitrocellulose has been cut into strips in kits for indirect EIA for patient antibody.

Perform an indirect EIA for patient antibody.

Substrate precipitates to form a colored line. Compare strip to control strip to determine molecular weight of proteins that reacted with patient antibody.

■ **FIGURE 7.5**   Western blot. In the first step, (1) a preparative polyacrylamide gel electrophoresis is performed to separate the proteins of the virus or other pathogen. Next, (2) the separated proteins are transferred to a nitrocellulose paper that binds protein well. The nonspecific binding sites of the nitrocellulose paper are blocked by the addition of nonfat dried milk. (3) The paper is cut into strips, and each strip is used to diagnose 1 patient. The next steps (3–5) are to perform an indirect enzyme immunoassay in which the patient sera containing the primary antibody to the viral proteins is added (3). After washing, (4) a secondary labeled antibody is added and after washing again, (5) the substrate is added.

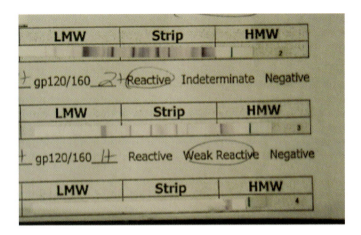

■ **FIGURE 7.6** A Western blot for confirmatory HIV diagnosis. After an enzyme immunoassay has been performed and determined to be positive, a Western blot will be performed for confirmatory analysis. For this diagnosis, the specificity is increased due to the requirement for multiple lines to be present. At each line is a different HIV antigen and its corresponding patient antibody. A strongly positive reaction is seen in the line on the top, a weak but positive reaction is seen in the middle, and a negative reaction is seen on the bottom. *Source:* Rittenhouse-Olson K. HIV testing and confidentiality. ASCP TechSample. Chicago, IL: ASCP; 2004.

of the multiple reactions required to determine the assays's positivity and for the requirement for the binding to occur at the appropriate molecular weight.

For the diagnosis of hepatitis C, an assay called **recombinant immunoblot assay (RIBA)** has been developed. It is a strip immunoblot which has some but not all of the characteristics of a Western blot. A nitrocellulose strip is prepared by the manufacturer which has multiple purified viral antigens each placed on a different spot. An indirect immunoassay is performed by the clinical laboratory on the strip, testing for patient's antibody to the different antigens on the strip and comparing it to the control. The difference between the RIBA and a Western blot is in how the antigens are placed on the strip. In the RIBA the antigens are not electrophoretically separated, but are recombinant antigens and synthetic peptides bearing the important viral epitopes that were prepared, purified, and placed onto the strips in separate spots. Except for this initial step, the strip immunoblot proceeds like a Western blot (8).

This assay format is called RIBA, strip immunoblot, or a line immunoassay. It has recently been developed as a line immunoassay called Immco-stripe to test for auto-antibody to heat shock proteins 70 (HSP70) which has been linked to sensorineural hearing loss. This assay is shown in Figure 7.7 ■

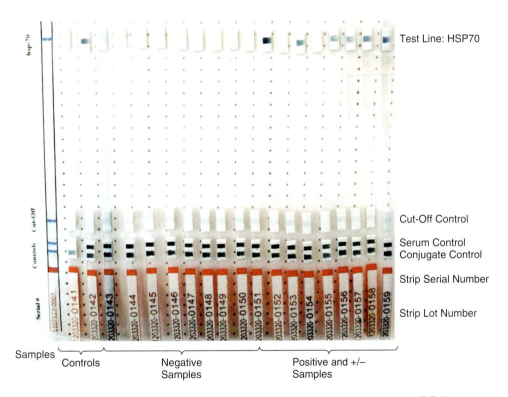

■ **FIGURE 7.7** Line immunoassay (LIA), also called recombinant immunoblot assay (RIBA) and Immuno-stripe, is similar to a Western blot in its membrane enzyme immunoassay format, but the antigens were not electrophoresed, but instead were made by recombinant methods and placed on the membrane. In this assay the test antigen, HSP70, is on the top, a cut-off control is next, then a control which will be positive if patient serum was added is next, followed by a control which will be positive if functional enzyme labeled anti-human antibody is added. *Source:* Immco Diagnostics, Inc. Buffalo, NY, USA

with controls on every strip. At the top, the test antigen line contains recombinant HSP70, next is the cut-off control, then a control that contains anti-human immunoglobulin which will be positive if the patient's serum has been added, which is followed by a conjugate control that contains human immunoglobulin which will be positive if the conjugate has been added and is functional.

FLOW CYTOMETRY

Flow cytometry combines either a direct or an indirect immunofluorescent assay with a cell sampling and cell optics system that enables the analysis of the individual labeled cells or particles one at a time. Flow cytometry (Figures 7.8 ■ and 7.9 ■) is most commonly used for analysis of CD4/CD8 ratios for HIV patient monitoring. This assay is performed by a direct immunofluorescent assay. The patient's white blood cells are incubated with fluorescently labeled antibodies to CD45, CD3, CD4, and CD8, and each antibody is labeled with a different color of fluorochrome. CD45 selects for white blood cells, antibody to CD3 ensures that the compared cells will be T cells, anti-CD4 and anti-CD8 are used to determine helper and cytotoxic T-cell numbers and ratio. After washing, the cells are introduced by vacuum into the flow cytometer in a sheath fluid that allows their movement in a single file through laser light. The laser light contains the excitation wavelength needed to excite the fluorochromes. Light is also scattered by the cells, and the amount scattered is used to identify the various cell types in the blood on the basis of their characteristic properties (9). From this point, several things, including the forward scatter, side scatter, and amount of emitted light from each of the fluorochromes, are measured. The forward light scatter is a measure of the cell size and the side scatter is a measure of the cell granularity. These 2 parameters are important to ensure the analysis of the correct cell population and to exclude cell aggregates. At this point in the analysis, the operator can elect to analyze further only those cells of the correct size and granularity and that are CD3 positive. The amount of each

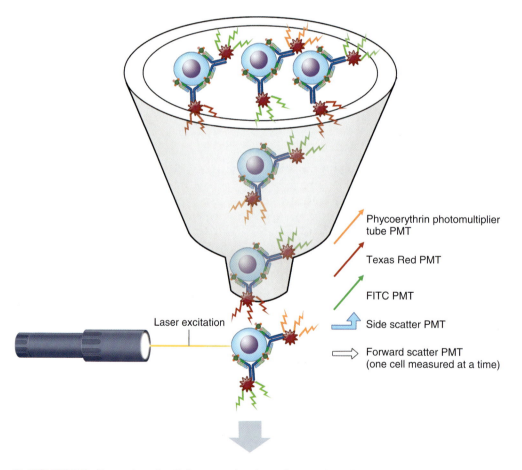

■ **FIGURE 7.8**   Flow cytometry. Cells expressing the surface markers CD4, CD8, and CD3 are labeled in a direct immunofluorescent technique with an antibody labeled with a fluorochrome. Anti-CD3 is labeled green with fluorescein isothiocyanate, anti-CD4 is labeled red with Texas Red, and anti-CD8 is labeled orange with phycoeryrthrin. Cells are processed single file and passed through an excitation wavelength and then through a detector that measures the amount of light at each emission wavelength. Also measured are forward scatter as a determination of cell size and side scatter as a determination of cell granularity.

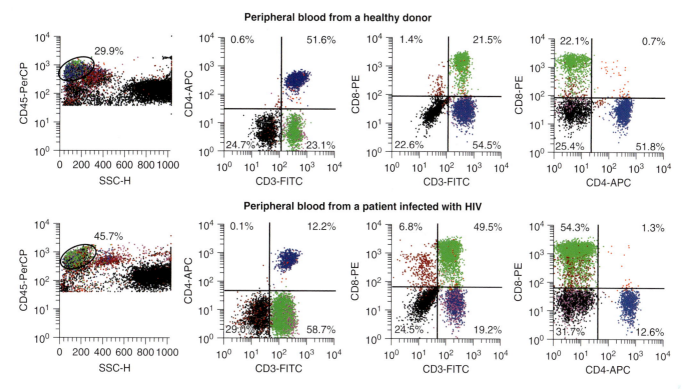

■ FIGURE 7.9   Flow data for a healthy donor (top panel) and a HIV positive patient. CD3 is a T-cell marker, CD4 is on helper T cells, and CD8 is on cytotoxic T cells. The number of CD3+ CD4+ dual positive cells is dramatically decreased in HIV patients. *Source:* Reprinted by permission of Paul Wallace and the Departmant of Flow Cytometry.

color emitted by the fluorochromes is measured by detectors and amplified to a digital signal using photomultiplier tubes (PMT). The data on the chosen cellular subset are presented as a 4-quadrant graph (Figure 7.9), which shows the percentage of the negative CD4 and CD8 cells, of dual positive CD4 and CD8 cells, and of those that are positive either for CD4 or CD8 but not both. Individuals without HIV (Figure 7.9 top) almost always have a CD4/CD8 ratio that is more than or equal to 1:1 whereas the ratio for HIV patients (Figure 7.9 bottom) is lower, and a drop in the ratio can indicate a worsening disease (9).

MULTIPLEXED FLUORESCENT MICROBEAD ASSAYS

Multiplexed fluorescent microbead assay is a new methodology that is an adaptation of flow cytometry which has recently been developed to respond to a need that is seen in some clinical diagnoses. In some cases, the clinical picture may indicate that several assays should be performed. For example, in autoimmune antibody screening, a positive antinuclear antibody result would indicate a need for follow-up (reflex) assays for antibody to the associated antigens SS-A, SS-B, Sm, RNP, Scl-70, Jo-1, dsDNA, centromere B, and histone (see Chapter 10 for a complete description of these antigens). In infectious disease testing, multiple analyses performed simultaneously are important in testing for stage and

prognosis of hepatitis B, as screening for levels of hepatitis B surface antigen, hepatitis B e antigen, and antibodies to them are all relevant indicators (see Chapter 17). In allergy testing multiple analyses for IgE to a panel of respiratory allergens simultaneously can speed discovery and avoidance of the allergen (10).

These simultaneous tests can be performed using a modification of the direct immunofluorescent flow cytometry assay described. In a multiple analyte assay, tiny color-coded beads that have a discreet fluorescent color code associated with a particular surface antigen have been prepared. The assay is performed in microtiter plates. The patient's serum is added to the beads in microtiter plates and is incubated, and then the beads are washed. Next a fluorescently labeled anti-human immunoglobulin is added, and the beads are washed. Analysis occurs in an instrument that uses flow cytometric methodology. The beads are passed through a laser to excite the fluorochromes, and then both the bead's internal color-coded fluorescence and the presence or absence of surface fluorochrome due to the indirect fluorescent immunoassay (patient antibody and fluorochrome-conjugated anti-human antibody binding) are measured. A pattern determining which of the colored beads (with a particular surface antigen) have fluorescently labeled anti-human immunoglobulin conjugate attached is found. Thus, the amount of a patient antibody reacting to up to 100 antigens at a time can be determined in 1 assay (10) (Figure 7.10 ■).

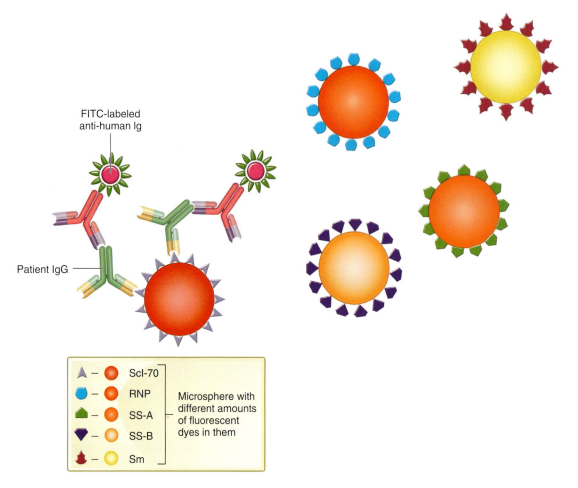

FITC-labeled
anti-human Ig

Patient IgG

▲	–	🔴	Scl-70
⬡	–	🔴	RNP
⬟	–	🔴	SS-A
▼	–	🟠	SS-B
✦	–	🟡	Sm

Microsphere with different amounts of fluorescent dyes in them

■ **FIGURE 7.10** Multiplexed fluorescent microbead assays. Multiplex analysis for the ENA antigens, Sm, RNP, SS-A, SS-B, and Scl-70. Each antigen is attached to a bead with a different fluorescence. The patient's antibody is shown binding to the bead that has Scl-70 on its surface. The use of a FITC labeled anti-human immunoglobulin makes the presence of this binding apparent.

► LABELS FOR HETEROGENEOUS ASSAYS

Heterogeneous assays can be performed utilizing any type of labels. The choice of radioactive, enzyme, fluorescent, chemiluminescent, or colloid particle labels is based on many factors, including the equipment available, cost, ease of use, sensitivity, and personal preference. The details of the different methods are discussed next.

RADIOIMMUNOASSAY

Radioimmunoassays were the first labeled immunoassays developed and they were thought to be ideal because linking small radioactive molecules to either antigen or antibody causes no steric effects. However, it was later determined that the addition of enzymatic labels usually had little or no steric effect on the antigen and antibody reaction either (2).

The difficulties with radioactive waste disposal and the general safety issues when working with radiochemicals led to decreased use of these labels. In addition, assay stability was limited by the radioactive half-life of the label used. The radiolabel most often utilized was ^{125}I with a half-life of 59.6 days. Occasionally, hospital clinical laboratories use assays that require radiolabels because these assays are highly sensitive. For example, a competitive radioimmunoassay is currently available for testosterone, and a capture radioimmunoassay is available for CA-125, an ovarian cancer tumor marker. Additionally, assays utilized in specialty laboratories may require the use of radiolabels.

ENZYME IMMUNOASSAYS: ENZYMES AND SUBSTRATES

Enzymes are the most often used labels for labeled immunoassays. The most frequently used are horseradish peroxidase and alkaline phosphatase (11, 12, 13). Less commonly used enzymes include glucose oxidase, β-galactosidase, and glucose-6-phosphate dehydrogenase. Horseradish peroxidase (HRP) is chosen often because it is inexpensive, stable, and produces a good yield of chromogenic products. It catalyses the oxidation of a variety of substrates by hydrogen peroxide. Substrates commonly used with this enzyme in enzyme immunoassays include diaminobenzidine (DAB), 3,3', 5,5'-tetramethylbenzidine (TMB), 4-choloro-1-napthol, o-phenylenediamine (OPD), and 2,2'-azino-bis-(3-ethylbenzothiazoline sulfonate) (ABTS). DAB (a suspected carcinogen) is used in immunohistochemistry and yields an insoluble brown product. TMB (noncarcinogenic), which yields a blue product that is soluble in water and when acidified yields a yellow product, can be used in assays measured spectrophotometrically and creates a sensitive assay. In addition, because the blue product can also be precipitated on nitrocellulose or nylon membranes, it is utilized in Western blots; 4-choloro-1-napthol is also used for Western blots and strip immunoblots. OPD, which yields an orange-brown soluble product that becomes orange when the reaction is stopped with H_2SO_4, is less sensitive than TMB. ABTS yields a water-soluble green product and is the least sensitive of these water-soluble substrates but also yields a lower background (11, 12, 13).

Optical immunoassays are special adaptations of the peroxidase enzyme immunoassay that are visualized based more on a property of the solid phase of the reaction than on the substrate. Optical immunoassays are based on the change in the color of light reflected from the solid-phase polymer membrane when an antigen and an antibody are bound in comparison to the color when they are not bound. A silicon wafer is covered with an optical coating, which in turn is covered with a polymer coating that will absorb the antigen if present. An antibody-peroxidase conjugate and TMB are added, and the wavelength of light that is reflected through the complex is different from that of the unbound surface.

Horseradish Peroxidase

It is important to remember that HRP is sensitive to a number of inhibitors, so all buffers and solutions must be free of azides, sulfides, and cyanides. Substrate solutions are light sensitive, and many must be made just prior to use.

Alkaline Phosphatase

Alkaline phosphatase is also a commonly used enzyme label, it is inexpensive and stable, and produces a good yield of chromogenic product. Substrates commonly used in enzyme immunoassays with this enzyme include p-nitrophenyl phosphate (PNPP), which yields a soluble yellow product measured spectrophotometrically and 4-methylumbelliferyl phosphate, which yields a fluorescent product, 4-methylumbelliferyl. Nitroblue tetrazolium/5-bromo-4-chloro-3-indoylphosphate (NBT/BCIP) is used with an alkaline phosphatase conjugate to yield an insoluble dark blue product for Western blots (15, 16). A chemiluminescent substrate, adamantyl dioxetane, is available for use with alkaline phosphatase-labeled assays. Proprietary chemiluminescent substrates are also used. It is

important to review product inserts to determine whether both serum and plasma are suitable for the assay because anticoagulants used in the collection of plasma may adversely affect results with some substrates. Phosphates should be avoided in buffers for the alkaline phosphatase substrate and conjugate because their use can lower the assay's sensitivity. Cysteine, cyanides, arsenates, and divalent cation chelators can also impact the sensitivity of the alkaline phosphatase-labeled assay (11, 12, 13, 14).

FLUORESCENT IMMUNOASSAYS

Fluorescent labels are most often used for direct fluorescent immunoassays on tissues and cells, for flow cytometry, indirect immunoassays, autoimmunity and infectious disease testing, and multiplexed fluorescent microbead analysis. The direct fluorescent immunoassays are used for tissue biopsies or to look for viral antigens after patient samples have been added to tissue culture cells. The fluorochrome most often utilized is the apple green fluorescein isothiocyanate (FITC). Many different color fluorochromes are used for flow cytometry. Each different antibody is attached to a different colored fluorochrome so that the distinctive cell types can be identified through positivity for multiple color labels. Phycoerythrin (orange-yellow), PerCP (red), Texas Red (orange-red), and Alex-Fluor 488 (green) are a few of the many fluorochromes used in flow cytometry (9).

CHEMILUMINESCENT ASSAYS

Chemiluminescent assays are used for antibody or antigen detection. These assays use acridinium-labeled antibody or antigen conjugates (14). Various proprietary labels are used. These assays generally have lower background than colorimetric or fluorimetric assays and are sensitive with a large linear range of measurement. This assay is similar to the enzyme immunoassay with a chemiluminescent product, but the chemiluminescent product is directly linked to the antigen or antibody. Restrictions are that the conjugation step of the chemiluminescent compound to either antibody or antigen must not affect luminescence. Advantages are that fewer steps are involved and that endogeneous enzyme or enzyme inhibitors do not interfere with the analysis. The chemiluminescence is brought about by the addition of a trigger compound (14). Heparin can inhibit some of the chemiluminescent reactions, so it is important to observe the guidelines for the assay (15).

COLLOID IMMUNOCHROMATOGRAPHY

Colloid-labeled immunoassays are often used for immunochromatographic laboratory, point-of-care based, and home-based immunoassays. Their final reader is not a spectrophotometer, fluorimeter, or a gamma counter, but it is the human eye. However, in this assay, either the antibody or antigen is labeled with an easily visualized colloid or particle. Like all labeled immunoassays, colloid immunoassays have a sensitivity that is much improved from the early unlabeled assays that were visualized by eye. The immunochromatography method, which utilizes colloid labels, has already been described and pictured in Figure 7.3(b). The colloid labels utilized are simply described in the assay product inserts as either a red colloid or as immunocolloidal gold.

▶ TYPES OF HOMOGENEOUS ASSAYS

By definition, *homogeneous assays* do not require separation of bound analytes from free ones, so they are easier to perform than heterogeneous assays. The binding of an antibody to an antigen in homogeneous assays causes a change in the compound used for visualization that can be measured. These assays are used for small molecules such as drugs, including drugs of abuse and therapeutic drugs, to measure appropriate dose to reach therapeutic levels (14).

FLUORESCENCE POLARIZATION IMMUNOASSAY

In the **fluorescence polarization immunoassay,** a fluorescent label is placed on the small molecule that is the analyte. Small molecules rotate freely in solution, so when plane polarized light is used as an excitation wavelength for a fluorochrome attached to a small molecule, this free rotation results in the emission of the fluorescent light in a variety of directions so that the light is no longer in 1 plane. However, if a relatively large antibody molecule has bound this small molecule, the rotation is retarded, and when the fluorochrome is excited by plane-polarized light, the emission remains polarized. The polarized emission can be measured using an appropriately placed detector. This assay is a competitive immunoassay; the unlabeled drug in the patient's serum competes with the labeled drug supplied in the assay for binding to antibody. In this assay, the more drug in the patient's serum, the lower the amount of plane-polarized fluorescence. The amount of drug in the patient's serum is determined by comparing the polarization units of the patient's sample with a standard curve prepared with known amounts of drug (Figure 7.11 ■) (9, 14).

ENZYME IMMUNOASSAY

In a homogeneous enzyme immunoassay, an enzyme bound to the drug analyte can perform its enzymatic function when the drug is free in solution. However, when an antibody binds to the drug-enzyme complex, the enzyme is sterically inhibited from having its enzymatic effect. As a specific example, the assay for amphetamine and methamphetamine includes these drugs labeled with glucose-6-phosphate dehydrogenase and monoclonal antibodies

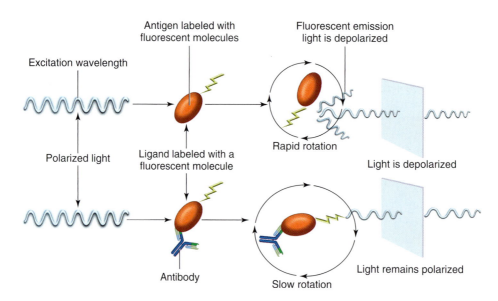

■ **FIGURE 7.11**   Flourescence polarization immunoassay. A florescently labeled analyte is excited with polarized light. When the analyte is bound to the antibody, the antibody rotates slowly, and the light is emitted in a polarized fashion. However, if the patient's serum contains the analyte, it competes for the antibody with the labeled analyte. Labeled analyte that is unbound moves freely in solution, so when the fluorochrome attached to it is excited, the emitted light is no longer polarized because of this free movement.

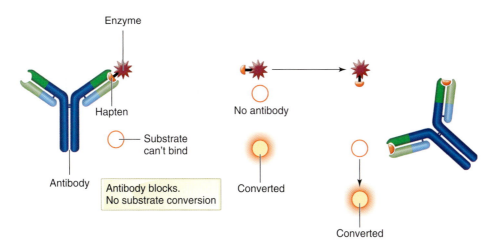

FIGURE 7.12 In a homogeneous enzyme immunoassay, antibody bound to the hapten conjugated to the enzyme prevents enzyme function by blocking the substrate interaction. When the patient serum contains the antigen, the enzyme-labeled antigen and the patient antigen complete the binding to the antibody and the enzyme function increases.

to both drugs. The presence of drug in the patient's urine decreases the amount of antibody available to bind to the enzyme-labeled drug and thus increases the amount of enzyme activity visualized. In this homogeneous assay, the amount of drug is directly related to the amount of enzymatic activity (Figure 7.12 ■) (13).

▶ INTERFERING SUBSTANCES

Some substances can interfere with individual proprietary tests. Certain assays are affected by using plasma from EDTA or heparin tubes, so serum must be used. Other interfering substances are patient specific and thus can specifically affect the test results of certain patients. This type of interference is more difficult to identify. The presence of rheumatoid factor (RF), heterophilic antibodies, and human anti-mouse antibody (HAMA) are examples of patient-specific characteristics that can affect the results of enzyme immunoassays.

RHEUMATOID FACTOR

Rheumatoid factor is antibody to the Fc region of the IgG immunoglobulin. It is usually, but not always, of the IgM class. In capture assays in which the antibody is the capture molecule, rheumatoid factor can bind to the Fc region of the capture immunoglobulin, and then other binding sites on the IgM rheumatoid factor will bind the Fc region of the detecting labeled antibody. Thus, unless controlled for, the rheumatoid factor could result in a false positive reaction for any capture assay. To explain the possible effect of rheumatoid factor on diagnoses, let's first look at an unaffected indirect enzyme immunoassay for IgM for toxoplasmosis—a disease where many people have had past infections but a current infection could have severe effects on the fetus

in a pregnant woman. The patient's serum is added to the microtiter well which has the toxoplasmosis antigen on its surface. The patient's IgG that developed during a past infection binds and the labeled anti-human IgM antibody does not bind the patient's IgG and the test result is negative for IgM to toxoplasmosis. In a similar patient with rheumatoid factor, after their IgG bound to the antigen, their rheumatoid factor would bind to their IgG. Next, when the anti-human IgM was added it would bind to their rheumatoid factor and the result would look positive for IgM to the toxoplasmosis antigen, when in fact, the patient had IgG due to a past infection, not IgM due to a current infection. To correct for such misdiagnoses, indirect assays for IgM can be corrected for the rheumatoid factor effect by removing the patient's IgG prior to the assay. Some capture assays may control for rheumatoid factor by using a serum diluent that contains excess IgG that does not react to the test antigen but would bind to the rheumatoid factor. In the selection of test kits for laboratory use, it is important to determine whether rheumatoid factor affects the assays and, if so, what should be included in the analysis to control for this interfering substance. In all cases, results from immunoassays should be interpreted by considering the patient's entire clinical picture (15, 16).

HUMAN HETEROPHILIC ANTIBODIES

Human heterophilic antibodies binding to animal immunoglobulin can be present in individuals who work with or are exposed to animals. These antibodies can cause false positive reactions in sandwich antigen capture immunoassays by forming an antibody-heterophile antibody-labeled antibody complex rather than the antibody-antigen-labeled antibody complex expected. This reactivity occurs because immunoassays commonly employ animal (goat, mouse, sheep) antibodies as reagents. The presence of heterophilic antibody is hard to predict, but it is important to note that because they are low-affinity antibodies, assay adaptations can be performed to minimize their effect. Heterophile antibodies show some Fc specificity because they have little or no effect if the capture and labeled antibodies used in the kit are $(Fab')_2$ rather than whole antibody molecules (15, 16). Again, in all cases, results from immunoassays should be interpreted with the patient's clinical data.

HUMAN ANTI-MOUSE ANTIBODY

Human anti-mouse antibody (HAMA) is a special type of heterophilic antibody whose presence is easier to predict. This antibody is produced by the immune response of a patient who has been treated with therapeutic or diagnostic mouse monoclonal antibody. HAMA is usually of a higher affinity than other heterophile antibodies. Addition of the mouse immunoglobulin, which does not react with the antigen in question, may inhibit this reaction, but it is important to use the entire clinical picture involved with any immunoassay results in interpreting the patient's clinical data (15, 16).

▶ SENSITIVITY COMPARISONS

In any immunoassay, the affinities of the antibodies utilized are major determinants in the assay's sensitivity. All labeled immunoassays have assay sensitivity at least 1000 times higher than the unlabeled assays. Homogeneous assays are inherently less sensitive than heterogeneous assays. The detection limit of indirect assays is higher than the direct assays because the anti-human immunoglobulin binds to more than 1 site on the human immunoglobulin, thus amplifying the reaction. The detection limit of capture assays is higher than those of the competitive assays. In general, radioimmunoassays have higher sensitivity than colorimetric enzyme immunoassays but have lower sensitivity than the enzyme immunoassays with a fluorescent or chemiluminescent product, which are the most sensitive labels.

⊘ CASE STUDY

A physician in your hospital is seeing a patient who has a respiratory infection. The cultures are negative, so the physician asks you to do a respiratory infection panel for IgM. You run several capture assays for patient IgM to different respiratory pathogens with a setup like that shown in Figure 7.3(b). The results are positive for every pathogen you tested!

1. What could have happened?
2. What could be done to correct the problem?

SUMMARY

Labeled immunoassays have increased the sensitivity of the detection of antibody and antigen when compared to unlabeled immunoassays. The original labeled assay was a radioimmunoassay closely followed and now largely supplanted by enzyme, fluorescent, colloid, and chemiluminescent immunoassays. These assays can be heterogeneous—requiring a separation step—or homogeneous—not requiring a separation step. The basic types of these assays are direct, indirect, sandwich, and competitive immunoassays. Adaptations of the basic solid-phase heterogeneous techniques include Western blotting, flow cytometry, and multiplexed fluorescent microbead analysis. A variety of different enzymes and substrate combinations can be measured either by spectrophotometry, fluorimetry, with a luminometer, or by eye. Many different fluorochromes are available for fluorescent immunoassays. Multiplexing using different color-coded fluorescent beads with different antigens on their surfaces may be the wave of the future, allowing multiple analyses to be performed at the same time on a small sample volume. Chemiluminescent reagents are generally the most sensitive assays and are increasing in use. Although these assays allow excellent sensitivity and specificity, some factors can affect their validity, so that each assay must be evaluated with regard to the rest of the clinical picture of the patient.

 Checkpoint! 7.5

What is the difference between a direct enzyme immunoassay and a direct radioimmunoassay?

 Checkpoint! 7.6

Comparing the labeled immunoassays to the unlabeled immunoassays discussed in Chapter 6, do you think that the labeled assays will show a prozone effect and a negative result when there is too much antibody like the unlabeled assays do?

REVIEW QUESTIONS

1. Enzyme immunoassay uses all of the following *except*
   a. Ab and Ag reaction
   b. washing steps
   c. separation of bound from free
   d. measurement of radioactivity

2. Which of the following characterizes homogeneous enzyme immunoassays?
   a. they use an enzyme that has been isolated from the same species that produced the Ab
   b. they require no separation step
   c. they require 2 antibody incubation steps
   d. they are used for large Ags only

3. Which of the following steps are performed in a Western blot?
   a. an Ouchterlony followed by electrophoresis
   b. a polyacrylamide gel electrophoresis followed by blotting followed by an enzyme immunoassay
   c. an enzyme immunoassay followed by a polyacrylamide gel electrophoresis
   d. agarose electrophoresis followed by blotting and then an enzyme immunoassay

4. In an indirect assay,
   a. antibody is always coated on the plate as a capture molecule
   b. only one antibody is used
   c. an anti-immunoglobulin that is labeled is used
   d. none of the above

5. In a sandwich assay,
   a. antibody is coated on the plate as a capture molecule
   b. only one antibody is used
   c. an anti-immunoglobulin that is labeled is always used
   d. none of the above

6. In a fluorescence polarization assay,
   a. Ag and Ab are labeled and produce a new color fluorescence together
   b. binding increases fluorescence
   c. binding increases the degree of the polarization of the emitted fluorescence
   d. none of the above

7. Which is the most sensitive?
   a. Ouchterlony
   b. a homogeneous EIA
   c. a heterogeneous chemiluminescence assay
   d. a heterogeneous colloid immunoassay

8. Flow cytometry measures the size of the cell by
   a. CD4 rhodamine fluorescence
   b. CD3 FITC fluorescence
   c. side scatter
   d. forward scatter

9. An assay to determine whether a patient has HCG incubates the patient sample with an antibody-coated plate and then adds a detecting antibody is best described as a(n)
   a. indirect EIA
   b. direct EIA
   c. sandwich EIA
   d. prozone EIA

10. In an indirect EIA, would the amount of color at the end be higher or lower if you forgot the washing step between (1) the conjugate and the addition of substrate or (2) the primary antibody and the conjugate but remembered it between the conjugate and the substrate?
    a. (1) higher, (2) lower
    b. (1) lower, (2) higher
    c. (1) lower, (2) lower
    d. (1) higher, (2) higher

REFERENCES

1. Yalow R. Radioimmunoassay: A probe for fine structure of biologic systems. Nobel lecture presented at: Stockholm Concert Hall, Stockholm, Sweden; December 8, 1977. http://gos.sbc.edu/w/yalow/yalow.html#fig5. Accessed December 18, 2008.
2. Engvall E, Perlman P. Enzyme-linked immunosorbent assay, Elisa 3. Quantitation of specific antibodies by enzyme-labeled anti-immunoglobulin in antigen-coated tubes. *J. Immunol.* 1972;109(129).
3. Inverness Medical Professional Diagnostics. Clearview HCG Combo II. Product Insert. http://www.invernessmedicalpd.com/point_of_care/womens_health/acceava%c2%ae_hcg_urine_ii.aspx. Accessed April 7, 2011.
4. Focus Diagnostics. West Nile Virus IgM Capture DxSelect™. Product insert. http://www.focusdx.com/focus/packageInsert/EL0300M.pdf. Accessed April 7, 2011.
5. Siemens Medical Solutions Diagnostics. Homocysteine Immunolite 2500. Product manual. http://diagnostics.siemens.com/siemens/en_GLOBAL/gg_diag_FBAs/files/package_inserts/immulite_2500/Anemia_n/pil5kho-5_siemens.pdf. Accessed July 5, 2011.
6. Abbott AxSym System HAVAB. http://www.abbottdiagnostics.com/webapp/index.cfm?event=getPDF&controlNumber=696582. Accessed April 7, 2011.
7. Bio-Rad Human Immunodeficiency Virus Type I GS HIV-1 Western Blot. Package insert. http://www.qualtexlabs.org/assets/pdfs/assays/506100a%20GS%20HIV-1%20Western%20Blot-stamped.pdf. Accessed April 7, 2011.
8. US Food and Drug Administration Hepatitis C Virus Encoded Antigen (Recombinant/Synthetic)(RIBA). Product insert. http://www.fda.gov/cber/label/hcvchir021199LB.pdf. Accessed April 7, 2011.

9. BD Biosciences. Customer Training: Introduction to Flow Cytometry. http://bdbiosciences.com/immunocytometry_systems/support/training/online. Accessed April 7, 2011.

10. Luminex. About xMAP Technology. http://www.luminexcorp.com/technology/index.html. Accessed April 7, 2011.

11. Worthington Biochemical Corporation. Enzyme Manual. Peroxidase http://www.worthington-biochem.com/HPO/default.html. Accessed July 5, 2011.

12. Worthington Biochemical Corporation. Alkaline Phosphatase. Enzyme Manual. http://www.worthington-biochem.com/BAP/default.html. Accessed July 5, 2011.

13. Abbott AxSym System. Amphetamine/Methamphetamine. http://www.abbottdiagnostics.com/webapp/index.cfm?event=getPDF&controlNumber=344988R14. Accessed July 5, 2011.

14. Lumigen, Inc. Chemiluminescent Detection in Biomedical Assays. http://www.lumigen.com/documents/assays.shtml. Accessed April 7, 2011.

15. Chaitoff K, Armbruster D, Maine G, Kuhns, M. Abbott Learning Guide Immunoassay. http://www.abbottdiagnostics.com.au/viewFile.cfm?file=learning_immunoassay.pdf. Accessed April 28, 2012.

16. Bjerner J, Børmer OP, Nustad K. The war on heterophilic antibody interference. *Clinical Chemistry*. 2005;51:9–11

PEARSON
myhealthprofessionskit™

Visit www.myhealthprofessionskit.com to access the interactive Companion Website for this textbook. Simply select "Clinical Laboratory Science" from the choice of disciplines. Find this book and log in by using your user name and password to access additional learning tools.

8

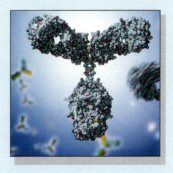

Serology Laboratory Math

■ OBJECTIVES—LEVEL I

After this chapter, the student should be able to:

1. Precisely and accurately calculate the amount of solute and diluent needed in the preparation of various simple and compound dilutions.
2. Calculate final dilution of a sample after being given the initial dilution and subsequent dilution(s) performed.
3. Calculate the amount of buffer that must be added to achieve a dilution ratio.
4. Calculate the amount of serum needed to make a defined volume of a defined dilution.
5. Calculate sensitivity.
6. Calculate specificity.
7. Move easily from the use of 1 unit to another using the metric prefixes kilo-, deca-, deci-, centi-, milli-, micro-, nano-, pico-, femto-, atto-, zepto-.

■ OBJECTIVES—LEVEL II

After this chapter, the student should be able to:

1. Calculate efficiency.
2. Calculate positive predictive value.
3. Calculate negative predictive value.

KEY TERMS

2-fold serial dilution
compound dilution
diluent
dilution
efficiency
negative predictive value
positive predictive value

sensitivity
serial dilution
serology
solute
specificity
titer

► LABORATORY DILUTIONS

Determining levels of *antibody* in a patient's blood is important in the diagnosis of infectious disease, allergy, and autoimmune disease. Information concerning a patient's antibody concentrations are also important in predicting whether that patient will be protected by the levels of antibody she or he currently has or if vaccination or revaccination is indicated. Similarly, determining levels of an *antigen* in the patient's serum, urine, or other body fluids is important in some infectious disease testing, cancer diagnosis, pregnancy testing, drug testing, and therapeutic drug concentration testing. **Serology** is the study of serum components of the blood. This science deals mostly with the *in vitro* measurement of antibody and antigen reactions in serum or plasma. In the clinical immunology laboratory, the relative level or titer of antibody or antigen is often determined by measuring the outcome of *in vitro* tests using serial dilutions of the serum or other body fluid. **Titer** is defined as the reciprocal of the last dilution that yields a positive test in the assay and is used to compare the relative amounts of antibody or antigen in different samples. A **serial dilution** is a sequence of dilutions made to the serum using the same ratio or fold-dilution.

Serial dilutions are referred to by the -fold difference between the tubes. For instance in a **2-fold serial dilution,** the first dilution tube might be a 1-part to 2-part final dilution (1:2), the next tube would be a 1:4 (1:4) dilution, the next a 1:8 dilution (1:8), and the next a 1:16 dilution from the original serum tube. Each of these tubes is related to the previous tube by the 1/2 dilution factor, which can be symbolized by the following equations:

1/2 (1/2) = 1/4, 1/4 (1/2) = 1/8, 1/8 (1/2) = 1/16

Each **dilution** contains the solute and the diluent. The **solute** is the material being diluted, and the **diluent** is the solution (usually buffer) in which it is being diluted. A dilution is expressed as a fraction of the beginning volume of the material being diluted over the final volume, so a 1/2 dilution means 1 part solute plus 1 part diluent equals 2 parts total. The amount of solute involved is the number at the top of this fraction (the numerator), and the *total volume* is placed on the bottom (the denominator). Please note that the total volume is placed in the denominator of this fraction and that the total volume equals the amount of diluent plus the amount of solute.

Some examples of simple dilutions follow.

Example 1: 2 ml of a 1:10 dilution is needed to run an assay. To make this, we set up the ratio we want, 1/10, and set it equal to the ratio we are making, using x to represent our unknown quantity of our solute and the known final volume of 2 ml. We then cross-multiply to determine the unknown part of the equation.

$$\frac{1}{10} = \frac{x}{2\ ml},\ so\ 10x = 2\ ml,\ x = 0.2\ ml$$

Thus, 0.2 ml of serum is needed, and 2 ml minus 0.2 ml = 1.8 ml of diluent is needed.

Remember that the equation is the beginning amount over final total amount!

Example 2: How can you make a 1:5 dilution if you have 0.1 ml of serum?

$$\frac{1}{5} = \frac{0.1\ ml}{x},\ so\ 0.1\ ml \times 5 = 1(x),\ x = 0.5\ ml$$

Thus, 0.5 ml final volume minus 0.1 ml serum (initial volume) equals 0.4 ml diluent.

 Checkpoint! 8.1

A 1:10 dilution is required. If we need 4 ml, how much of the serum do we need? How much of the diluent do we need?

A **compound dilution** is defined as a process in which several dilutions are made to arrive at the desired final dilution; it is used to make very dilute solutions. A compound dilution allows for an accurate final dilution to be made without using an amount of the solute that is too small to measure accurately or an amount of diluent that is too large to be practical.

Example 3: We need 1 ml of a 1/10 000 dilution. Using only a simple dilution, we would have to make the following:

1/10 000 = x/1, so x = 0.0001 ml

or 0.1 microliter in 1 ml (0.1 microliter is impractical to measure accurately in the serology lab).

Instead, we could make excess by making 1 ml into 9999 ml to make 10 liters, but we need only 1 ml, so this would be wasteful. Using a compound dilution, we could make a 1/200 dilution followed by another 1/50 dilution and the final dilution would be

$$\frac{1}{200} \times \frac{1}{50} = \frac{1}{10\ 000}$$

The 1/200 dilution could be made by using 0.1 ml in 20 ml final.

Example 4: Instead of putting 1 ml plus 499 ml to make a 1:500 dilution, we make a 1:50 and than a 1:10 from it. To determine the dilution factor, we multiply each dilution.

$$\frac{1}{50} \times \frac{1}{10} = \frac{1}{500}$$

In many immunologic assays, a series of dilutions is used to determine the titer of antibody in the serum. For a

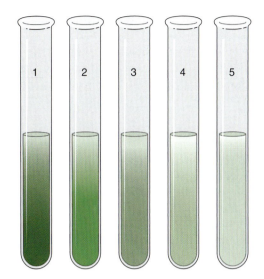

■ **FIGURE 8.1** A 2-fold serial dilution showing the result of moving 0.2 ml of green food coloring successively into tubes containing 0.2 ml of buffer. .

serial dilution, a series of tubes is set up to yield the same dilution from one tube to the next with the same amount of diluent in each. Common serial dilutions utilized in the serology/immunology lab are 2-fold, 3-fold, 5-fold, and 10-fold.

Example 5: In the serial dilution example (see Figure 8.1 ■), each tube contains 0.2 ml of buffer to start, and we add 0.2 ml of green food coloring to tube 1. Why does this result in a 1:2 dilution?

The dilution equals the starting volume over final volume, so this is:

$$\frac{0.2}{0.2 + 0.2} = \frac{0.2}{0.4}$$

So, 0.2 ml dye (0.2 ml dye plus 0.2 ml buffer) or 0.2/0.4.

We simplify this result to have a whole number (usually 1 as the numerator) so that both the numerator and the denominator are multiplied by 5 to set the numerator to 1.

$$\frac{0.2}{0.4} \times \frac{5}{5} = \frac{1}{2}$$

If we move 0.2 ml from tube 1 to tube 2, 0.2 ml from tube 3 to tube 4, 0.2 ml from tube 4 to tube 5, what is the dilution in each tube?

The dilution in each tube is the previous dilution multiplied by the dilution that was just performed on it. So, a 1:2 dilution of a 1:2 dilution is a 1:4 dilution. These are read in this way: a 1-to-2 dilution of a 1-to-2 dilution is a

1-to-4 dilution. Next, 1:2 of a 1:4 equals a 1:8 dilution, and a 1:2 dilution of a 1:8 dilution is a 1:16 dilution; finally, a 1:2 dilution of a 1:16 dilution is a 1:32 dilution.

Sometimes in the laboratory you may need to be flexible in how you approach making a dilution depending on sample or test requirements, but the basic ratios and equations remain the same.

Example 6: Imagine a common scenario: A patient's blood has been drawn and then she or he has gone home. Several people realize that they need some of the serum so only 0.2 ml is now available to you. You know that you need to make 1 ml of a 1:10 dilution, but you wonder whether you have enough.

You need a 1:10 dilution, so you need to set up the ratio as follows:

$$\frac{1}{10} = \frac{0.2}{x} \text{ (ie, the amount you have)}$$

Cross multiply, and 10(0.2) = x, 2 = x, which means you have enough to make 2 ml at the required dilution, so you have enough!

✓ **Checkpoint! 8.2**

You have just set up an assay and have room for 1 more sample. A sample comes in labeled stat *(a common abbreviation for the Latin term* statim, *which means immediately). You read the kit instructions, which says that the samples must be added within 30 minutes. It has been 20 minutes, so time should be no problem. You have 10 minutes to make this last dilution. You need 1 ml of a 1:10 000 dilution. However, you notice that you only have 2 ml of buffer left. How do you make this dilution? The smallest pipet in the lab is 10 microliters.*

We express the result obtained at the end of the assay using serial dilutions as the titer. The titer is the reciprocal of the last dilution that is positive in the assay. Consider a patient after treatment whose serum was assayed for rheumatoid factor. In this assay, the last dilution that was positive for rheumatoid factor was a 1/80 dilution; therefore, the patient's titer for rheumatoid factor was 80. The serum of this patient drawn prior to treatment showed the last positive result in the tube diluted to 1/2560 for a titer of 2560. In comparing the patient's titers, the post-treatment titer of 80 shows much less rheumatoid factor than the pretreatment titer of 2560. The use of the reciprocals of the last positive dilution provides a comparison in which the larger number indicates more of the measured antibody or antigen.

Sometimes an assay is used with a standard reference curve, and to find a value within the working linear range of the assay standard curve, the patient's sample is diluted. In this case, the value obtained for the sample from the standard reference curve must be corrected for the dilution made to the sample. To make this correction, the value obtained must be multiplied by the reciprocal of the dilution made. So, if a value of 2 microgram/ml of IgE was obtained for a sample that was diluted 1:100, then the factor by which to multiply the result is 100, and the reported result for IgE, would be 200 micrograms/ml (1).

► SENSITIVITY AND SPECIFICITY DETERMINATIONS

Assays currently available in the clinical immunology laboratory are very accurate clinically. Thus, when the result shows that a patient has high enough levels of the antigen or antibody in question to be considered positive, the result usually correlates with the clinical determination that the patient does have the disease. When the results are below a certain cutoff, the patient usually does not have the disease.

However, no assays are perfect, so there are measures that determine how often an assay is correct. An assay's **specificity** is the percentage of times in which there is a true negative test result divided by the number of total true negatives when the total negatives equal tested true negatives plus false positives. This gives us a measurement of the assay's accuracy in terms of how often a true negative sample will yield a negative test result. The higher the percentage of specificity, the less likely we are to tell a patient who does not have the disease in question that he or she does have it. The higher the specificity the fewer the number of false positives.

Example 7: In an oral test for HIV, the true negative results were 999 cases of a total of 1000 negative patients who were analyzed.

$$\text{Specificity} =$$

$$\frac{\text{True negatives (TN)}}{\text{True negatives} + \text{False positives (FP)}} \times 100\%$$

Another way to think of this is

$$\text{Specificity} = \frac{\text{Tested true negatives}}{\text{Total true negatives}}$$

$$= \frac{\text{TN}}{\text{TN} + \text{FP}}$$

Where tested true negatives are those samples that are negative for the disorder and that test negative divided by the number of samples from patients that were truly negative for the disorder.

The specificity of this oral test is 999/1000, or 99.9%; that is, 999 patients of every 1000 who are negative will test negative. One patient of every 1000 who appears positive in this assay would be a false positive (2). In addition,

$$\text{Specificity} = 100\% - \% \text{ false positives.}$$

Sensitivity of an assay gives us a measure of how often the assay will diagnose the disease or condition in question in a group of patients who have the disease or condition. This is the number of tested true positive results divided by the number of positive individuals analyzed. The number of positive individuals analyzed equals the number of tested true positive plus the number of false negatives. So in a new assay for pregnancy, 2 days after conception, of 100 pregnant patients tested, 85 test positive; in the same assay, 4 days after conception, 100 of every 100 pregnant women test positive. For this pregnancy test, the sensitivity is 85% at 2 days after conception and 100% at 4 days afterward. This helps us understand how often we can miss a diagnosis because the patient has levels of the antibody or antigen lower than the cutoff in the assay.

$$\text{Sensitivity} =$$

$$\frac{\text{True positives}}{\text{True positives} + \text{False negatives}} \times 100\%$$

$$= \frac{\text{TP}}{\text{TP} + \text{FN}}$$

Thus, sensitivity is the number of positive samples that test positive (true positives) divided by the number of true positives plus the false negatives.

In addition,

$$\text{Sensitivity} = 100\% - \% \text{ false negatives}$$

► EFFICIENCY

The **efficiency** of a test (that is, the total number of times the test obtained the correct results) can also be calculated:

$$\text{Efficiency} = \frac{\text{The true positives} + \text{The true negatives}}{\text{Total analyzed}}$$

The total analyzed is the true negatives plus the true positives plus the false negatives plus the false positives. See the equation below:

$$\text{Efficiency} = \frac{\text{The true positives} + \text{The true negatives}}{\text{The true negatives} + \text{The true positives} + \text{The false negatives} + \text{The false positives}} = \frac{\text{TP} + \text{TN}}{\text{TP} + \text{TN} + \text{FN} + \text{FP}}$$

Example 8: A new assay developed for cervical human papilloma virus testing for cervical cancer risk may replace the previous assay, the PAP smear, but has been found to have a higher sensitivity and a lower specificity. The overall efficiency was then compared.

For the new assay:

- The number of true positives was 90, and the number of false negatives was 10.
- The number of true negatives was 850, and the number of false positives was 50.

$$\text{Efficiency new test} = \frac{90 + 850}{90 + 850 + 10 + 50} = \frac{940}{1000},$$

or 94%

For the old assay:

- The number of true positives was 75 and of the false negatives was 25.
- The number of true negatives was 860 and of false positives was 40.

$$\text{Efficiency new test} = \frac{75 + 860}{75 + 860 + 25 + 40} = \frac{935}{1000},$$

or 93.5%

So the new test is slightly better than the old one in terms of overall efficiency.

Remember, however, that more than just efficiency goes into the choice of an assay. What creates a more serious clinical problem in this case: a false negative or a false positive? A false negative could result in increased time for the dysplasia to progress whereas a false positive would lead to additional testing or unnecessary patient procedures such as biopsy (2).

▶ POSITIVE AND NEGATIVE PREDICTIVE VALUES

The usefulness of a test depends on the test parameters including sensitivity and specificity as well as the characteristics of a population, such as how often the target population tested has the disease or condition in question.

Example 9: The same HIV test with a 99.9% specificity described here was used for a group of individuals donating blood in the United States where the incidence of HIV is 0.001, or 1 in every 1000 individuals, and for a group of individuals from Lesotho, where the incidence of HIV is 0.232. From the 99.9% specificity of the assay already discussed, when testing every 1000 individuals, 1 false positive result was obtained. In testing 1000 individuals in the US group, 1 true positive was found whereas when testing 1000 individuals in Lesotho, 232 true positive results were obtained. The **positive predictive value** is the percentage of time there is a true positive result of the obtained positive results for a certain population.

Positive predictive value

$$= \frac{\text{True positive results}}{\text{True positive} + \text{False positive}} \times 100\%$$

$$= \frac{\text{TP}}{\text{TP} + \text{FP}}$$

The positive predictive value of the assay in the United States is

$$\frac{1}{2} \times 100\% = 50\%$$

with 1 true positive, 1 false positive, and a positive predictive value of 50%.

The positive predictive value of the assay in Lesotho is

$$\frac{232}{233} = 99.57\%$$

with 232 true positive results and 1 false positive result.

It is also important to determine the negative predictive value of an assay.

Negative predictive value

$$= \frac{\text{True negative results}}{\text{True negative} + \text{False negative}} \times 100\%$$

$$= \frac{\text{TN}}{\text{TN} + \text{FN}}$$

This gives us the percentage of time that a negative value was truly negative for the disease in question.

Example 10: In a group of 1000 children who come in with sore throats and are tested using a rapid test for Strep throat, 600 test positive and 400 test negative. For the 400 that test negative, the gold standard culture test is performed; 40 were positive by culture, and the remaining 360 were negative. The negative predictive value would be

$$= \frac{360}{(360 + 40)} = \frac{\text{True negative}}{\text{True negative} + \text{False negative}}$$

That is, 90% of the time when the rapid test found someone to be negative, that person was negative.

The clinical value of an assay depends on its characteristics, sensitivity and specificity, and the characteristics of the population being tested. To obtain clinical results most appropriate for the diagnosis of an intended target population, the assay with the characteristics most important to the diagnostic picture should be chosen to yield the best positive predictive value. For example, in the HIV screening assay described, if in the United States the population chosen for screening had been a high-risk population with clinical symptoms, the number of true positive values per 1000 would be higher (2).

► SHORT REFRESHER ON UNITS

Making serial dilutions allows samples to be run at a range of concentrations; thus, it is important for clinical immunologists to review the terms used in the metric system so they can easily perform calculations using metric units with prefixes such as kilo-, deca-, deci-, centi-, milli-, micro-, nano-, pico-, femto-, atto-, and zepto (Table 8.1). If a sample has been diluted 1:10 000 and the diluted sample has 50 mcg of immunoglobulin, the original undiluted sample had a concentration equal to 50 micrograms times the dilution factor of (10 000) thus having a concentration equal to 500 000 micrograms. Because we would like to express this value in terms of milligrams, we would multiply it by the fact that there is 1 milligram per every 1000 micrograms.

500 000 micrograms (1 milligram/1000 micrograms)

= 500 milligrams

Clearly, in this equation, the units of microgram cancel and the final units become milligrams. In turn, if we would like to express this as grams, we would multiply as follows:

500 milligrams (1 gram/1000 milligrams) = 0.5 grams

If a patient has multiple myeloma and we are measuring the concentration of the immunoglobulin after therapy to see whether the original values of 5.4 g/dL have decreased, we would run the serum in the assay neat and dilute to a concentration in which the 5.4 g/dL was within the test range in case the therapy had not resulted in a change in values. The normal range for immunoglobulin in human serum is 600 to 1800 mg/dL, and all samples within the normal range are within testable range in the radial immunodiffusion assay. How much would we have to dilute a 5.4 g/dL sample to be sure it was within range?

First, let us convert g/dL to mg/dL.

5.4 g/dL (1000 mg/g) = 5400 mg/dL

The sample is 5400 mg/dL, and 1800 mg/dL is the maximum value for the assay, so we must dilute the sample at least as follows

(5400 mg/dL)/1800 mg/dL = 3

so we must dilute the sample *at least* 1/3 to bring it to this range.

✓ **Checkpoint! 8.3**

You have a sample that contains 0.1 mg, and your friend has a sample that contains 10 000 ng. Who has more?

 CASE STUDY

You are happily married and are trying to start a family. You decide to do an over-the-counter pregnancy test and go to the drugstore to pick one up. Two tests are available; one costs $28 and the other $7. You look at the side of the test boxes and Test A, the one that is $28, is 98% sensitive and 99.9% specific at 1 week after your last menstrual period. Test B, the one that is $7, is 90% sensitive and 99.9% specific at 1 week after your menstrual period and has the same sensitivity and specificity as Test A if you test after 2 weeks.

1. Explain what these values mean for each test.

SUMMARY

Determination of the value to assign the titer of a patient's antibody or the amount of antigen in a patient's serum depends on the ability to easily perform a variety of dilutions. A patient's titer is the reciprocal of the last positive dilution of the patient's serum. This value depends on the amount of antibody in the patient's serum and on the sensitivity of the assay.

The sensitivity, specificity, efficiency, and positive and negative predictive values are test characteristics that the laboratory scientist and the physician should understand to select the best test for the patient population and disease in question. In a screening test, false positive results lead to additional testing prior to diagnosis; thus, in a screening, false positive test results would be more acceptable than in the final diagnostic assay. These mathematical concepts are as key to proper laboratory analysis and diagnosis as are the basic vocabulary of scientific units.

✪ **TABLE 8.1**

Review of Metric Prefixes	
kilo-	1000 10^3
deca-	10
deci-	0.1 10^{-1}
centi-	.01 10^{-2}
milli-	0.001 10^{-3}
micro-	0.000001 10^{-6}
nano-	10^{-9}
pico-	10^{-12}
femto-	10^{-15}
atto-	10^{-18}
zepto-	10^{-21}

LABORATORY EXERCISE

INSTRUCTIONAL OBJECTIVES

At the conclusion of this lab, the student will be able to:

AFFECTIVE DOMAIN

1. Observe and adhere to safety and dress code requirements in the laboratory.
2. Realize the importance of arriving punctually for this and all future laboratory experiences.
3. Realize the importance of keeping and leaving their laboratory area neat and properly disinfected.
4. Discuss and comply with requirements for laboratory safety.

COGNITIVE DOMAIN

1. Define serology.
2. Define *titer*.
3. Discuss the basic principle of Beer's Law.
4. Compare and contrast 2 ways of calibrating pipettes.
5. Discuss the effect of wavelength on absorbance and how the appropriate wavelength of sample measurement is determined (ie, would a blue sample be measured at the same wavelength as a red sample?)

PSYCHOMOTOR DOMAIN

1. In performance of all laboratories in this course demonstrate proper universal safety precautions.
2. Properly choose the correct size test tube and the correct pipette for this and subsequent laboratory experiments.
3. Demonstrate the correct use of a pipet with a bulb and with a pipette aid.
4. Accurately prepare various simple dilutions.
5. Perform a 2-fold serial dilution and analyze the accuracy of a prepared dilution by spectrophotometry.
6. Apply Beer's law to data obtained from a spectrophotometer.
7. Apply the principle of Beer's law to different samples and spectrophotometers with different pathlengths.
8. Perform use of a simple spectrophotometer to obtain accurate absorbance data. This will include knowledge of the 0 and the 100% transmittance adjustment on the spectrophotometer for use.
9. Analyze the accuracy of a pipette using a commercial kit and a standard curve, which they prepare, utilizing Beer's Law.
10. Calculate final dilution of a sample, after being given the initial dilution and subsequent dilution(s) performed.
11. Calculate the amount of buffer that must be added to achieve a dilution ratio.
12. Calculate the amount of serum needed to make a defined volume of a defined dilution.

The accuracy of pipetting and preparation of a serial dilution can be measured spectrophotometrically by using Beer's law. *Beer's law* states that the amount of light (represented by A in the equation) that gets through a tube with colored fluid in it depends on (b) the width of the tube (how long a path the light must take), (c) how concentrated the color is, and a property that is specific to the compound that is making the color called its *extinction coefficient* (a) (Figure 8.2 ■). This yields the simple equation:

$$A = abc$$

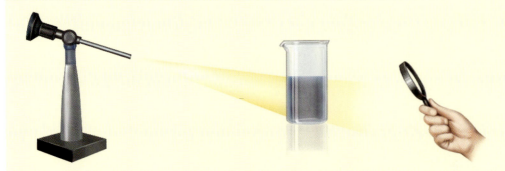

■ **FIGURE 8.2**   Beer's law. The amount of light A that gets through a sample depends on the concentration of the solution c, how long the path length is b (the width of the tube), and a property of the chemical, the extinction coefficient a.

The amount of light that gets through the tube can be measured in a spectrophotometer, and the plot of concentration on the x-axis (c in the equation) versus the Absorbance or optical density (A in the equation) on the y-axis will be a straight line.

EXERCISE

Prepare 2 sets of test tubes, one to practice pipetting and the second to measure and determine the accuracy of a serial dilution by plotting the results.

PRACTICING PIPETTING

Use of Fast Release Pipet Pumps (Figure 8.3 ■)

Choose the appropriate *pipet and pump* for the volume of fluid you want to deliver. Insert the pipet into the white area of the pump, holding the pipet toward the top. Be sure that the pipet fits securely.

To pipet, start with the shaft about $\frac{1}{2}$ inch up (Figure 8.4 ■), place the pipet in the liquid, and rotate the wheel downward to bring liquid up into the pipet. Stop rotating when the desired

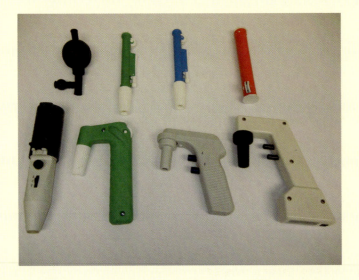

■ **FIGURE 8.3**   Different types of pipet aids.

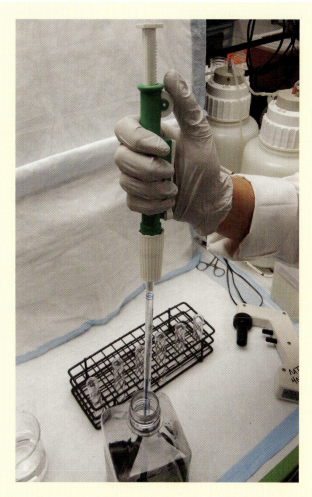

■ **FIGURE 8.4** With this type of fast release pipet pump, start with the top rolled up a little bit. This will allow the little extra push to get the remaining solution from a blow-out pipet.

volume is in the pipet. Note in Figure 8.5 ■ the way that most pipets are labeled with the 0 at the top and the maximum number at the bottom, bringing liquid in a 5 ml pipet to the 2 would give you 3 (5 − 2 = 3) ml. Some pipets are labeled both ways, so if you turn it, you will see that on the other side it is numbered with the 0 at the bottom; bringing liquid in this side to the 3 mark will give you 3 (3 − 0 = 3) ml. If the level of the fluid does not stay in the pipet, adjust the way the pipet is fitted into the pipet aid. If the pipet continues to leak, its opening may have gotten worn so the pipet aid may no longer be useful. Try a new pipet aid.

To release the liquid drop by drop, roll the wheel upward. To release the liquid all at once, squeeze the fast release bar on the side of the pipet aid.

Use of Drummond Pipet Aid

Choose the appropriate pipet for the volume you will be pipetting.

Insert the pipet into the black nosepiece.

Press the top black button to aspirate fluid to desired volume. *Be careful not to aspirate too fast because letting the fluid in too fast may force fluid up into the nosepiece. If this happens, the Pipet Aid will no longer work until the filter in the nosepiece is changed.*

Press the bottom black button to release fluid.

LABORATORY EXERCISE *(continued)*

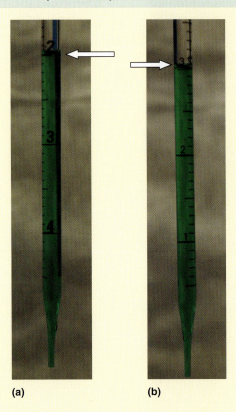

(a)   (b)

■ **FIGURE 8.5** (a) Most pipets are labeled with the 0 at the top and the maximum number at the bottom, so bringing a 5 ml pipet to the 2 would give you 3 (5 − 2 = 3) ml. (b) Some pipets are labeled both ways, so if you turn them, the second side is numbered with the 0 at the bottom. Bringing this side to the 3 will give you 3 (3 − 0 = 3) ml.

PIPETTING PRACTICE

A green food coloring stock solution is prepared by making a 1:200 dilution from a green standard food color bottle obtained in any grocery store.

1. Prepare the following 4 simple dilutions and 1 complex dilution of the green food coloring stock solution in 3 ml tubes. First determine how much of the diluent and how much of the green food dye you will add to each.
   a. 1:2 dilution in a final volume of 2 mL
   b. 1:4 dilution in a final volume of 2.4 mL
   c. 1:10 dilution in a final volume of 2 mL
   d. 1:20 dilution in a final volume of 2 mL
   e. 1:50 dilution in a final volume 2 mL using the 1:10 dilution from tube c, and note that this tube is a compound dilution

2. Perform dilutions. Place water in tubes first with 1 pipet and then place green dye in the tubes. Generally, the buffer is added before the solute. Usually less of the solute is added and the solute can be in such low volumes that the sample can dry and become damaged before the diluent is added. Use a different pipet for the water and the green food coloring.

   Check these dilutions before you proceed to the next part of the laboratory. Compare them with those in Figure 8.6 ■.

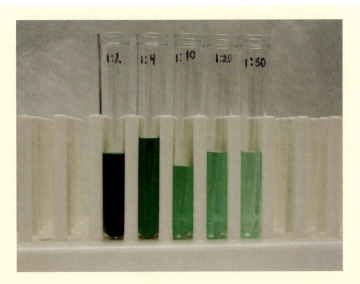

■ **FIGURE 8.6**   Practice dilution tubes should look like these. Note that the tubes get lighter in color from left to right as the dilution is increases. Also note that the 1:2, the 1:20, and the 1:50 tubes contain exactly the same volumes and that the second tube contains the highest volume.

SERIAL DILUTION

See Figure 8.7 ■ for photographs of the serial dilution.

   Create a 2-fold serial dilution of the green food coloring stock starting with a 1:2 dilution and continuing until you have a 1:64 dilution.

1. Label six 10 ml test tubes: 1:2, 1:4, 1:8, 1:16, 1:32, and 1:64.

2. Using 1 pipet, add 2 mL of diluent to each tube.

3. Using a new pipet, add 2 mL of the green food coloring stock to tube 1, and mix. Note that in a serial dilution, only the first tube receives any solution from the stock.

4. Using the same pipet, transfer 2 mL from tube 1 to tube 2 and mix.

5. Continue to transfer 2 mL with mixing from tube 2 to tube 3, from tube 3 to 4 and tube 4 to 5.

6. Check to see whether all your tubes contain equal volumes.

To apply Beer's law to determine how well you pipetted, measure the *Absorbance* of light at 630 nm for each tube, using the spectrophotometer as follows:

1. Turn on and allow the spectrophotometer to warm up.

2. Set the wavelength to 630 nm. This is the optimal wavelength for absorption by the green food coloring.

3. Zero on the cuvette containing diluent only.

4. Put the highest dilution, 1:64, into the cuvette and then put this first sample cuvette into the spectrophotometer. Always read the most dilute sample first. Read and record the absorbance, the optical density reading for the y-axis.

5. Place sample back in tube. It is a good policy to save your samples when you have finished an assay until you are sure that all the steps have worked properly.

6. Repeat for the other 4 samples, moving from highest to lowest dilution.

7. Plot your samples using 100% on the x-axis for the 1:2 dilution, 50% for the 1:4, 25% for the 1:8, 12.5% for the 1:16 , 6.25% for the 1:32, and 3.125% for the 1:64.

8. Check your line. Is 1 point above the line or below the line? If so, what must have happened?

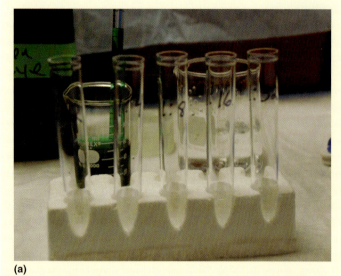
(a)

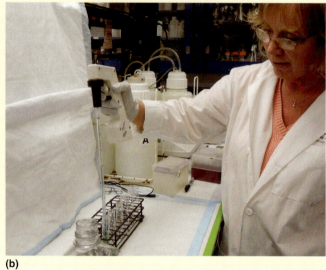
(b)

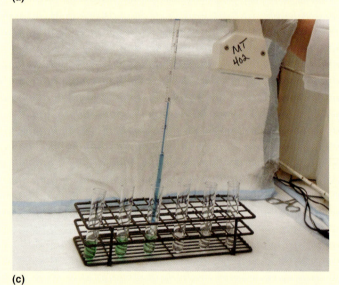
(c)

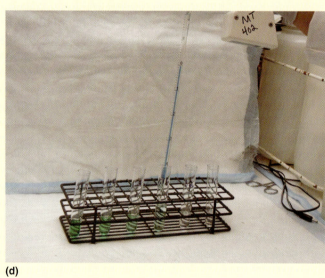
(d)

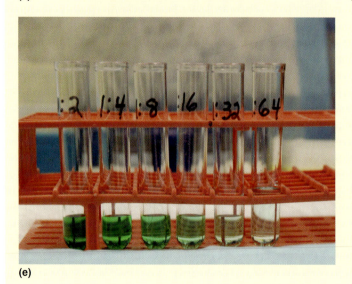
(e)

■ **FIGURE 8.7**   (a) The serial dilution: 2 ml of buffer is in each labeled tube; (b) 2 ml of the diluted green food coloring stock is added to the tube labeled 1:2 and mixed, and the 2 ml from this tube is added to the second tube to make the 1:4 dilution, and mixed. This process is repeated throughout all of the tubes in (c) and (d). (e) A finished serial dilution: A 2-fold serial dilution performed to make the 1:2, 1:4, 1:8, 1:16, 1:32, and 1:64 dilutions.

LABORATORY QUESTIONS

1. You added 0.5 ml serum to 2.5 ml phosphate-buffered saline (PBS). What dilution is this?

2. To the tube referred to in Question 1 you now add 3 ml. What dilution is it now?

3. You have 3 ml of urine. You want to make a 2-fold serial dilution to 128. Show how to make each tube.

4. You need to make a 2-fold serial dilution starting at 1:100 and ending at 1:3200. You need 2 ml in each tube when you are finished. You have 40 microliters of serum. Do you have enough?

5. You do a 1:5 of a 1:10 dilution. What is your final dilution?

6. How would you make a 1:50 starting with 2 ml of serum?

REVIEW QUESTIONS

1. I removed 3 ml of a 1:10 dilution and added 9 ml of diluent to it. What is the final dilution?
   a. 1:18
   b. 1:6
   c. 1:21
   d. 1:40

2. The first tube of a 3-fold serial dilution is 1:3. What is it in the 3rd tube?
   a. 1:6
   b. 1:9
   c. 1:27
   d. 1:54

3. You have 4 ml of a 1:10 dilution. How much buffer do you need to add to make it a 1:40 dilution?
   a. 12
   b. 16
   c. 20
   d. 4

4. In a tube test, we add 0.75 ml of saline to 0.25 ml of serum. Then from this, we remove 0.5 for the next tube and keep 0.5 in tube 1. Into tube 2, we now add 0.5 ml of buffer. What is the final dilution of the serum in tube 2?
   a. 1:4
   b. 1:8
   c. 1:7.5
   d. 1:16

5. Add 5 ml of diluent to 5 ml of a 1:10 dilution. What is your new dilution?
   a. 1:15
   b. 1:17
   c. 1:20
   d. 1:50

6. The first tube in a 2-fold serial dilution is 1:2. What is it in the fourth tube?
   a. 1:10
   b. 1:6
   c. 1:16
   d. 1:32

The following information applies to Questions 7 to 10. A newly developed assay that would save your laboratory money is being marketed, so you are looking at the product specifications. The following information is listed:

Number of Patients Tested	Number of True Positives	Number of True Negatives	Number of False Positives	Number of False Negatives
1000	500	400	60	40

7. What is the specificity of this assay?
   a. 87%
   b. 93%
   c. 90%
   d. 89%

8. What is the positive predictive value of this assay in the population tested?
   a. 87%
   b. 93%
   c. 90%
   d. 89%

REVIEW QUESTIONS (continued)

9. What is the sensitivity of the assay?
   a. 87%
   b. 93%
   c. 90%
   d. 89%

10. What is the efficiency of the assay?
    a. 87%
    b. 93%
    c. 90%
    d. 89%

11. A solution is 1 g/ml and was diluted 1/100. What is its concentration now?
    a. 0.1 g/ml
    b. 100 mg/ml
    c. 100 mcg/ml
    d. 10 mg/ml

REFERENCES

1. Solberg HE. Establishment and use of reference values. In: Tietz NW, ed. *Textbook of Clinical Chemistry.* Philadelphia, PA: WB Saunders; 1986:356–386.

2. Current information on rapid diagnostic tests. http://www.rapid-diagnostics.org/accuracy.htm. Accessed May 2, 2010.

PEARSON
myhealthprofessionskit

Visit www.myhealthprofessionskit.com to access the interactive Companion Website for this textbook. Simply select "Clinical Laboratory Science" from the choice of disciplines. Find this book and log in by using your user name and password to access additional learning tools.

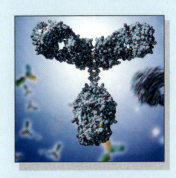

PART 3
SEROLOGY OF NONINFECTIOUS CLINICAL DISORDERS

9

Hypersensitivity Reactions

■ OBJECTIVES—LEVEL I

After this chapter, the student should be able to:

1. List and describe the 4 types of hypersensitivity reactions as described by Gell and Coombs.

2. Compare and contrast the role of antibody (and their different immunoglobulin classes), T cells, macrophages, neutrophils, and complement in each of the hypersensitivity reactions described. Be sure to know the numerical number associated with each hypersensitivity type.

3. Define the terms *hypersensitivity, allergy,* and *allergen.*

4. Describe the roles of IgE, cross-linking, and mast cells in type I hypersensitivity.

5. Describe the roles of antibody and complement in type II hypersensitivity.

6. Describe the roles of immune complexes, complement, and phagocytes in type III hypersensitivity.

7. Diagram the chain of immunological events that leads to type IV hypersensitivity.

8. Diagnose each form of hypersensitivity from clinical manifestations.

9. Give an example of a clinical condition that is characteristic of each form of hypersensitivity.

10. Describe clinical and laboratory methods used to detect and/or evaluate hypersensitivity.

11. Describe prophylactic and therapeutic approaches for each type of hypersensitivity.

12. Diagram the 3 phases of type I hypersensitivity: sensitization, activation, and effector.

13. Relate the range of clinical aspects of hypersensitivity from a mosquito bite to death due to anaphylaxis following a bee sting and describe the mediators produced.

14. Identify the organs affected in the various manifestations of hypersensitivity and the different times of effect.

15. Discuss different types of intervention in type I hypersensitivity including environmental, pharmacologic, and immunologic (hyposensitization and desensitization).

16. Discuss nonpathologic biologic function of IgE.

■ **OBJECTIVES—LEVEL II**

After this chapter, the student should be able to:

1. Compare and contrast the RIST and RAST tests and then compare each of them with the newer enzymatic allergy assays.

2. Correlate the size of the skin test reaction to the amount of IgE that the patient has produced.

3. Evaluate the symptoms and diagnoses for the 4 types of hypersensitivity, and the laboratory tests used for each.

4. Diagram the problems and the solution when an Rh negative mother is carrying an Rh positive child.

5. Categorize the mediators released from basophils and mast cells when an allergic reaction takes place.

6. Describe other things that can cause mast cell degranulation.

7. Compare and contrast other factors involved and their function:

   a. eosinophil chemotactic factor

   b. neutrophil chemotactic factor

   c. leukotrienes

   d. prostaglandins

   e. platelet activating factor

   f. serotonin

   g. early and late mediators

KEY TERMS

allergen
allergy
anaphylactic
Arthus reaction
contact dermatitis
Gell and Coombs classification
erythroblastosis fetalis

hypersensitivity
Mantoux test
radioallergosorbent test (RAST)
radioimmunosorbent
  test (RIST)
serum sickness
tolerization

▶ INTRODUCTION

In a system as complex as the immune system, many things can go wrong, and the effects caused by things going wrong depend on which component or components of the system fail to function properly. For example, a problem in the function of either a single aspect of the immune system or its total function can create partial or total immunodeficiency. Failures in the recognition of self and nonself, on the other hand, can lead to autoimmunity. However, even a properly functioning immune system acting against a foreign entity or antigen can create problems for the host. This is the case for **hypersensitivity** reactions including **allergy** when the effector mechanisms that the immune system selects to defend the host from a perceived threat are more damaging to the host than the perceived threat itself. In a way, hypersensitivity can be characterized as the "friendly fire" of the immune army. In this chapter, we describe the different mechanisms of the various forms of hypersensitivity, their consequences to the host, and examples of pathology associated with each form. We also discuss different laboratory and diagnostic techniques to evaluate hypersensitivity as well as therapeutic approaches.

▶ HYPERSENSITIVITY REACTIONS

Hypersensitivity reactions are immune responses that are overtly injurious to the host. They occur in subjects previously exposed to an antigen who have developed an immune response to it (sensitization). The clinical manifestations observed in hypersensitivity reactions depend on the host's response, not the nature of the antigen (1).

✪ TABLE 9.1

Gell and Coombs Classification of Hypersensitivity Reactions

Type	Features	Sample Condition
Type I	IgE mediated, mast cell degranulation	Asthma, hay fever
Type II	Antibody-mediated cell surface reactions that cause cytotoxicity, complement activation	Hemolytic anemia, HDFN
Type III	Immune complex mediated, complement activation	Arthus reaction
Type IV	Cell mediated, sensitized T cells, activated macrophages	Contact dermatitis

In 1963, Philip Gell and Robin Coombs classified the different hypersensitivity reactions into 4 major groups, depending on the mechanism responsible for that particular reaction. This is now known as the **Gell and Coombs classification** of hypersensitivity (2). See Table 9.1 ✪ for the different classifications and the basic mechanisms associated with them.

✓ Checkpoint! 9.1

For the hypersensitivities how can you remember which one is which? Remember the mnemonic ACID

Type I	***A****naphylaxis*
Type II	***C****ell or surface bound antibody*
Type III	***I****mmune complex mediated*
Type IV	***D****elayed type hypersensitivity*

Technically, the word *allergy* refers to 2 of the 4 forms of hypersensitivity: type 1 (also called *immediate hypersensitivity*) and type 4 (also called *delayed type hypersensitivity*). Allergic reactions are quite common in humans as a result of an immune response to an otherwise harmless antigen. The clinical manifestations of allergic reactions are designed to contain, fight, or expel a potential invading microorganism, especially parasites; however, these reactions often occur against innocuous antigens. Common allergens can include dust, pollen, and animal dander as well as food and various medications. Various substances that come in contact with the skin, such as certain metals (for example, components of a watch band or bracelet), plant compounds, latex components, or components of certain cosmetics, can also cause allergic reactions. The venom of certain stinging insects, such as bees and wasps, can also cause allergic reactions (1, 3). Classic type I allergic reactions include eczema, hay fever, asthma, hives, and food allergies. See Figure 9.1 ■ for an example of outcomes of hypersensitivity reactions based on the organ

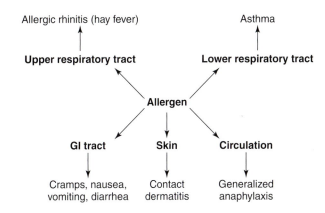

■ **FIGURE 9.1** Hypersensitivity reactions and different target organs.

system they affect. Most allergic reactions are not life threatening and can be treated with proper control and therapy; however, they can be troublesome and affect and influence everyday life and, in extreme cases, can be fatal as in the case of systemic anaphylaxis (4).

✓ Checkpoint! 9.2

Remember types I, II, and III involve antibody, while type IV involves a cell mediated response.

▶ TYPE I (IMMEDIATE) HYPERSENSITIVITY

Type I (**anaphylactic**) hypersensitivity is also know as *immediate hypersensitivity,* which refers to the timing between allergen exposure and the clinical manifestations of the reaction relative to other forms of hypersensitivity reactions that take longer between exposure and clinical manifestation. Type IV hypersensitivity, called *delayed hypersensitivity,* takes longer than type I. Refer to Figure 9.2 ■ for typical times for the different hypersensitivity reactions.

Type I hypersensitivity reactions are mediated by IgE; the clinical manifestations of such reactions result from the release of either preformed or newly synthesized mediators from mast cells and basophils (Figure 9.3 ■), and the effects can be either localized or generalized (ie, systemic). Contact uticaria is an example of localized type I hypersensitivity

Type I (Mediated by IgE)	2–30 min
Type II (Antibody-mediated cytotoxicity)	5–8 hr
Type III (Mediated by immune complexes)	2–8 hr
Type IV (cell-mediated)	24–72 hr

■ **FIGURE 9.2** Different time courses of hypersensitivity reactions.

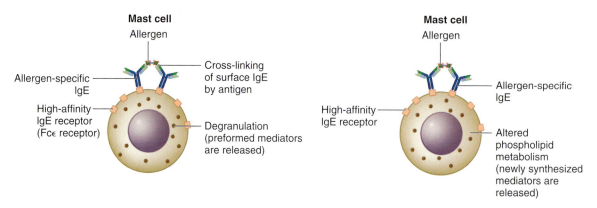

■ **FIGURE 9.3**   Release of preformed and newly synthesized (de novo) mediators from mast cells.

(Figure 9.4 ■). In type I hypersensitivity reactions, antigens stimulate an antibody-dependent immune response by causing the activation of the Th2 helper T-cell subsets discussed in Chapter 4. When activated, these cells produce certain cytokines that cause a class switch to the IgE isotype and that can activate allergy-related cells such as mast cells and basophils. Harmless antigens that can specifically stimulate an IgE response are called **allergens.** Although people are exposed to a wide variety of innocuous antigens on a daily basis, it is unclear why certain ones stimulate an immune response in which IgE predominates (5).

CLINICAL MANIFESTATIONS AND MOLECULAR MECHANISMS

The clinical manifestations of type I hypersensitivity are the result of the release of preformed and newly synthesized mediators from mast cells and basophils and are designed to drive out potential parasitic pathogens or prevent their

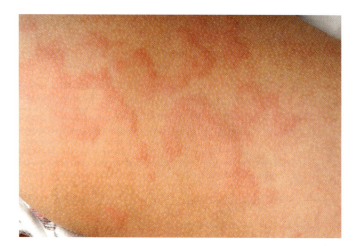

■ **FIGURE 9.4**   Uticaria, a skin rash caused by type I hypersensitivity. *Source:* Levent Konuk/Shutterstock.com.

entry. Examples include clearing the gastrointestinal tract via vomiting and diarrhea, contracting or blocking airways, and even increasing fluids and blood flow to allow better access to immune and inflammatory components to the site of an attack. However, in places where parasitic infections are rare, the result of an IgE-mediated response ranges from bothersome to life threatening.

When first experiencing an allergic reaction and considering what he or she has been exposed to, the patient frequently looks for something that he or she had never before eaten or been exposed to. However, allergic reactions cannot occur upon first exposure to the antigen. During this first exposure large amounts of IgE are produced; these antibodies then bind to mast cells and basophils that have large numbers of receptors for the Fc portion of IgE on their surfaces. This is called the *sensitization phase.* These high-affinity receptors for IgE, called *FcεRI*, can bind IgE without the immunoglobulin being bound to an antigen. Once bound, the IgE remains on the surface of the cell, which is activated only when a second exposure to the allergen occurs, causing it to attach to these cell-bound IgE molecules and cross-link different FcεRI receptors. Thus, the first exposure to an allergen "arms" a cell by coating it with IgE specific to that particular allergen, and a subsequent exposure activates the cell and leads to a cascade of biochemical and cellular events that ultimately lead to the allergic reaction. This is what differentiates IgE and its Fc receptors from other immunoglobulin isotypes; in general, immune cells that are activated by antibodies respond to antibody–antigen complexes that bind and cross-link their Fc receptors after the antibody has bound to an antigen. However, mast cells and basophils bind free-circulating IgE via the FcεRI. The binding of antigen and subsequent cross-linking of surface FcεRI by antigen binding to bound IgE is called the *activation phase* of the allergic reaction (6, 7, 8).

Different molecular mechanisms are activated at different times in the mast cell, so type I hypersensitivity reactions have an early and a late phase. These reactions that occur when the substances released by the mast cell have their biologic effect are called the *effector phase* of the allergic reaction.

Preformed Mediators of Mast Cells	
Mediator	**Action(s)**
Histamine ECF-A	Increased permeability of capillaries; contraction of smooth muscle
Serotonin	Increased permeability of capillaries; contraction of smooth muscle
HMW-NCF	Recruitment of neutrophils
Proteases (eg, tryptase)	Degradation of basal membranes; cleave complement proteins

(a)

Newly Synthesized Mediators of Mast Cells	
Mediator	**Action(s)**
Leukotrienes (C, D, and E)	Increased permeability of capillaries; contraction of smooth muscle
Platelet-activating factor (PAF)	Platelet aggregation; contraction of smooth muscle
Prostaglandin D2	Constriction of bronchial smooth muscle
Cytokines (IL-4, -5, -6)	Many different actions

(b)

■ **FIGURE 9.5** (a) Preformed mediators released by mast cells and their actions. (b) Newly synthesized mediators released by mast cells and their actions.

Once activated, mast cells and basophils immediately go through the process of degranulation in which contents of cellular granules are released into the surrounding environment. In this early phase, preformed mediators stored in the cell granules are released; these include histamines, prostaglandins, eosinophil chemotaxins, serotonin, and various proteases. A later phase involves the synthesis and secretion of various cytokines and some chemokines and leukotrienes (1, 9, 10). The majority of the more severe clinical manifestations of type I hypersensitivity are the result of the early phase response. However, late-phase responses play a major role in more chronic and often very serious manifestations of type I hypersensitivity, for example, chronic asthma, a condition that can be long lasting and cause problems sometimes even in the absence of the original allergen. See Figure 9.5 ■ for examples of preformed and newly synthesized mediators that play a role in type I hypersensitivity (11).

In general, the effects of both early and late responses tend to be localized around the area of allergen exposure because the action of the various mediators tends to be short lived. However, in some cases, the allergen can enter the systemic circulation and activate mast cells in the blood vessels at different and multiple anatomical sites. This can occur when certain allergenic medications are administered systemically to an allergic individual as in the case of the injection of venom by a stinging insect or the absorption of an allergen into the gut very rapidly. This can lead to systemic responses such as systemic anaphylaxis, and the effects that are usually localized become widespread, sometimes with catastrophic consequences. For example, when localized, increased blood vessel permeability can have limited effects but systemic permeability can result in a disastrous loss of blood pressure and cardiovascular collapse. Smooth muscle contraction can lead to extreme respiratory difficulties, and severe swelling of the upper airway can lead to asphyxia. Common allergens that can cause systemic anaphylaxis are venom from bees and wasps, food products containing peanuts or peanut-derived

components, certain other nuts, some shellfish, and various antibiotics such as penicillin (3). In the latter case, penicillin, although a very small molecule, can link to host cells or proteins, thus functioning as a hapten (see Chapter 3). As such, it can activate IgE-coated mast cells and basophils in allergic individuals and generate a systemic response. The severity of such reactions depends on a particular individual's levels of allergen-specific IgE, the amount of allergen, and the site or route through which the allergen has been introduced (1, 5).

Fortunately, the majority of type I hypersensitivity reactions are localized, and the clinical manifestations depend on the anatomical site of allergen exposure or entry. Because the great majority of allergens are inhaled, the respiratory system is the most common portal of entry for various allergens. Even within that system, the clinical manifestations of allergic reactions depend on the anatomical site of allergen exposure. For example, an allergen encounter in the upper respiratory tract can lead to allergic rhinitis, a condition also called *hay fever,* in which the allergen activates mast cells in the nasal passages. This results in the typical sneezing, watery nose, mucosal plugging, and irritation of the nasal airways and the eyes. An allergen that gets deeper and into the lower respiratory tract can lead to a condition called *allergic asthma* (12). The main symptoms of this condition, which can vary in severity from mild and episodic to life threatening, are airway constriction and obstruction, increased airway resistance, swelling of mucosa, mucus secretion, and mild to severe difficulty breathing. There has been some suggestion that smaller particles go more deeply into the lungs and are more likely to cause asthma than rhinitis. Refer to Figures 9.6 ■ and 9.7 ■ for examples of early and late responses in allergic asthma.

Certain foods can also cause both systemic and localized allergic reactions. In most cases, the reaction to foods is localized to the digestive tract where mast cells reacting to the particular allergen release mediators that cause biochemical events that result in diarrhea and vomiting. Food allergens can also cause systemic reactions, ranging from urticaria (hives)

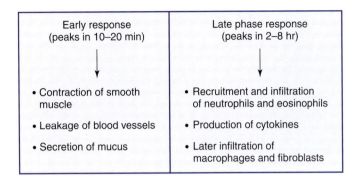

Early response (peaks in 10–20 min)	Late phase response (peaks in 2–8 hr)
• Contraction of smooth muscle • Leakage of blood vessels • Secretion of mucus	• Recruitment and infiltration of neutrophils and eosinophils • Production of cytokines • Later infiltration of macrophages and fibroblasts

■ **FIGURE 9.6**   Early and late responses in allergy.

to systemic anaphylaxis, but the precise mechanisms are still under investigation. Foods that can cause life-threatening reactions include peanuts and peanuts byproducts, certain nuts, and shellfish.

WHY ARE ONLY CERTAIN PEOPLE ALLERGIC?

The susceptibility of different individuals to allergic reactions has a genetic basis; allergic individuals tend to be more prone to the stimulation of Th2 cells than nonallergic individuals under the same immunological stimuli. In addition, allergic individuals have a higher level of circulating IgE than nonallergic individuals. In general, these features are associated with a particular individual's genetic composition (1, 13).

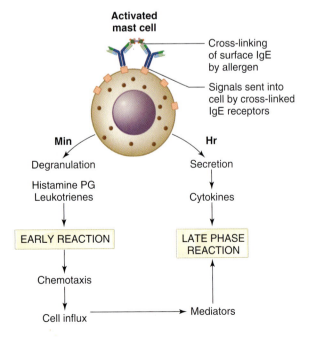

■ **FIGURE 9.7**   Cell activation in early and late responses.

Allergic people are also called *atopic individuals* and this is interesting because *atopic* is Greek for unusual, but atopy or allergy is not really that unusual. Atopic individuals seem to have particular combinations of MHC haplotypes that favor a strong Th2 response. Some have specific genetic variations that encode for cytokines that promote or favor an IgE-selected antibody response. For example, a genetic variation in the IL-4 gene has been reported for certain atopic individuals and is associated with higher levels of IL-4 in these individuals. Other cytokine genes include Il-3, IL-5, IL-9, IL-13, and granulocyte/monocyte colony-stimulating factor (GM-CSF), all of which can favor a Th2 response. Others have shown an association of certain variations in the gene encoding for the high-affinity FcεRI IgE receptor with strong allergic responses. Sometimes these genetic traits are associated with a higher response to a particular allergen; for example, the MHC class II allele DRB1-1501 has been associated with a strong allergic response to the pollen of certain plants. Thus, certain class II molecules are more likely to bind and present allergens, causing production of IgE. So, if other members of your family have allergies, you are more likely to have them, and if your mother is allergic to strawberries, you are more likely to be allergic to them. This association is such that when a child in a family has a severe peanut allergy, the recommendation is to keep all children in the family away from peanuts. In addition to the genetic link in antigen presentation, there also appears to be a difference in mucosal permeability in individuals with allergic respiratory reactions; for example, inhaled pollen, which becomes wet in the nose, releases some proteins into the mucus, which enter the mucosa and become antigens available for presentation.

In places where parasitic infections are common, allergic reactions are rare, perhaps because the FcεRI on the mast cells are already fully occupied with IgE antibody that reacts with the parasite.

WHY ARE SOME ANTIGENS ALLERGENIC?

It has been suggested that very small protein antigens that are carried on dry particles such as pollen grains come in contact with the mucosa and elute protein into it. Very low concentrations of these proteins (often in the form of enzymes) tend to stimulate an IgE response. Because an IgE response is usually generated against various parasites and because certain parasites use particular enzymes to break down and penetrate the host tissue, it has been proposed that the IgE response to these allergenic proteins may be caused by an enzyme recognition mechanism originally designed to fight parasites. For example, the allergen in the feces of the common dust mite (a very common allergen) is very similar in structure to the enzyme papain. Of course, not all allergens are enzymes, so other mechanisms must be involved.

In addition, because IgE responses are designed to fight parasitic infections, immune components committed to an

IgE response tend to be localized to sites that are likely entry points of parasites, such as the mucosa-associated lymphoid tissue (MALT), at epithelial surfaces in the airways, in the mucosa of the digestive system, and under the skin (14). The immune cells at these sites are programmed to initiate a Th2 response and IgE production by secreting cytokines that steer the immune response to an antibody-mediated IgE response. So, when an antigen comes in contact with the immune system at these sites, allergy results. Production of IL-4 and IL-13 can stimulate B cells to selectively produce large amounts of IgE against the allergen.

In addition, IL-4 and IL-5 can stimulate the activation of mast cells. Modulation of receptors for the Fc portion of IgE on mast cells and basophils can also contribute to the strength of an IgE-mediated response. Once an IgE response is generated, it stimulates mast cells and basophils, which can amplify this response themselves by secreting IgE-stimulating cytokines such as IL-4 (11).

TESTING FOR TYPE I HYPERSENSITIVITY

Testing for hypersensitivity involves 2 basic approaches: evaluating levels of components of the immune response to an allergen, for example, total IgE or allergen-specific IgE; or evaluating the actual physiological reaction of an individual to a particular allergen, such as in skin testing. Two early tests that exemplify the first approach are the **radioimmuno-sorbent test (RIST)** and the **radioallergosorbent test (RAST).** The RIST evaluates total serum levels of IgE regardless of its antigen specificity. In this test, antibodies specific for human IgE are linked to a solid matrix such as a test tube, and test serum from an individual is allowed to react with the matrix-bound anti-IgE to capture the IgE present in the individual's serum. After washing the unbound material, radiolabeled antibodies against human IgE are allowed to react with the remaining mixture; the unbound radioactive anti-IgE is then washed off, and the amount of bound radioactive label reflects the amount of IgE that originally bound to the matrix. From this, an extrapolation about the amount of IgE present in the individual's serum can be made. Although levels of total serum IgE vary among different individuals and can be affected by factors such as age, gender, genetics, and environmental factors such as smoking, levels of IgE beyond certain values (ie, age dependent but 100 international units in adults) can indicate the person's propensity for the development of IgE-mediated allergies. The RAST, on the other hand, evaluates levels of IgE specific for a particular allergen. In this test a solid matrix is coated with a specific test allergen; the subject's serum is then allowed to react with the allergen-coated matrix, and the unbound material is then washed off. Radiolabeled antibodies against human IgE are then added and after washing the unbound material again, the amount of radioactive anti-IgE antibodies bound to the matrix indicates the amount of IgE stuck to the allergen and, therefore, a reflection of the levels of IgE specific for that allergen in the

Radioimmunosorbent test (RIST)
(measures total serum IgE level)

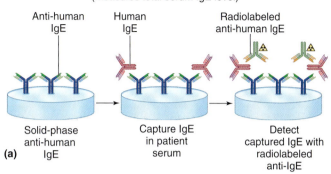

(a)

Radioallergosorbent test (RAST)
(measures allergen-specific IgE activity)

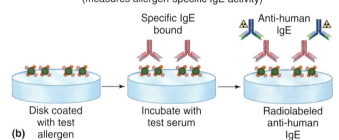

(b)

■ **FIGURE 9.8** (a) Radioimmunosorbent test (RIST); (b) radioallergosorbent test (RAST).

subject's serum (15). See Figure 9.8 ■ (a) and (b) for diagrams of RIST and RAST.

The radioactive methods to measure IgE have generally been replaced by enzymatic and colorimetric methods that avoid the use of radioactive reagents, but the basic assay principles remain the same. A common new method is a chemiluminescent enzyme immunoassay (Figure 9.9 ■). More recently, large microwell arrays have been developed to test thousands of different allergens at once. Again, a particular allergen in minute amounts is linked to a matrix, the patient's serum is allowed to react with the allergen-matrix complex, and then, after washing the unbound material, an antibody against human IgE with a fluorescence label is allowed to react with the bound IgE. As in the radioactive assay, after washing again, the amount of fluorescence remaining reflects the presence and amount of allergen-specific IgE.

SKIN TESTING

Although RIST, RAST, and similar tests evaluate levels of IgE (either total or allergen specific) in an individual, skin tests evaluate the person's *in vivo* response to a test allergen. The advantage of this approach is that it is a simple and easy method, is very sensitive, is very specific to a particular allergen, and examines the final reaction of an individual to that allergen *in vivo*. Currently, 2 skin tests are used to determine allergy to specific allergens. The most common test is

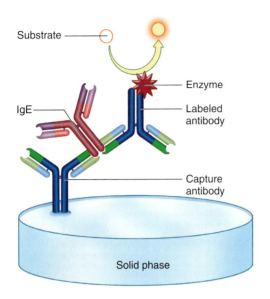

Substrate

Enzyme

IgE

Labeled antibody

Capture antibody

Solid phase

■ **FIGURE 9.9** Chemiluminescent test for IgE.

the results are no different than the saline negative control but there is still a suspicion that the individual tested may be allergic to a particular allergen, an intradermal test can be performed. This test uses a much lower does of the allergen than the prick test (anywhere from 100 to 1000 times less) but is injected between the different layers of the skin. In this case, however, great caution must be exercised not to stimulate an anaphylactic reaction; to avoid this, the intradermal test is usually administered on a limb such as an arm, which can be isolated with a tourniquet to avoid spreading the allergen systemically. Both types of skin testing employ a negative saline control and a positive histamine control. The purpose of the negative control is to show how the patient's skin reacts after injection of the saline buffer under the skin as a baseline, and the positive histamine control is performed to ensure that the patient's test results are not affected by any residual antihistamines that they may have taken. The results are reported by measuring the size of the wheal and flare (the raised red response to the allergen).

PROPHYLAXIS AND TREATMENT

The most basic and self-evident method of prevention of allergic reactions is allergen avoidance; in other words: if you are allergic to cats, do not get a cat. However, for most allergens, this is easier said than done because many allergens such as dust, pollen, mites, insects, and certain food products are practically ubiquitous. The avoidance method used depends on the nature of the allergen. For example, if dust is at issue, special furnace filters and ventilation ducts are available to control its amount. People allergic to stinging insects are advised to avoid potential encounters with such insects, for instance, by avoiding wooded areas or places where these insects are likely to nest. Various allergen-proof materials to cover mattresses and pillows to decrease dust mite exposure are on the market, and people allergic to certain metals usually avoid purchasing jewelry or other personal items that may contain those metals. Finally, people allergic to certain food or food products such as peanuts must adjust their diet with specially prepared and carefully screened food.

the "prick" test, where a small amount of sample allergen is injected into the skin and the area of the injection is then observed for a localized reaction. The reaction is then compared to a negative control injection, usually saline without the allergen (16, 17). This method can test for several different allergens on a large surface of skin, such as an arm or the back (Figure 9.10 ■). A positive reaction is usually indicated within 15 to 30 minutes by the appearance of an area of redness and inflammation at the site of the injection. If

Clinical approaches to hypersensitivity have concentrated mostly on treatment methods, which have, in turn, focused on decreasing symptoms rather than the finding of a specific "cure." In extreme cases such as systemic anaphylaxis, rapid administration of epinephrine can control the most severe effects of such reaction. Because the mechanisms of action of hypersensitivity are inflammatory in nature, many treatments for hypersensitivity are anti-inflammatory agents. For example, treatment of asthma, depending on its severity, can range from the use of antihistamines such as Benadryl and inhaled β2 agonists to oral corticosteroids (Figure 9.11 ■).

The method of hyposensitization has been reasonably successful in preventing certain reactions (eg, hypersensitivity to insect stings). In hyposensitization, extremely small amounts of allergen are administered to an allergic individual. This is

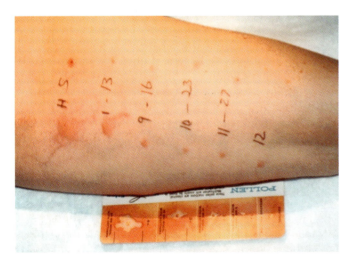

■ **FIGURE 9.10** Skin testing. Note the spot labeled H, which is the positive histamine control, and the spot labeled S, which is the negative saline control. A definite allergic reaction is seen at the spot labeled 1. Note also the ruler under the patient's arm that is used for reporting the amount of the response. Different size spots are reported as 1+ to 4+.

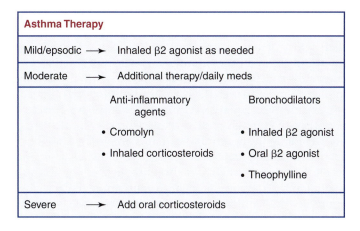

Asthma Therapy	
Mild/epsodic →	Inhaled β2 agonist as needed
Moderate →	Additional therapy/daily meds

Anti-inflammatory agents	Bronchodilators
• Cromolyn	• Inhaled β2 agonist
• Inhaled corticosteroids	• Oral β2 agonist
	• Theophylline

Severe →	Add oral corticosteroids

■ **FIGURE 9.11** Asthma treatments.

repeated over a long period of time during which the amount of allergen gradually increases (18). This, in turn, is thought to change the individual's response to that allergen from an IgE response to an antigen to an IgG response, thus avoiding an IgE-mediated anaphylactic reaction. The mechanisms involved are still being investigated, but the long-term administration of antigen is thought to generate IgG-blocking antibodies that cover the antigen and block it from binding with IgE. In addition, it has also been suggested that the repeated administration of antigen may stimulate regulatory T cells to downregulate the response to that antigen, a process known as **tolerization.** Another recent approach has been the use of antibodies against human IgE. Monoclonal anti-IgE is thought to bind to IgE, thus preventing it from attaching to mast cells. This, in turn, prevents the "arming" of the mast cells described earlier.

▶ TYPE II HYPERSENSITIVITY

Type II hypersensitivity is mainly mediated by the complement-activating antibodies IgG and IgM. The classic mechanisms involved in type II hypersensitivity are cellular destruction as the result of antibody- and complement-mediated lysis, antibody- and complement-mediated opsonization, and antibody-directed cellular cytotoxicity (ADCC). Cells and tissues from different organ systems can be targeted, but most commonly affected are blood cells, lungs, and kidneys. The basic commonality among type II hypersensitivity reactions is the deposition of IgG and IgM antibodies on cells and tissues as well as the subsequent activation of complement and recruitment of inflammatory cells, ultimately resulting in cell or tissue destruction. The antigens that are targeted can be either self-antigens that may have undergone some alteration and now look foreign or truly endogenous antigens. The major players in this type of hypersensitivity are antibody, complement, and phagocytes. Activation of complement, in turn, can cause cell lysis and further recruitment of additional phagocytes (eg, via its

C3b component). Antibody deposited on the surface of a tissue or cell can recruit phagocytic cells such as neutrophils and macrophages, which, in turn, can result in cell or tissue damage (1). Classical clinical conditions that are examples of type II hypersensitivity reactions are transfusion reactions, hemolytic anemias, and a condition called hemolytic disease of the fetus and newborn (HDFN, also known as **erythroblastosis fetalis**).

TRANSFUSION REACTIONS

Transfusion responses are hemolytic reactions that can occur when large amounts of blood are transfused between individuals with incompatible blood groups (1). Blood groups and transfusions are covered in more detail in Chapter 14; briefly, blood groups are defined by the nature and presence of certain antigens on the surface of red blood cells. A large number of different blood groups are divided into several different families, but the ones that have a major clinical relevance are the ABO system and the Rhesus, or Rh, groups. Although different blood group antigens have clinical relevance, the ABO system is the one with the most relevance when dealing with transfusions because people have naturally occurring antibodies to these antigens. These antibodies develop as a result of exposure to cross-reactive antigens from various natural sources, for example, certain bacteria. People do not generate antibodies to their own blood type because of the immunological tolerance mechanisms described in Chapter 4. However, people do generate antibodies to other blood groups. For example, an individual of blood type A generates antibodies to blood antigen B; likewise, an individual with blood type B generates antibodies to blood type A. This becomes an issue with a blood transfusion. If a significant amount of blood from a person is transfused into an ABO-incompatible individual (ie, an individual with a different blood group than the donor), a transfusion reaction can occur. In this case, circulating antibodies in the recipient can attack the donor's red blood cells. The severity of this reaction depends on several factors, including the titer of antibodies in the recipient serum, the amount of blood transfused (ie, the number of red blood cells that act as antigen), and whether the recipient has been transfused with the ABO-incompatible blood for the first time or for a subsequent time. ABO incompatibility transfusion reactions can occur very quickly from within a few minutes to hours. Responses are usually characterized by the reaction of IgM antibodies against the incompatible red blood cells and in the most severe cases can be fatal. The binding of IgM to the incompatible red blood cells can activate the complement cascade and cause almost immediate hemolysis of the red blood cells.

This hemolysis can start a cascade of events such as the activation of coagulation factor XII (Hageman factor), which, in turn, activates the kinin system, thus causing increased capillary permeability, dilation of arterioles, and hypotension. Hageman factor and free incompatible erythrocyte stroma activate the intrinsic clotting cascade, resulting in disseminated intravascular coagulation, systemic hypotension with renal vasoconstriction, and the formation of intravascular thrombi leading to renal failure. Because of this, determining ABO compatibility between donors and recipients is a must before blood transfusions and is done on a routine basis in most clinical settings. Although the ABO blood antigens are the major antigens of concern in blood transfusions, others, such as the Kell and Duffy antigens and the Rh antigens, can also be clinically significant when dealing with exposure to these other blood antigens for a second or subsequent time. The antibody response in this case is predominantly of the IgG class, the response occurs later (ie, weeks after exposure), and the clinical manifestations (mild anemia and fever) are not severe.

HEMOLYTIC ANEMIA

Deposition of antibodies on the surface of red blood cells is the main cause of hemolytic anemia caused by type II hypersensitivity. Antibodies of the IgG and IgM class can activate complement and, in turn, destroy the red blood cells to which they are attached (19, 20). Some different examples of anemia will be discussed in Chapter 11 covering autoimmunity. Certain medications, such as penicillin and some sulfonamides, can attach to the surface of red blood cells and induce antibody formation that ultimately results in cell destruction. Long-term exposure to certain chemicals such as formaldehyde can "alter" the structure of red blood cell components, making these components appear "foreign," resulting in an autoantibody response to the cells.

HEMOLYTIC DISEASE OF THE FETUS AND NEWBORN

Hemolytic disease of the fetus and newborn (HDFN) occurs when a pregnant woman makes antibodies against the red blood cells of her fetus as the result of the incompatibility of blood antigens between mother and fetus. These antibodies can cross the placenta and damage the fetal red blood cells (1, 21). The most common antigen involved in HDFN is the D antigen belonging to the Rh blood groups. Within this group, the D antigen is highly immunogenic and can stimulate a strong IgG response in an individual who does not have that antigen. *Rh positivity* refers to the presence of the RhD antigen on the surface of red blood cells. Because of the genetic makeup of a man and a woman, a situation may occur in which an RhD negative woman (ie, one who does not have the RhD antigen on the surface of her red blood cells) conceives and carries a fetus that is Rh positive (ie, has the RhD antigen on the surface of his or her red blood cells). Because of the physiological mechanism of childbirth, during such process, some of the fetal red blood cells leak back through the placenta and into the mother's circulation. If enough of these Rh positive cells (ie, that have the RhD antigen on their surface) enter the circulation of the mother who is not Rh positive, the mother's immune system sees them as foreign and treats them as any other antigen. In this case, the mother is "immunized" or sensitized against the RhD antigen, which generates memory B cells against the antigen. This does not affect the first Rh-positive child, who is born before the mother's immune system has a chance to mount a response against the RhD antigen. The problem surfaces, however, if a second or subsequent child is also RhD positive. In this case, the immunized mother produces antibodies of the IgG class against the RhD antigen. Maternal IgG crossing the placenta is a natural phenomenon designed to transfer some natural passive immunity to the fetus; however, in the case of the HDFN, if the second child is Rh positive, the antibodies crossing the placenta can attack the fetal red blood cells, causing hemolytic anemia in the fetus and newborn, often with devastating consequences, ranging from anemia and jaundice to fetal death (Figure 9.12 ■). Two types of tests for this disease are available, one for the woman's blood for antibody to the Rh antigen and the second for the baby's red blood cells to see whether they are coated with antibody. Testing the mother's serum is done using an *indirect antiglobulin test (IAT)*. The woman's serum is incubated with Rh-positive red blood cells and then anti-human immunoglobulin is added to facilitate hemagglutination, which is observed after centrifugation. Testing of the baby's red blood cells is performed using the direct antiglobulin test (DAT); the anti-human globulin is added directly to the cells and if the red blood cells are coated with anti-Rh antibodies, the red blood cells will agglutinate.

In recent decades, administration of anti-RhD antibodies to the mother has achieved prevention of HDFN (22). A pregnant woman who is Rh negative is given a preparation of anti-RhD immunoglobulin (commercially called *Rhogam*) at approximately 6 months of gestation and 24 to 72 hours after delivery. It is proposed that these antibodies react with the few red blood cells leaking from the baby and destroy them, thus preventing the mother from being immunized by them. Incompatibility between mother and fetus can also involve the ABO system; however, the response to such antigens generates a predominantly IgM response, an antibody isotype that cannot cross the placenta, so these antibodies are not involved in hemolytic disease of the newborn. In some cases, however, the IgG antibodies created by ABO incompatibility between mother and fetus can, indeed, cross the placenta. In this condition, known as *ABO hemolytic disease of the newborn (ABO HDN)*, these IgG antibodies can cause hemolysis of fetal red blood cells, resulting in anemia in the fetus. However, the actual development of symptomatic ABO HDN is very rare, and only a very small number of fetuses, most often from a mother of blood group O, develop it.

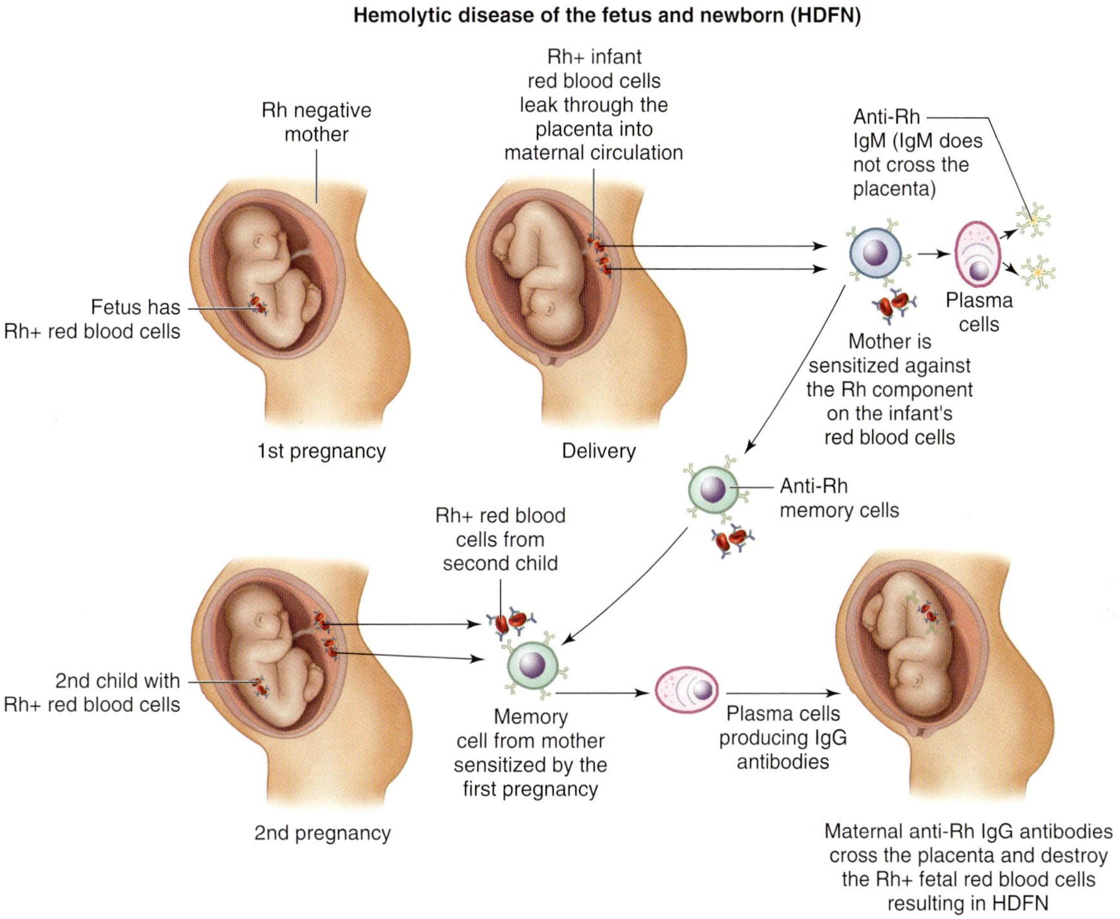

Hemolytic disease of the fetus and newborn (HDFN)

■ **FIGURE 9.12**   Erythroblastosis fetalis.

▶ TYPE III HYPERSENSITIVITY

The major players in type III hypersensitivity are immune complexes formed when soluble antigens and antibodies in the right concentrations form large structures or lattices that, if large enough, can precipitate out of solution (see Chapter 2 and immunopreciptation reaction). Unlike a type II response, the immune response in type III hypersensitivity is to an antigen in solution rather than on a particular cell or tissue. These immune complexes can get stuck at various anatomical filtering sites and initiate an inflammatory response there. The response and subsequent damage of the tissue on which these immune complexes are deposited result primarily in the activation of complement and the recruitment of a variety of immune and inflammatory cells. As with other forms of hypersensitivity, the antigens involved are usually innocuous and not deleterious to the host; the immune and inflammatory responses are designed to clear these immune complexes that cause the tissue damage seen in this form of

hypersensitivity. In general, phagocytic cells can usually clear these complexes without much damage to the host. However, if the precipitated complexes are in enough quantities and of the required size, they can be deposited on various filtering tissues where they can activate complement, recruit phagocytes such as neutrophils, and cause tissue damage (23). Typical target tissues are blood vessel walls, kidneys (glomerular basement membrane), and tissues in the joints (filtering area for joint fluid) and lungs.

Maurice Arthus first observed results of this mechanism in the early 1900s; he immunized laboratory animals so that they would develop high titers of antibodies against a particular antigen (24). After developing the antibody response, the animals were injected intradermally with the same antigen, and a localized reaction appeared within a few hours. This reaction was characterized by localized swelling, redness of the skin, localized increased blood flow, and in more severe cases, tissue necrosis and ulceration. Now known as the **Arthus reaction,** this result is caused by immune complexes generated by IgG that

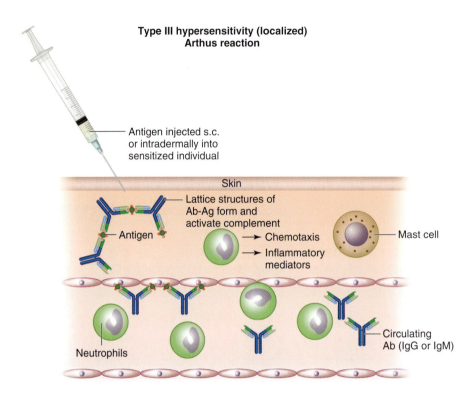

**Type III hypersensitivity (localized)
Arthus reaction**

Antigen injected s.c.
or intradermally into
sensitized individual

Skin

Lattice structures of
Ab-Ag form and
activate complement

Antigen

Chemotaxis

Inflammatory
mediators

Mast cell

Neutrophils

Circulating
Ab (IgG or IgM)

■ **FIGURE 9.13**   Immunologic and inflammatory mechanisms of the Arthus reaction.

has infiltrated the tissues combining with the antigen injected intradermally. These complexes, in turn, cause a multiplicity of inflammatory events composed mainly of the activation of complement as well as platelet aggregation and increased capillary permeability; increased permeability, in turn, allows a greater influx of inflammatory and phagocytic cells such as neutrophils, to the site, causing the tissue damage observed at the site of the reaction. See Figure 9.13 ■ for an illustration of the biological mechanisms of the Arthus reaction.

Whereas the Arthus reaction was performed to experimentally demonstrate the mechanisms involved in type III hypersensitivity, a different real-life example of type III hypersensitivity in humans is serum sickness. Before the development of specific antibiotics and successful vaccines, certain infections were treated by passive transfer of antibody. An example of this is the treatment of human pneumonia by the administration of large quantities of anti-pneumococcal antibodies raised in a different species, for example, a horse. The rationale was that by administering large amounts of "immune" serum from another species, the antibodies contained in that serum would supplement the inadequate response of the patient, thus clearing the offending organisms before permanent damage was achieved. However, the administration of such serum often resulted in a systemic (ie, generalized) reaction characterized by fever, chills, generalized rash, arthritis and, sometimes, kidney damage. The transfusion of serum that generated such reaction was called **serum sickness.** Because serum, not just antibodies, were

administered to the infected person, many of the other components of such serum, particularly soluble proteins in large quantities, played a major role in the reaction. These proteins act as powerful immunogens and cause the production of antibodies in the host, which, in turn, form immune complexes with the proteins throughout the host's body. As in any other immune complex-mediated immune response, these complexes can activate complement, recruit inflammatory cells such as leukocytes, and cause tissue damage. Serum sickness is usually a self-limiting event; once clearance of the complexes is achieved, its clinical manifestations disappear. Subsequent injection of serum from the same species could, however, cause shock and death.

The mechanisms involved in type III hypersensitivity can also take place in certain forms of autoimmunity, for example, rheumatoid arthritis and systemic lupus erythematosus. Unlike serum sickness, these forms of type III hypersensitivity are not self-limiting and can cause significant morbidity and mortality. These conditions are discussed in more detail in Chapter 10.

▶ TYPE IV HYPERSENSITIVITY

Type IV hypersensitivity is also known as *delayed-type hypersensitivity;* the word *delayed* refers to the time between antigen exposure and reaction when compared to the other types of hypersensitivity. The main difference between type IV

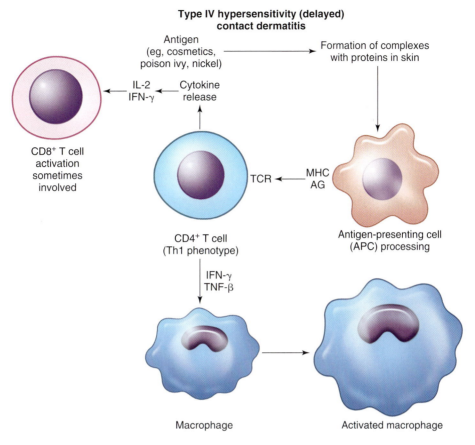

**Type IV hypersensitivity (delayed)
contact dermatitis**

■ **FIGURE 9.14**   Basic molecular mechanisms of delayed-type hypersensitivity.

hypersensitivity and the other types is that whereas the other types are mediated mainly by antibodies (ie, IgE, IgG, and IgM and/or antibody-antigen immune complexes), type IV hypersensitivity is mediated by Th1 T cells and CD8-positive cytotoxic cells (1). This was demonstrated by the fact that, unlike in the other forms of hypersensitivity that could be transferred with antibody, type IV hypersensitivity could be transferred from one experimental animal to another by transferring T cells sensitized to that allergen. Transfer of serum could not transfer the response. As with type I hypersensitivity, the clinical manifestations of type IV hypersensitivity occur upon a second or subsequent exposure to the allergen. The molecular mechanisms involved in type IV hypersensitivity are essentially those involved in cell-mediated immunity and T-cell activation described in Chapter 4. Specifically, the first step in these reactions is exposure to the allergen in the sensitization phase of the reaction, in which antigen-presenting cells, after uptake of the antigen, migrate into the lymphoid system and present the antigen to Th1 cells, thus generating memory T cells. In the second (elicitation) phase, introduction of the antigen at a specific site is followed by uptake of the allergen by local antigen-presenting cells at the site of exposure. If Th1 cells that were previously sensitized to

that allergen arrive at the site, antigen processing and presentation to these Th1 cells follow. Only Th1 cells that have clonally expanded as the result of previous exposure to the allergen will be activated, and it may take some time for the necessary Th1 cells to arrive at the site; this is one of the reasons that it takes a much longer time for type IV hypersensitivity to result in clinical manifestations than the other types of hypersensitivity. Once activated, however, these cells can release cytokines that can activate endothelial cells and can recruit inflammatory cells at the site of allergen exposure. At this point, a localized inflammatory response is characterized by fluid buildup, accumulation of macrophages, and localized tissue damage (Figure 9.14 ■).

Although delayed-type hypersensitivity can target different areas of the body, the classical example of it is **contact dermatitis** (1, 25), which is usually initiated by small substances that are in contact with the skin and penetrate it. Once absorbed into the skin, these molecules can attach to host proteins acting as haptens, forming hapten-protein complexes, and rendering those self-proteins "foreign looking" and thus immunogenic. Many small compounds can cause contact dermatitis: examples include various plant compounds such as urushiol in poison ivy or poison oak; certain components of commonly used cosmetics; some metals used in jewelry, for example, nickel in a watch band or ring; and several different topical medications such as a local antiseptic or anesthetic. In certain cases, occupational exposure favors delayed-type hypersensitivity to a particular allergen. For example, health care workers are more prone to develop latex hypersensitivity, a reaction to certain components of natural rubber, because of their continuous use of latex products such as medical gloves. The clinical manifestations of contact dermatitis involve mild to severe localized inflammation, mainly as the result of the action of activated macrophages. The skin may present with redness, blisters, edema, intense itching, and peeling (Figure 9.15 ■). The intensity of the reaction depends on the

concentration of allergen and the degree of sensitization to it. The duration of the reaction varies and can range from several days to several weeks after the allergen's removal. This type of allergic reaction can be tested with patch testing, which involves placing the chemical against the skin using paper tape. The area is read 72 to 96 hours later for signs of contact dermatitis.

✓ Checkpoint! 9.3

A young man has developed a rash of unknown origin on his arm. Because he has had this rash before, he thinks it is due to a hypersensitivity reaction rather than the response to an infectious condition. What would be a test to distinguish between the 2 scenarios?

Interestingly enough, type IV hypersensitivity is used as a diagnostic tool in medicine, specifically in the **Mantoux test** based on the fact that individuals exposed to *Mycobacterium tuberculosis* develop a T-cell immune response to that organism whose soluble components can elicit a delayed-type hypersensitivity to those components. If soluble components of *mycobacterium tuberculosis* (usually purified cell wall components) are injected intradermally and the individual has been exposed to the microorganism, a localized type IV hypersensitivity reaction develops at the site of the injection. The area tested is raised and red and does not pit with pressure because it contains fibrin (Figure 9.16 ■). Appearance of the reactions indicates a positive tuberculin test. It must be emphasized that a positive tuberculin test does not indicate active or even past tuberculosis but the test is based on the concept of cross-reacting antigens discussed in Chapter 3. The result means that the individual has been exposed to components that share antigenic determinants with *mycobacterium tuberculosis*. However, it does indicate the possibility that the individual was exposed to *mycobacterium tuberculosis* itself, and more testing is warranted. The Mantoux test has largely replaced an older test, called the *tine test,* which used small, multiple punctures instead of a single intradermal injection.

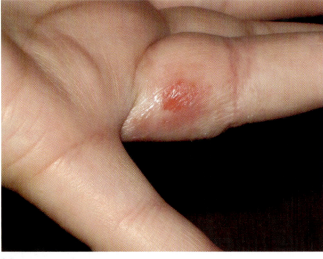

(a)

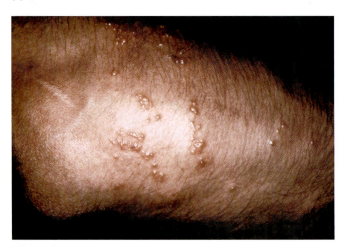

(b)

■ **FIGURE 9.15** (a) Type IV hypersensitivity reaction, contact dermatitis as the result of reaction to the nickel in a ring. (b) Type IV hypersensitivity reaction as the result of poison ivy. *Source:* © CDC.

✓ Checkpoint! 9.4

A difference between immediate hypersensitivity and delayed hypersensitivity is, as the names imply, a difference in the time between exposure to the allergen and the clinical manifestation of the reaction to it. Why do you think it takes much longer to develop a reaction in delayed hypersensitivity than in immediate hypersensitivity?

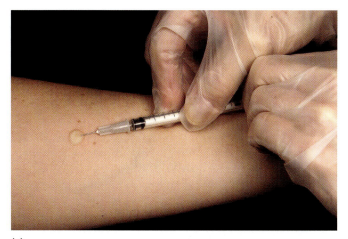

(a)

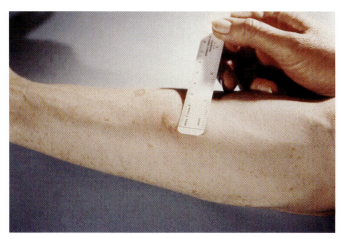

(b)

■ **FIGURE 9.16** The Mantoux tuberculin skin test. (a) Injection of antigen. *Source:* © CDC. (b) Positive reaction. *Source:* CDC/ Donald Kopanoff.

CASE STUDY

Lauren, a college sophomore, has joined her friends at a Chinese restaurant. She has recently found out that she has a severe allergy to shrimp, so she avoids the shrimp dishes. She has the chicken cashew dish that is next to the shrimp lo mein. Unfortunately, the student in front of her has used the shrimp spoon for the chicken cashew. Lauren eats the chicken cashew and notices a seafoodlike taste but ignores it. Twenty minutes later, she begins to have difficulty breathing, and her face and neck swell and become quite red.

Lauren recovers, and in the summer, she volunteers with a group called Unite for Sight that helps fit people in Africa for donated glasses. She does some additional travel while she is there and goes to the Nile Delta region in Northern Africa where she contracts schistosomiasis (a very severe parasitic infection). She returns from Africa and is treated with antiparasitic drugs. Upon returning home,

Lauren's Aunt Nelly gives her krill oil, a health food supplement that contains antioxidants to help her feel better. Unfortunately, this supplement is related to shrimp and contains the same allergen.

1. What type of hypersensitivity do you think Lauren experienced at the Chinese restaurant?

2. What do you think should have been done to treat Lauren at the Chinese restaurant?

3. Assuming that the allergen in krill oil is the same and at a concentration similar to the amount in her dinner at the Chinese restaurant, would Lauren's allergic reaction be more or less severe than the one at the restaurant? Why?

SUMMARY

Hypersensitivity reactions are immune reactions to a usually harmless antigen (allergen) when the reaction causes more damage to the host than the antigen itself. Reactions occur in subjects previously exposed to an antigen and who developed an immune response to it, a process called *sensitization.* The Gell and Coombs classification assigns hypersensitivity reactions to 4 different groups: I, II, III, and IV, according to the molecular and immunological mechanisms involved in the reaction. Type I hypersensitivity is also called *immediate hypersensitivity,* which refers to the short time between allergen exposure and reaction when compared to the other types. Type I hypersensitivity is mediated by IgE, which, when bound to immune cells such as mast cells and basophils, can attach to allergens and cross-link IgE Fc receptors on the surface of these cells. This, in turn, causes the degranulation of the cells and the release of performed mediators that have various biological effects. The activation of these cells also stimulates the de novo synthesis of other mediators such as cytokines, which have other biological effects. Preformed mediators include histamines, prostaglandins, eosinophil chemotaxins, serotonin, and various proteases. Mediators synthesized in addition to various cytokines include chemokines and leukotrienes. The combined effects of these mediators cause increased capillary permeability, recruitment of inflammatory cells, airway constriction, and mucus secretion. Their effects depend on the anatomical location of the reaction. Most type I hypersensitivity reactions are localized and include atopic dermatitis, rhinitis, asthma, diarrhea, and vomiting; in rare cases, however, they can become systemic and life threatening such as in systemic anaphylaxis. Testing for type I hypersensitivity involves evaluating levels of IgE either total or specific for a particular allergen or in vivo testing of an individual response to a particular allergen. The total level of IgE can be measured with the RIST test and tests using chemiluminescence. IgE to a specific allergen can be tested with the RAST test and, more recently, microwell assays. In vivo tests include the skin or "prick" test used to determine an individual's reaction to an allergen by observing a localized skin reaction to that allergen.

Type II hypersensitivity is mediated by IgG and IgM to cell surface antigens and by the activation of complement. The tissue destruction observed in type II hypersensitivity is as the result of antibody- and complement-mediated lysis, antibody- and complement-mediated opsonization, and antibody-dependent cellular cytotoxicity. The most commonly affected targets are blood, lungs, and kidneys. Typical examples of type II hypersensitivity are transfusion reactions, hemolytic anemia, and hemolytic disease of the fetus and newborn (HDFN). Tests for HDFN include ABO and Rh blood typing, checking a woman's blood for antibody to the Rh antigen, and testing of a baby's red blood cells for the presence of anti-Rh antibodies.

Type III hypersensitivity is characterized by the presence of immune complexes deposited at various anatomical sites. The immune reaction to these complexes causes tissue damage in type III hypersensitivity. Unlike a type II response, the immune response in type III is to an antigen in solution rather than one appearing on a particular cell or tissue. Immune complexes deposited on a tissue activate complement and recruit phagocytic and inflammatory cells to the site. Typical target tissues of type III hypersensitivity are blood vessel walls, glomerular basement membrane, and tissues in the joints and lungs.

Type IV hypersensitivity (*delayed hypersensitivity*) takes a longer period of time from exposure to reaction when compared to other types. Type IV hypersensitivity is primarily cell mediated rather than antibody mediated and involves the activation of Th1 T cells, CD8-positive cytotoxic cells, and macrophages. An example of type IV hypersensitivity is contact dermatitis, which is a localized inflammatory reaction to various different allergens, resulting in redness, blisters, edema, intense itching, and peeling of the skin. These allergens can include substances from various plants such as poison ivy and poison oak, cosmetics, latex products, and certain metals in jewelry items.

The most common approach to preventing type I and type IV hypersensitivities is allergen avoidance; however, hyposensitization (allergy shots) to prevent type I hypersensitivity is also employed. To prevent type II hypersensitivity, administration of anti-Rh antibodies (Rhogam) to an Rh-negative pregnant woman to prevent HDNB is the preventative method.

REVIEW QUESTIONS

1. Opsonization, activation of complement, and antibody-dependent cellular cytotoxicity (ADCC) are features of
   a. immediate hypersensitivity
   b. type II hypersensitivity
   c. type I hypersensitivity
   d. delayed hypersensitivity

2. The radioallergosorbent test (RAST) measures
   a. total amount of allergen
   b. total serum IgE levels
   c. type III hypersensitivity
   d. IgE specific for a particular allergen

3. Release of newly synthesized and preformed mediators from mast cells and basophils are characteristics of
   a. delayed hypersensitivity
   b. type I hypersensitivity
   c. type II hypersensitivity
   d. type III hypersensitivity

4. The major classes of immunoglobulins that participate in type II (cytolytic) and type III (immune complexes) hypersensitivity are
   a. IgE and IgD
   b. IgG and IgM
   c. IgE
   d. IgA and IgD

5. Rhesus (also called Rhogam) prophylaxis is used in the prevention of erythroblastosis fetalis. Which of the following are administered to the mother to obtain such prophylaxis?
   a. anti-RhD antibodies
   b. mother's red blood cells coated with father's antibody
   c. Rh-compatible red blood cells (ie, same as the mother)
   d. father's red blood cells

6. IgE plays its most important role in
   a. delayed-type hypersensitivity
   b. type I hypersensitivity
   c. type III hypersensitivity
   d. type II hypersensitivity

7. The radioimmunosorbent test (RIST) measures
   a. total amount of allergen
   b. total serum IgE levels
   c. type II hypersensitivity
   d. IgE that is specific for a particular allergen

8. Sensitized T cells and activated macrophages are characteristic of
   a. anaphylaxis reactions
   b. type II hypersensitivity
   c. type III hypersensitivity
   d. delayed type hypersensitivity

9. A direct test
   a. measures the amount of antibody in the RH negative pregnant woman that reacts with the RH positive fetal red blood cells
   b. determines whether anti-RH is already present on the newborn's red blood cells
   c. measures the amount of antibody produced by the fetus to the mother's red blood cells
   d. uses cross-linking antibodies of the IgD type

10. A male model for *GQ* magazine came into the doctor's office after a photo shoot for an American jewelry company. He had done a photo shoot involving 14 karat gold necklaces, bracelets, and an earring. All these areas were covered with a rash 48 hours after the session. The rash was caused by T cells. This young man was experiencing
    a. type I hypersensitivity
    b. type II hypersensitivity
    c. type III hypersensitivity
    d. type IV hypersensitivity

REFERENCES

1. Murphy K. *Janeway's Immunobiology.* 8th ed. New York, NY: Garland Publishing; 2012.

2. Gell PGH, Coombs RRA, eds. *Clinical Aspects of Immunology.* Oxford, England: Blackwell; 1963.

3. Kay AB. Overview of allergy and allergic diseases: With a view to the future. *Br Med Bull.* 2000;56(4):843–864.

4. Neugut AI, Ghatak AT, Miller RL. Anaphylaxis in the United States: An investigation into its epidemiology. *Arch Intern Med.* 2001;161(1):15–21.

5. Corry DB, Kheradmand F. Induction and regulation of the IgE response. *Nature.* 1999;402:B18.

6. Boyce JA. The biology of the mast cell. *Allergy Asthma Proc.* 2004;25:27.

7. Kinet JP. The high-affinity IgE receptor (FcεRI): From physiology to pathology. *Annu Rev Immunol.* 1999;17:931.

8. Stone KD, Prussin C, Metcalfe DD. IgE, mast cells, basophils, and eosinophils. *J Allergy Clin Immunol.* 2010;125:S73.

9. Akdis CA, Jutel M, Akdis M. Regulatory effects of histamine and histamine receptor expression in human allergic immune responses. *Chem Immunol Allergy.* 2008;94:67.

10. Lieberman P. Biphasic anaphylactic reactions. *Ann Allergy Asthma Immunol.* 2005;95(3):217–226.

11. Lombardi V, Singh AK, Akbari O. The role of costimulatory molecules in allergic disease and asthma. *Int Arch Allergy Immunol.* 2010;151:179.

12. Kumar V, Abbas AK, Fausto N, et al. *Robbins and Cotran Pathologic Basis of Disease.* 8th ed. Philadelphia, PA: Saunders; 2010.

13. Grammatikos AP. The genetic and environmental basis of atopic diseases. *Ann Med.* 2008;40:482–495.

14. Gould H, et al. The biology of IGE and the basis of allergic disease. *Annu Rev Immunol.* 2003(21):579–628.

15. Hamilton RG, Adkinson NF Jr. Clinical laboratory methods for the assessment and management of human allergic diseases. *Clin Lab Med.* 1986;6:117.

16. Ten RM, Klein JS, Frigas E. Allergy skin testing. *Mayo Clin Proc.* 1995;70:783–784.

17. Orovitg A, Guardia P, Barber D, et al. Enhanced diagnosis of pollen allergy using specific immunoglobulin E determination to detect major allergens and panallergens. *Investig Allergol Clin Immunol.* 2011;21:253–259.

18. Rank MA, Li JT. Allergen immunotherapy. *Mayo Clin Proc.* 2007;82:1119–1123.

19. Gehrs BC, Friedberg RC. Autoimmune hemolytic anemia. *Am J Hematol.* 2002;69:258–271.

20. Shoenfield Y, et al. *Diagnostic Criteria in Autoimmune Disease.* Totowa, NJ: Humana Press; 2008.

21. Gruslin AM, Moore TR. Erythroblastosis fetalis. In: Martin R, Fanaroff A, Walsh M, eds. *Neonatal-Perinatal Medicine.* Philadelphia, PA: Mosby Elsevier; 2006.

22. Bowman J, et al. Rh-immunization during pregnancy: Antenatal prophylaxis. *Canadian Med Ass J.* 1978;118:623–627.

23. Shmagel KV, Chereshnev VA. Molecular bases of immune complex pathology. *Biochemistry (Mosc).* 2009;74:469.

24. Arthus M. Injections répétées de serum du cheval chez le lapin. *Comptes rendus des séances de la Société de biologie et de ses filiales.* 1903;55:817–820.

25. Kimber I, Basketter DA, Gerberick GF, et al. Allergic contact dermatitis. *Int Immunopharmacol.* 2002;2:201–211.

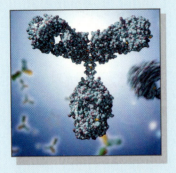

10

Systemic Autoimmunity

■ OBJECTIVES—LEVEL I

After this chapter, the student should be able to:

1. Discuss the role of genetics, gender, and environmental factors in the etiology of autoimmunity.
2. Describe the mechanisms of immunopathology that cause disease in autoimmunity.
3. Describe the etiology of systemic lupus erythematosus and its clinical manifestations.
4. List and describe different tests for the diagnosis of systemic lupus erythematosus.
5. Describe the etiology of rheumatoid arthritis and its clinical manifestations.
6. Describe the cellular and molecular mechanisms of immunopathology and tissue destruction in rheumatoid arthritis.
7. Name and describe different diagnostic tests for the diagnosis of rheumatoid arthritis.
8. Name and describe laboratory tests that are common to different systemic autoimmune diseases.

■ OBJECTIVES—LEVEL II

After this chapter, the student should be able to:

1. Discuss the basic immunologic mechanisms that may cause autoimmunity.
2. Describe possible biological mechanisms that may lead to systemic lupus erythematosus.

KEY TERMS

antinuclear antibodies (ANA)
apoptosis
central tolerance
endocarditis
hematuria
immunologically privileged site
knockout mice
molecular mimicry
myocarditis
pannus
pericarditis

peripheral tolerance
pleuritis
polyarthritis
proteinuria
rheumatoid factor (RF)
self-reactivity
self-tolerance
superantigen
synovitis
vasculitis

▶ INTRODUCTION

The ability to recognize one's own environment is critical for the survival and function of most organisms. Although this ability may be taken for granted, all species from microorganisms to mammals, including humans, use it. Bees and ants must recognize their own hives or nests and be able to keep away individuals from different hives or nests. We use this ability to find directions, food, shelter, and mates, and for self-protection. This is also true at the molecular level; the immune system is our mechanism of cellular and molecular recognition. It is designed to promote communication and function and, most importantly, distinguish friends from foe. *Autoimmunity* occurs when the immune army turns against itself instead of recognizing itself from nonself. In this chapter, we discuss autoimmunity as a dysfunction of the immune system. We cover potential mechanisms that may be involved in these dysfunctions, some mechanisms of tissue injury, and clinical examples of autoimmune disease that affect an individual systemically. The forms of autoimmunity that affect specific tissues or organs are covered in Chapter 11. In addition, diagnostic methods for systemic autoimmunity are discussed in this chapter.

▶ MECHANISMS OF AUTOIMMUNITY

Much remains unknown about the causes and development of autoimmunity, but several possibilities have been proposed, including a failure of mechanisms that maintain **self-tolerance.** Genetics, environmental factors, infections, and gender are also thought to contribute to the development of autoimmunity. Autoimmunity affects 5 to 7% of the population. In Chapter 4, we discussed the concept of immunological self-tolerance, a mechanism designed to eliminate or suppress potentially self-reactive immune cells. This mechanism is necessary because, as we discussed in Chapter 3, the repertoire of recognition molecules such as immunoglobulins and T-cell receptors is generated randomly, that is, it is based on the creation of a very large repertoire of different randomly selected patterns to ensure that such antigen receptor molecules have all specificities that may be required to recognize a particular pathogen at a particular point in time. Because of this randomness of specificity, an immunoglobulin or a T-cell receptor molecule may by chance express a random specificity that can recognize self-antigens; this, of course must be prevented, and this is where the mechanism of self-tolerance comes into play. However, this mechanism is not perfect and, at times, can fail.

The development of self-tolerance relies on several different mechanisms, each with a particular purpose. These mechanisms range from the elimination of self-reacting cells from the immune repertoire to the downregulation of immune responses that may react with an individual's own antigens. Mechanisms such as positive and negative selection,

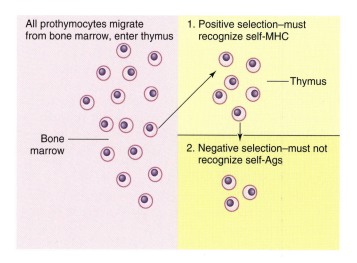

■ **FIGURE 10.1** Review of central tolerance.

which compose in part **central tolerance,** are described in Chapter 4 and reviewed in Figure 10.1 ■. Unfortunately, these processes are not perfect and do not eliminate all self-reactive T cells. For example, negative selection depends on many factors including the accessibility of developing T cells to self-antigens, the combined avidity of TCR and CD4/CD8 molecules for MHC and self-antigens, and the identity of the cells presenting self-antigens. Therefore, autoreactivity must also be kept in check during **peripheral tolerance** by regulating self-reacting immune responses that have escaped deletion by the mechanisms of central tolerance. The prevention of autoreactivity also involves other regulatory mechanisms including regulatory T cells that play a major role in the downregulation of any potentially reactive T cell that may have escaped negative selection. In addition, B cells may also acquire **self-reactivity** through reaction with cross-reactive antigens (ie, antigens that may share antigenic determinants with self-antigens). For instance, exposure of B cells to polyclonal activators such as lipopolysaccharides (LPS) or Epstein-Barr (EBV) infection may nonspecifically activate B cells that recognize self-antigens. These cells must also be downregulated beyond central tolerance. Experimental evidence has shown that the development of autoimmunity may involve defects in either of these regulatory mechanisms (1).

CTLA-4 is an inhibitory receptor on T cells that downregulates T-cell signaling response and prevents T-cell activation. CTLA-4 **knockout mice** (ie, mice that have been genetically manipulated to have a particular gene deleted from its genome, in this case, CTLA-4) develop fatal autoimmunity. Likewise, the loss of T regulatory (suppressor) cells and their inhibitory cytokines (IL-10, TGFβ) may contribute to autoimmunity, as IL-10 KO and TGFβ knockout mice experience autoimmune syndromes. Although different regulatory mechanisms may be implicated in autoimmunity, malfunctions in peripheral tolerance are thought to be major contributors to it.

▶ GENETIC FACTORS

Genetics plays an important role in the susceptibility of an individual to autoimmune diseases. Not surprisingly, genes that are involved in the immune response are the major players, so major histocompatibility complex (MHC) and human leukocyte antigen (HLA) loci are frequently linked to certain autoimmune diseases. The possible reason for this is that presumably a self-antigen is particularly well presented by a particular MHC haplotype following the mechanisms described in Chapters 3 and 4. Therefore, an individual with that particular haplotype may present self-antigens better or more efficiently, thus increasing chances for an autoimmune response. For example, when looking at the HLA-DQb1 gene, most people have aspartic acid at position 57, but patients with type 1 diabetes mellitus (T1DM) more often have valine, serine, or alanine at that position. Perhaps because of this, autoantigens are better presented in those individuals than in people having aspartic acid at the same position, resulting in a higher incidence of autoimmune diabetes in this latter group. See Table 10.1 ✪ for examples of the association between certain HLA haplotypes and autoimmune diseases (2).

▶ GENDER

Gender also plays a large role in the susceptibility to autoimmune diseases as indicated by the fact that they affect females generally much more severely and more often than men. This has been shown to be true in both humans and mice when castrated male mice become more susceptible to autoimmunity, and, conversely, androgen treatment of female mice reduces such incidence. Hormonal influences thus clearly play a role in this association. In fact, it has been suggested that estrogen may stimulate immune responses by enhancing B-cell activation while downregulating suppressor T cells. Females tend to mount stronger inflammatory responses to different antigens than men, which may translate into larger inflammatory responses to self-antigens too. Additional indications that estrogen may play a role in autoimmunity are the variabilities in autoimmune diseases during fluctuations in hormonal changes as in menstruation and pregnancy, or when using oral contraceptives.

▶ INFECTION AND ENVIRONMENTAL FACTORS

In Chapter 3, we introduced the concept of immunological cross-reactivity (ie, the reaction of an antibody with an antigen other than the one that induced its formation). Epitopes are shared in nature, and at times foreign epitopes can be very similar to self-epitopes and trigger an immune response that reacts with self. This can occur during an infection by a process called **molecular mimicry,** a situation in which microbial antigens cross-react with the host's self-antigens. In this case, the immune response generated against a particular microorganism also reacts with components of the host's tissues. For example, streptococcal infections can cause the development of antibodies that also recognize heart muscle antigens, which, in turn, can cause severe cardiac damage. Thus, infection can also play a role in the development of autoimmunity.

In addition, environmental factors may also contribute to or exacerbate an autoimmune condition. For example, smoking can increase the severity of diseases in many cases; the disease fatalities in Goodpasture's syndrome are associated with kidney failure and/or pulmonary hemorrhage, the latter of which is seen most often in patients who smoke. Finally, trauma can also cause autoimmunity if it releases self-antigens that are sequestered in **immunologically privileged sites,** such as the anterior chamber of the eye. Damage to this area can release antigens never "seen" by the immune response and thus immunize the host against them as it occurs in sympathetic opthalmia.

✪ TABLE 10.1	
Association of Different HLA Alleles and Increased Susceptibility to Autoimmune Diseases	
HLA Alleles	**Diseases with Increased Risk**
HLA-B27	Ankylosing spondylitis
	Acute anterior uveitis
HLA-DR2	Goodpasture's syndrome
	Multiple sclerosis
HLA-DR3	Grave's disease
	Myasthenia gravis
	Autoimmune hepatitis
	Type 1 diabetes mellitus
	Systemic lupus erythematosus
	Primary Sjögren's syndrome
HLA-DR4	Type 1 diabetes mellitus
	Rheumatoid arthritis
	Pemphigus vulgaris
HLA-DR5	Hashimoto's thyroiditis

 Checkpoint! 10.1

Molecular mimicry becomes an important issue when considering the development of a vaccine. Why is this?

► MECHANISMS OF PATHOLOGY

Autoimmunity is an immune reaction to self-antigens so, not surprisingly, the mechanisms that the immune system uses to destroy pathogens can also cause pathology and tissue destruction in autoimmunity. These mechanisms include immune complex-mediated injury as well as anti-tissue antibodies and cell-mediated immunity. Immune complexes with autoantigens can be deposited on tissues such as blood vessels where these complexes can activate complement and/or recruit inflammatory cells such as neutrophils, thus causing tissue destruction and **vasculitis.** Likewise, antibodies can also directly bind to self-tissues and cause destruction by these mechanisms. Cytotoxic T cells are also involved in the pathology of autoimmunity. The clinical manifestations of such destruction depend, of course, on the nature of the tissue being destroyed, ultimately leading in some functional loss of the tissue or organ affected. For instance, in type 1 diabetes mellitus auto-antibodies to pancreatic β cells in islets of Langerhans cause the destruction of these cells, resulting in decreased production of insulin and therefore increased blood glucose and subsequent metabolic problems. In addition, dysfunction also can arise when tissue damage is not the main problem. Autoantibodies can also be stimulating or blocking; for example, in myasthenia gravis, antibodies to acetylcholine receptors prevent acetylcholine from binding their receptors by blocking them, thus interfering with receptor activation and, ultimately, interfering with muscle activation and function. Conversely, in Grave's disease, antibodies to the thyroid-stimulating hormone receptor mimic the hormone and can activate the receptor, resulting in hyperstimulation of the thyroid and hyperthyroid syndrome. Type 1 diabetes mellitus, myasthenia gravis, and Grave's disease are discussed in Chapter 11.

► TYPES OF AUTOIMMUNE DISEASES

Autoimmune diseases can be divided into 2 major groups: organ specific and systemic. The distinction relates to the target of the autoimmune response; the target in organ-specific autoimmune diseases is usually a specific type of cell, organ, or tissue (ie, the response is to a target antigen whose expression is restricted to a particular organ or tissue). On the other hand, systemic autoimmune diseases are due to the formation of immune complexes that travel in the circulation and deposit in several different tissues and organs and cause damage. See Table 10.2 ✪ for the different diseases in each category. Chapter 11 will discuss organ-specific autoimmune diseases. This chapter focuses on examples of systemic autoimmune diseases.

✪ TABLE 10.2

Examples of Different Autoimmune Diseases

Systemic Diseases	Organ-Specific Diseases
Systemic lupus erythematosus	Hashimoto's thyroiditis
Rheumatoid arthritis	Type 1 diabetes mellitus
	Myasthenia gravis
	Grave's disease
	Addison's disease
	Autoimmune hemolytic anemia

► SYSTEMIC LUPUS ERYTHEMATOSUS

If there were ever a quintessential example of an immune complex autoimmune disease, it would be systemic lupus erythematosus (SLE). Lupus erythematosus is a name given to a group of somewhat different yet similar conditions in which there is antibody formed to nuclear antigens that have been released into the blood stream as the result of the cell death. The antinuclear antibody and the nuclear antigens form immune complexes (3). Because the immune complexes travel throughout the body and become trapped and affect different organs, tissues, cells, and molecules, the word *systemic* is used. Areas with filtering functions like the kidney, the synovium, and other serous linings are most affected by the immune complex deposition. This systemic form of SLE is most often seen, but it can also manifest itself in a purely cutaneous form as in the case of acute cutaneous lupus erythematosus. Tissues and organs affected include kidneys, joints, blood cells, blood vessels, skin, lungs, liver, the nervous system, and heart; whereas SLE is the most common and most severe of these conditions, other form of lupus, namely, discoid lupus, drug-induced lupus, and neonatal lupus, have also been described.

The incidence of SLE is 10-fold higher in women than men, and it is more prevalent in persons of non-European lineage, African Americans, and Hispanics. Europe has approximately 40 cases per 100 000, but the incidence can be as high as 159 cases per 100 000 among those of Afro-Caribbean descent. No single cause or single gene for SLE has been identified. However, SLE does have a genetic basis and tends to run in families. It has been suggested that several different genes play a role in the susceptibility to SLE; not surprisingly, HLA genes are among them. Environmental factors have also been suggested to be implicated in either the onset or the exacerbation of SLE. These include medications, stress, hormones such as estrogen, infection, and exposure to sunlight (3). Although there is no known cure for SLE, survival rates in the western world are good (ie, 95% at 5 years, 90% at 10 years, and almost 80% at 20 years).

SIGNS AND SYMPTOMS

Because of the multiplicity of autoimmune targets, the fact that SLE has a wide variety of clinical signs and symptoms should not be surprising. In fact, SLE is often misdiagnosed because some of its signs and symptoms mimic those of a variety of different clinical conditions. The fact that the course of SLE is erratic and irregular with periods of symptoms followed by periods of remission also complicates diagnosis, and in some cases, patients with SLE can experience unexplained symptoms for years without a clear diagnosis of their condition. The pathology of SLE and rheumatoid arthritis are both based, at least in part, on the effects of inflammation caused by circulating and depositing immune complexes (3, 4).

Areas of the body where deposition or filtering of immune complexes occurs, such as the kidneys and the joint spaces, can be damaged by these complexes and this damage can cause symptoms. In a kidney biopsy, immunofluorescence shows deposition of these immune complexes in a lumpy bumpy pattern as in a sieve entrapping the immune complex clumps. In Goodpasture's disease, the kidney is also affected but a biopsy would show a linear or ribbon pattern showing antibody binding to an antigen in the basement membrane. Symptoms caused by immune complex deposition include fever, painful joints, tiredness and fatigue, photosensitivity, muscle pain, loss of appetite, confusion, proteinuria, and a decrease in cognitive capabilities (Figure 10.2 ■). Specifically, however, different signs and symptoms associated with SLE can be divided into categories depending on the body system that is affected. Dermatological manifestations are common; as much as 50% of SLE patients can exhibit a classic facial rash called *butterfly rash* or *malar rash*, because of its shape (Figure 10.3 ■). In fact, the term *lupus*, which is Latin for "wolf," refers to this facial rash, which resembles the pattern seen on a wolf's face. Hair loss, scaly patches, lesions of the skin, and ulcers in the mouth, nose, and vagina are also common manifestations. Painful joints are another common manifestation of SLE with smaller joints (eg, hands, wrists) usually affected more often than others. Muscle pain is also a manifestation of SLE; in general, however, these symptoms are usually not severe, and the tissue destruction of joints in

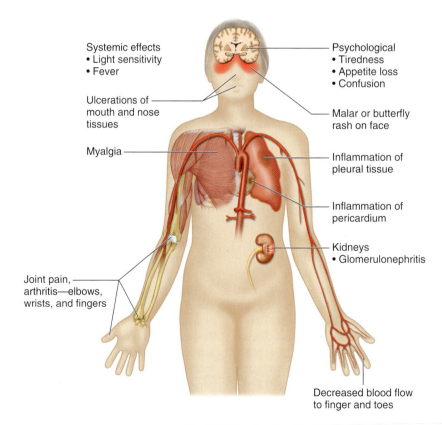

■ **FIGURE 10.2**   Most common symptoms of systemic lupus erythematosus (SLE).

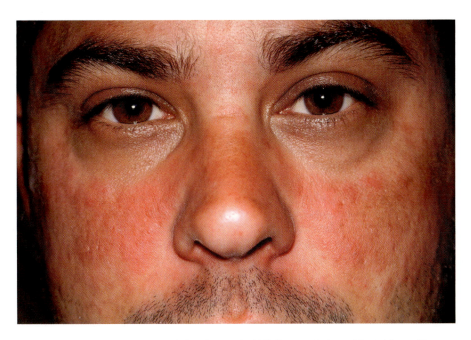

■ **FIGURE 10.3**   Typical "butterfly" rash seen in SLE. *Source:* Science Photo Library/Custom Medical Stock Photo, Inc.

rheumatoid arthritis is usually not seen in patients suffering from SLE. Because erythrocytes are one of the cells affected by SLE, anemia and iron deficiencies are reported in about half of SLE cases (3, 4, 5).

Cardiac manifestations of SLE include **pericarditis, myocarditis,** and **endocarditis** involving the heart valves, particularly the mitral and tricuspid valves. Pulmonary involvement in SLE includes **pleuritis,** pulmonary hypertension, emboli, pleural effusion, and pulmonary hemorrhage. Blood in the urine (**hematuria**) and protein in the urine (**proteinuria**) are renal manifestations of SLE and in some severe cases (eg, lupus nephritis), SLE can lead to renal failure (6). SLE can also be associated with neurological and psychological manifestations; because the central and peripheral nervous systems can be targeted, various signs and symptoms can be observed, the most common one being headache (7). However, neuropsychiatric manifestations can include mood changes, confusion, cognitive problems, anxiety, seizures, and, in extreme cases, psychosis. To help in the diagnosis of SLE, the American College of Rheumatology (ACR) in 1982 developed 11 criteria ranging from malar rash to photosensitivity to serositis. For the complete list see: http://www.rheumatology.org/practice/clinical/classification/SLE/sle.asp. The diagnosis for SLE should be considered when a person meets 4 or more of these criteria. This diagnostic approach has a sensitivity of 85% and a specificity of 95% for SLE.

✓ **Checkpoint! 10.2**

Why is SLE so difficult to diagnose initially?

PATHOPHYSIOLOGY

Although the autoimmune response in SLE can target many cells and tissues, the antigens for this response are components of the cell nucleus. The antibodies seen against these antigens are called **antinuclear antibodies (ANA).** It is thought that the exposure to the immune system of these components for various reasons makes some people mount an immune response to them. One of the factors that may contribute to autoimmune reactions is abnormality in **apoptosis,** the process by which a sequence of events results in the elimination of old cells, cells that are no longer necessary, or cells that may be unhealthy, and in the clearance of these apoptotic cells (8, 9, 10). It is one way in which the body keeps healthy cells and replenishes old and sick ones; in fact, it is estimated that the body replaces more than 1 million cells every second. Abnormalities in apoptotic mechanisms can contribute to autoimmunity in different ways. For example, apoptosis eliminates many autoreactive B and T cells; deficiencies in this process may allow these cells to persist and generate autoimmune responses.

In addition, and just as critical, is the fact that having undergone apoptosis, dead cells or cell debris, especially nuclear components that could mimic viral antigens, must be removed because some of this debris could be seen as "foreign." Complement and phagocytic cells are involved in clearing apoptotic cells by phagocytic "clearing" cells such as macrophages, which recognize dying cells. Part of the process of apoptosis involves the dying cell's secreting a "find-me" signal for the clearing cells. The binding of this signal to receptors on the clearing cell causes it to undergo chemotaxis. In addition, apoptotic cells also display an "eat-me" signal on their surface, so that when clearing cells following the find-me signal arrive, they respond to the eat-me surface component and engulf the dying or dead cell. Once the clearing cells have ingested the dead cells, the clearing cells break down the resulting cell debris back into basic building blocks, such as amino acids, nucleotides, sugars, and others, which are then recycled to make new cell molecules. So, the function of these clearing cells is crucial in the elimination of cellular debris and prevents its accumulation. Should there be a dysfunction in this clearing activity, cellular debris would accumulate without breaking down. This accumulation, in turn, could trigger an immune response to this debris. Experimental evidence has shown that this does occur; mice deficient in the engulfment of apoptotic cells develop SLE-type autoimmune diseases. In addition, deficient degradation of the chromosomal DNA from engulfed cells in mice activates macrophages, leading to lethal anemia in embryos and chronic arthritis in adults. These observations indicate that the dead cells and the nuclei expelled from erythroid precursor cells need to be swiftly cleared for animals to maintain homeostasis.

Therefore, the inefficient clearing of dying cells and the resulting accumulation of cell remnants is considered an intrinsic defect that results in continuous or permanent presence of cell debris and the subsequent initiation of systemic autoimmune diseases such as SLE. The antigens involved in SLE are complex and contain nucleic acids that can look like opsonized viral antigens to the immune system, leading to the production of type 1 interferon, something that is commonly seen in SLE. Ultimately, the constant presence of these antigens leads to the polyclonal activation of B cells, increased production of antibodies, and increased presence of a wide variety of immune complexes. These immune complexes are not cleared efficiently and accumulate in different tissues, triggering immune complex injury via the recruitment of inflammatory cells and the activation of complement, ultimately resulting in tissue destruction.

DIAGNOSIS AND TESTING

As we have discussed, common autoantigens in SLE are components of the cell nucleus such as DNA or nuclear proteins such as histones. Not surprisingly, a logical approach in testing for SLE is detecting the presence of ANA (3), a group of antibodies that react to different nuclear, nucleolar, or perinuclear antigens such as nucleic acids, histones, chromatin, and nuclear and ribonuclear proteins. Testing for ANA and anti-extractable nuclear antigen (anti-ENA) are common approaches for the diagnosis of SLE. More than 95% of SLE patients have a positive ANA, but ANA can also be found in other conditions, such as scleroderma, Sjögren's syndrome, and rheumatoid arthritis, and some healthy individuals may also exhibit ANAs. Therefore, many people with a positive ANA test do not actually suffer from SLE. Higher titers are more definitive for SLE.

The classical and widely used initial test for ANA has been indirect immunofluorescence (11). Specifically, the method involves testing various dilutions of a patient's serum against a cell substrate to observe the presence or absence of antibody that binds to the nucleus and, if it is present, to observe the staining pattern of the immunofluorescence. A commonly used cell substrate is HEp-2 cells (a human laryngeal epithelioma cancer cell line); in a monolayer on a spot on a microscope slide the different patterns of indirect immunofluorescence staining can suggest a particular autoimmune disease; commonly seen patterns include homogenous, diffuse, speckled, and peripheral (called *rim*). The pattern of staining is important because some are characteristic of different diseases or prognostic conditions and can be used to narrow subsequent testing for proper diagnosis. Examples of different immunofluorescence patterns and related diseases are shown in Figure 10.4 ■.

A diffuse or homogeneous pattern of staining occurs with antibodies against deoxyribonucleoprotein, histones, or dsDNA and is suggestive of SLE whereas a speckled pattern of staining indicates that the patient has either antibodies to Smith antigen, which indicates SLE; antibodies to SS-A and SS-B antigens, which indicate Sjögren's syndrome; or antibodies to Scl-70, which may suggest progressive systemic scleroderma, or antibodies to ribonucleoprotein, which indicates mixed connective tissue disease or SLE. Nucleolar staining indicates that the patient has antibody to nucleolar RNA and may have SLE or scleroderma. Centromere staining indicates that the patient may have limited scleroderma (formerly called CREST) a subset of systemic sclerosis. To narrow diagnosis for a speckled staining pattern, enzyme-linked immunosorbant assays (ELISA) are routinely used to determine which antibody is involved. ELISA is also used to confirm the antibodies suggested by the other patterns of staining. The principles and methodologies of immunofluorescence and ELISA are discussed in Chapter 7.

ELISA provides improved specificity over the immunfluorescence analysis, allowing determination of whether the antinucleua staining seen is due to anti-Smith antibodies and anti-double-stranded DNA antibodies (anti-dsDNA), which are associated with SLE, anti-histone antibodies, which are linked to drug-induced lupus, anti-SS-A (Ro), anti-SS-B (La), anti-Rnp, or anti-Scl-70 (11).

Staining	Antigen	Disease
Diffuse or homogeneous	Deoxyribonucleoprotein, histone, ds DNA	Systemic lupus erythematosus (SLE)
Peripheral or rim	ds DNA	SLE
Speckled	saline extractable antigens Sm	SLE
	SS-A, **SS**-B	**S**jögren's **S**yndrome
	Scl-70	Progressive systemic **scl**erosis
	RNP	Mixed connective tissue disease, SLE
Nucleolar	Nucleolar RNA	SLE, scleroderma
Centromere	Centromere/kinetochore region of chromosome	Crest subset of systemic sclerosis

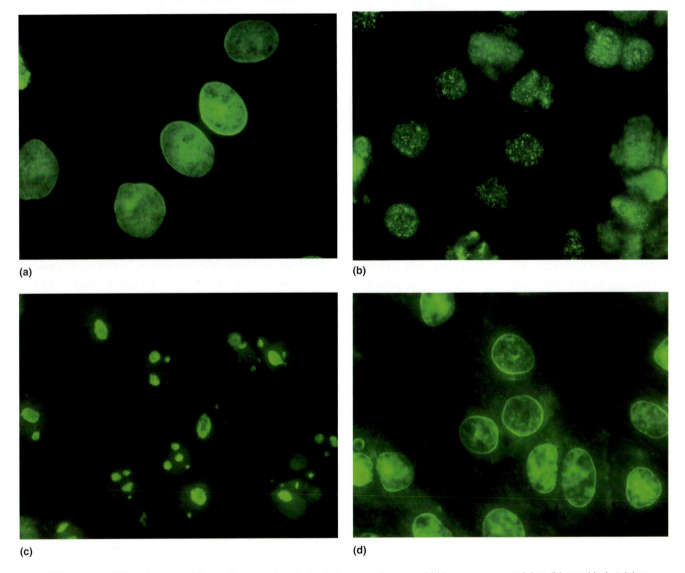

(a) (b) (c) (d)

■ **FIGURE 10.4** Different ANA staining patterns and related autoimmune diseases. (a) Homogeneous staining, (b) speckled staining, (c) nucleolar staining, and (d) peripheral staining. *Source:* Courtesy of Wade J. Sigurdson.

SUBSETS OF ANA

Some of the most specific ANA for SLE are anti-dsDNA anti-bodies, which are valuable diagnostic and prognostic markers for the disease. Anti-dsDNA antibodies are associated with renal damage perhaps because the charge of this antigen is more likely to cause immune complex deposition and entrapment with associated inflammation in the kidneys. Because lower levels of anti-dsDNA antibodies can also be detected in conditions such as certain forms of hepatitis and rheumatic disease, the titers are important in the correct diagnosis of SLE. Titers of more than 80 usually have reliable diagnostic value. Immunofluorescence assays for anti-dsDNA antibodies rely on protozoan called *Crithidia luciliae,* which contains dsDNA in certain intracellular organelles. Binding of a patient's IgG to these organelles indicates the presence of anti-dsDNA antibodies in the patient's serum. In the case of ELISA, dsDNA is bound to the ELISA plate and the patient's serum is tested for the presence of anti-dsDNA antibodies following standard ELISA procedures (11). Anti-dsDNA antibodies are found in more than 70% of SLE patients but in less than 1% in subjects without SLE.

Anti-Sm antibodies are found almost exclusively in SLE because they are not commonly seen in other autoimmune conditions. However, only 10 to 25% of SLE patients have anti-Sm antibodies, so their absence does not exclude SLE. Anti-histone antibodies, as the name implies, react to histones, the nuclear proteins that are the main components of chromatin. Almost three quarters of patients with SLE have anti-histone antibodies, and this percentage rises to more than 95% in patients with drug-induced lupus erythematosus. ELISA detects anti-histone antibodies.

Other autoantibodies in SLE include antibodies to the SS-A (Ro) and SS-B (La) antigens. The SS-A antigens are polypeptides complexed to RNA. Antibodies to SS-A antigens are found in 10 to 50% of patients with SLE and are strongly associated with certain subtypes of SLE, including subacute lupus erythematosus and drug-induced subacute lupus erythematosus and in patients with hereditary C2, C4, or C1q deficiency with lupus or lupuslike disease, but antibodies to SS-A indicate Sjögren's syndrome because about 70% of patients with it have these antibodies. SS-B (La) is a single extractable nuclear antigen, and antibodies to SS-B are observed in about 10% of patients with SLE and are found in about 60% of patients with Sjögren's syndrome. Both SS-A and SS-B have also been shown to be risk factors for heart conduction block in neonatal lupus.

Antibodies to RNP are also found in SLE. Of patients with SLE, 20 to 40% exhibit anti-RNP antibodies, although they are also found in Sjögren's syndrome and other autoimmune conditions. Antibodies to topoisomerase are also found in different autoimmune conditions. Topoisomerase is an enzyme that unwinds DNA; anti Scl-70 is an antibody against topoisomerase 1. Testing for anti-Scl-70 is also of diagnostic value because it is more prevalent in progressive systemic sclerosis and scleroderma. Other tests for SLE include the evaluation of the levels of complement components; inflammatory responses can "use up" these components as part of the immunological mechanisms of inflammation, and thus low levels of these components may be associated with SLE.

 Checkpoint! 10.3

Why would patients with SLE be recommended to avoid intense sunlight?

TREATMENT

There is no known cure for SLE; however, survival rates are encouraging. Because of the complexity of symptomology and clinical involvement in SLE, treatment modalities can vary from one individual to another and, in general, are directed to decrease the clinical manifestation of the disease itself. Anti-inflammatory drugs such as corticosteroids are commonly used; in the case of lupus nephritis (eg, as diffuse proliferative glomerulonephritis), the use of cytotoxic drugs such as cyclophosphamide or mycophenolate may be required. Disease-modifying anti-rheumatic drugs (DMARDs) can be used to reduce the incidence of flares. Because pain is a common symptom in SLE, analgesics, treatment from over-the-counter NSAIDs (eg, ibuprofen) to prescription analgesics such as hydrocodone are commonly indicated. Behaviorally, avoiding sunlight is recommended because cell death due to ultraviolet (UV) exposure supplies antigen for immune complex formation. In severe cases, such as end-stage renal disease, renal transplantation is also indicated.

▶ RHEUMATOID ARTHRITIS

Rheumatoid arthritis (RA) is a destructive inflammatory disease that primarily affects the synovial joints (1, 12) including carpal, wrist, elbow, shoulder, knee, ankle, feet, and hip joints. The inflammation in RA can also affect the tissues associated with the lungs and heart. Nodular lesions underneath the skin can be seen in RA, as can skin ulcerations, dry eyes, dry mouth, pulmonary nodules, and pulmonary interstitial fibrosis. RA affects about 1% of the population and occurs throughout the world. It tends to be more prevalent as people age with its frequency being more common at the ages of 40 to 50 (although it can manifest itself at any age), and, as is often the case for autoimmune diseases, it affects women 3 times more than men.

Like other autoimmune diseases, RA has a genetic basis; subjects with the HLA DR4 alleles have the strongest association with RA (see Table 10.1). RA is a **polyarthritis** with diverse clinical manifestations; people most commonly experience symmetrical joint swelling and pain, stiffness, tiredness, and a general feeling of discomfort. Uncontrolled RA eventually

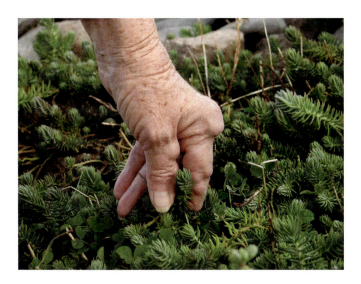

■ **FIGURE 10.5** Deformation of the hand from rheumatoid arthritis. *Source:* Sue McDonald/Shutterstock.com.

leads to joint damage, deformity, and disability. A deformation of the hand from RA appears in Figure 10.5 ■, and a radiograph of joint damage and deformity is in Figure 10.6 ■. These are typical of RA and are due to synovial inflammation and destruction of the joints of the fingers and wrist joints. Swelling of the area is also common as is a localized feeling of warmth and tenderness. Functionally, the range of motion and the strength of handgrip decrease with time (12).

PATHOPHYSIOLOGY

No single specific cause of RA has been described; in fact, little is known about the factors that may be directly involved in the development of RA. It has been proposed that environmental factors, along with hormonal factors, infections,

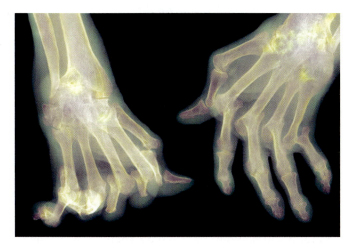

■ **FIGURE 10.6** Joint deformities from rheumatoid arthritis. *Source:* CNRI/Photo Researchers, Inc.

and **superantigens,** may play a role in its development in a genetically susceptible individual. Some microorganisms have been suggested to play a role in the development of autoimmunity in RA through molecular mimicry, but this remains controversial, and large epidemiological studies have not confirmed it. The molecular mechanisms involved in the clinical manifestations of the disease are the classical mechanisms of a chronic inflammatory condition. Pro-inflammatory cytokines such as IL-1, IL-6, IL-8, IL-15, IL-18, and TNF-α, are commonly found in the synovial fluid of RA patients.

A **pannus** (a general medical term for a granuloma tissue deposited due to inflammatory processes) eventually forms in the joints and overruns the cartilage; cells that are associated with the pannus include CD4+ T cells, CD8+ T cells, B cells, plasma cells, macrophages, and neutrophils. The complex network of these cells and proinflammatory cytokines creates an environment that results in a continuous state of chronic inflammation. The starting spark that initiates these processes is the presence of immune complexes that become deposited in the joints and start the inflammatory cascade.

The role of autoantibodies in the pathogenesis of RA is still debated; however, a common finding in RA is the presence of IgM antibodies (although they can also be of different isotypes) reacting to the Fc portion of IgG, resulting in the formation of immune complexes. This anti-IgG antibody has been termed **rheumatoid factor (RF)** and is found in more than 70% of all RA subjects. However, it is also found in a small percentage of healthy subjects and in up to 20% of subjects over the age of 65. Therefore, the presence of RF indicates rheumatoid arthritis but is not a conclusive diagnosis. The deposition of these immune complexes in the joints activates the classical complement pathway (see Chapter 5), initiating a cascade of events that ultimately result in the inflammatory damage. Activation of complement results in the production of chemoattractants that recruit macrophages and neutrophils at the site. These cells can cause both tissue destruction as well as propagation of the inflammatory response. Activation of macrophages results in the generation of proinflammatory cytokines, which, in turn, recruit additional cells and amplify the response. Antigen presentation and T-cell activation further expand the reaction; in fact, a recently developed strategy for treating RA is based on blocking T-cell co-stimulation by antigen-presenting cells, suggesting an important role of activated T cells in the pathological mechanisms of RA.

In addition to inflammation, physical changes contribute to the damage: the pannus generated from the synovial membrane proliferates, invading the cartilage and eventually the bone. The cartilage is destroyed, the bone under the joint is eroded, and ligaments become lax. Some of the cytokines released stimulate osteoclasts to cause bone erosion, and eventually osteoporosis in the areas of the joints occurs. The question remains as to what the original antigen that results in the formation of immune complexes is.

Components that have been identified as important antibodies for diagnosis are antibodies to cyclic citrullinated peptides, which are circular peptides containing the amino acid citrulline; antibodies against cyclic citrullinated peptides (anti-CCP) recognize antigens that contain arginyl converted to citrullyl residues by the enzyme peptidylarginine deiminase. This enzyme is found in various cells including neutrophils and macrophages, and cyclic citrullinated peptides may be produced upon the death of these cells. The overproduction of these cyclic citrullinated peptides may cause an autoimmune response in certain susceptible individuals. Studies have demonstrated that anti-CCP antibodies can be found in over two-thirds of RA patients with a specificity of more than 95%. In fact, for the past several years, anti-CCP antibodies have become a highly specific and fairly sensitive diagnostic test for RA. Interestingly, the presence of RF and anti-CCP antibodies can be detected without the presence of clinical symptoms and often well before these clinical symptoms become evident. This suggests that the events leading to the pathology seen in RA can start well before there is clinical evidence of it.

 Checkpoint! 10.4

Given the importance of activated T cells in the pathological mechanisms of RA, why are superantigens suspected as a factor in RA?

DIAGNOSIS AND TESTING

Some time ago the American College of Rheumatology developed a set of 7 criteria for the classification of RA. See: http://www.rheumatology.org/practice/clinical/classification/ra/ra.asp for complete list. For RA to be considered, a patient should have at least 4 of the 7 criteria. Criteria 1 through 4 must be present for at least 6 weeks. This classification system was not designed to diagnose RA but to evaluate a patient suspected of suffering from RA. The criteria were to be used by clinicians to narrow the diagnosis and follow up with more specific testing. A much more comprehensive set of criteria has recently updated this classification (13). Although the clinical manifestations of RA are characteristic of the disease, diagnosis can be difficult, especially in its early stages. Therefore, diagnosis of RA depends on a combination of medical history, physical observations, symptomology, radiographic analysis, and laboratory tests. In the early stages of RA, no drastic physical changes may be observed either by visual or x-ray inspection. Later, some osteopenia may be observed along with localized swelling and a decrease of space in the area of the joints. In the later stages bone erosion, deformation and joint dislocation are observed (Figures 10.5 and 10.6). In recent years, in addition to x-rays, techniques such as magnetic resonance and ultrasounds have been used in subjects with RA. Doppler and power Doppler ultrasound can be used to detect actual active **synovitis,** which has been a good predictor of joint damage.

Laboratory tests for RA include assessing for rheumatoid factor (Figure 10.7 ■) and for anti-CCP antibodies (12, 14). As mentioned, RF can suggest the presence of RA; however, RF is also found in normal individuals and in some other conditions such as Sjögren's syndrome, and certain forms of hepatitis, so a positive RF test per se does not always indicate RA. Likewise, roughly 15% of subjects with RA are not positive for the RF test, especially in the early stages of the disease, so a negative RF test does not exclude RA. Anti-CCP antibodies are present in about 70% of RA cases but are rarely seen in subjects without RA, giving them a specificity of roughly 95%.

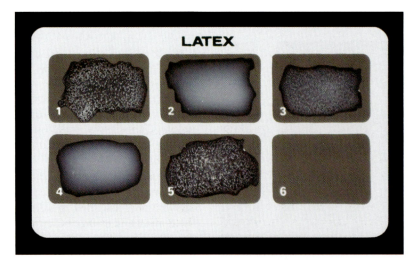

■ **FIGURE 10.7** A latex agglutination test for rheumatoid factor. A positive control at 1. A negative control at 2. A positive patient at 3 and 5. A negative patient at 4.

TREATMENT

As with SLE, there is no cure for RA. Physical and occupational therapy along with analgesics are common palliative treatments for RA. As expected, anti-inflammatory drugs including NSAIDs and steroids are used; in addition, disease-modifying antirheumatic drugs (DMARDs) are used in an attempt to diminish the autoimmune inflammatory reactions and diminish tissue damage (15). Because TNF-α is a pivotal inflammatory cytokine in RA, approaches that block its actions are used in the treatment of RA. These include the use of monoclonal antibody preparations against TNF-α (eg, infliximab) and etanercept, a recombinant fusion protein engineered to link a TNF receptor to an immunoglobulin molecule. This large, synthetic molecule binds to TNF-α and interferes with its function.

► OTHER COMMON TESTS

Because autoimmune diseases are inflammatory in nature, tests for common markers of inflammation are also performed for the different diseases (14) to monitor inflammation levels after diagnosis. These procedures include measuring erythrocyte sedimentation rates (ESR) and levels of C-reactive protein (CRP). CRP, an acute phase reactant (see Chapter 1) was so named because when first identified, it reacted to the C-polysaccharide of *Streptococcus pneumoniae*. ESR measures how many red blood cells precipitate in a tube as a function of time. This, in turn, depends on the concentration of various other serum proteins in the blood sample to be tested. Because inflammation is usually associated with a decrease in the serum concentration of these proteins, red blood cells tend to precipitate faster; therefore, inflammation relates to an increase in ESR. Thus, ESR can be used to monitor levels of inflammation and the relationship of the levels to either disease progression or effectiveness of therapeutic approaches. Caution must be exerted in the interpretation of results because single factors such as age, gender, and concentrations of hemoglobin and immunoglobulins can affect ESR.

Proinflammatory cytokines can also stimulate the liver to produce certain acute phase proteins such as CRP, fibrinogen, and haptoglobin. CRP is an opsonin that can activate the complement cascade and can contribute to the elimination of dead cells and of some microorganisms by binding to phosphocholine on the surface of a dying cell or a bacterium. In addition to activating complement, the binding of CRP to the dying cell or bacterium attracts phagocytes, which, in turn, phagocytose them. The levels of CRP can rise as much as several thousandfold during an acute inflammatory episode and therefore is used as a diagnostic parameter to monitor inflammation. Levels of CRP of more than 1 mg/dl are considered to be markers of either an infection or ongoing inflammation. CRP is also elevated in inflammatory cardiovascular diseases,

and it is usually measured using a high-sensitivity solid phase chemiluminescent assay.

⊘ CASE STUDY

In your immunology laboratory course, your professor always has used her serum as a negative control for the antinuclear antibody test. She had only 0.4 ml remaining, so she aliquoted 0.2 ml for the dilutions to be made for the students sitting at tables 1 and 2 in the lab class. For the students at table 3, her blood was drawn and new serum was prepared. Table 2 also used an aliquot of the new serum to have a second negative control because students at it had a well remaining. Although your professor's samples from last year were negative, this year, both table 2 and table 3 see speckled staining at a 1:64 dilution of the professor's serum sample.

1. What should be done?

SUMMARY

Autoimmune diseases are conditions in which, for various reasons, the immune system has a dysfunction in its ability to distinguish self versus nonself and result in an immune reaction against self-antigens. Factors that may cause autoimmunity are under investigation; the causes often remain unknown. However, several possibilities have been proposed, including a failure of mechanisms of central tolerance and, more likely, those of peripheral tolerance including regulatory mechanisms that usually prevent self-reactivity. Genetics and gender play a major role in the susceptibility to autoimmunity, and autoimmune diseases tend to be more prevalent in women than men. Environmental factors also contribute to autoimmunity, and immunological cross-reactivity with certain microbial antigens, a phenomenon termed *molecular mimicry*, can cause autoimmunity. The tissue destruction or altered functions seen in autoimmunity are caused by the same immunological mechanisms of a normal response against nonself-antigens; these can include destructive antibodies, immune complexes deposition, cytotoxic T cells, complement, and recruitment of inflammatory cells. In addition, antibodies can also be agonistic or antagonistic, resulting in either hyperstimulation or blocking of a particular organ function.

Autoimmune diseases can be functionally divided into systemic and organ or tissue specific. Systemic autoimmune diseases involve immune complexes that form in various parts of the body and travel in the circulation causing inflammation wherever they are deposited. On the other hand, organ or tissue-specific autoimmune diseases, as the name implies, target antigens that are expressed on a specific organ or tissue. A quintessential example of a systemic autoimmune disease is systemic lupus erythematosus (SLE), a condition that is characterized by autoantibodies to nuclear antigens including nucleic acids and nuclear proteins, with immune complex formation that can affect blood cells, blood vessels, skin, joints, lungs, kidneys, liver, the nervous system, and the heart. No single cause for SLE has been found; however, abnormalities in apoptosis and defective clearance of apoptotic cells have been proposed as possible causes. There is no cure for SLE; however, survival rates are good. Treatment usually focuses on anti-inflammatory drugs and analgesics. Diagnostic tests include evaluation of antinuclear antibodies and their subsets by immunofluorescence and ELISA. Rheumatoid arthritis (RA) is a destructive inflammatory disease that primarily affects the synovial joints, although it can also affect the lungs, heart, and skin. As is the case with SLE, RA is more common in women than men. No single cause of RA is known, but molecular mimicry has been suggested as a potential one. Diagnosis and testing for RA involve medical history, physical observation, radiographs, and laboratory testing for rheumatoid factor, certain ANA, and anti-CCP antibodies. Treatment for RA includes the use of anti-inflammatory drugs, disease-modifying antirheumatic drugs (DMARDs), and analgesics along with physical therapy. Because autoimmune diseases are inflammatory in nature, other common tests include markers of inflammation such as erythrocyte sedimentation rates (ERS) and levels of C-reactive protein (CRP).

LABORATORY EXERCISE

OBJECTIVES

AFFECTIVE DOMAIN

1. In this laboratory and all others, behave in a manner that shows respect for the patient's sample.

COGNITIVE DOMAIN

1. Discuss rheumatoid factor and its disease associations.
2. Discuss 4 methods of detecting and quantitating rheumatoid factor.

PSYCHOMOTOR DOMAIN

1. Perform and interpret the results of a latex agglutination slide test for detection of rheumatoid factor.
2. Create an experiment to show whether a negative result seen at a low dilution was caused by a prozone effect.

RHEUMATOID FACTOR

Rheumatoid factor (RF) is an autoantibody (usually of the IgM class) directed against the Fc portion of IgG. It can be found in 70 to 80% of the cases of rheumatoid arthritis, and in several other diseases. RF is found in SLE, scleroderma, Sjögren's syndrome, hepatitis, syphilis, and patients with TB. Chronic presence of immune complexes in chronic infections or autoimmune diseases increases the likelihood of developing rheumatoid factor. Of healthy individuals, 1 to 4% may also have RF but at low titers (less than 20). The highest titers of RF are found in individuals with the most severe disease.

LABORATORY

MATERIALS

1. Sure-Vue RF Rapid latex beads coated with human IgG
2. Positive control serum (human)
3. Negative control serum (human)

4. Disposable latex agglutination slides

5. Wooden stir sticks

6. Patient's serum diluted 1:40

PROCEDURES

1. With a partner, add 1 drop of the positive control to the first section. Add 1 drop of the negative control to the second section. Add 1 drop (or 50 microliters) of your diluted patient's serum to the third section, and have your partner add 1 drop of the second patient's diluted serum to the next section.

2. Mix the latex-globulin reagent using gentle inversions of the container. Using the dropper, add 1 drop of the reagent to each section. Mix each section separately using a new stirrer. Discard stirrers in sharps containers. Spread the fluid in the section.

3. After the last section has been mixed, rotate the slide for 1 minute. At the end of 1 minute, observe the slide for agglutination. You will see aggregation of the particles, which will result in clearing of the milky suspension of the particles to form a clear solution with white aggregates. Reaction time is important; after a prolonged period, the rate of false positives will increase. *Note:* The positive control should show agglutination while the negative control should not.

4. It is possible to quantitate the positive sera by preparing a serial 2-fold dilution of the sera in the recommended diluent, starting at 1:40, and reacting each dilution with 1 drop of the latex-globulin reagent. The titer is the reciprocal of the highest dilution that exhibits definite agglutination. A titer of greater than 80 is considered a positive reaction. A titer of 20 or 40 is considered a weakly positive reaction.

LABORATORY EXERCISE

OBJECTIVES

ANTINUCLEAR ANTIBODY

AFFECTIVE DOMAIN

1. Always use fresh reagents and cells for analysis of ANA to lessen the chance of misinterpretation of patient results.

COGNITIVE DOMAIN

1. Explain the principles of direct and indirect immunofluorescence and the advantages of the latter.

2. List several diseases associated with a positive ANA.

3. Discuss 6 methods of detecting antinuclear antibody.

4. Discuss the heterogeneity of antinuclear antibody.

5. Describe the 4 patterns of fluorescence.

6. Explain the importance of washing after each step in the procedure.

7. Compare and contrast excitation light and emission light

8. Discuss ANA antibodies in terms of staining pattern seen and the disease with which it is associated.

LABORATORY EXERCISE *(continued)*

PSYCHOMOTOR DOMAIN

1. Prepare serial dilutions of a patient's serum for ANA analysis.

2. Prepare an ANA slide using a commercially prepared substrate and perform an assay of various patient sera.

3. Interpret what is seen under the fluorescent microscope for each of the 4 main staining patterns for ANA. Develop the expertise to evaluate patients' serum samples in relation to the presence or absence of these 4 patterns of staining.

Antinuclear antibody (ANA) is actually a family of *autoantibodies* directed against various component antigens in the nucleus. Patients with autoimmune diseases (formerly called *collagen vascular diseases*) have a high incidence and high titer of ANA. Therefore, the ANA assay can be used as a screening test for these diseases, particularly SLE, in which 95% of patients are positive for ANA.

Antinuclear antibodies are measured in this test on tissue culture fibroblasts (Hep-2 cell line). The nuclear antigen must be accessible to the serum antibody, must be present in sufficient concentration, and must maintain reactivity after processing.

The *conjugate* used in the indirect test was prepared by first immunizing a goat with human immunoglobulin. The fluorochrome substance conjugated to antibody is a fluorescent compound. Its electrons can absorb ultraviolet light energy, jump to a high-energy orbital, and then return to the ground state, emitting light energy of a longer wavelength and heat energy. The fluorescent microscope used to examine the slide can use a light source to provide the excitation light. A filter is in place so that through the ocular of the microscope, only the emission wavelength is observed.

To test for antinuclear antibody, sections of Hep-2 are used as the antigen substrate. When this substrate is overlaid with the patient's serum, ANA antibodies, if present, will bind to nuclear antigens in the Hep-2 cells.

After incubation with the cell substrate, the excess serum is removed by washing, and fluorescein-isothiocyanate (FITC) labeled anti-human IgG is added. After incubation, the slide is washed to remove unbound FITC labeled anti-IgG and observed under the fluorescence microscope.

The first wash step is important because there are many other immunoglobulins present in the serum, and without a thorough wash step, the FITC-anti-human globulin would bind the nonbinding immunoglobulin, decreasing the reaction with the bound antibodies. The second wash step is important because failure to adequately remove unbound FITC-anti-human IgG could result in high background and even a false positive result.

The presence of ANA in the serum sample is demonstrated by green fluorescence in the nucleus when observed under a fluorescence microscope. The serum is initially screened at 1:40 dilution to avoid prozone and nonspecific fluorescence. Positive sera are then serially diluted and tested again to determine a titer. The titer is the reciprocal of the highest dilution that shows fluorescence. ANA can be seen on many different cell types, but for clinical consistency, titers are obtained using HEp-2 cells.

LABORATORY

MATERIALS

1. ImmuGloAutoantibody test system from Immcodiagnostics

2. Fluorescence microscope

3. ANA Positive patients serum

4. Negative control

5. Moist chamber

6. Buffered diluent, pH 7.1

PROCEDURES

1. To avoid damaging cells, carefully remove the substrate slide from the foil bag that has been allowed to reach room temperature.

2. Label the slide on the frosted end and place the slide in the moist chamber.

3. Place 50 μL of positive control into circle 1 and 50 μL of negative control into circle 2.

4. Place 50 μL of a 1:40 dilution of each sample into the remaining circles.

5. Place the lid on the moist chamber and incubate the slide for 30 minutes at room temperature.

6. Remove the slide from chamber and rinse it with phosphate-buffered saline, and then wash 10 minutes in PBS bath in Coplin jar.

7. Tap the edge of the slide on the paper towel to remove excess phosphate-buffered saline. Replace the slide in the moist chamber and immediately add 1 drop of anti-human IgG conjugate per well. *Do not allow the slide to dry.*

8. Replace the lid on the moist chamber and incubate the slide with anti-human IgG conjugate for 20 minutes at room temperature.

9. Remove the lid from the chamber, remove the slide, and rinse it with 10 ml of phosphate-buffered saline. Transfer slide to a Coplin jar containing PBS with 3 drops of Evans Blue counterstain for 10 minutes.

10. Remove the slide from the Coplin jar and tap it on the paper towel to remove excess moisture. Put 3 drops of mounting medium at the lower edge of the slide, add the cover slip, and allow the air bubbles to escape.

11. Examine the slide under the fluorescence microscope under high power. Read the slide within 48 hours.

Fluorescent staining of the nucleus may be classified by pattern as follows:

- A *diffuse* (homogenous) pattern is defined as a uniform, solid fluorescent stain throughout the nucleus.

- A *peripheral* pattern has a characteristic fluorescent staining of the rim or edge of the nucleus.

- A *nucleolar* pattern refers to fluorescent staining of the nucleolus.

- A *speckled* pattern has numerous, discrete specks of fluorescent staining throughout the nucleus.

- If a patient does not have ANA, the section will look dark, so it is important to check that you are in focus. Turn on the white light, and you should observe the Evans Blue–stained cells in focus.

- More than 1 staining pattern may be seen in the same sample.

The ANA *titer* is important clinically. A titer of 40 is borderline, 80 is low positive, and greater than 160 is high positive.

REVIEW QUESTIONS

1. Rheumatoid arthritis is
   a. more common in whites than in blacks
   b. most common in people with Asian backgrounds
   c. most commonly initially diagnosed in individuals 30 to 50 years of age
   d. most common initially diagnosed in individuals over 70 years of age

2. A 40-year-old black female sees her physician with complaints of pains in the joints of both her right and left wrists. She has a rash on both cheeks. On physical examination, edematous swelling of her joints is noticeable. Her rheumatoid factor is positive to a titer of 2. Her lab results show an elevated sedimentation rate and some proteinuria. An ANA is performed, and homogeneous staining of the nuclei is seen with a titer of 640.
   a. The patient's symptoms and lab results suggest SLE.
   b. The patient's symptoms and lab results suggest Lyme disease.
   c. The patient's symptoms and lab results are suggest rheumatoid arthritis.
   d. All of the above.

3. A 45-year-old woman reported to the hospital with swelling in her wrists, knees, and fingers. She reported that her family had a history of SLE. An ANA was performed, and her sera showed homogeneous staining with a titer of 1:20. Latex agglutination for rheumatoid factor was performed, and her titer was 8000. She had proteinuria.
   a. The patient's symptoms and lab results suggest SLE.
   b. The patient's symptoms and lab results suggest Lyme disease.
   c. The patient's symptoms and lab results suggest rheumatoid arthritis.
   d. None of the above.

4. Systemic lupus erythematosus is
   a. a disease that involves linear deposition of IgG in the kidney and, thus, kidney failure develops
   b. a disease that involves lumpy bumpy deposition of IgG and, thus, kidney failure develops
   c. diagnosed solely based on the presence or absence of anti-dsDNA Ab
   d. diagnosed by kidney biopsies that show immunofluorescent staining for human immunoglobulins

5. Which of the following is *not* related to the cause of death for SLE patients?
   a. kidney lesions
   b. glomerulonephritis
   c. dsDNA-Ab complexes
   d. LE cells

6. Rheumatoid arthritis patients have an antibody called *rheumatoid factor*. Which of the following do *not* also express rheumatoid factor?
   a. hepatitis
   b. mononucleosis
   c. tuberculosis
   d. neonates

7. Rheumatoid factor is present in
   a. rheumatoid arthritis patients only
   b. patients with rheumatoid arthritis and with chronic infections
   c. rheumatoid arthritis patients and neonates
   d. patients with rheumatoid arthritis and with DiGeorge's syndrome

8. SLE patients show
   a. hypercomplementemia
   b. species-specific antibody
   c. organ-specific antibody
   d. increased sun sensitivity

9. A speckled pattern in ANA testing indicates
   a. antibody to double-stranded DNA or histones
   b. antibody to nucleolar RNA
   c. antibody to Sm, SS-A, SS-B, Scl-70, or RNP
   d. antibody to dsDNA

10. A rim pattern in ANA testing indicates
    a. antibody to double-stranded DNA or histones
    b. antibody to nucleolar RNA
    c. antibody to Sm, SS-A, SS-B, Scl-70, or RNP
    d. antibody to dsDNA

REFERENCES

1. Janeway CA, Travers P, Walport M, et al. *Immunobiology.* 6th ed. New York, NY: Garland Publishing; 2005.

2. Klein J, Sato A. The HLA system: Second of two parts. *N Engl J Med.* 2000;343:782–786.

3. Rahman A, Isenberg DA. Systemic Lupus Erythematosus. *N Engl J Med.* 2008;358(9):929–939.

4. Bartels CM, Muller D. Systemic lupus erythematosus: Differential diagnoses & workup. eMedicine. 2010. http://emedicine.medscape.com/article/332244-diagnosis. Acessed 3/17/2012

5. Mendoza-Pinto C, García-Carrasco M, Sandoval-Cruz H, et al. Risk factors of vertebral fractures in women with systemic lupus erythematosus. *Clin Rheumatol.* 2009;28:579–585.

6. Asanuma Y, Oeser A, Shintani AK, et al. Premature coronary-artery atherosclerosis in systemic lupus erythematosus. *N Engl J Med.* 2003;349:2407–2414.

7. The American College of Rheumatology nomenclature and case definitions for neuropsychiatric lupus syndromes. *Arthritis Rheum.* 1999;42:599–608.

8. Cohen PL. Apoptotic cell death and lupus. *Springer Sem Immunol.* 2006;28:145–152.

9. Muñoz LE, Lauber K, Schiller M, et al. The role of defective clearance of apoptotic cells in systemic autoimmunity. *Nat Rev Rheumatol.* 2010;6:280–289.

10. Nagata S, Hanayama R, Kawane K. Autoimmunity and the clearance of dead cells. *Cell.* 2010;140:619–630.

11. Castro C, Gourley M. Diagnostic testing and interpretation of tests for autoimmunity. *J Allergy Clin Immunol.* 2010;125:S238–S247.

12. Majithia V, Geraci SA. Rheumatoid arthritis: Diagnosis and management. *Am J Med.* 2007;120:936–939.

13. Aletaha D, et al. 2010 Rheumatoid Arthritis Classification Criteria. *Arthritis & Rheumatism.* 2010;62:2569–2581.

14. Wener MH. *Educational Review Manual in Rheumatology.* 4th ed. New York, NY: Castle Connolly Graduate Medical Publishing; 2007:1–42.

15. Joseph A, Brasington R, Kahl L, et al. Immunologic rheumatic disorders. *J Allergy Clin Immunol.* 2010;125:S204–S215.

PEARSON
myhealthprofessionskit

Visit www.myhealthprofessionskit.com to access the interactive Companion Website for this textbook. Simply select "Clinical Laboratory Science" from the choice of disciplines. Find this book and log in by using your user name and password to access additional learning tools.

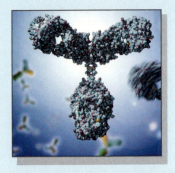

11

Organ and Tissue Specific Autoimmunity

Lucy D. Mastrandrea, M.D., Ph.D.

■ OBJECTIVES—LEVEL I

After this chapter, the student should be able to:

1. Define *organ-specific autoimmunity.*
2. Discuss the utility of screening tools in the diagnosis of autoimmune disorders.
3. Discuss the management of primary autoimmune disorders of the endocrine system.
4. Compare the clinical presentation and causes and effects of autoimmune thyroid diseases.
5. Describe the biologic assays used in the diagnosis of autoimmune hyperthyroidism.
6. Discuss the causes and effects of type 1 diabetes and describe the metabolic abnormalities associated with type 1 diabetes.
7. Describe the autoantibodies associated with the development of type 1 diabetes.
8. Discuss the diagnosis and management of type 1 diabetes.
9. Describe the causes and effects of celiac disease.
10. Discuss screening tools used to identify an individual at risk for celiac disease.
11. Discuss the role of dietary and self-antigens in the development of celiac disease.
12. Discuss role of gluten-free diet in the management of celiac disease.
13. Compare and contrast ulcerative colitis and Crohn's disease.
14. Discuss autoantibodies associated with inflammatory bowel disease.
15. Describe the difference between pemphigus and pemphigoid disorders.
16. Discuss skin pathology associated with celiac disease.
17. Describe the causes and effects of myasthenia gravis.
18. Discuss the autoantibodies associated with myasthenia gravis.
19. Describe the clinical spectrum associated with the diagnosis of multiple sclerosis.
20. Describe the causes and effects of Goodpasture's disease.
21. Discuss the role of autoantibodies in the diagnosis and management of Goodpasture's disease.

KEY TERMS

anorexia
ataxia
cholestasis
exophthalamos
follicle
glomerulonephritis
granulomas
hyperpigmentation
immunologically privileged site

megaloblastic anemia
microsome
oligodendrocyte
plasmapheresis
postsynaptic membrane
primary adrenal insufficiency
sepsis
single nucleotide polymorphism

▶ INTRODUCTION

In Chapter 10 we discussed immune complex mediated autoimmune diseases that affect a variety of organs and tissues, and are thus classified as systemic autoimmune diseases. In this chapter, we will focus on autoimmune conditions that target either specific tissues or specific organ systems.

▶ ENDOCRINE SYSTEM

Three of the top 10 most common autoimmune disorders involve the endocrine system: Graves' disease (autoimmune hyperthyroidism), Hashimoto's thyroiditis (autoimmune hypothyroidism), and type 1 diabetes (Table 11.1 ✪) (1, 2). These diseases are commonly diagnosed in young and middle-aged individuals, significantly impacting the health of those affected. This section reviews those diseases and discusses autoimmune disorders of the adrenal glands and gonads (Table 11.2 ✪).

In most cases, the autoimmune process causes destruction of the gland with concomitant failure of the gland to produce

✪ TABLE 11.1

Prevalence and Sex Distribution of Top 10 Autoimmune Diseases Diagnosed in the United States

Disease	Prevalence per 100 000	Female:Male
Hashimoto's thyroiditis*	1324	90:10
Graves' disease	1259	88:12
Rheumatoid arthritis†	1008	70:30
Vitiligo	400	52:48
Type 1 diabetes	192	48:52
Pernicious anemia	151	67:33
Multiple sclerosis	54	63:37
Glomerulonephritis	40	33:67
Systemic lupus erythematosis	24	88:12
Addison's disease	14	93:7

Prevalence represents the number of individuals with a disease at a given period of time.

*Ages 10 years and older.

†Includes individuals with juvenile rheumatoid arthritis.

⭐ **TABLE 11.2**

Summary of Autoimmune Diseases Involving the Endocrine System

Organ System	Organ	Disease	Type of Immune Response	Antigen	Assay for Diagnosis	Clinical Effects
Endocrine	Thyroid	Hashimoto's thyroiditis	Cellular and antibody	Thyroglobulin Thyroperoxidase TSH-binding inhibitory antibody	Elevated TSH Low thyroxine Thyroglobulin and thyroperoxidase antibodies • IFA • ELISA • Passive Hemaglutinin	Poor energy Fatigue Weight gain Cold intolerance Enlarged thyroid Dry skin Hair loss Constipation
		Graves' disease	Antibody	Thyroid-stimulating hormone receptor antibody Thyroperoxidase	Suppressed TSH Elevated thyroxine Antibody to thyroid-stimulating hormone receptor (TSI) • Biologic assay • Radiobinding	Weight loss Anxiety Difficulty sleeping Rapid heart rate Heat intolerance Protruding eyes Enlarged thyroid Tremor
	Pancreas	Type I diabetes mellitus	Cellular	Pancreatic β cells Insulin	Elevated blood sugars Glucose in urine Pancreatic β-cell antibodies • Glutamic acid decarboxylase-65 (GAD-65) • Insulin–associated antigen Insulin • ELISA • IFA • Radiobinding • RIA	Weight loss Increased thirst Increased appetite Increased urination Bedwetting
	Adrenal	Addison's disease Primary adrenal insufficiency	Cellular and antibody	Adrenal cortex steroidogenic cells	Low cortisol Elevated ACTH Low sodium 21-hydroxylase antibody • Radiobinding • ELISA Adrenal cortex antibodies • IFA	Poor energy Weight loss Poor appetite Bronzing of skin Salt craving Dehydration Low blood pressure
	Ovary	Primary ovarian failure	Cellular and antibody	Steroidogenic cells	Low estradiol Elevated gonadotropins Ovarian antibodies • IFA	Amenorrhea Osteoporosis Infertility Delayed puberty

⊘ **TABLE 11.2**

Summary of Autoimmune Diseases Involving the Endocrine System *(continued)*

Organ System	Organ	Disease	Type of Immune Response	Antigen	Assay for Diagnosis	Clinical Effects
	Testicular	Primary testicular failure	Cellular and antibody	Steroidogenic cells	Low testosterone Elevated gonadotropins Low sperm counts Steroidal cell antibodies • IFA	Infertility Impotence Poor energy Bone loss
	Sperm	Low sperm count	Antibody	Sperm	Low sperm counts Sperm antibodies • Immunobead agglutinization	Infertility

adequate amounts of the corresponding hormone, although in Graves' disease, the autoimmune process actually causes increased production of the associated hormone. Failure of the gland to produce the corresponding hormone is exemplified when a child develops type 1 diabetes mellitus because autoimmune destruction of the β cells within the pancreatic islet of Langerhans leads to decreased release of insulin. As a result, cells are not able to take up glucose and high blood glucose, or hyperglycemia, develops. Increased blood glucose causes symptoms of increased thirst and urination. Reliance on alternate energy sources (fat and protein) causes accumulation of free fatty acids and ketones, resulting in acetone-scented breath and urine ketones. These are both signs of newly diagnosed or poorly controlled type 1 diabetes.

THYROID GLAND

The thyroid gland located in the front of the neck is a shield-shaped organ that is composed of **follicles** lined with cuboidal epithelial cells and filled with a colloid. The colloid contains thyroglobulin, a glycoprotein from which thyroid hormones T3 and T4 are synthesized. Every cell in the body has a nuclear receptor for thyroid hormone; thus, this hormone is essential for a multitude of cellular functions, including neuron development, bone metabolism, cholesterol metabolism, normal linear growth, muscle contractility, and basal metabolic rate. The production of thyroid hormone is driven by a feedback system in which the pituitary produces thyroid-stimulating hormone (TSH), which binds to receptors on the thyroid and leads to increased production of thyroid hormones (thyroxine) T3 and T4. Thyroxine, in turn, by feedback inhibition can downregulate production of TSH by the pituitary (Figure 11.1 ■). Autoimmune thyroid disease represents a family of organ-specific disorders that affect thyroid gland function. Understanding the feedback pathways between the pituitary gland and thyroid gland can aid in the diagnosis of autoimmune thyroid disease.

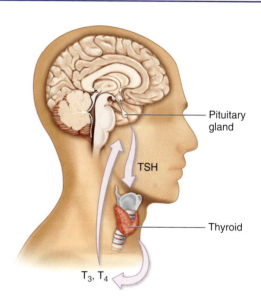

■ **FIGURE 11.1** Thyroid hormone production—Relationship between pituitary and thyroid glands. Thyroid hormone synthesis is primarily mediated by thyroid stimulating hormone (TSH), which is secreted by the pituitary in response to thyrotropin-releasing hormone (TRH) by the hypothalamus. Thyroid hormone (T4 and T3) is released into the serum in free form or bound to thyroid-binding globulin (TBG). Free thyroxine (free T4) exerts negative feedback at both the level of the pituitary and hypothalamus to decrease TSH release.

Autoimmune Thyroid Disease

Thyroid autoimmunity represents one of the most common organ-specific autoimmune diseases, affecting ~12% of the general population. The hallmark of autoimmune thyroid disease is the presence of serum autoantibodies against thyroglobulin or thyroid peroxidase. An individual with serologic evidence of autoimmunity may present in one of three biochemical states: hypothyroid, hyperthyroid, or normal thyroid function. The latter state, characterized by normal thyroid function tests with the presence of positive thyroid antibodies, is the most common clinical scenario. This particular diagnosis affects 5 to 10% of the general population. Autoimmune thyroid disease is more common in females, and prevalence tends to increase with age (3).

There is a strong genetic component to autoimmune thyroid disease with clustering of hypothyroidism (Hashimoto's disease) and hyperthyroidism (Graves' disease) within families. Genetic susceptibility genes to autoimmune thyroid disease have been linked to HLA-DR3 and HLA-DR5 alleles (4). In addition, specific polymorphisms in the cytotoxic T lymphocyte-associated antigen-4 (CTLA-4) gene are strongly linked to autoimmune hyperthyroidism whereas others are associated with increased risk of hypothyroid disease. The CTLA-4 gene protein product is an important negative regulator of T-cell immune response. CTLA-4 is expressed on the surface of T cells and is responsible for modulating the differentiation of T cells that recognize self-antigens. Therefore, polymorphisms that lead to mutations in the protein product may result in proliferation of T cells capable of inducing autoimmune disease. An additional genetic risk factor for the development of autoimmune thyroid disease is the protein tyrosine phosphatase 22 (PTPN22) gene. It is hypothesized that mutations in this enzyme allow self-reactive T cells to proliferate. A **single nucleotide polymorphism** has been linked to increased risk of Graves' disease.

Chronic Autoimmune Thyroiditis

Also known as Hashimoto's thyroiditis, chronic autoimmune thyroiditis is characterized by elevated TSH levels with either normal (compensated) or low thyroxine levels and positive thyroid antibodies. Autoimmune thyroiditis is caused by activation of CD4 T-helper lymphocytes that react to specific thyroid antigens (5). These activated CD4 cells recruit CD8 cytotoxic T cells that are responsible for the destruction of the gland. The antibodies associated with Hashimoto's thyroiditis are antithyroglobulin, antithyroid peroxidase (formerly called *thyroid microsomal antigen*) and TSH-binding inhibitory antibody among others. Although measurement of autoantibodies is important for diagnosing the disease, antibody titer does not correlate with disease activity.

Autoimmune hypothyroidism is suspected in individuals with a goiter or enlarged thyroid gland (Figure 11.2 ■). If thyroid hormone levels are low, the patient may have low energy levels, weight gain, dry skin, brittle hair, constipation, cold intolerance, and apathy. Women may also experience menstrual irregularity or infertility. Severe hypothyroidism in children is associated with growth failure, which resolves when normal thyroid hormone levels are restored. Individuals with hypothyroidism have elevated TSH, low thyroid levels, and positive thyroid antibodies. Hypothyroidism is treated with daily oral thyroxine replacement based on TSH levels.

Graves' Disease

Autoimmune-mediated hyperthyroidism, also known as *Graves' disease*, is diagnosed in 1% of individuals with autoimmune thyroid disease and is more common in women than

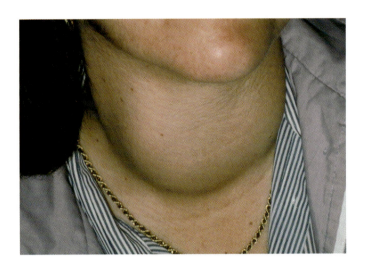

■ **FIGURE 11.2**   Goiter as commonly seen in autoimmune thyroid disease. *Source:* SPL / Photo Researchers, Inc.

in men. Individuals with Graves' disease have signs of thyroid hormone excess: weight loss, anxiety, difficulty sleeping, rapid heart rate, heat intolerance, and tremor. Patients, particularly children, may also have difficulty concentrating, so hyperthyroidism may interfere with school success. Physical exam findings that are consistent with the hyperthyroid state include goiter (enlarged thyroid gland with swelling in the neck), increased heart rate and blood pressure, tremor, restlessness, brisk reflexes, and muscle weakness. **Exophthalmos,** which is manifested by stare and prominent bulging of the eye, is a physical finding associated with Graves' disease (6).

Laboratory diagnosis of Graves' disease is made by measuring TSH, which will be suppressed, and thyroid hormone levels, which will be elevated. Antithyroglobulin and thyroperoxidase antibodies are often elevated but are not specific for Graves' disease. The hyperthyroid state is the result of a biologically active autoantibody, thyroid-stimulating immunoglobulin (TSI), which binds to the TSH receptor on thyroid follicular cells and stimulates thyroid hormone release independent of TSH.

Graves' disease is treated by controlling both high blood pressure and elevated heart rate and decreasing thyroid hormone production. Patients are treated initially with drugs to block thyroid hormone production. Definitive therapy involves surgical resection or radioablation of the gland with ^{131}Iodine followed by thyroid hormone replacement. Interestingly, Graves' disease resolves spontaneously within 2 years of diagnosis in about 30% of the cases (7). However, these patients may evolve to an autoimmune-mediated hypothyroid state and require thyroxine replacement. Therefore, thyroid function tests should be followed on a regular basis in this population.

Measurement of Thyroid Autoantibodies

The major categories of thyroid autoantibodies include those that recognize proteins involved in thyroid hormone production and those that recognize the TSH receptor. Thyroglobulin is the glycoprotein that supports thyroid hormone synthesis and serves as a reservoir for thyroid hormone. Tyrosine residues in the polypeptide backbone are iodinated and coupled to form thyroid hormone, which, in turn, is released from the follicle upon stimulation by TSH (8). Thyroperoxidase is the enzyme responsible for oxidation of iodine prior to its linkage to thyroglobulin. It is estimated that 11% of the population has autoantibodies against thyroperoxidase with the prevalence of autoantibodies as high as 26% in middle-aged women (3). Detection of thyroglobulin and thyroperoxidase antibodies is highly specific for Hashimoto's disease and can be performed by indirect immunofluorescence assay (IFA), enzyme-linked immunosorbent assay (ELISA), or immunoprecipitation assays (8, 9). Although it has been demonstrated that thyroperoxidase antibodies can inhibit enzyme function *in vitro*, hypothyroidism develops in patients with Hashimoto's disease as a result of thyroid gland destruction by infiltrating reactive T cells.

As discussed, although individuals with autoimmune hyperthyroidism often have serologic evidence of antibodies directed against thyroperoxidase and thyroglobulin, the hyperthyroid state is mediated by the bioactive TSI, which binds to the TSH receptor, increasing thyroid-stimulating hormone synthesis. This occurs independently of regulation by feedback at the level of the pituitary gland, resulting in elevated thyroid hormone production. TSI can be detected by two different methods. Bioassay techniques detect the presence and activity of autoantibodies by quantitating stimulation of the TSH receptor. This technique treats tissue culture cells with serum from a patient with suspected Graves' disease, and cyclic adenosine monophosphate (cAMP) released into culture media is quantitated by chemiluminescence (10, 11). The activity is expressed as a TSI percentage and correlates with the relative bioactivity of the autoantibody. TSI is also detected by competitive radiobinding assays that measure the competition between radiolabeled TSH and serum autoantibodies for binding to the TSH receptor. However, the presence of TSI by competitive binding assay does not always predict bioactivity of the antibody; therefore, clinical correlation with thyroid function testing is warranted (12).

 ## Checkpoint! 11.1

How do thyroid stimulating immunoglobins (TSI) differ from thyroperoxidase and thyroglobulin antibodies?

PANCREAS

The pancreas is located behind the stomach and serves two main functions. The exocrine pancreas secretes enzymes that participate in the digestive process. The endocrine pancreas function is mediated by the pancreatic islets of Langerhans, which are small clusters of cells scattered throughout the entire gland. The islet is made up of at least three major types of cells, each of which is responsible for the secretion of a different hormone into the blood stream. Insulin, which regulates uptake of glucose into cells, is secreted by β cells, glucagon is secreted by α-cells, and somatostatin is secreted by δ-cells. Autoimmune disease of the pancreas is isolated to destruction of pancreatic β cells with subsequent loss of insulin production.

Type 1 Diabetes Mellitus

Type 1 diabetes mellitus (T1DM) is an autoimmune disease of the endocrine pancreas. When β-cells of the pancreatic islets are destroyed, insulin secretion decreases. As a result, patients develop significant hyperglycemia and have lifelong dependence on subcutaneous insulin. This is a relatively common autoimmune disorder with a prevalence of 1:500, and, although most cases are diagnosed before age 20, some individuals develop autoimmune diabetes as late as the third and fourth decades of life. Unlike most autoimmune disorders, males and females are equally affected. The disease is most common in Caucasians, and the lowest rate of disease is in Asian populations. The incidence of T1DM has increased over the last 40 years, particularly in European nations.

Susceptibility to development of T1DM is multifactorial with a genetic component that is associated with HLA class II alleles DR and DQ, the major histocompatibility complex (MHC) I-related gene (MIC-A), and the cytotoxic T lymphocyte associated antigen-4 (CTLA-4) (13). The overall likelihood of developing T1DM is about 0.2%; however, individuals with certain genetic profiles have an increased absolute risk up to 6.7% (14). Although more than 90% of individuals with T1DM carry some gene associated with the development of the disease, the risk for T1DM cannot be attributed completely to genetic factors. Even in the case of monozygotic twins, the likelihood of both twins being affected is only 30% (15). The current model is that T1DM develops when an individual with a susceptible genetic background is exposed to an environmental agent that triggers the activation of autoreactive T cells to attack β cells. Environmental exposures that have been associated with increased risk of T1DM include timing of introduction of cereal in infancy, early exposure to cow's milk, and viral infections (16, 17). The viral exposures most frequently associated with increased risk include cytomegalovirus, rubella, and Coxsackie B4 virus, and it is suggested that viral antigens are recognized as molecular mimics of self-antigens associated with the β cell, triggering antibody production and activation of T cells.

T1DM develops when there is loss of more than 80% of the pancreatic β cells. Over a period of weeks to months, the patient develops clinical symptoms including increased thirst, increased urination, and weight loss. The disease is diagnosed based on elevated serum blood sugars, increased urine glucose, and, in some cases, elevated serum ketones, which signal an insulin-deficient state and breakdown of fatty acids as an alternative energy source. The diagnosis of autoimmune diabetes is confirmed by the presence of serum autoantibodies against proteins within the pancreatic β cell including glutamic acid decarboxylase-65 (GAD-65), insulin-associated antigen, and insulin itself. Radioimmunoassay, indirect immunofluorescence, and radiobinding assays are used to detect the autoantibodies and are highly specific for the disease once an individual has clinical signs of diabetes (18). Individuals at high risk for developing T1DM based on their genetic background may have circulating autoantibodies many years prior to the presentation of the disease (19). In fact, the type, number, and titer of autoantibodies can predict the likelihood that an individual will develop T1DM. Currently, ongoing trials are aimed at preventing T1DM in targeted populations at high risk for the disease (20).

T1DM is treated with insulin, which must be administered subcutaneously because oral insulin is not stable to digestive enzymes. The goal in management of diabetes is to achieve nearly normal glucose levels while minimizing the risk of the most significant side effect of insulin therapy, hypoglycemia. To achieve this goal, daily therapy with 3 to 5 insulin injections is recommended. Long-acting insulin is injected once to twice a day to control blood sugars during fasting and between meals, and short-acting insulin is administered with meals to cover carbohydrate intake. An alternate strategy involves administering insulin via continuous subcutaneous infusion using an insulin pump. This therapy mimics biologic release of insulin by the pancreas, allowing patients to achieve blood glucose levels near normal.

T1DM is strongly associated with other autoimmune disorders, including autoimmune thyroid disease, celiac disease, and adrenal insufficiency (21), all of which have the potential to impact glucose control. Thus, an individual with T1DM may have more than one autoimmune disease. Management of these patients includes careful attention to signs and symptoms of these other diseases as well as recommended screening tests to identify individuals at risk prior to the development of poor diabetes control.

ADRENAL GLAND

The adrenal glands are located on top of the kidneys. (Figure 11.3 ■). The gland can be divided into two distinct areas, the adrenal cortex and the adrenal medulla. The adrenal medulla secretes catecholamines in response to sympathetic nervous system stimulation. The adrenal cortex plays a role in regulating both carbohydrate metabolism and fluid and electrolyte balance through production of cortisol (glucocorticoid) and aldosterone (mineralocorticoid).

Primary Adrenal Insufficiency

In the mid-19th century, Thomas Addison described a clinical syndrome with fatal outcomes resulting from the pathological destruction of the adrenal gland. When Dr. Addison described primary adrenal failure, infections, usually the result of tuberculosis, were the most common cause. Today the disease affects approximately 1:10 000 individuals, and

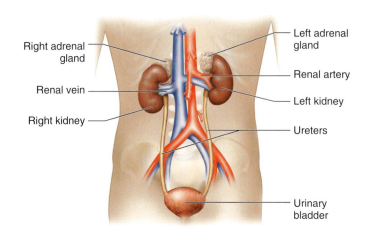

■ **FIGURE 11.3**   Adrenal gland.

the most common cause in the general population is autoimmune destruction of the adrenal cortex (22). As a result, cortisol and aldosterone deficiency develop, leaving patients with symptoms of fatigue, weakness, **anorexia** (loss of appetite), weight loss, and, in some cases, salt craving. In times of significant physiologic stress, such as injury or illness, the adrenal cortex normally responds by increasing cortisol production. However, in **primary adrenal insufficiency,** inability of the gland to increase cortisol results in low blood pressure, dehydration, and low blood sugar, all of which may progress to shock and even death. Treatment of adrenal failure involves lifelong replacement of both glucocorticoids and mineralocorticoids. Patients require "stress dose" hydrocortisone replacement under conditions of physiologic stress, such as fever, trauma, or surgery when the adrenal glands cannot respond appropriately with a rise in cortisol.

As with T1DM, risk for developing autoimmune adrenal insufficiency is associated with HLA class II alleles, including HLA-DR3/4, HLA-DR3-DQ2, and HLA-B8. Additional risk factors include polymorphisms in the MIC-A and CTLA-4 genes. The rate of autoimmune adrenal failure is 0.5% in patients with T1DM, with women more likely to be diagnosed with both disorders, while in the general population the rate of adrenal failure is equal between males and females.

The classic physical exam finding for diagnosing primary adrenal insufficiency is **hyperpigmentation,** or darkening of the skin, resulting from overexpression of melanocyte-stimulating hormone (part of the preprohormone secreted when pituitary adrenocorticotropin ACTH) increases to stimulate the adrenal cortex to produce cortisol. In the pediatric population, growth failure and weight loss are physical findings consistent with adrenal insufficiency. Once the diagnosis of adrenal insufficiency is suspected, elevated serum ACTH and plasma renin levels confirm deficiencies of cortisol and aldosterone. Serologic markers for autoimmune adrenal disease include autoantibodies targeting the adrenal cortex and the 21-hydroxylase enzyme. Adrenal cortex antibodies can be detected by IFA, and 21-hydroxylase antibodies are detected by radiobinding or immunoabsorption assay. Screening for adrenal autoantibodies is performed in individuals at high risk for developing adrenal insufficiency before the onset of outright adrenal dysfunction (23). Therefore, serologic identification of adrenal autoantibodies is an important risk factor for the development of adrenal disease.

✓ Checkpoint! 11.2

What is the most specific test for primary adrenal insufficiency?

REPRODUCTIVE ORGAN FAILURE

Autoimmune primary reproductive organ (gonadal) failure is rare and generally occurs in conjunction with other autoimmune disorders. The presentation and biochemical diagnosis depends on the sex of the affected individual, and treatment must be individualized.

Autoimmune Ovarian Failure

Premature ovarian failure represents a class of disorders in which estrogen deficiency and elevated serum gonadotropins occur before the age of 40. Women with premature ovarian failure may present with delayed puberty, primary or secondary amenorrhea, infertility, or osteoporotic fractures as a result of estrogen deficiency. The prevalence of premature ovarian failure is 1% with 0.2% of cases caused by autoimmune disease. Elevated follicle-stimulating hormone (FSH) levels in conjunction with low estradiol levels are diagnostic of premature ovarian failure. Autoimmune ovarian failure is associated with autoantibodies against steroid cells, which are detected by IFA. However, IFA sensitivity is very low, and not all individuals with suspected autoimmune ovarian dysfunction have detectable autoantibodies. Primary adrenal failure is diagnosed in up to 10% of individuals with autoimmune ovarian failure, and 25% of this population also has evidence of thyroid autoimmunity (24). Autoimmune ovarian failure is treated with estrogen replacement therapy.

Autoimmune Testicular Failure

Autoimmune gonadal failure is rarer in males than females. The testes contain two major cells types: Leydig cells, which synthesize testosterone, and the Sertoli cells, which participate in sperm production. Patients with autoimmune testicular failure present with infertility and/or low testosterone levels. Two major categories of autoantibodies contribute to gonadal failure. Patients may have steroid cell autoantibodies that indicate Leydig cell failure, leading to decreased testosterone production and elevated luteinizing hormone (LH). In addition, sperm counts are low due to testosterone deficiency. Individuals with steroid cell autoantibodies often have codiagnosis of adrenal failure or autoimmune thyroid disease. Detection of

steroid cell autoantibodies has been described. Patients are treated with testosterone; however, infertility may persist.

The second category of autoimmune testicular failure involves autoantibodies directed against sperm. Diagnostic testing shows normal testosterone levels, elevated FSH levels, and low sperm counts. Antibodies directed against sperm may be of the IgA or IgG subclass and are detected by immunobead technology. In this test, sperm are mixed with latex beads coated with either anti-IgA or anti-IgG, and the degree of agglutination is measured. These patients are infertile; the disorder occurs in men who have had testicular trauma or vasectomy reversal (25). It is believed that anti-sperm antibodies develop as a result of compromise of the testis as an **immunologically privileged site.**

✓ Checkpoint! 11.3

What components of the immune system mediate autoimmune endocrine failure?

▶ DIGESTIVE SYSTEM

Autoimmune disorders of the digestive system include diseases that affect the gastrointestinal tract (intestinal diseases) and those that affect liver function (hepatic diseases) (Table 11.3 ✪).

INTESTINAL DISEASES

Autoimmune diseases that affect the intestinal tract include celiac disease, pernicious anemia, and inflammatory bowel disease. These diseases can result in significant nutritional deficiencies. Symptoms and manifestations associated with diseases of the gastrointestinal system can guide the clinician during the diagnostic process.

Celiac Disease

Celiac disease is an autoimmune disorder in which genetically susceptible individuals develop intolerance to dietary gluten, a protein present in wheat, barley, and rye. As a result there is inflammation of the small intestine (Figure 11.4 ■), leading to poor absorption of nutrients. The prevalence of celiac disease in the Western population is 0.5 to 1%, and those at highest risk include women, first-degree relatives of those with celiac disease, and Caucasians of western European descent (26). Patients with celiac disease have weight loss, bloating, cramping, diarrhea, and, occasionally, constipation. Other signs and symptoms that should alert clinicians to the diagnosis of celiac disease include growth failure in pediatric patients, low calcium levels, vitamin D deficiency, anemia, osteoporosis, and a related autoimmune skin disorder called *dermatitis herpetiformis* (see Figure 11.5 ■). However, most individuals with celiac disease are asymptomatic, and screening is performed for those in a high-risk category. In addition to individuals with first-degree relatives with celiac

✪ TABLE 11.3

Summary of Autoimmune Diseases Involving the Digestive System—Intestinal Diseases

Organ System	Organ	Disease	Type of Immune Response	Antigen	Assay for Diagnosis	Clinical Effects
Digestive system	Small intestine	Celiac	Cellular and antibody	Tissue transglutaminase Endomysium Gliadin	Biopsy, blunted villi Tissue transglutaminase Gliadin and Endomysium antibodies • ELISA • IFA	Weight loss Diarrhea Constipation Abdominal pain Vitamin D deficiency Osteoporosis Failure to thrive Anemia Dermatitis herpetiformis
	Stomach and terminal ileum	Pernicious anemia Autoimmune atrophic gastritis	Antibody and cellular	Intrinsic factor Gastric parietal cells	Megaloblastic anemia B12 deficiency Intrinsic factor antibodies • ELISA Parietal cell antibodies • IFA • ELISA	Fatigue Paleness Anemia
		IBD	Cellular Cytokine		Endoscopy and histopathology	Abdominal pain Bloody diarrhea Fevers Weight loss
	Large intestine (spares anus)	Ulcerative colitis		Neutrophil cytoplasmic antigens (ANCA) myeloperoxidase and proteinase 3	pANCA • ELISA • IFA	Constipation Poor appetite
	Entire intestine (mouth to anus)	Crohn's disease		Saccharomyces cerevisiae antigens (Crohn's)	Antibodies to saccharomyces cerevisiae • ELISA	

disease, populations with a higher likelihood of developing celiac disease include those with other autoimmune disorders such as T1DM, autoimmune thyroid disease, and selective IgA deficiency and certain genetic syndromes, such as Turner syndrome, Down syndrome, and Williams syndrome (27).

Celiac disease develops when a susceptible individual consumes gluten-containing foods. During digestion, gluten is modified by tissue transglutaminase, an enzyme which deamidates the gliadin component of gluten. The modified polypeptides are then presented to T cells within the intestinal wall, stimulating an immune response (Figure 11.6 ■). Screening for celiac disease is performed in symptomatic and high-risk individuals and is based on the observation that individuals with celiac disease have IgA autoantibodies against gliadin, tissue transglutaminase (TTG-IgA) (28), and endomysium, a component of the connective tissue lining smooth muscle within the intestine (EMA-IgA) (29). The initial screen for celiac disease in high-risk and symptomatic individuals is serum TTG-IgA and serum IgA to rule out IgA deficiency. TTG antibodies and EMA antibodies are detected by ELISA and immunofluorescence techniques. All screening should be performed while the patient is on a gluten-containing diet because antibodies decline with elimination of gluten from the diet.

If screening indicates that the individual is likely to have celiac disease or if screening is negative yet symptoms are consistent with the disease, endoscopy with proximal small bowel biopsy is performed to confirm the disease. Once histologic diagnosis is made, the individual is counseled to follow a gluten-free diet, eliminating all wheat-, rye-, and barley-containing foods (Figure 11.7 ■). Response to the diet is monitored by resolution of clinical symptoms, improvement of nutritional deficiencies, and declines in titers of TTG-IgA and EMA-IgA antibodies.

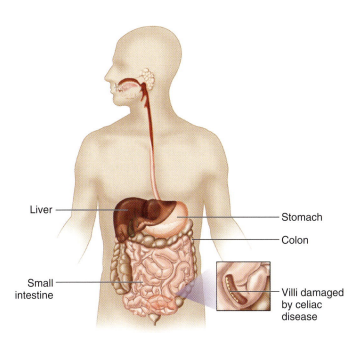

Liver

Stomach

Colon

Small
intestine

Villi damaged
by celiac
disease

■ **FIGURE 11.4**   Celiac disease affects the small intestine.

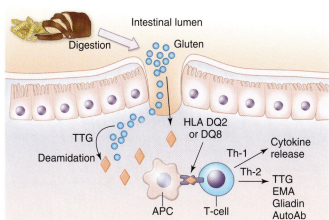

■ **FIGURE 11.6**   Pathophysiology of celiac disease. In susceptible
individuals, gluten-containing foods are digested, and gluten
moves between the intestinal cells into the space below them.
Here, tissue transglutaminase (TTG) deamidates gluten,
creating peptides that are efficiently presented to CD4 T cells by
HLA-specific antigen-presenting cells (APCs). Cytokine release
promotes inflammation and direct toxicity to the intestinal cells.
Additional B-cell expansion produces autoantibodies against TTG,
endomysium (EMA), and gliadin. *Source:* Adapted with permission
of Dr. Daniel Gelfond, Buffalo, New York.

PERNICIOUS ANEMIA

Pernicious anemia is an autoimmune cause of nutritional
megaloblastic anemia that is the result of cobalamin (B12)
deficiency (30). Megaloblastic anemia is defined by low red
blood cell counts and red cells with a mean corpuscular volume more than 100 femtoliter (fL). B12 deficiency is rarely
due to poor dietary intake because total body stores are high.

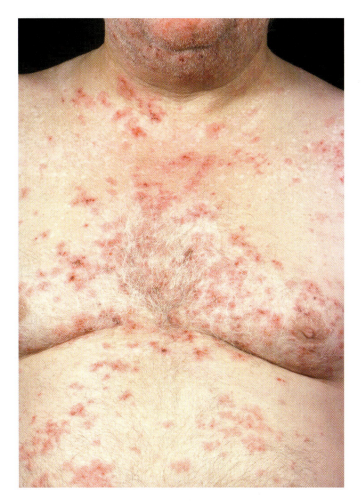

■ **FIGURE 11.5**   Dermatitis herpetiformis is a blistering skin condition
associated with celiac disease. *Source:* © Medical-on-Line/Alamy.

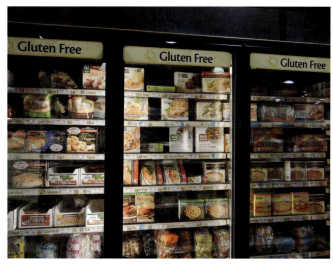

■ **FIGURE 11.7**   Patients with celiac disease must maintain a
gluten-free diet. Many gluten-free items are widely available.

Rather, the deficiency results from abnormalities in the release and absorption of cobalamin from meat and dairy products. The process by which dietary B12 enters the circulation depends on production of stomach (gastric) acid and the binding of cobalamin to intrinsic factor, a protein produced by parietal cells in the stomach. The intrinsic factor-cobalamin complex travels to the terminal ileum where specific receptors are present, allowing cobalamin to enter the circulation.

Two pathologic abnormalities lead to the development of pernicious anemia. First, autoantibodies against intrinsic factor decrease intrinsic factor levels or block the binding of the intrinsic factor-cobalamin complex to receptors in the terminal ileum. These antibodies are detected in up to 70% of individuals with the disease. The second defect is caused by chronic gastritis resulting from autoantibodies directed against the gastric parietal cells.

The diagnosis of pernicious anemia is suspected when a patient has megaloblastic anemia. In long-standing cobalamin deficiency, patients may develop neurologic abnormalities including **ataxia,** dementia, and cognitive decline due to defects in myelin formation. Once it is determined that the patient has cobalamin deficiency, autoantibodies against intrinsic factor and gastric parietal cells will confirm the diagnosis of pernicious anemia. Intrinsic factor autoantibodies are measured by ELISA, and antigastric parietal cell antibodies are measured either by IFA or ELISA (31). Because instrinsic factor autoantibodies are highly predictive, levels of these antibodies can be measured in individuals at high risk for developing pernicious anemia in order to prevent the signs and symptoms of cobalamin deficiency. Patients with pernicious anemia are treated with monthly intramuscular B12 injections to ensure adequate replacement. Resolution of anemia demonstrates that the deficiency is corrected.

INFLAMMATORY BOWEL DISEASE

Inflammatory bowel disease (IBD) is a class of chronic diseases of the gastrointestinal tract. Ulcerative colitis and Crohn's disease represent the two categories of IBD in which individuals are classified. The disease is typically diagnosed between the ages of 15 to 40 and occurs with equal prevalence in men and women. There is a familial component to the disease; up to 25% of affected individuals have a first-degree relative with the disease. The etiology of these diseases is still being debated with genetic, environmental, and immune factors all playing a role. Risk of IBD is associated with the major histocompatibility complex haplotypes HLA-DR3-DQ2, HLA-B27, and HLA-DR2 (32, 33).

Symptoms of IBD include poor appetite, abdominal pain, weight loss, intermittent fevers, diarrhea with or without blood, and constipation, particularly in those affected by ulcerative colitis. The two disorders are distinguished both endoscopically and pathologically (34). Endoscopic evaluation indicates that ulcerative colitis is characterized by mucosal inflammation of the entire colon that spares the anus.

On the other hand, Crohn's disease affects any region of the digestive tract, including the anus and mouth with the most commonly affected areas being the colon and the terminal ileum. It is associated with "skip" lesions in which areas of normal intestine are adjacent to mucosa that is friable and has a cobblestone appearance. Intestinal biopsy of affected areas shows severe mucosal inflammation with epithelial cell damage and occasional mucosal erosions. These findings are confined to the rectum and the large intestine. The key identifying microscopic feature of Crohn's disease is the presence of **granulomas,** or collections of macrophages and monocytes associated with inflammation within any layer of the intestinal wall. Other histologic findings typically seen in Crohn's disease are ulcerations of the mucosal layer and inflammation that affects the entire wall of the intestine (Figure 11.8 ■).

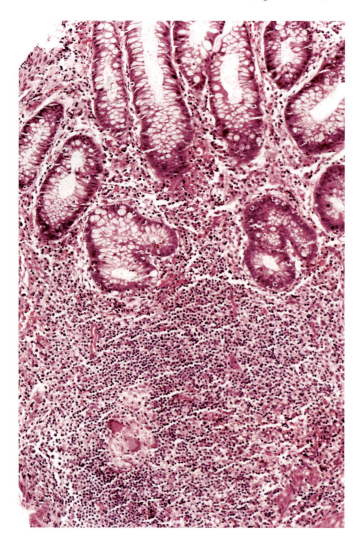

■ **FIGURE 11.8** Histopathologic findings in Crohn's disease. A high magnification micrograph of a colonic biopsy of mucosa affected by Crohn's disease demonstrates crypt branching and active inflammation (H&E stain). Crypt branching is a sign of a chronic crypt destructive process. *Source:* Biophoto Associates /Photo Researchers, Inc.

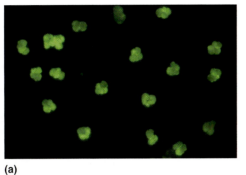 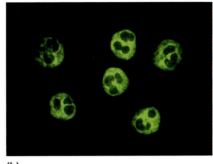

(a)   (b)

■ **FIGURE 11.9**   Antineutrophil cytoplasmic antibody staining patterns. Indirect immunofluorescence of ethanol-fixed human neutrophils demonstrates either (a) perinuclear (pANCA) or (b) cytoplasmic (cANCA) staining patterns. pANCA staining is more commonly seen in patients with ulcerative colitis and vasculitis whereas cANCA staining is associated with Wegener's granulomatosis. The differentiated staining pattern is specific for ethanol-fixed neutrophils; antibodies that demonstrate pANCA staining in ethanol-fixed cells have a diffuse cytoplasmic staining pattern in formalin fixed neutrophils. *Source:* Immco Diagnostics, Inc. Buffalo, NY, USA.

Diagnosis of IBD is made based on clinical presentation, endoscopic findings, and histopathology. Additional serologic tools can be used to differentiate between Crohn's disease and ulcerative colitis. Autoantibodies associated with IBD include antineutrophil cytoplasmic antibodies (ANCA; see Figure 11.9 ■ and the following section on vasculitis), which are more commonly seen with ulcerative colitis. These can be detected by ELISA or IFA. In addition, it has been observed that individuals with Crohn's disease have serologic evidence of antibodies against the yeast species Saccharomyces cerevisiae, which can be detected by ELISA (35). Although not autoantibodies, it is hypothesized that molecular mimicry plays a role in the development of these antibodies and the disease.

Management of IBD relies primarily on decreasing the inflammatory component of the disease. Another important component of IBD treatment involves careful attention to diet to decrease the risk of malnutrition as well as vitamin and mineral deficiencies. Finally, patients with IBD require frequent endoscopic surveillance because there is a higher risk of epithelial dysplasia and carcinoma in this population.

HEPATIC DISEASES

Autoimmune hepatic disease can affect both the hepatocyte (liver cell) and the biliary tree involved in the drainage of bile from the liver to the intestinal tract.

Autoimmune Hepatitis

Autoimmune hepatitis is a chronic disease that affects individuals of all ages and is characterized by a broad clinical spectrum ranging from subclinical asymptomatic disease to fulminant liver failure (36). Asymptomatic individuals are usually identified based on routine blood work demonstrating elevated liver enzymes. In spite of the lack of symptoms in this group, biopsy reveals significant liver damage. At the other end of the spectrum are those with acute liver disease who present with signs of liver failure such as jaundice (yellowing of the skin and eyes), elevated liver enzymes, and clotting disorders. Liver biopsy in these patients reveals a chronic necrotic inflammatory picture more indicative of long-standing disease. It is believed that this subgroup of patients has a subclinical component to their disease, reflected as constitutional symptoms, namely fatigue, anorexia, and abdominal pain, that were not attributed to hepatic disease.

Autoimmune hepatitis is suspected in an individual with evidence of hepatic failure when other forms of chronic liver disease, particularly viral hepatitis and alcoholism, have been excluded. The disease can be divided into two subtypes based on the serology of autoantibodies (37). Type 1 disease is characterized by antinuclear antibodies (ANA) and antismooth muscle antibodies. Individuals with type 2 disease have antibodies against liver and kidney **microsomes** and liver cytosol antigen. Autoantibodies are detected by IFA and ELISA. Although autoantibody detection is important for clarifying the etiology of hepatitis, they are not specific for the disease. In addition, the antibodies are not thought to be pathogenic and do not predict disease severity or response to therapy. Another diagnostic feature of autoimmune hepatitis is high serum IgG titers. Diagnosis of autoimmune hepatitis is made based on a scoring system that considers the presence and titer of autoantibodies, IgG levels, liver histology, and exclusion of viral hepatitis (38).

Initiation of treatment for autoimmune hepatitis is based on liver enzyme levels and hepatic pathology with glucocorticoids used as first-line therapy. Serologic remission, as defined

✪ TABLE 11.4

Summary of Autoimmune Diseases Involving the Digestive System—Hepatic Diseases

Organ System	Organ	Disease	Type of Immune Response	Antigen	Assay for Diagnosis	Clinical Effects
Hepatic system	Liver	Autoimmune hepatitis	Cellular	Nuclear and smooth muscle antigens Liver and kidney cytosol and microsome antigens	Elevated liver enzymes and bilirubin Liver biopsy High IgG levels ANA Smooth muscle antibodies Liver/kidney microsome and liver cytosol antibodies • IFA • ELISA	Fatigue Jaundice Poor appetite Abdominal pain Bleeding
		Primary biliary sclerosis	Cellular	Mitochondria	Elevated liver enzymes and bilirubin Abnormal clotting times Liver biopsy Anti-mitochondrial antibodies • IFA • ELISA	Jaundice Itching Abdominal pain Xanthomas Enlarged liver Weight loss Poor appetite Bleeding Cirrhosis

by declines in liver enzymes and improvements in bilirubin levels, generally precedes histologic improvement by 6 to 12 months. Therefore, treatment should be continued until biopsy demonstrates resolution of inflammation and necrosis.

Primary Biliary Cirrhosis

Primary biliary cirrhosis (PBC) is a rare autoimmune disease that causes inflammation of the bile ducts within the liver. Over time, scarring and destruction of the biliary network occurs blocking the flow of bile from the liver (cholestasis). At end stage, the disease progresses to cirrhosis and liver failure. PBC predominantly affects Caucasian women between the ages of 35 to 70, and there is a strong familial component. Some studies have suggested an association between certain HLA haplotypes and PBC; another study showed an association between PBC and the cytotoxic T lymphocyte-associated antigen-4 (CTLA-4) gene (39).

Individuals generally present with nonspecific systemic symptoms including fatigue and pruritus (itching). As the scarring of the biliary system progresses, affected individuals may have abdominal pain localized to the right upper quadrant, dry mouth and eyes, and joint pain. Physical exam may reveal enlarged liver and spleen, and skin findings including excoriations as a result of severe pruritus, xanthomas (small yellow fat deposits within the skin), and jaundice.

The diagnosis of PBC is made by measuring serum tests of liver function including liver enzymes, total and direct bilirubin, and coagulation profiles. The most sensitive and specific diagnostic test for the disease is serum levels of antimitochondrial antibodies, which are present in more than 95% of individuals with the disease (40). The antibodies are detected by IFA or ELISA. Some evidence indicates that measurable antimitochondrial antibodies may predict the development of the disease in asymptomatic individuals. However, currently there are no recommendations for screening high-risk subjects, including first-degree relatives with the disease. Management of PBC is aimed at relief of symptoms, control of cholestasis, and management of cirrhosis (Table 11.4 ✪).

▶ INTEGUMENTARY SYSTEM

Skin is composed of three major layers (Figure 11.10 ■). The outer layer, or epidermis, is made up of squamous epithelial cells and provides a protective barrier. The middle layer, or dermis, contains the cushioning connective tissue and is where sweat glands, hair follicles, nerve endings, and blood vessels are located. The deepest layer, or hypodermis, is the area that anchors skin to the muscle and bone beneath. Autoimmune skin diseases occur when immune attack of structural

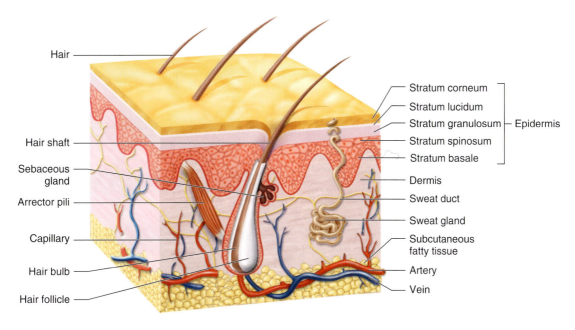

■ **FIGURE 11.10** Skin.

proteins interferes with cell–cell and cell–matrix interactions that are essential for the integrity of the skin layers. They may affect the skin and mucous membranes. The location and extent of the lesions, associated clinical symptoms, and immunohistologic findings aid in focusing the diagnosis. In certain conditions, the degree of skin affected may be significant, placing the patient at risk for secondary bacterial infections, poor nutrition, and dehydration (Table 11.5 ✪).

✪ **TABLE 11.5**

Summary of Autoimmune Diseases Involving the Skin

Organ System	Organ	Disease	Type of Immune Response	Antigen	Assay for Diagnosis	Clinical Effects
Skin	Skin	Pemphigus vulgaris	Antibody	Desmoglein Epidermal antigen	Skin biopsy Antidesmoglein antibodies • Direct IF • IFA • ELISA	Large blisters in mouth and on scalp, chest, axilla, and groin Skin infections Dehydration Hypothermia
		Bullous pemphigoid	Antibody	Hemidesmosome antigens Bullous pemphigoid (BP) antigens 1 and 2 Epidermal/Dermal junction	Skin biopsy Anti-BP antbodies • Direct IF • IFA • ELISA	Large blisters on lower abdomen, groin, axilla, between fingers Skin infections Dehydration Hypothermia
		Dermatitis herpetiformis	Antibody	Epidermal tissue transglutaminase	Skin biopsy Diagnosis of celiac disease Tissue transglutaminase antibodies • ELISA • IFA	Small blisters on erythematous base located on torso and extensor surfaces of extremities Strong association with celiac disease

PEMPHIGUS AND PEMPHIGOID DISORDERS

Pemphigus and pemphigoid diseases are autoimmune blistering diseases of the skin (41). The diseases are differentiated by the skin layer affected. The disorders are characterized by blisters or bullae (blisters greater than 1cm in diameter) filled with clear fluid accompanied by reddening of the skin (erythema), erosion around the blister, and pruritus. The autoantibodies associated with these diseases recognize specific antigens within the skin layers disrupting the integrity of the skin. Although these disorders are rare, they cause significant disfigurement and are associated with increased morbidity and mortality (42).

Pemphigus vulgaris is one of the most common of the autoimmune blistering skin disorders. Women are affected more than men, and the disease rate increases with age. Pemphigus vulgaris is characterized by blisters within the epithelial layer of the skin (Figure 11.11 ■). Affected individuals have both cutaneous and mucosal lesions, predominantly in the areas of the oral cavity, scalp, chest, axilla, and groin. The blisters rupture easily, leaving a raw area of skin that is susceptible to secondary bacterial infection. Autoantibodies responsible for pemphigus vulgaris are directed against desmoglein, an epidermal adhesion molecule. The antibodies are pathogenic as demonstrated by the formation of intraepithelial blisters in neonatal mice injected with autoantibodies isolated from affected patients. Diagnosis is made by taking a biopsy of an area of skin adjacent to a fresh lesion. Antidesmoglein antibodies are detected by direct immunofluorescence, which demonstrates intercellular antibody deposition; see Figures 11.12(a) ■ and 11.12(b). Alternatively, serum autoantibodies are detected by ELISA or IFA techniques. First-line therapy for pemphigus vulgaris is systemic glucocorticoids.

In contrast to pemphigus vulgaris, the blisters associated with bullous pemphigoid are below the epidermis, disrupting

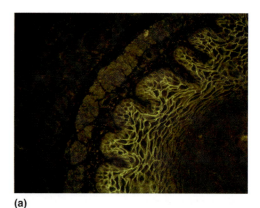

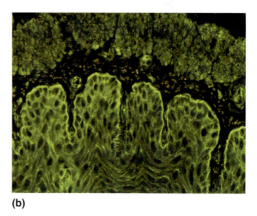

(b)

■ **FIGURE 11.12** Immunofluorescent staining patterns of pemphigus and pemphigoid diseases. Indirect immunofluorescent techniques detect antidesmoglein antibody (associated with pemphigus vulgaris) and antibodies against hemidesmosmal proteins (associated with bullous pemphigoid). (a) The intercellular staining pattern that is diagnostic for pemphigus vulgaris. (b) Linear deposition of antibodies along the dermal–epidermal junction is diagnostic for bullous pemphigoid. *Source:* Immco Diagnostics, Inc. Buffalo, NY, USA.

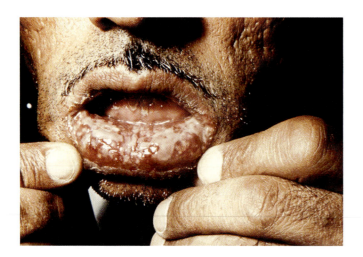

■ **FIGURE 11.11** Blisters seen in pemphigus. *Source:* CDC/ Dr. J. Lieberman; Dr. Freideen Farzin, Univ. of Tehran.

the basement membrane zone between the epidermal/dermal junction (43). The blisters are large and are located in the lower abdomen, groin, axilla, and between the fingers with minimal involvement of mucosal regions. The autoantibodies associated with bullous pemphigoid are directed against two hemidesmosmal proteins: bullous pemphigoid antigen 1 (BP230) and bullous pemphigoid antigen 2 (BP180) (44). The hemidesmosome is a component of the basement membrane that participates in anchoring the epidermal layer to the dermal layer. Diagnosis is made by performing biopsy at the edge of an intact bulla. Direct immunofluorescent microscopy of an affected region shows deposits of antibody along the epidermal-dermal junction; see Figure 11.12(b). Additionally, serum autoantibodies against BP180 and BP230 can be detected either by IFA or ELISA. Patients with extensive involvement of skin are at risk for dehydration, hypothermia, and **sepsis** and should be treated similarly to burn victims in a hospital setting. Management of the autoimmune component of bullous pemphigoid is similar to pemphigus vulgaris.

Checkpoint! 11.4

What immunodiagnostic test demonstrates deposition of antibodies in skin biopsies of pemphigoid blisters?

DERMATITIS HERPETIFORMIS

Dermatitis herpetiformis is an autoimmune blistering skin condition characterized by small blisters on an erythematous base distributed over the trunk and extensor surfaces of the extremities (see Figure 11.5). It is accompanied by significant itching with subsequent erosion of the blisters. Dermatitis herpetiformis is strongly associated with celiac disease. Approximately 85% of individuals with the skin disease have biopsy-proven intestinal disease whereas ~25% of adults with celiac disease have skin manifestations (45). Similar to celiac disease, affected individuals have elevated serum TTG autoantibodies, which recognize epidermal transglutaminase. In fact, for individuals with symptoms typical of celiac disease accompanied by dermatitis herpetiformis and serologic evidence of gluten autoimmunity, intestinal biopsy is not required to make a diagnosis of celiac disease. Direct immunofluorescence of affected lesions reveals IgA deposits at the dermal papillae and linear IgA deposits at the dermal–epidermal junction. Serum detection of autoantibodies is similar to that for celiac disease (see the earlier discussion). Most individuals have resolution of the skin lesions when gluten is eliminated from the diet.

▶ MUSCULOSKELETAL SYSTEM

Locomotion, strength, and control of bodily functions, such as swallowing and breathing, are important functions of the musculoskeletal system. The principal autoimmune disease that affects the musculoskeletal system is myasthenia gravis. This disease impacts transmission of neural signaling to the muscles, affecting a wide variety of functions.

MYASTHENIA GRAVIS

Myasthenia gravis is an autoimmune disease affecting the neuromuscular junction. Onset of the disease may be acute or may develop over a prolonged period of time. Patients present with weakness and easy fatigability that worsens with activity and resolves with rest. Skeletal muscle groups are most often affected, and patients complain of double vision, difficulty climbing stairs or carrying objects, and trouble with talking or swallowing. Respiratory failure due to respiratory muscle weakness is a significant life-threatening symptom. Patients with isolated eye abnormalities are diagnosed as having ocular myasthenia gravis whereas those with more systemic symptoms have generalized disease (Figure 11.13 ■).

Myasthenia gravis is the result of antibody-mediated destruction of the acetylcholine receptor at the **postsynaptic**

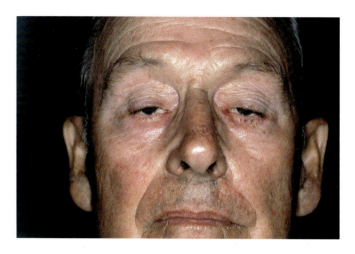

■ **FIGURE 11.13**   Muscle weakness caused by myasthenia gravis is evident in the eyes of this patient. *Source:* © Hercules Robinson/Alamy.

membrane of the neuromuscular junction (46). As a result, acetylcholine released by the neuron fails to initiate signaling (Figure 11.14 ■). T cells also play a role in the pathophysiology of the disease, likely by stimulating B-cell antibody production and through altered activity of regulatory T cells. Serologic tests for binding or blocking autoantibodies are performed when the disease is suspected, and antibodies against the acetylcholine receptor are present in greater than 80% with the disease (47). In patients who lack acetylcholine receptor autoantibodies, antibodies directed against the muscle-specific

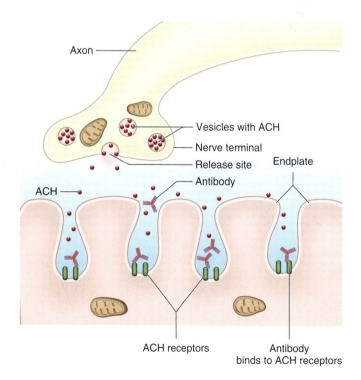

■ **FIGURE 11.14**   Antibodies in myasthenia gravis block the acetylcholine receptors at the neuromuscular junction.

receptor tyrosine kinase may be present. Autoantibodies are measured by radioimmunoassay and are very specific for the disease.

Management of myasthenia gravis targets several aspects of the disease. First, patients can be treated with acetylcholinesterase inhibitors to increase the concentration of acetylcholine within the neuromuscular junction (48). Second, to address the autoimmune component, patients can be treated with immunosuppressive drugs, such as glucocorticoids (49). Although autoantibody titers do not correlate with disease severity, titers tend to decline in those who respond successfully to immunotherapy. In severe, generalized myasthenia gravis, particularly with respiratory failure, **plasmapheresis** is performed to decrease acetylcholinesterase receptor antibody titers.

▶ ## NERVOUS SYSTEM

The nervous system consists of the central nervous system—brain, spinal cord—and the peripheral nervous system responsible for receiving and transmitting signals to and from the central nervous system. The complexity of neural pathways and functional control contributes to the presentation of diseases of the nervous system.

MULTIPLE SCLEROSIS

Multiple sclerosis is a chronic neurologic disease of the central nervous system (CNS) caused by inflammatory destruction of the myelin sheath surrounding nerves. It is widely held that multiple sclerosis is an autoimmune disease mediated by autoreactive T cells. Rates of multiple sclerosis are highest in the Western hemisphere and lowest in the equatorial regions. The prevalence varies from 0.8 to 150:100 000, depending on the geographic location (50). Similar to other autoimmune diseases, multiple sclerosis is more common in women and usually presents in the 3rd to 4th decades of life. In addition, there is a strong association between multiple sclerosis and other autoimmune disorders, including autoimmune thyroid disease, T1DM, and inflammatory bowel disease. Individuals with the HLA-DRB1 allele are at high risk for developing the disease (51).

The presentation of multiple sclerosis depends on the region of the CNS affected. Symptoms associated with the disease include, but are not limited to, double vision, weakness, gait abnormalities, dizziness, pain, and the sensation of electric shocks with movement of the neck (Figure 11.15 ■). Multiple sclerosis is categorized as relapsing-remitting or progressive, depending on the clinical progression of symptoms and may follow a benign or rapidly progressive course.

The exact etiology of multiple sclerosis is unclear, but the most widely held hypothesis is that of a CD4+ T cell mediated autoimmune reaction against myelin or glial cell antigens. An alternative hypothesis points to a viral-mediated inflammatory response triggering molecular mimicry against self-antigens. Regardless of the precipitating event, the disease is characterized by significant inflammatory response within the white matter with both lymphocytes and cytokines implicated in causing the disease (52). The hallmark pathologic findings are plaques within the CNS that can be

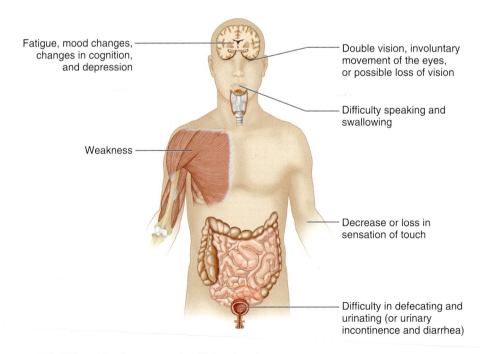

■ **FIGURE 11.15** Symptoms of multiple sclerosis.

identified by magnetic resonance imaging (MRI). Many individuals with the disease have serum autoantibodies against myelin basic protein and other **oligodendrocyte** antigens (53). However, diagnosis of multiple sclerosis is not based on serum autoantibodies because the clinical presentation and MRI findings are usually sufficient to establish the diagnosis.

First-line therapy for relapsing-remitting multiple sclerosis are the beta-interferons, which work by modulating cytokine production and reducing disease flairs (54). Other therapies suppress autoreactive T cells (55). These therapies are not completely effective in preventing relapses, nor do they have an effect on existing neurologic defects. When acute exacerbations occur, glucocorticoids are used to lessen the severity and duration of the attack. A significant treatment component of multiple sclerosis involves occupational and physical therapy to preserve strength and allow the affected individual to continue with an independent life.

▶ VASCULAR SYSTEM

The cardiovascular system is made up of the heart and blood vessels through which blood transports gases (oxygen and carbon dioxide) and nutrients to and from tissues/cells. Autoimmune diseases of the vascular system may affect either the blood vessels themselves (vasculitis) or may alter the flow of blood throughout the body (thrombotic disease).

VASCULITIS

Vasculitis is defined as inflammation within the walls of the blood vessels. A large number of disorders are associated with vasculitis, many of which are not autoimmune in origin. In addition, some systemic diseases have vasculitis as part of the clinical spectrum, including systemic lupus erythematosis, rheumatoid arthritis, and other connective tissue diseases (see Chapter 10). Inflammation of blood vessels causes constriction and/or rupture, which can lead to tissue death and hemorrhage. The size of vessels and tissue affected determine the signs and symptoms of the disease.

Antibodies directed against antineutrophil cytoplasmic antigens (ANCA) are associated with some forms of vasculitis, and identification of these autoantibodies aids in the diagnosis and classification of vasculitic diseases (56). For example, Wegener's granulomatosis is a systemic vasculitic disease affecting medium and small arteries. Approximately 90% of individuals with Wegener's disease have ANCA antibodies (57). The disease primarily affects blood vessels of the respiratory tract and kidneys and is characterized by necrotic granulomas. As a result, individuals present with bloody nasal discharge, bloody cough, and urine containing blood or protein.

ANCA autoantibodies predominantly recognize two neutrophil antigens: myeloperoxidase and proteinase 3 (58). Antibodies are identified in serum by ELISA or IFA with IFA

offering greater sensitivity. Two patterns of immunofluorescent staining are generally identified: pANCA is characterized by perinuclear staining pattern whereas cANCA has cytoplasmic staining pattern. Antibodies that yield a cytoplasmic pattern usually recognize proteinase 3, whereas perinuclear staining is generally due to myeloperoxidase staining (see Figure 11.9). Staining patterns are not specific for individual diseases, although cANCA autoantibodies are more often demonstrated with vasculitic diseases (59).

In addition to Wegener's granulomatosis, ANCA autoantibodies are detectable in other conditions such renal-limited vasculitis, Goodpasture's disease (discussed later), certain drug-induced vasculitic disorders, and inflammatory bowel disease (see earlier discussion). Because ANCA autoantibodies are not specific for a particular disease and results are not standardized, they should not be used for screening. In summary, a positive ANCA result supports a clinical diagnosis that should be confirmed by biopsy of affected tissue.

THROMBOTIC DISEASE

Diseases associated with abnormal activation of the coagulation cascade lead to the inappropriate formation of clots (thrombosis). As a result, patients are at risk for deep venous thrombosis (clots within the deep blood vessels), pulmonary embolism (clots that migrate to the lungs), and strokes. Although many conditions and drugs place an individual at risk for thrombotic disease, anti-phospholipid syndrome is an autoimmune disease associated with recurrent venous and arterial clots. Individuals may also have low platelet counts, and women may have recurrent miscarriages (60). There is a strong association of the syndrome with systemic lupus erythematosis (see Chapter 10).

Two major criteria are necessary to diagnosis antiphospholipid syndrome (61). First, there must be at least one clinical feature consistent with the disease. Second, there must be persistent serologic evidence of antiphospholipid antibodies. These antibodies represent a class of autoantibodies that recognize plasma proteins bound to phospholipids. The major categories of antiphospholipid antibodies are lupus anticoagulant, anticardiolipin antibodies, antibodies against beta-2 glycoprotein-1, and antibodies against specific phospholipids, such as phosphatidylserine and phosphatidylinositol. Many of these antibodies bind to proteins involved in the coagulation cascade, acting to increase the risk of clotting either by initiating thrombosis, activating platelets, or inhibiting fibrin clot breakdown.

Although antiphospholipid syndrome is associated with thrombosis, paradoxically, the activated partial thromboplastin time (aPTT) is often prolonged in an individual with the disease. In fact, prolonged aPTT may initiate the workup for antiphospholipid syndrome in an unaffected individual. The inhibitory antibodies bind to activated phospholipid complexes of the coagulation cascade, interfering with the intrinsic coagulation pathway during this *in vitro* test.

Identification of antiphospholipid antibodies is performed by either immunochemical techniques or functional assays. ELISA detects anticardiolipin and anti-beta 2-glycoprotein 1 antibodies. Functional assays must be performed to detect lupus anticoagulant autoantibodies because not all of these antibodies have clinical activity (62). In these assays, serum from the affected patient is mixed with normal serum. If the coagulation parameters are not corrected by the addition of normal serum, then inhibitors in the test serum are interfering with coagulation. This inhibition is then corrected by adding phospholipid to the serum in question to absorb the autoantibodies that are negatively impacting the clotting time.

Individuals with antiphospholipid syndrome who have suffered a major clotting event must be treated aggressively with anticoagulation therapy using either heparin or warfarin. In cases of repeated deep venous thrombosis, a filter may be placed in the inferior vena cava to decrease the risk of pulmonary emboli. In those who have been diagnosed but are asymptomatic, treatment is aimed at preventing clots by counseling to eliminate secondary risk factors, including smoking, use of oral contraceptive pills, and high lipid levels. In addition, these individuals are counseled to avoid prolonged periods of inactivity, particularly after surgical intervention. Prophylactic aspirin therapy may also be considered (63).

✓ Checkpoint! 11.5

Are functional clotting studies or autoantibody titers more specific for diagnosing antiphospholipid syndrome?

▶ PULMONARY AND RENAL SYSTEMS

GOODPASTURE'S DISEASE

Goodpasture's disease, also referred to as *Goodpasture's syndrome,* is a rare autoimmune cause of **glomerulonephritis** (64). The disease affects approximately 1 per 1 million in the general population and is diagnosed in less than 20% of individuals with acute glomerulonephritis. The disease is characterized by acute onset of blood and protein in the urine with rising creatinine levels, indicative of renal failure. Approximately 60% of affected individuals also have signs and symptoms of pulmonary disease, including cough, shortness of breath, and pulmonary hemorrhage. Unlike other autoimmune disorders, Goodpasture's disease is more common in young men. The disease is sometimes preceded by a viral infection. Because the risk of chronic renal failure and mortality rate are high if not treated, it is imperative to make a diagnosis early in the presentation of the disease.

Autoantibodies against the glomerular basement membrane (GBM) precipitate the damage to the glomeruli. In contrast to many other autoimmune disorders, the development of GBM autoantibodies occurs acutely and titers decay rapidly. Infusion of GBM antibodies into experimental animals induces acute glomerulonephritis, indicating that the antibodies are in part pathogenic. The autoantibodies recognize epitopes in the noncollagenous domain of the alpha-3 chain of type IV collagen. As the autoantibodies bind, immune complexes form, activating the complement cascade, which destroys the GBM. Renal biopsy followed by direct immunofluorescence demonstrates antibody deposition in a linear fashion along the glomerular capillaries.

Goodpasture's disease is diagnosed in an individual with acute renal failure accompanied by bloody urine and respiratory symptoms. ELISA, RIA, and IFA are technologies used to identify anti-GBM antibodies in serum. High titers of serum anti-GBM correlate with this rapidly progressive, aggressive disease. When Goodpasture's disease is strongly detected yet serologic testing is non-diagnostic, renal biopsy followed by direct immunofluorescence is recommended. Once the diagnosis of Goodpasture's disease is made, first-line therapy is plasmapheresis to remove the circulating autoantibodies, and immunosuppressive therapy. The goal is to lower the titer of anti-GBM antibodies until remission of the disease occurs. Early recognition and initiation of therapy decrease the likelihood that the patient will go on to chronic renal failure and long-term dialysis (Table 11.6 ✪).

▶ EXOCRINE GLANDS

SJÖGREN'S SYNDROME

Sjögren's syndrome (SS) is a fairly common autoimmune disease. It is characterized by an autoimmune inflammatory reaction affecting mostly the exocrine glands such as salivary and lacrimal glands. Figure 11.16 ■ demonstrates the signs and symptoms experienced by an individual affected by Sjögren's syndrome. SS affects less than 1% of the world population, but the female-to-male ratio of occurrence is 9:1. Its incidence is the highest in people between 40 and 50 years old (although it can occur at any age), and many SS patients also have other autoimmune diseases. Because the lacrimal and salivary glands are most affected, the most common clinical symptoms are dry eyes and dry mouth, and these are associated with difficulty in eating and eye discomfort. Reduced salivary flow promotes an environment that favors oral bacterial growth; thus, subjects with SS have an increase in dental caries and periodontal disease. They also suffer from vision disturbances and risk of corneal ulcerations due to the lack of ocular lubrication and the absence of a film of tears.

Other symptoms of SS include dry skin, purple discoloration of the skin, joint pain, and hives. SS can also affect the

⊙ TABLE 11.6

Summary of Autoimmune Diseases Affecting Musculoskeletal, Nervous, Vascular, Pulmonary, and Renal Systems

Organ System	Organ Affected	Disease	Type of Immune Response	Antigen	Assay for Diagnosis	Clinical Effects
Musculoskeletal system	Neuromuscular junction Skeletal muscles	Myasthenia gravis	Antibody Cellular	Acetylcholine receptor	Acetylcholine receptor antibodies • RIA	Fatigue Weakness Double vision Respiratory failure
Nervous system	Central nervous system Myelin	Multiple sclerosis	Cellular	Myelin basic protein Glial antigens	MRI Myelin basic protein antibodies • RIA • ELISA	Weakness Gait problems Dizziness Double vision Pain Fatigue
Vascular system	Blood vessels	Vasculitis Example: Wegener's disease (lungs and kidney)	Cellular	Neutrophil cytoplasmic antigens	Biopsy of affected tissue Antineutrophil cytoplasmic antigen antibodies • IFA • ELISA	Bleeding Hypertension Pain Fever Wegener's disease • Bloody nasal discharge • Bloody cough • Blood in urine • Kidney failure
	Clotting system	Antiphospholipid syndrome	Antibody	Phospholipids β2-glycoprotein-1 Cardiolipin Lupus anticoagulant	Prolonged partial thromboplastin time Antiphospholipid antibodies • IFA • ELISA • Mixing studies	Deep venous thrombosis Pulmonary embolus Stroke Recurrent miscarriage
Pulmonary and renal systems	Kidney and lungs	Goodpasture's disease	Antibody	Glomerular basement membrane Type IV collagen	Kidney biopsy Antiglomerular basement membrane antibodies • Direct IF • ELISA • IFA	Acute renal failure Blood and protein in urine Cough Shortness of breath Pulmonary hemorrhage

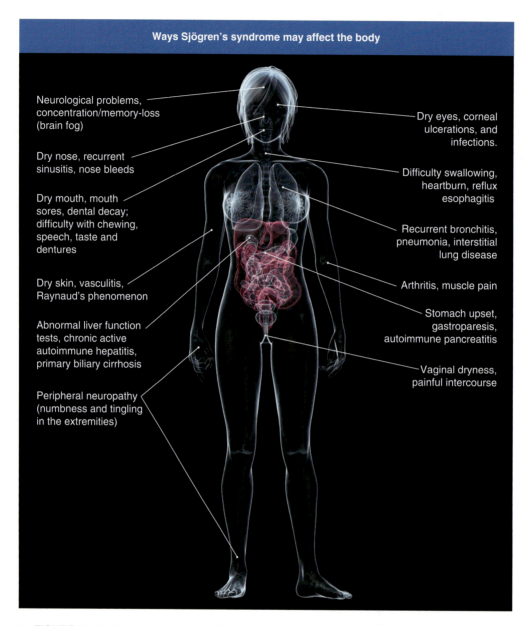

Ways Sjögren's syndrome may affect the body

Neurological problems, concentration/memory-loss (brain fog)

Dry nose, recurrent sinusitis, nose bleeds

Dry mouth, mouth sores, dental decay; difficulty with chewing, speech, taste and dentures

Dry skin, vasculitis, Raynaud's phenomenon

Abnormal liver function tests, chronic active autoimmune hepatitis, primary biliary cirrhosis

Peripheral neuropathy (numbness and tingling in the extremities)

Dry eyes, corneal ulcerations, and infections.

Difficulty swallowing, heartburn, reflux esophagitis

Recurrent bronchitis, pneumonia, interstitial lung disease

Arthritis, muscle pain

Stomach upset, gastroparesis, autoimmune pancreatitis

Vaginal dryness, painful intercourse

■ **FIGURE 11.16**   Physical features of Sjögren's syndrome. *Source:* Ways Sjogren's Syndrome May Affect the Body, www.sjogrens.org. Reprinted by permission.

lungs with resulting dry airways, hyperreactive airway disease, and pulmonary hypertension. The pathophysiology of SS is still under investigation, but recent studies have shown that glandular epithelial cells release proinflammatory cytokines and chemokines that recruit inflammatory cells into the affected glands, thus causing the localized inflammatory reactions. The nature of the antigen that may stimulate an autoimmune response is unclear (although alpha-fodrin has been suggested); however, viral infections have been suspected as playing a role in the autoimmune response in SS. ANA and RF can also be found in 60 to 80% of SS patients; therefore,

ANA testing is also a part of differential diagnosis between different autoimmune conditions such as SLE, RA, and SS (see Chapter 10). Many individuals with SS have antibodies to SS-A (Ro) and SS-B (La): anti-SS-A antibodies are present in about 40% of subjects with SS. In addition, approximately 33% of subjects with SS also have serum antibodies to microsomal and gastric parietal cells.

Diagnostic approaches include the Schirmer test. This involves the placement of a strip of paper between the eyeball and the eyelid. Presence of 5 mm of wetness on the strip in less than 5 minute indicates a positive tests. Additionally, decreased salivary flow is part of the diagnosis: If less than 1.5 ml of whole saliva is collected in 15 minutes, diagnosis of SS is considered. There is no cure for SS. Most treatment is designed to replace moisture in the eyes in the form of artificial tears; cyclosporine is also used as an immunosuppressant to reduce inflammation. Drugs that stimulate salivary flow, such as cevimline or pilocarpine are also used. Oral hygiene and preventive dental care are of critical importance to prevent caries and periodontal disease.

CASE STUDY 1

Your grandma has been feeling quite tired. She has not mentioned it to anyone because she just is not a complainer, but you notice that she is walking up the stairs to her room more slowly and that her eyelids are rather droopy. You give her a gift of a coffee table book on her favorite subject of gardening, and you see as she attempts to carry the book upstairs to her room that it just seems too much for her.

1. For what disease do you think she should be checked?
2. What autoantibody may be present?
3. How should she be treated?

CASE STUDY 2

In your wedding pictures you and your husband look great, but now 5 years later, the contrast is getting ridiculous! He has gotten a lot thinner, and you hate to admit it, but you have gotten quite a bit heavier. That is not all. You and he used to agree about everything, but now he is always hot but you are always cold; he does not want to go to sleep, but you are always tired! Your skin is dry and you just don't seem to care that much anymore. Your neck is funny with a swelling at the front. Meanwhile your husband is restless and his eyes are bugging out!

1. What disease do you think that your husband may have?
2. What disease do you think that you might have?
3. For what antibodies should you and your husband be checked?

SUMMARY

Autoimmune diseases represent a wide array of disorders that result when the immune system recognizes self-antigens as foreign. Targets of the immune system can include the endocrine system, the digestive system, the musculoskeletal system, the skin, the nervous system, the vascular system, and the pulmonary and renal systems. As a result, wide arrays of symptoms and pathologies can occur. The factors that contribute to the development of autoimmune diseases include genetics, immune cell biology, and environmental agents. In this chapter, we discussed many organ-specific autoimmune diseases and described the causes and diagnosis of the diseases. In many cases, direct or indirect immunofluorescent staining is involved in the diagnosis; in some cases, radioimmunoassays or enzyme immunoassays are also utilized. As researchers continue to understand the relationships between the different factors that lead to the failure of self-tolerance, strategies to prevent or ameliorate autoimmune diseases will be developed.

REVIEW QUESTIONS

1. Which of the following assays is used for the detection of autoantibodies associated with organ-specific autoimmune disorders?
   a. enzyme linked immunosorbant assay
   b. radioimmunoassay
   c. indirect immunofluorescence
   d. all of the above

2. A 17-year-old female presents to her primary physician with a 2-month history of rapid heart rate, increased appetite, weight loss, and anxiety. On physical exam, she is noted to have an enlarged thyroid, tremor, and tachycardia. What is the likely diagnosis?
   a. Addison's disease
   b. Hashimoto's disease
   c. Graves' disease
   d. anorexia

3. Antibodies directed against which of the following thyroid antigens contributes to the development of Graves' disease?
   a. thyroperoxidase
   b. thyroglobulin
   c. thyroid-binding globulin
   d. thyroid-stimulating hormone receptor

4. Pernicious anemia affects the absorption of which of the following nutrients?
   a. iron
   b. cobalamin
   c. hiamin
   d. vitamin D

5. A 9-year-old female presents with a vesicular rash on the extensor surfaces of her forearms. Review of her medical record reveals that she has a history of failure to thrive. Which of the following laboratory tests would be useful in diagnosing the cause of her growth failure and persistent rash?
   a. serum IgG levels
   b. tissue transglutaminase antibodies
   c. antibodies against bullous pemphigoid antigen
   d. positive immunofluorescent staining of the dermal–epidermal junction

6. Which of the following pairs is *not* correct?
   a. myasthenia gravis and antibodies to acetylcholine receptors
   b. Graves' disease and thyroid-stimulating immunoglobulin
   c. Goodpasture's disease and anti-basement membrane antibodies
   d. Crohn's disease and gliadin antibodies

7. Peter comes to his physician's office complaining of being cold all the time, having poor energy, and gaining weight. He mentions to the physician that his sister has the same symptoms. A section of monkey thyroid incubated with the patient's serum shows staining that is not nuclear. The titer of serum that yields positive staining is 1:25 000. He has a cellular infiltrate in the affected organ. What disease do Peter and his sister have?
   a. Graves' disease
   b. Hashimoto's disease
   c. multiple sclerosis
   d. myasthenia gravis

8. Peter's brother has different symptoms than those of his siblings. Bob feels hot all the time and has difficulty sleeping. He has a large appetite yet has been losing weight. His eyes are protruding. On physical exam, his heart rate is fast and his blood pressure is very high. What disease does Bob have?
   a. Graves' disease
   b. Hashimoto's disease
   c. multiple sclerosis
   d. myasthenia gravis

9. What is the primary immunologic contributor to Bob's disease?
   a. antibodies
   b. T cells
   c. antibodies and T cells
   d. macrophages

10. A 10-year-old girl complains of increased thirst and frequent urination. She has elevated glucose in her blood stream and her breath smells fruity. She is diagnosed with type 1 diabetes. Which of the following is true regarding type 1 diabetes?
    a. There is a genetic component to the disease.
    b. It may be related to a past viral infection.
    c. It is the result of autoimmune destruction of pancreatic cells.
    d. All of the above are correct.

11. Which of the following is associated with multiple sclerosis?
    a. ANA
    b. rheumatoid factor
    c. antimyelin antibody
    d. cold agglutinins

12. A young man presents to his doctor's office with a complaint of bloody cough. He is found to have protein in his urine. If a biopsy were performed on both his lungs and kidneys, ribbonlike deposits would be seen at the basement membrane of both organs. What disease does this patient have?
    a. antiphospholipid syndrome
    b. Wegener's disease
    c. systemic lupus erythematosis
    d. Goodpasture's disease

REFERENCES

1. Jacobson DL, Gange SJ, Rose NR, et al. 1997 Epidemiology and estimated population burden of selected autoimmune diseases in the United States. *Clin Immunol Immunopathol.* 1997;84:223–243.

2. Cooper GS, Stroehla BC. The epidemiology of autoimmune diseases. *Autoimmun Rev.* 2003;2:119–125.

3. Hollowell JG, Staehling NW, Flanders WD, et al. Serum TSH, T4, and thyroid antibodies in the United States population (1988 to 1994): National Health and Nutrition Examination Survey (NHANES III). *J Clin Endocrinol Metab.* 2002;87:488–499.

4. Tandon N, Zhang L, Weetman AP. HLA Associations with Hashimoto's thyroiditis. *Clin Endocrinol.* 1991;34:383–386.

5. Dayan CM, Daniels GH. Chronic autoimmune thyroiditis. *N Engl J Med.* 1996;335:99–107.

6. Stiebel-Kalish H, Robenshtok E, Gaton DD. Pathophysiology of Graves' ophthalmopathy. *Pediatr Endocrinol Rev.* 2010;7:178–181.

7. Glaser NS, Styne DM for the Organization of Pediatric Endocrinologists of Northern California Collaborative Graves' Disease Study Group. Predicting the likelihood of remission in children with Graves' disease: A prospective, multicenter study. *Pediatrics.* 2008;121:e481–488.

8. Rousset BA, Dunn JT. Thyroid hormone synthesis and secretion. http://www.thyroidmanager.org/Chapter2/2-framehtm. Accessed May 15, 2010.

9. http://www.esoterix.com. Accessed June 2, 2010.

10. http://www.immcodiagnostics.com/products/default.aspx. Accessed August 3, 2010.

11. https://www.labcorp.com/wps/portal/provider/testmenu. Accessed June 29, 2010.

12. http://www.thyroidmanager.org/Chapter6/Ch-6-6.htm. Accessed August 25, 2010.

13. Mehers KL, Gillespie KM. The genetic basis for type 1 diabetes. *Br Med Bull.* 2008;88:115–129.

14. Onengut-Gumuscu S, Concannon P. The genetics of type 1 diabetes: Lessons learned and future challenges. *J Autoimmun.* 2005;25:Suppl:34–39.

15. Hyttinen V, Kaprio J, Kinnunen L, et al. Genetic liability of type 1 diabetes and the onset age among 22,650 young Finnish twin pairs: A nationwide follow-up study. *Diabetes.* 2003;52:1052–1055.

16. Norris JM, Barriga K, Klingensmith G, et al. Timing of initial cereal exposure in infancy and risk of islet autoimmunity. *JAMA.* 2003;290:1713–1720.

17. Akerblom HK, Knip M. Putative environmental factors in type 1 diabetes. *Diabetes Metab Rev.* 1998;14:31–67.

18. http://www.questdiagnostics.com/hcp/qtim/testMenuSearch.do. Accessed June 30, 2010.

19. Orban T, Sosenko JM, Cuthbertson D, et al. Pancreatic islet autoantibodies as predictors of type 1 diabetes in the Diabetes Prevention Trial–Type 1. *Diabetes Care.* 2009;32:2269–2274.

20. http://www.clinicaltrials.gov/ct2/show/NCT00419562?term=TrialNet&rank=3. Accessed September 15, 2010.

21. Not T, Tommasini A, Tonini G, et al. Undiagnosed coeliac disease and risk of autoimmune disorders in subjects with Type I diabetes mellitus. *Diabetologia.* 2001;44:151–155.

22. Betterle C, Dal Pra C, Mantero F, et al. Autoimmune adrenal insufficiency and autoimmune polyendocrine syndromes: Autoantibodies, autoantigens, and their applicability in diagnosis and disease prediction. *Endocr Rev.* 2002;23:327–364.

23. Coco G, Dal Pra C, Presotto F, et al. Estimated risk for developing autoimmune Addison's disease in patients with adrenal cortex autoantibodies. *J Clin Endocrinol Metab.* 2006;91:1637–1645.

24. Welt CK. Autoimmune oophoritis in the adolescent. *Ann NY Acad Sci.* 2008;1135:118–122.

25. Haas GG, Cines DB Jr, Schreiber AD. Immunologic infertility: Identification of patients with antisperm antibody. *N Engl J Med.* 1980;303:722–727.

26. Fasano A, Berti I, Gerarduzzi T, et al. Prevalence of celiac disease in at-risk and not-at-risk groups in the United States: A large multicenter study. *Arch Intern Med.* 2003;163:286–292.

27. Mastrandrea LD. Autoimmune disorders associated with type 1 diabetes mellitus. Diagnosis and implications for diabetes control. In: Aucoin L, Prideaux T, eds. *Handbook of Type 1 Diabetes Mellitus: Etiology, Diagnosis, and Treatment Chapters* New York: Nova Science.

28. Dieterich W, Laag E, Schopper H, et al. Autoantibodies to tissue transglutaminase as predictors of celiac disease. *Gastroenterology.* 1998;115:1317–1321.

29. Chorzelski TP, Beutner EH, Sulef J, et al. A 1984 IgA anti-endomysium antibody. A new immunological marker of dermatitis herpetiformis and coeliac disease. *Br J Dermatol.* 1984;111:395–402.

30. Toh B, Van Driel IR, Gleeson PA. Mechanisms of disease: Pernicious anemia. *N Engl J Med.* 1997;337:1441–1448.

31. http://www.pathology.med.umich.edu/handbook/details.php?testID=714. Accessed June 3, 2010.

32. Scaldaferri F, Correale C, Gasbarrini A, et al. Mucosal biomarkers in inflammatory bowel disease: Key pathogenic players or disease predictors? *World J Gastroenterol.* 2010;16:2616–2625.

33. Lees CW, Satsangi J. Genetics of inflammatory bowel disease: Implications for disease pathogenesis and natural history. *Expert Rev Gastroenterol Hepatol.* 2009;3:513–534.

34. http://www.med-info.nl/Literatuur/Crohn_CU_IBS.pdf. Accessed July 21, 2010.

35. Peeters M, Joossens S, Vermeire S, et al. Diagnostic value of anti-Saccharomyces cerevisiae and antineutrophil cytoplasmic autoantibodies in inflammatory bowel disease. *Am J Gastroenterol.* 2001;96:730–734.

36. Krawitt EL. Autoimmune hepatitis. *N Engl J Med.* 2006;354:54–66.

37. Czaja AJ, Freese DK. Diagnosis and treatment of autoimmune hepatitis. *Hepatology.* 2002;36:479.

38. Manns MP, Czaja AJ, Gorham JD, et al. AASLD Practice Guidelines: Diagnosis and management of autoimmune hepatitis. *Hepatology.* 2010;51:1–31.

39. Gregory WL, Bassendine MF. Genetic factors in primary biliary cirrhosis. *J Hepatol.* 1994;20:689–692.

40. Muratori L, Granito A, Muratori P, et al. Antimitochondrial antibodies and other antibodies in primary biliary cirrhosis: Diagnostic and prognostic value. *Clin Liver Dis.* 2008;12:261–276.

41. Schmidt E, Zillikens D. 2010 Modern diagnosis of autoimmune blistering skin diseases. *Autoimmunity Reviews.* In press.

42. Patrício P, Ferreira C, Gomes MM, et al. Autoimmune bullous dermatoses: A review. *Annals of the New York Academy of Sciences.* 2009;1173:203–210.

43. Yancey KB, Egan CA. Pemphigoid: Clinical, histologic, immunopathologic, and therapeutic considerations. *JAMA.* 2000;284:350–356.

44. http://www.mbl.co.jp/e/ivd/pdf/7613e.pdf. Accessed July 1, 2010.

45. Abenovali L, Prioetti I, Leggio L, et al. Cutaneous manifestations in celiac disease. *World J Gastroenterol.* 2006;12:843–852.

46. Drachman DB. Myasthenia gravis. *N Engl J Med.* 1994;330:1797–1810.

47. Drachman DB, Adams RN, Josifek LF, et al. Functional activity of autoantibodies to acetylcholine receptors and the clinical severity of myasthenia gravis. *N Engl J Med.* 1982;307:769–775.

48. Punga AR, Stålberg E. Acetylcholinesterase inhibitors in MG: To be or not to be? *Muscle & Nerve*. 2009;39:724–728.

49. Saperstein DS, Barohn RJ. Management of myasthenia gravis. *Semin Neurol*. 2004;24:41–48.

50. Rosati G. The prevalence of multiple sclerosis in the world: An update. *Neurol Sci*. 2001;22:117–139.

51. The International Multiple Sclerosis Genetics Consortium. Risk alleles for multiple sclerosis identified by a genomewide study. *N Engl J Med*. 2007;357:851–862.

52. Barnett M, Parratt J, Pollard J, et al. MS: Is it one disease? *International MS Journal*. 2009;16:57–65.

53. Archelos JJ, Storch MK, Hartung HP. The role of B cells and autoantibodies in multiple sclerosis. *Annals of Neurology*. 2000;47:694–706.

54. Dubucquoi S, de Seze J, Lefranc D, et al. Interferon beta in multiple sclerosis: Relationship between sustained serum IgG levels and clinical outcome. *J Neuroimmunol*. 2002;129:232–236.

55. Duda P, Schmied M, Cook S, et al. Glatiramer acetate (Copaxone) induces degenerate, Th2-polarized immune responses in patients with multiple sclerosis. *J Clin Invest*. 2000;105:967–976.

56. Seo P, Stone JH. The antineutrophil cytoplasmic antibody-associated vasculitides. *Am J Med*. 2004;117:39.

57. van der Woude FJ, Rasmussen N, Lobatto S, et al. The TH 1985 Auto-antibodies against neutrophils and monocytes: Tool for diagnosis and marker of disease activity in Wegener's granulomatosis. *Lancet*. 1985;1:425–429.

58. Hoffman GS, Specks U. Antineutrophil cytoplasmic antibodies. *Arthritis Rheum*. 1998;41:1521–1537.

59. Han WK, Choi HK, Roth RM, et al. Serial ANCA titers: Useful tool for prevention of relapses in ANCA-associated vasculitis. *Kidney Int*. 2003;63:1079–1085.

60. Asherson RA, Khamashta MA, Ordi-Ros J, et al. The "primary" antiphospholipid syndrome: Major clinical and serological features. *Medicine*. 1989;68:366–374.

61. Wisløff F, Jacobsen EM, Liestøl S. Laboratory diagnosis of the antiphospholipid syndrome. *Thromb Res*. 2002;108:263–271.

62. Lupus anticoagulant working party on behalf of the BCSH haemostasis and thrombosis task force. Guidelines on testing for the lupus anticoagulant. *J Clin Pathol*. 1991;44:885–889.

63. Erkan D, Yazici Y, Peterson MG, et al. A cross-sectional study of clinical thrombotic risk factors and preventive treatments in antiphospholipid syndrome. *Rheumatology*. 2002;41:924–929.

64. Bolton WK. Goodpasture's syndrome. *Kidney Int*. 1996;50:1753–1766.

12

Tumor Immunology

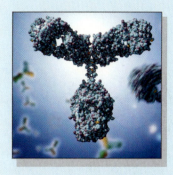

■ OBJECTIVES—LEVEL I

After this chapter, the student should be able to:

1. Define and explain *benign, malignant, invasive, metastasis, cancer, carcinoma, adenocarcinoma, sarcoma, leukemia, lymphoma, myeloma, grade,* and *stage.*
2. Define *tumor immunology* and *tumor-associated antigens.*
3. State the potential clinical uses for tumor-associated antigens.
4. Give information concerning currently used tumor markers.
5. Explain criteria for screening.
6. List costs and benefits of screening for tumors.
7. List criteria for immunologic screening using tumor markers.
8. State the use for and limitations of Bence-Jones proteins, immunoglobulin, AFP, human chorionic gonadotropin (hCG), prostate-specific antigen (PSA), and CA-125.
9. Draw curves associated with monitoring a tumor patient through treatment.
10. Describe the clinical importance of tumor antigen monitoring.
11. Describe the criteria that would allow a tumor marker to be a good monitoring marker.
12. List the antigens currently being used for monitoring.
17. List possible staging markers for cancer.
18. List tumor markers for which serum levels are predictive of outcome.
20. List major areas of diagnostic usefulness of immunohistochemistry for solid tumors.

■ OBJECTIVES—LEVEL II

After this chapter, the student should be able to:

1. Give examples of genetic screening.
2. Name a common marker for epithelial tumors.
3. Name a common marker for tumors of mesenchymal origin.
4. Name a common marker for tumors of hematopoietic origin.
5. Describe the estrogen receptor, progesterone receptor, and HER-2 marker and their importance.
6. Discuss the basic limitations involved for a tumor associated-antigen to be useful in radioimmunolocalization.
7. Discuss the clinical purpose of radioimmunolocalization.
8. Discuss the difference between active and passive immunotherapy.
9. Describe the requirements for an antigen to be used as a target for monoclonal antibody based tumor therapy.

■ **OBJECTIVES—LEVEL II** *(continued)*

10. Describe the currently available antibodies for tumor radioimmunolocalization and tumor radioimmunotherapy.
11. Describe active immunotherapy for cancer.
12. Describe immunosurveillance.

KEY TERMS

adenocarcinoma
alpha 1-fetoprotein (AFP)
Bence-Jones proteins
benign tumors
beta-2 microglobulin
Bexxar
BRCA1
BRCA2
CA 15-3
CA 27-29
CA 19-9
CA 125
cancer
carcinoembryonic antigen (CEA)
carcinomas
CD45
central nervous system cancers
confirmatory diagnosis
cytokeratins
estrogen receptors
free to total PSA
Gardasil
grade
Herceptin

immunolocalization
HER-2 marker
human chorionic gonadotropin (hCG)
leukemias
lymphomas
malignant tumors
metastasize
monitoring
monoclonal immunoglobulin
myelomas
progesterone receptors
prostate-specific antigen (PSA)
Prostascint
Provenge
PSA velocity
radioimmunotherapy
sarcomas
screening
stage
tumor
tumor-associated antigens
tumor immunology
vimentin
Zevalin

▶ INTRODUCTION

The word **tumor** can mean either a benign or a malignant abnormal growth of cells. **Benign tumors** are not cancer, they do not grow into other tissues, nor do they spread to other parts of the body, and they usually are not life threatening. When a benign growth (Figure 12.1 ■) is surgically removed, it usually does not grow back. **Malignant tumors** are cancer, and they can invade and grow into other organs and spread throughout the body (Figure 12.2 ■). Tumors that invade surrounding tissues are called invasive (Figure 12.3 ■). The ability to spread throughout the body is called the ability to **metastasize** (Figure 12.4 ■). The origin of the tumor is called the *primary site of the tumor,* and other areas into which the tumor spreads are called *metastatic sites.* The place of origin of the tumor is the type of tumor the patient has, so that a breast tumor that has traveled and is now in the liver

is still a breast tumor, not a hepatoma or tumor of the liver (1, 2, 3, 4, 5, 6).

Cancer is a group of diseases that begin with the abnormal and uncontrolled proliferation of 1 cell. The uncontrolled spread of the progeny of this 1 cell can impinge and affect the functioning of normal organs throughout the body. The effect of the cancer cells on the normal organs, if left uncontrolled, can cause death. Cancer is second only to cardiovascular disease in the list of the 15 leading causes of death (7, 8). Because of the prevalence of cancer, many of you will find the information in this chapter useful not only in your careers but also as you help friends and acquaintances understand their diagnosis and therapy. Cancer is one of the many instances that you will find that your knowledge can help others arm themselves with the strength of understanding their disease. **Carcinomas** are tumors that arise from epithelial tissue; an **adenocarcinoma** is a tumor arising from epithelial cells that

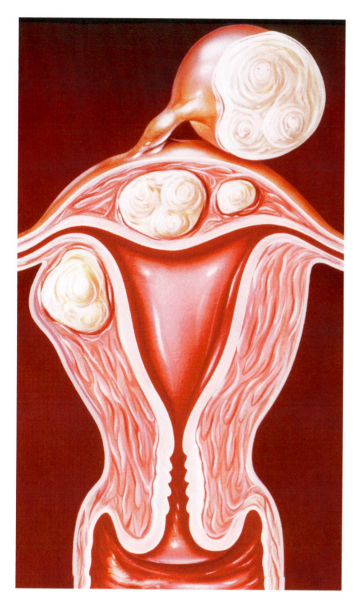

formed glandular structures. **Sarcomas** are cancers that arise from supportive or connective tissue such as muscle, bone, cartilage, fat, and blood vessels. **Leukemias, lymphomas, and myelomas** are cancers of the white blood cells. **Central nervous system cancers** can arise in either the brain or the spinal cord (1, 2, 3, 4, 5, 6).

✓ Checkpoint! 12.1

Two patients have a tumor on their chest. In Fred, the tumor origi- nated from cells of the rib, but in Velma, the tumor originated in the breast. What type of tumor does Fred have? What type of tumor does Velma have?

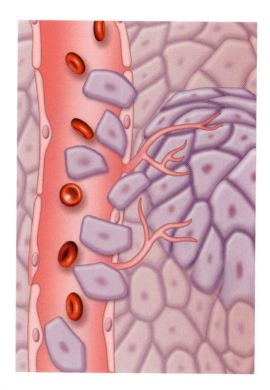

■ **FIGURE 12.2** Metastatic process: Tumor leaving primary site to travel to other distant organs to grow.

Various risk factors are associated with cancer, but people without known risk factors can have the disease and people with risk factors can remain disease free. The following are commonly associated with increased risk for cancer: age, tobacco use, sunlight, tanning booths, family history of certain types of cancer (breast, colon), alcohol use, certain hormones, exposure to certain chemicals called *carcinogens*, ionizing radiation, certain viruses and bacteria, poor diet, lack of physical activity, and obesity (1, 2, 3, 4, 5, 6) (Figure 12.5 ■).

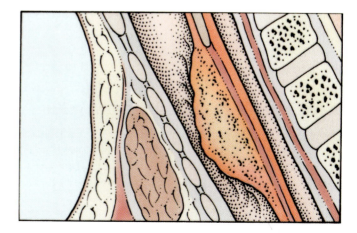

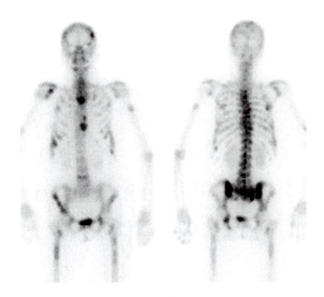

■ **FIGURE 12.4**   Metastatic spread of the tumor shown with imaging techniques. *Source:* Courtesy of Dr. Dominick Lamonica and the Nuclear Medicine Service of the Roswell Park Cancer Institute, Buffalo, NY, U.S.A.

A normal cell is said to have been transformed when its proliferation results in the formation of a tumor cell. Tumor cells differ from normal cells in several ways, but a key difference is that tumor cells proliferate independently of normal growth signals or controls. This usually results in a higher than normal proliferation rate with an increased amount of

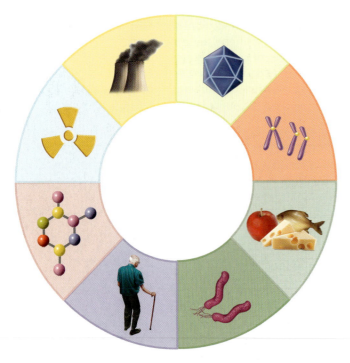

■ **FIGURE 12.5**   Cancer risks: Ionizing radiation, pollution, viruses, genetic predisposition, diet (obesity, poor nutrition), bacteria, age, and carcinogens.

DNA in each cell, possibly due to a higher number of cells about to divide. The increased growth rate can also result in increased cellular acidity due to a higher metabolic rate. Transformation is thought to be caused by 2 or more mutations in the same cell. Another key difference in a cancer cell involves dedifferentiation of the cell so that it becomes more like the embryonic precursor of the organ type rather than the fully differentiated cells of the organ (1, 2, 3, 4, 5, 6).

This change in differentiation leads to a tool for the clinical evaluation of the tumor, which is called the **grade** of the tumor. In grading a tumor, the term G1 is well differentiated, G2 is moderately differentiated, G3 is poorly differentiated, and G4 is undifferentiated. These terms are used to relate how much the tumor looks like the tissue of origin with very similar called *well differentiated* and very dissimilar called *undifferentiated*. In general, the more dissimilar the tumor is from the tissue of origin, the worse the prognosis. An additional prognostic indicator is the tumor's **stage;** with this clinical nomenclature, the physician defines how far the tumor has grown and spread. Three different letters are used in describing cancer: T for tumor size, N for number of lymph nodes involved, and M for whether distant metastases are found. T0 indicates no evidence of tumor, Tis indicates the tumor is *in situ* and has not spread, and T1, T2, T3, and T4 indicate progressively larger tumor size. N0 indicates that no lymph nodes are involved, Nx indicates that the clinician is unable to define nodal involvement, and N1, N2, and N3 indicate increased amount of nodal involvement. M0 indicates that no distant metastasis were found, Mx indicates that metastatic involvement cannot be evaluated, and M1 indicates that distant metastasis were found. The T, N, and M information is summarized as a stage number, from stage 0, I, II, III, to IV. This information helps the physician choose the therapeutic regimen and the patient understand her or his prognosis (1, 2, 3, 4, 5, 6).

✓ **Checkpoint! 12.2**

There is a chemotherapeutic drug that works better at a pH slightly lower than most normal cells, so the side effects with this drug are lower. But why would this work against cancer cells?

Cellular changes such as dedifferentiation can lead to changes in the markers on the cell surface, and changes in growth controls can lead a cell to secrete a product into the blood stream that was originally secreted into the gland's lumen. These changes can lead to measurable substances in the blood and on the tumor cell surface. These substances, which are expressed more in the tumor than in normal tissue, are called **tumor-associated antigens.** Changes related to dedifferentiation can cause the reoccurrence of antigens that were lost after embryonic tissues developed to adult tissues on the surface of the tumor cell; these tumor-associated antigens are called *oncofetal antigens*. Tumor-associated antigens can also be antigens that are present on the normal cell surface, such as growth factor receptors, but that are present in much higher concentration on the tumor cell surface. Tumor-associated antigens can also be of viral origin, such as the human papilloma virus associated with cervical cancer and the Epstein Barr virus associated with Burkitt's lymphoma, but most human tumors have not been found to have a viral origin. These antigens are called *tumor-associated* rather than *tumor-specific antigens* because other than the viral-associated antigens, these antigens are also found in lower levels in some normal human tissues. Measurement of tumor-associated antigens is part of a science called *tumor immunology* (1, 2, 3, 4, 5, 6).

 ### Checkpoint! 12.3

What are the 2 words in this chapter that make evident the similarities between fetal tissues and tumor tissues? We have already learned about one, what is it? Keep an eye out for the second word.

In addition to being the study of the antigens associated with the tumor, **tumor immunology** involves the study of the patient's immune response to the tumor, the study of the use of the immune system to destroy the tumor, and the study of the effect of the tumor on the patient's immune status. Paul Ehrlich coined the term *immunosurveillance* to explain why more tumors do not occur even though a huge number of cell divisions are required throughout our lifespan and errors normally occur during cell division that would result in a higher number of tumors if nothing was effecting the rate. The theory of immunosurveillance postulates that the immune system must be preventing many of these cancers. T cells, NK cells, lymphokine-activated killer cells, and antibodies may all be involved in immune elimination of abnormal cells, so any tumor that does form must have only weakly immunogenic tumor antigens or it would have been destroyed. Many of these tumor antigens are present in small amounts on normal tissues; thus, the patient would be tolerant to these antigens, but they are still useful clinically. The study of the markers associated with the tumor can help in diagnosis, staging, monitoring, tumor metastasis localization, pathologic evaluation of biopsies, and immunotherapy of the tumor (1, 2, 3, 4, 5, 6).

▶ DIAGNOSIS AND SCREENING

In general, the more quickly cancer is diagnosed, the more likely it is that the patient will have a positive outcome. **Screening** involves testing for cancer in a population when no symptoms of the cancer exist, allowing for earlier diagnosis. A tumor generally grows with 30 doubling times from 1 tumor cell to 1 billion tumor cells (1 cm tumor) in 5 to 8 years, but takes only 10 more doublings, or 1.6 to 3 years, to reach a lethal size of 1 kg. Diagnosis could occur during the early years of cancer growth and would allow less aggressive therapy with fewer side effects if the tumor has not metastasized (1, 2, 3, 4, 5, 6).

However, for screening to be cost effective and have a high positive and negative predictive value (see Chapter 8) so that few patients are told that they have the cancer when they do not compared to the number whose cancers were detected and few cancers are missed, the tumor and the patient population must meet certain criteria. The tumor for which the screening is performed must be an important health problem, and there must be an early recognizable symptom or risk factor that would lead to selection of the group of patients to test. For screening to be important for the patient's prognosis, the treatment of the tumor at an earlier stage must be more beneficial than treatment at a later stage either in terms of reduced morbidity or decreased mortality. Because cancer is relatively common, screening individuals without symptoms is done for some cancers if patient populations that represent a higher risk group can be selected. This higher risk group may be set by familial incidence and, thus, genetic risk or just by age risk. Screening tests are available only for the most common cancers because they carry higher risks. These common cancers include breast, prostate, colon, cervical, skin, and testicular. Nonserologic screening techniques include breast self-exams (Figure 12.6 ▪) and mammograms for screening for breast cancer (Figure 12.7 ▪), testicular self-exams for those at high risk for testicular cancer, fecal occult blood tests for early colorectal cancer, digital rectal exam for prostate cancer, and colonoscopy and sigmoidoscopy for colorectal cancer. Cancer markers can also be used as diagnostic aids when clinical signs and symptoms exist (1, 2, 3, 4, 5, 6).

For a screening test to be utilized, it must be acceptable to the population; for example, a mammogram test with tissue compression (Figure 12.7) would not be acceptable for testicular examination nor would a screening test that included evaluation of the cerebral spinal fluid be acceptable for low-risk patients. The costs of the screening, both in monetary terms and in increased testing caused by false positive results, must be acceptable. The costs due to increased testing and anxiety caused by false positive results led the 2010 U.S. Preventative Services Task Force to recommend mammography beginning at age 50 rather than 40 and every other year rather than every year as recommended by the American Cancer Society. In this controversial difference in opinion, the Preventative Services Task Force emphasized the costs resulting from false positive mammograms, both from the actual costs of the additional sonograms and possible biopsies and from the psychological costs of the tentative false positive for the patient. This remains a controversial difference (1, 2, 3, 4, 5, 6).

For a tumor antigen to be used in a serological assay for diagnosis or screening for a cancer, the antigen must be absent from or in low levels in most individuals without the disease

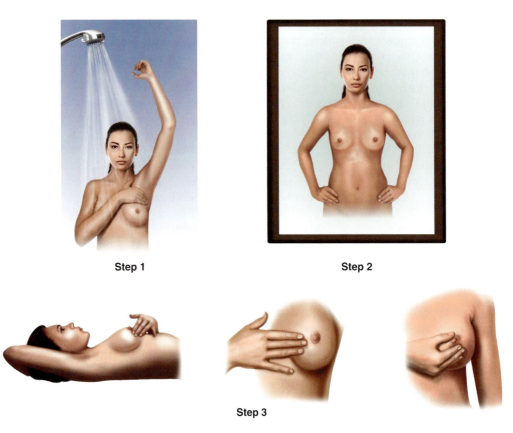

Step 1

Step 2

Step 3

■ **FIGURE 12.6**   Steps of screening test: breast self-exam. Early detection can find cancer when it is most curable. See the American Cancer Society website for complete instructions as well as instructions for testicular self-exam for men at high risk.

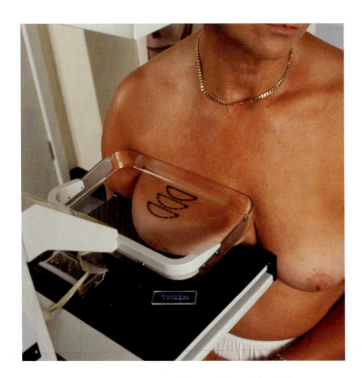

■ **FIGURE 12.7**   Mammogram. *Source:* Chris Priest / Photo Researchers, Inc.

(low false positive rate), and must be elevated in most individuals with the disease (low false negative rate). In addition, the marker must be secreted into a fluid that can be assayed easily, and it must be elevated while the disease is in a treatable stage. Diagnosis can also include the use of tumor markers to confirm a diagnostic conclusion drawn from the clinical symptoms of the patient. The use of tumor markers in this capacity is for a **confirmatory diagnosis.** In this use, the positive predictive value for most tumor markers is quite high (1, 2, 3, 4, 5, 6).

▶ MONITORING PATIENTS FOR RESPONSE AND RECURRENCE

Serological analysis for a tumor marker can also be used for **monitoring** the patient's therapeutic response. The serum levels of markers used this way change relative to tumor size because they are produced by the tumor cells, secreted into the serum, and have a biological half-life fast enough to decrease with decreasing tumor burden and slow enough to increase with increasing tumor burden. If serum levels of a tumor marker in a patient undergoing therapy go down after a chemotherapeutic regime has begun, the treatment is likely to be working and killing tumor cells. If serum levels of a tumor marker go up after a chemotherapeutic regime has begun; the treatment is likely to be unsuccessful and should be changed (Figure 12.8(a) ■). Serum levels of the marker in a patient with no evidence of disease can be used to determine whether the tumor has recurred. The levels are measured during doctor visits, and if 2 consecutive increases are seen and the levels go above baseline, the physician will do further testing to determine the presence of a recurrence (Figure 12.8(b)). The baseline is set at a level in which the marker value in almost all healthy individuals is lower than the baseline (1, 2, 3, 4, 5, 6).

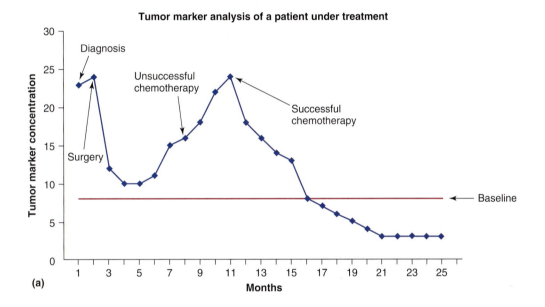

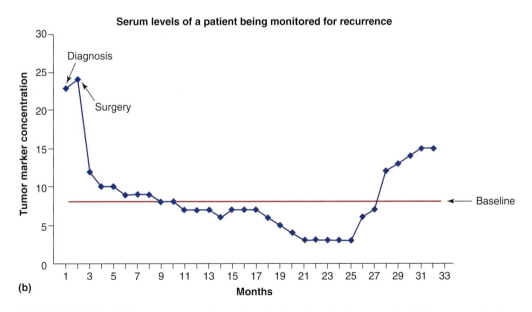

■ **FIGURE 12.8**   (a) Tumor marker analysis of a patient undergoing therapy, who (1) after surgery had residual disease and levels of the marker above baseline, (2) during the first chemotherapy, which was unsuccessful, had increasing levels of the marker, and (3) during successful chemotherapy had decreasing levels of the marker that went below baseline at which time the patient had no evidence of disease. (b) Tumor marker analysis of a patient with no evidence of disease monitored for tumor recurrence. The tumor was shown by serum marker levels to have recurred at ~29 months.

▶ STAGING USE OF TUMOR MARKERS IN BLOOD OR TISSUES

For some tumor types, the TNM system for tumor staging can be supplemented by the serum levels of tumor markers at diagnosis or at the beginning of therapy. In addition, antibodies to tumor markers are utilized in screening lymph nodes, and blood and bone marrow aspirates to detect tumor cells. The presence of the tumor marker on cells in these areas indicates a worse prognosis because these results indicate that the tumor has spread. In blood or bone marrow aspirates, the presence of tumor antigen positive cells can be measured either by flow cytometry using a fluorescent-labeled antibody to the tumor-associated antigen, by other immunocytochemical techniques, and by molecular techniques including fluorescent *in situ* hybridization (FISH) or quantitative real-time polymerase chain reaction (qPCR). The presence of cells in the blood or in bone marrow aspirates is called the presence of *disseminated tumor cells*. Immunohistochemical staining of fixed sections of the lymph nodes can indicate in a sensitive fashion whether the tumor has spread to the lymph nodes by enhancing the ability to see the tumor cells (1, 2, 3, 4, 5, 6, 9).

SERUM MARKERS FOR SCREENING, DIAGNOSIS, MONITORING, AND STAGING

Bence-Jones Proteins and Monoclonal Immunoglobulins

Bence-Jones proteins and **monoclonal immunoglobulins** are used to confirm diagnosis in patients with multiple myeloma. These tests are performed for patients who are already presenting a clinical picture that indicates a diagnosis of myeloma. Bence-Jones proteins are immunoglobulin light chains that are found in the urine of patients with multiple myeloma. One of the first tumor markers discovered, it was reported in 1846 (9).

Although immunoglobulins are produced in significant levels by all healthy people and in elevated levels in people with infectious disease and autoimmunity, it is the monoclonality and the high concentration that make monoclonal immunoglobulin a tumor marker for myeloma. These antigens and myeloma will be discussed more in Chapter 13, which describes the hematopoeitic malignancies including leukemia, lymphoma, and myeloma (9, 10).

Beta-2 Microglobulin

Beta-2 microglobulin is a component of the class I molecule and as such is on all nucleated cells. However, serum levels of beta-2 microglobulin are elevated in and used in the diagnosis of multiple myeloma, chronic lymphocytic leukemia, and some lymphomas. Beta-2 microglobulin levels that are high at diagnosis indicate poor prognosis and the

concentration is used in staging. Beta-2 microglobulin can also be used to monitor multiple myeloma to determine whether the therapy is effective (9, 10, 11).

Alpha 1-Fetoprotein

Alpha 1-fetoprotein (AFP) is a tumor marker that is elevated in about 60% of nonseminomatous testicular cancers (but not elevated in seminomatous testicular cancer), 50 to 70% of people with liver cancer (hepatoma), and some rare germ cell tumors. It is used for a differential diagnosis in testicular cancer and is useful in diagnosis of hepatoma as well. It is also used in the evaluation of serum of pregnant women to assess for open neural tube defects of their fetus in the second trimester of pregnancy. Understanding the production of AFP helps in understanding these apparently very different diagnostic roles. AFP is produced initially by the fetal yolk sac, then by the fetal liver, and finally by the liver and the gastrointestinal tract. It is a major protein in fetal serum. AFP is very important in monitoring the response of both testicular and hepatocellular carcinoma patients' response to therapy. Levels of this marker are a sensitive indicator of a change in tumor size and thus are very useful in evaluating therapeutic response (9, 12).

AFP and liver ultrasound are used for screening for hepatoma. A screening program with AFP in China of individuals at risk for hepatoma due to chronic Hepatitis B infection was shown to decrease death due to hepatoma by 37%. Other people at risk for hepatocellular carcinoma are those with hepatitis C infections, alcoholics, those exposed to aflatoxin, and individuals with certain rare genetic diseases. As mentioned, AFP levels are used for monitoring the therapeutic response in hepatomas, and AFP is included in some (but not all) of the staging systems used for hepatomas (9, 12).

A glycoform of AFP called *AFP-L3* is associated with cancer whereas the glycoform AFP-L1 is associated with benign disease of the liver. *Glycoforms* are molecules with the same protein structure but with differing amounts of glycosylation. Thus, the degree of glycosylation on this molecule that is, the amount of an additional alpha 1-6 linked fucose on the AFP molecule, may improve diagnosis by helping differentiate benign from malignant liver disease. The measurement involved compares the percentage of AFP-L3 to the total AFP. At the time of this publication, the AFP-L3 test had not yet gained widespread use but was gaining acceptance in evaluating the risk of hepatocellular carcinoma in individuals with benign liver disease. More recent studies show that elevated AFP-L3 percentages are also seen in testicular cancer (9, 12).

Human Chorionic Gonadotropin

Human chorionic gonadotropin (hCG) is a tumor marker that, like AFP, is elevated in nonseminomatous testicular cancer. It is used in conjunction with AFP for diagnosis and monitoring of nonseminomatous testicular cancer. It is elevated in gestational trophoblastic tumors and germ cell tumors. Elevation of hCG is also used as a diagnostic tool for pregnancy. hCG is produced by cells of the placenta, which accounts for its rise quickly after fertilization. It is a very sensitive indicator of trophoblastic tumors. To decrease the false negative rate, AFP and hCG are used together for confirmatory diagnosis of nonseminomatous testicular cancer. hCG, AFP, and lactate dehydrogenase (LDH), a marker for cell turnover, are used together to stage nonseminomatous testicular cancer; with lower levels indicating a better prognosis than higher levels (9, 12, 13).

CA 15-3 and CA 27-29

Assays for the breast cancer markers **CA 15-3** and **CA 27-29** measure different epitopes on the MUC-1 molecule and differ not only in the epitope that they measure but also because the clinical assays for CA 15-3 are sandwich assays whereas the assays for CA 27-29 are competitive. Screening with these molecules is not possible because elevated levels are not found in cancer patients with early disease, are only seen in 70% of patients with advanced disease, and elevations can occur in benign breast conditions and hepatitis. However, these molecules are useful in monitoring the course of disease because levels drop with a decrease in tumor burden. Care must be taken in monitoring therapy with these markers because as cancer cells die and release their contents, the CA 15-3 levels (and perhaps CA 27-29 levels) increase temporarily. Clinically, a 25% increase in the marker concentration indicates disease progression, and a 50% decrease indicates successful therapy (9, 14, 15, 16, 17).

CA 19-9

Assays for **CA 19-9** are used in monitoring the course of disease in patients with pancreatic cancer and hepatobiliary cancer (bile duct). Not all patients who have these tumors are positive for this marker, and it is used only for following the course of treatment of patients who are positive at initiation of treatment. Any obstruction of the bile duct causes elevations in CA 19-9 levels, so CA 19-9 can be elevated without tumor occurrence. Its levels can also be elevated in stomach cancer (~50%) and colorectal cancer (30% of cases). High levels of CA 19-9 at diagnosis indicate a poor prognosis but are not generally used in staging. CA 19-9 is a monosialoganglioside and Lewis a and b negative individuals may not make this antigen. The American Society of Clinical Oncologists (ASCO) recommends that CA 19-9 measurements be used for monitoring pancreatic cancer therapy and used for screening only for the return of cancer with confirmatory biopsies or imaging tests. Because CA 19-9 is usually negative in early stage pancreatic cancer and it can be negative even in more advanced pancreatic cancer patients, its use as a screening tool would cause excessive false negative results. Because CA 19-9 can be elevated in pancreatitis patients and in any benign blockage of the bile duct, use of its levels for diagnosis could cause too excessive positive results. ASCO also does not recommend use of this marker for staging (9, 18).

CA 125

CA 125 is a tumor marker used to follow the response to surgery and therapy of women with ovarian cancer. It is elevated in about 90% of women with advanced ovarian cancer and can be monitored in these women during therapy. The fact that CA 125 levels are elevated in about half of the patients whose cancer is still localized to the ovary has spurred studies on its use as a screening or diagnostic tool. Although its diagnostic use in women with symptoms or those who are at familial risk as well as postmenopausal women is done, this use is not currently supported by the NCCN. Uterine fibroids, endometriosis, pelvic inflammatory disease, and even menstruation can elevate levels of CA 125, decreasing its diagnostic utility in premenopausal women (19). It is clinically used in the differential diagnosis of pelvic masses.

Carcinoembryonic Antigen

As its name implies, **carcinoembryonic antigen (CEA),** is an oncofetal antigen. Like CA 15-3, CA 19-9, and CA 125, it is a mucin (a heavily glycosylated protein) that is elevated in the serum of patients with certain cancer types. Originally described as a tumor-associated antigen for colorectal cancer, it has also been found to be elevated in the serum of some patients with breast, lung, pancreas, stomach, and ovarian cancers. CEA levels are also elevated in smokers and in a variety of noncancerous conditions such as inflammatory bowel disease. Elevations in these individuals without cancer would yield excessive false positive results, and some tumors are negative, so the combination of these 2 problems precludes the use of CEA as a screening marker. It is, however, elegantly predictive of recurrence and response to therapy and is used in serial monitoring of colorectal cancer every 3 months for 3 years if no recurrence is detected. When chemotherapy or radiation therapy causes a large amount of tumor cell death, a transient rise in CEA levels may occur before the decrease. High CEA levels at diagnosis indicate poor prognosis and are used in staging (20).

Prostate-Specific Antigen

Prostate cancer is the most common cancer in men other than skin cancer, and 1 of every 6 men will be diagnosed with prostate cancer, and 1 of 30 will die of prostate cancer, so diagnosis of this disease has important health implications. Discovered by T. Ming Chu and collaborators in 1979, **prostate-specific antigen (PSA)** is released into the serum by prostate cancer cells. It is a protease in seminal fluid, enhancing sperm motility by its effects on semen fluidity. PSA is present in low amounts in the serum of normal men, and the normal serum concentration of PSA increases as the size of the prostate increases with age (17, 21).

The use of PSA as a screening molecule has been quite controversial. Using a cutoff of 4 ng/ml, an elevated level of PSA is 2 of 3 times a false positive result, however the higher the PSA level, the more likely the patient is to have prostate cancer. In addition, 1 of 7 men who have prostate cancer have PSA values below 4 and these would yield a false negative result. Finally, the controversy also includes the fact that many of the cancers that are detected are slow growing, and their detection results in treatment, which is thought of as overtreatment because the slow-growing prostate tumor would not have caused significant morbidity for the individual. Overtreatment is particularly the case in tumors detected in men over the age of 75. PSA has been used for years as a screening marker but because of the controversy, a large randomized trial was recently done and the utility of PSA as a screening marker was shown. The European Randomized Study of Screening for Prostate Cancer randomized 180 000 men between 50 and 74 to screening every 4 years or no screening for PSA and found that the death rate due to prostate cancer of the screening group was 20% less than the control group (17, 21).

The result of all the information garnered is that PSA levels can be used in diagnosis, but should be used in a rather complex protocol, so that the PSA testing has the best positive and negative predictive value. The National Comprehensive Cancer Network (NCCN) recommends that men have baseline PSA testing at 40 and if the PSA level is above 1.0 ng/ml or if the individual is African American, they should get annual PSA and digital rectal exam (DRE) screening. African Americans are selected for more proactive screening protocols because prostate cancer occurs earlier in these men. If the PSA is under 1.0, the next PSA analysis is recommended to be 5 years later at 45. If the PSA values are still under 1 at this screening, the patient should be offered annual screening starting at age 50. If the PSA values at 40 or 45 are over 1 ng/ml, the patient should have annual DRE and PSA screening. In any case when the DRE is positive, a biopsy should be done (21).

If DRE is negative, the PSA is less than 2.5 ng/ml, and the PSA velocity has increased less than 0.35 ng/ml/year, the patient should have annual DRE and PSA screening. **PSA velocity** is the amount of increase in the PSA levels from the previous year. With lower initial PSA values, 1 velocity cutoff is used, and with higher initial PSA values, a higher velocity cutoff is used. If the DRE is negative, the PSA is 2.6 to 4 ng/ml or the PSA velocity is greater than 0.35, and the PSA levels are less than 2.5 ng/ml, the patient and the physician should consider a biopsy (21).

If the PSA level is 4–10 and the patient is healthy, a biopsy should be performed. If the patient with the PSA value of 4–10 is not otherwise healthy, then another PSA screening test should be done, comparing the **free to total PSA.** PSA circulates in the serum either complexed to endogenous protease inhibitors or as free PSA. The percent of PSA that circulates as free PSA is lower in cancer patients, with a cutoff of equal to or less than 25% indicates that the patient has prostate cancer. The use of free to total PSA has been helpful in reducing the number of unnecessary biopsies. The converse of free PSA, the amount of PSA that is complexed to alpha-1 antichymotrypsin is also measured. The higher the percent of PSA complexed, the more likely the patient is to have prostate cancer (21).

A few additional facts help to understand these guidelines. Prostate cancer is diagnosed with PSA, DRE, and biopsy and is treated with surgery, radiation, or watchful waiting. In men over 75, watchful waiting is often used because the slow growth rate of some of these tumors makes it unlikely that significant morbidity will occur as a result of these cancers during the patient's lifetime (21).

There are patient-related issues that can affect the serum levels of PSA that must considered. More than 20% of men in the age group screened using PSA levels take herbal medicines such as saw palmetto that may contain varying levels of phytoestrogens. Phytoestrogens can affect PSA levels and may give these individuals falsely negative values. In addition, about 10% of men take drugs for lower urinary tract symptoms that lower PSA levels by about 50%, and this should be considered in analysis. Prostatitis, an inflammation of the prostate, causes elevations in PSA, but these elevations usually decrease with antibiotic therapy, so in a young man with elevated PSA levels, antibiotic therapy should follow a measurement of an elevated PSA level. A repeat PSA value should be taken after the course of the antibiotic to determine whether prostatitis rather than cancer was the cause of the elevation (21).

TISSUE MARKERS BY IMMUNOHISTOCHEMISTRY AND FLUORESCENCE *IN SITU* HYBRIDIZATION

The laboratory at an area cancer hospital performs about 200 different tumor marker tests in their pathology laboratory either by immunohistochemistry or by fluorescence *in situ* hybridization. Covering all of these antigens is beyond the scope of this chapter, but the general uses and a few examples follow. These analyses include a group of markers that help differentiate the general origin of a tumor (including cytokeratins, vimentin, and CD45), a group that is related more specifically to the tissue origin of the tumor (including PSA, AFP, and hCG), and a group that is related to the therapeutic response of the tumor (such as the estrogen receptor, the progesterone receptor, and HER-2 marker for breast cancer).

Differentiating Unknown Tumor Origin by Class: Sarcoma, Melanoma, Lymphoma, or Carcinoma

Sometimes it is not easy to tell where the primary origin of a patient's tumor is, so immunohistochemical testing of tumor samples must be used for this determination. Carcinomas (cancers of breast, lung, prostate, germ cell, thyroid, gastrointestinal tract, endocrine, and liver) can be detected by immunohistochemical analysis by the presence of **cytokeratins** in these tumors. Mesenchymal tumors (tumors of melanocyte, muscle fibrous, endothelium, nerve, paraganglioma, synovium, or cartilage origin) can be detected by immunohistochemical analysis by the presence of **vimentin** in them.

Hematopoietic tumors (leukemias, lymphomas, myelomas) can be detected when using immunohistochemical analysis by the presence of **CD45** (4, 5, 6).

Differentiating Tumor Origin Based on More Specific Tumor Reactions

To further differentiate a tumor of unknown primary origin, tumor-associated markers that are more tissue specific can also be used. Some of the tumor markers that have already been mentioned in the discussions above concerning serum analysis are also utilized as tumor markers in tissue analysis to find a more specific answer to the question of tumor origin. These react in immunohistochemistry to the same tumor types described in the serum analysis; examples include PSA, AFP, and hCG among many others.

Differentiating Between Treatment Options

Ligand binding, enzyme immunoassays, and immunohistochemical assays of tumor tissue for **estrogen receptor** and **progesterone receptor** are routinely done in all newly diagnosed breast cancer cases. The presence of these markers on the tumor tissue indicates that the tumor is likely to respond to endocrine therapy. The **HER-2 marker** is measured to determine whether the tumor will be susceptible to monoclonal antibody treatment with the anti-HER-2 antibody, Herceptin. The amount of HER-2 can also be utilized to predict responsiveness to anthracycline therapy (a type of chemotherapeutic drug). Only tumors with high levels of HER-2 are responsive to this therapy type. HER-2 is measured either by immunohistochemistry or fluorescence *in situ* hybridization (FISH) (9, 14, 15, 16, 17).

✓ Checkpoint! 12.4

Matching

1. Breast cancer   A. CA 15-3
2. Pancreatic cancer   B. CA 125
3. Ovarian cancer   C. CA 19-9
                       D. CA 27-29

▶ DETECTION OF CIRCULATING OR DISSEMINATED TUMOR CELLS

Cancer death is almost always due to metastasis, and the presence of circulating tumor cells in the blood stream indicates the ability of the patient's tumor to metastasize. Presence of tumor cells in the bone marrow indicates that the tumors cells have disseminated. The detection of circulating or disseminated tumor cells indicates the need for more aggressive treatment in cases where otherwise metastases were not detected. Different methods are available for detection of circulating tumor cells and detection of circulating tumor cells is recommended by the American Society of Clinical Oncology (22).

Circulating tumor cells from carcinomas are present in very low numbers in the blood stream, so methods of detecting them must be sensitive and specific so that a false positive signal is not seen with the 1 to 10 million-fold higher concentration of leukocytes. Cell detection methods can utilize fluorescent labeled monoclonal antibodies for epithelial markers such as cytokeratin or organ-specific markers such as CEA or PSA and scanning using either fiber-optic array scanning, laser scanning cytometry, or flow cytometry. Cell detection methods can also use detection by polymerase chain reaction (PCR). Cell enrichment methods include density gradient centrifugation based on the lighter density of tumor cells, cell filtration based on the usually large cell size of tumor cells, and immunomagnetic separation using magnetic bead-labeled antibodies that react with either the normal leukocytes or tumor cells (22).

Detection and enrichment methods can be combined, and currently only 1 diagnostic test for circulating tumor cells is approved by the FDA. Anti-EpCAM antibodies (antibodies that react with carcinomas) bound to ferric particles are used to enrich tumor cells from the blood, and magnets are used to separate these cells. The specificity is increased through the use of a second antibody, a fluorescent labeled anticytokeratin, which reacts with carcinomas to detect tumor cells. To further increase specificity, a third antibody, anti-CD45, which reacts with leukocytes and is fluorescently labeled with a different color, is used. For a cell to be considered a tumor cell, it must be isolated by the anti-EpCAM, stained with the anti-CK, and negative for the anti-CD45 labeling. Flow cytometric methods are used to separate cells labeled with the different fluorochromes (22).

▶ IMMUNOLOCALIZATION AND RADIOIMMUNOTHERAPY

Immunolocalization involves the intravenous injection of radiolabeled monoclonal antibody followed by patient imaging to determine the presence or absence of tumor metastasis. For a radiolabeled antibody to be used this way, the target antigen must be on the tumor cell surface in much higher amounts than on normal tissues. Circulating levels of the antigen should not be elevated in the serum or the antibody would bind there before it reached the tumor. Importantly, all tumor metastases should express the antigen. Currently, 3 monoclonal antibodies are used clinically for these determinations. **Prostascint** is an antibody to prostate-specific membrane antigen (PSMA). This antibody is used after prostatectomy to detect distant metastasis. It cannot be used before surgery because the normal prostate also contains this antigen and would act as a sink for the monoclonal antibody.

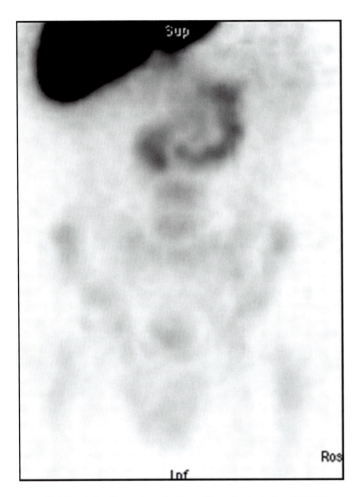

■ **FIGURE 12.9** Tumor localization with radiolabeled anti-PSMA
Source: Courtesy of Dr. Dominick Lamonica and the Nuclear
Medicine Service of the Roswell Park Cancer Institute, Buffalo,
NY, U.S.A.

The other 2 antibodies used for radioimmunolocalization are used primarily for radioimmunotherapy (Figure 12.9 ■) (23). **Radioimmunotherapy** is the transfer of radiolabeled antibodies at a level high enough to have a therapeutic effect on the tumor. Radioimmunotherapy is done with 2 different antibodies (different manufacturers), both of which react with the CD20 antigen that is present on B-cell non-Hodgkin's lymphomas. You may remember that CD20 is also present on normal B cells, and a predose of unlabeled antibody is given to reduce targeting of the spleen. Tumor cells are destroyed and normal B cells are dramatically decreased, but the normal B-cell numbers begin to recover by 12 weeks. These 2 antibodies are called **Bexxar,** an [131]Iodine-labeled antibody which is used in a dosimetric concentration followed by a therapeutic concentration, and **Zevalin,** which uses [111]Indium-labeled for imaging and [90]Yttrium-labeled for therapy. At 12 weeks, both of these agents show an overall tumor response rate between 60 to 83% and a complete response rate of 15 to 52% (23).

IMMUNOTHERAPY

For antibody-mediated immunotherapy to be successful, the antibody must bind to a tumor cell, and not to any normal cells which would be affected by binding of the antibody. Immunotherapeutic modalities in addition to radioimmunotherapy have recently achieved success. These therapies can be either passive or active immunotherapy. Passive immunotherapy, the transfer of monoclonal antibody to the tumor antigen, includes the successful monoclonal antibody **Herceptin,** which reacts with HER-2 antigen. Herceptin is used with chemotherapy. The HER-2 antigen is a growth factor receptor and is present in about 25% of breast cancer cases (16).

Active immunotherapy includes the vaccine **Gardasil,** which is used to prevent human papilloma virus (HPV)-associated cervical cancer. **Provenge** is a prostate cancer vaccine that received FDA approval in 2010. In this vaccine patient antigen-presenting cells are isolated and in culture are loaded with a tumor antigen called *prostatic acid phosphatase.* After they become activated and proliferate, these antigen-presenting cells are returned to the patient and stimulate the patient's T cells to make a response (21).

Cytokine therapy is performed to help a cancer patient make an immune response to his or her tumor. Interferon alpha is used in hairy cell and chronic myeloid leukemia, melanoma and Kaposi's sarcoma, kidney cancer, and non-Hodgkin's lymphoma. IL-2 is used to enhance the immune response in patients with melanoma and those with kidney cancer. In addition, cellular therapy using cells incubated and allowed to proliferate in culture with IL-2 is performed. Lymphokine-activated killer (LAK) cells are expanded and infused back into the patient. An improvement of cellular therapy using similarly expanded lymphocytes isolated from inside the removed tumor tissue, called *tumor-infiltrating lymphocytes (TIL),* has been performed with some success. TIL infusion is utilized along with IL-2 infusion of patients for cancer therapy (24).

New modalities are reaching the clinic at an impressive rate, but only time will tell whether their use is as successful as it is currently hoped.

GENETIC MARKERS

A small percentage of cancer cases has been found to be genetically linked, but in these defined cases, genetic testing can play a role.

There is a strong genetic link in about 10 to 15% of breast cancer cases, and the associated genetic mutation can be detected by looking for certain mutations in the breast cancer susceptibility genes **BRCA1** and **BRCA2.** The cumulative risk of breast cancer to age 80 with a BRCA1 mutation is about 90%, and with a BRCA 2 mutation is 41%. The cumulative risk of ovarian cancer for women with a BRCA1 mutation is 16 to 60% and with a BRCA 2 mutation 16 to 27%. Genetic counseling is an important part of understanding the risks and the options for these individuals (25).

A type of colon cancer that accounts for about 1% of new cases can be detected genetically also. This type of cancer, called *familial adenomatous polyposis,* actually has 100% penetrance, with every person with this mutation developing colon cancer by age 40 unless they have their colons removed.

CASE STUDY

Mr. Hernandez has developed blood in his stool and a change in bowel habits. A colonoscopy revealed a 0.5 cm tumor. During the surgery, a portion of the colon was removed as were the associated lymph nodes.

1. In immunohistochemistry, which marker could be used for staining tumor cells in the lymph nodes?
2. Which marker can be used for monitoring the course of Mr. Hernandez's treatment?
3. If Mr. Hernandez's diagnosis was T1, N0, M0 after the workup, what was the result of the immunohistochemistry of the tumor-associated lymph nodes?
4. For what other types of cancer can the marker that was used for Mr. Hernandez be used?
5. Can serum levels of this marker be used for staging?

SUMMARY

Cancers are the second most common cause of death. The word *cancer* indicates a group of diseases in which 1 cell has undergone transformation and now proliferates without control. The type of cancer is based on the specific organ in which this cell arose. Treatment of cancer is based on 4 elements: the organ in which the tumor arose, how far the tumor has spread, the degree of differentiation of the tumor cells, and whether these cells contain certain markers that would indicate they are susceptible to certain treatments. Tumor-associated antigens can be used to help to determine these factors (1, 2, 3, 4, 5, 6, 7, 8, 9) (Table 12.1).

Screening is an effort to find tumors early so that the patient has better prognosis with less morbidity. Screening involves testing for cancers in a population when no cancer exists; the criteria

for a screening marker to be used are very stringent because a small false positive rate could have a dramatic effect when large populations are being tested and the cancer occurs with a low incidence. Screening is more successful when a group at higher risk is selected. Confirmatory diagnosis involves testing individuals who have signs, symptoms, and possibly other testing results that indicate that a tumor is present. Screening can be by a variety of nonimmunologic means, but the immunologic means are the primary focus of this chapter. AFP (hepatoma) and PSA (prostate cancer) are used for screening. AFP (hepatoma, testicular cancer), hCG (testicular cancer), PSA (prostate cancer), Bence-Jones proteins (myeloma), immunoglobulins (myeloma), and Beta-2 microglobulins (multiple myeloma, chronic lymphocytic leukemia, lymphomas) are used for confirmatory diagnosis. Screening with PSA can include PSA serum levels, PSA velocity, and free to total PSA levels (9, 10, 11, 12, 13, 14, 15, 16, 17, 18, 19, 20).

Monitoring the course of the disease can be facilitated using levels of tumor antigens that rise and fall with the amount of tumor load. Monitoring is important because it can help the physician determine whether any tumor remains after surgery, if the tumor has recurred, and if the therapy is working or should be changed. The criteria for an antigen to be used this way are that the initial tumor was positive for the antigen, and the antigen has a half-life long enough to accumulate with increasing tumor burden and short enough that it decreases with decreasing tumor burden. The tumor-associated antigens that can be used this way include Bence-Jones proteins (myeloma), immunoglobulins (myelomas), AFP (testicular cancer, hepatoma), hCG (testicular cancer), Beta-2 microglobulin (myeloma, non-Hodgkin's lymphoma, lymphomas), CA 15-3, CA 27-29 (breast cancer), CA 19-9 (pancreatic cancer), CA 125 (ovarian cancer), CEA (colon cancer), and PSA (prostate cancer) (9, 10, 11, 12, 14, 15, 16, 17, 18, 19, 20, 21, 22, 23, 24).

Staging the cancer in terms of the patient's amount of tumor burden can be related to serum levels for Bence-Jones proteins (myeloma), immunoglobulins (myelomas), AFP (testicular cancer, hepatoma), hCG (testicular cancer), beta-2 microglobulin (myeloma, non-Hodgkin's lymphoma, lymphomas), and CA 19-9 (pancreatic cancer). Staging according to the presence of the antigen in sentinel lymph nodes is performed with CEA (colon cancer), and staging with the presence of the antigen in bone marrow aspirates and lymph nodes can be accomplished with PSA (prostate cancer) (9, 10, 11, 12, 14, 15, 16, 17, 18, 19, 20, 21, 22, 23, 24).

TABLE 12.1

Tumor Markers Involved in Screening, Confirmatory Diagnosis, Monitoring, and Staging

Antigen	Tumor Type(s)	Screening (S) or Confirmatory Diagnosis (CD)	Monitoring	Staging
Bence-Jones proteins	Myeloma	Yes (CD)	Yes	Yes
Immunoglobulin	Myeloma	Yes (CD)	Yes	Yes
AFP	Nonseminomatous testicular cancer Hepatoma	Yes (S), (CD)	Yes	Yes for nonseminomatous testicular cancer Yes for some staging systems for hepatoma

✪ TABLE 12.1

Tumor Markers Involved in Screening, Confirmatory Diagnosis, Monitoring, and Staging *(continued)*

Antigen	Tumor Type(s)	Screening (S) or Confirmatory Diagnosis (CD)	Monitoring	Staging
hCG	Nonseminomatous testicular cancer	Yes (S), (CD)	Yes	Yes for nonseminomatous testicular cancer
Beta-2 microglobulin	Myeloma Non-Hodgkin's lymphomas	Yes (CD) part of diagnostic workup	Yes	Yes amount at diagnosis used in staging
CA 15-3	Breast cancer	No	Yes*	No
CA 27-29	Breast cancer	No	Yes*	No
CA 19-9	Pancreatic cancer	No	Yes	Yes if no bile obstruction
CA 125	Ovarian cancer	No Some use for high-risk patients† Used to differentiate pelvic masses	Yes	No
CEA	Colon cancer	No	Yes	No with sera IHC of sentinel lymph node investigational
PSA	Prostate cancer	Yes (S), (CD)	Yes	No with sera Yes in bone marrow aspirates, lymph node by IHC

Some recent studies say that use is not validated.
†*Used in some centers, not recommended by NCCN 2010, but recommended by some expert groups.*

REVIEW QUESTIONS

1. A tumor normally grows
   a. from 1 cell to a billion cells in 1 year
   b. independent of normal growth signals and controls
   c. from a group of 10 different cells, so it is polyclonal in origin
   d. with a decrease in metabolic rate when compared to normal cells

2. Tumor markers that are elevated in testicular cancer are
   a. CEA and CA 19-9
   b. CA 125 and CEA
   c. AFP and hCG
   d. CA 15-3 and CA 27-29

3. Tumor markers that are elevated in breast cancer are
   a. CEA and CA 19-9
   b. CA 125 and CEA
   c. AFP and hCG
   d. CA 15-3 and CA 27-29

4. PSA is found free or complexed; if a patient has a tumor, the percent of free PSA should be
   a. less than 35%
   b. less than 25%
   c. more than 25%
   d. more than 35%

5. PSA velocity refers to
   a. how quickly PSA levels fall to background after a patient's surgery
   b. how quickly PSA levels fall to background after chemotherapy
   c. the biological half-life of PSA
   d. the amount that the patient's PSA has increased in a year

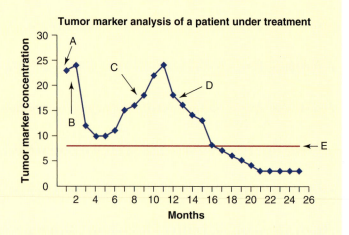

Tumor marker analysis of a patient under treatment

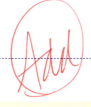

6. The point labeled B on the graph on the previous page could be
   a. the baseline
   b. a biopsy
   c. surgery
   d. unsucessful chemotherapy

7. The point labeled C on the graph could be
   a. the baseline
   b. a biopsy
   c. the diagnosis
   d. unsucessful chemotherapy

8. Looking for the expression of a tumor antigen in a tissue is done to aid the pathologist in making a diagnosis. This analysis can allow the pathologist to determine whether a tumor is
   a. a sarcoma, melanoma, lymphoma, or carcinoma
   b. a prostate tumor
   c. a tumor that will be responsive to endocrine therapy
   d. all of the above

9. Bexxar is
   a. a monoclonal antibody that reacts with the CD20 molecule on lymphomas and can be used for therapy
   b. a breast cancer antigen that can be used in screening breast cancer patients
   c. a type of surgery in which monoclonal antibody is injected around the tumor tissue
   d. used antibody radiolabeled with Yttrium

10. Genetic prediction of cancer
    a. is never utilized
    b. is possible and important with a small percentage of breast, ovarian, and colon cancers
    c. can be used in every patient
    d. is most important with testicular cancer

11. Active immunotherapy includes
    a. transfer of Bexxar to the patient
    b. transfer of Herceptin to the patient to treat breast cancer
    c. vaccination with Gardasil
    d. all of the above

12. AFP can be used for the diagnosis of
    a. pregnancy
    b. nonseminomatous germ cell tumors
    c. myelomas
    d. thyroid carcinoma

13. hCG is used in screening in conjunction with which of the following molecules?
    a. calcitonin
    b. CEA
    c. immunoglobulin
    d. AFP

14. Which is a common marker for epithelioid tumors?
    a. cytokeratins
    b. vimentin
    c. CD45
    d. PSA

15. *Grading* of a tumor refers to
    a. placing a rough edge against the tissue and abrading it
    b. determining how far the tumor has metastasized
    c. determining how many lymph nodes contain the tumor
    d. determining how well differentiated the tumor tissue is

16. A patient who has the following staging determination T_0, N_0, M_0
    a. probably does not have long to live
    b. will be relieved at this diagnosis
    c. has a primary tumor but no metastasis
    d. has not yet been examined

17. Which of the following is *not* used for staging with serum analysis?
    a. Bence-Jones proteins
    b. AFP
    c. hCG
    d. PSA

18. The pathologist uses all of the following for staging except
    a. PSA antigen levels in the primary tumor
    b. PSA antigen present in the bone marrow
    c. CEA in the lymph node
    d. cytokeratins in the lymph node

19. In monitoring the course of cancer,
    a. the antigen must be released from the tumor into the serum or other easily assayed fluid
    b. the half-life of the protein must be long enough so that concentrations become measurable
    c. the half-life of the protein must be short enough that along with a decrease in tumor burden there is a timely decrease in antigen levels
    d. all of the above

20. Which of the following is *not* a marker used for monitoring?
    a. CA 15-3
    b. carcinoembryonic antigen
    c. CA-125
    d. cytokeratin

REFERENCES

1. National Cancer Institute. What you need to know about cancer. http://www.cancer.gov/cancertopics/wyntk/cancer/allpages/print. Accessed May 18, 2010.

2. National Cancer Institute. Fact sheet cancer: Questions and answers. http://www.cancer.gov/cancertopics/factsheet/Sites-Types/general. Accessed June 4, 2010.

3. American Society of Clinical Oncology (ASCO). http://www.cancer.net/patient/All+About+Cancer. Accessed July 7, 2011.

4. National Cancer Institute. Fact sheet tumor markers: Questions and answers. http://www.cancer.gov/cancertopics/factsheet/Detection/tumor-markers/print?page=&keyword=. Acessed March 15, 2012.

5. American Cancer Society. Tumor markers. http://www.cancer.org/docroot/PED/content/PED_2_3X_Tumor_Markers.asp?sitearea=PED. Accessed March 15, 2012.

6. Sturgeon CM, Duffy MJ, Stenman U-H, et al. National Academy of Clinical Biochemistry Laboratory Medicine Practice Guidelines for use of tumor markers in testicular, prostate, colorectal, breast, and ovarian cancers. *Clin Chem.* 2008;54:e11–e7. 10.1373/clinchem.2008.105601

7. Center for Disease Control and Prevention. Faststats—Leading causes of death. www.cdc.gov/nchs/fastats/lcod.htm. Accessed March 15, 2012.

8. Center for Disease Control and Prevention. National vital statistics reports deaths: Final data for 2006. http://www.cdc.gov/nchs/data/nvsr/nvsr57/nvsr57_14.pdf. Accessed March 15, 2012.

9. National Academy of Clinical Biochemistry Laboratory Medicine Practice Guidelines. NACB: Tumor markers. http://www.aacc.org/EXPIRED/TumorMarkers/Pages/TumorMarkersPDF.aspx. Accessed March 15, 2012.

10. National Comprehensive Cancer Network. NCCN clinical practice guidelines in oncology (NCCN Guidelines™): Multiple myeloma. http://www.nccn.org/professionals/physician_gls/PDF/myeloma.pdf. Accessed March 15, 2012.

11. National Comprehensive Cancer Network. NCCN clinical practice guidelines in oncology (NCCN Guidelines™): Non-Hodgkin's lymphoma. http://www.nccn.org/professionals/physician_gls/PDF/nhl.pdf. Accessed June 4, 2010.

12. American Society of Clinical Oncology (ASCO). Testicular cancer: Staging. http://www.cancer.net/patient/Cancer+Types/Testicular+Cancer?sectionTitle=Staging. Accessed March 15, 2012.

13. National Comprehensive Cancer Network. NCCN clinical practice guidelines in oncology (NCCN Guidelines™): Hepatobiliary cancer. http://www.nccn.org/professionals/physician_gls/pdf/hepatobiliary.pdf. Accessed March 15, 2012.

14. Klee GG, Schreiber WE. MUC1 gene-derived glycoprotein assays for monitoring breast cancer (CA 15-3, CA 27.29, BR): Are they measuring the same antigen? *Arch Pathol Lab Med.* 2004;128(10):1131–1135.

15. Duffy MJ. Serum tumor markers in breast cancer: Are they of clinical value? *Clin Chem.* 2006;52(3):345–351. Epub January 12, 2006.

16. National Comprehensive Cancer Network. NCCN clinical practice guidelines in oncology (NCCN Guidelines™): Breast cancer. http://www.nccn.org/professionals/physician_gls/PDF/breast.pdf. Accessed March 15, 2012.

17. Esserman L, Shieh Y, Thompson I. Rethinking screening for breast cancer and prostate cancer. *JAMA.* 2009;302(15):1685–1692.

18. National Comprehensive Cancer Network. NCCN clinical practice guidelines in oncology (NCCN Guidelines™): Pancreatic adenocarcinoma. http://www.nccn.org/professionals/physician_gls/PDF/pancreatic.pdf. Accessed March 15, 2012.

19. National Comprehensive Cancer Network. NCCN clinical practice guidelines in oncology (NCCN Guidelines™): Ovarian cancer. http://www.nccn.org/professionals/physician_gls/PDF/nhl.pdf. Accessed June 4, 2010.

20. National Comprehensive Cancer Network. NCCN clinical practice guidelines in oncology (NCCN Guidelines™): Colon cancer. http://www.nccn.org/professionals/physician_gls/PDF/colon.pdf. Accessed March 15, 2012.

21. National Comprehensive Cancer Network. NCCN clinical practice guidelines in oncology (NCCN Guidelines™): Prostate cancer. http://www.nccn.org/professionals/physician_gls/PDF/prostate.pdf. Accessed March 15, 2012.

22. Gerges N, Janusz Rak J, Jabado N. New technologies for the detection of circulating tumour cells. *Br Med. Bull.* 2010;94(1):49–64; doi:10.1093/bmb/ldq01123.

23. Jacene HA, Filice R, Kasecamp W, et al. Comparison of 90Y-ibritumomab tiuxetan and 131I-tositumomab in clinical practice. *J Nucl Med.* 2007;48(11):1767–1776. Epub 2007 Oct 17.

24. Rosenberg SA, Packard BS, Aebersold PM et al. Use of tumor-infiltrating lymphocytes and interleukin-2 in the immunotherapy of patients with metastatic melanoma. *N Engl J Med.* 1988;319:1676–1680.

25. Lab Tests Online. Triple Screen or Quad Screen. http://www.labtestsonline.org/understanding/analytes/triple_screen/glance.html. Accessed March 15, 2012.

26. Tan DS, Rothermundt C, Thomas K, et al. "BRCAness" syndrome in ovarian cancer: A case-control study describing the clinical features and outcome of patients with epithelial ovarian cancer associated with BRCA1 and BRCA2 mutations. *J Clin Oncol.* 2008;26(34):5530–5536. Epub 2008 Oct 27.

13

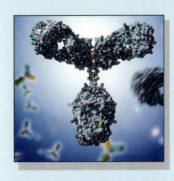

Immunoproliferative Diseases

■ OBJECTIVES—LEVEL I

After this chapter, the student should be able to:

1. Compare and contrast lymphoma and leukemia.
2. Compare and contrast Hodgkin's and non-Hodgkin's lymphoma.
3. Describe plasma cell dyscrasias including monoclonal gammopathy of undetermined significance.
4. Describe myelomas in terms of monoclonal versus polyclonal gammopathy, diagnosis, hyperviscosity, Bence-Jones proteins, organ damage, skeletal system damage, suppression of other Igs, and prognosis.
5. Describe heavy chain disease.
6. Describe light chain disease.
7. Describe macroglobulinemia in terms of categorization as a lymphoma, electrophoresis pattern, hyperviscosity and associated changes, rouleaux formation, organ changes, amyloidosis, and cryoglobulin.
8. Describe serum protein electrophoresis patterns of myeloma and macroglobulinemia. Describe this method and interpret serum protein electrophoresis (SPE) patterns.
9. Describe immunofixation electrophoresis. Describe this method and interpret immunofixation patterns.
10. Compare and contrast normal myeloma and macroglobulinemia serum protein patterns in percentages and in mg/dL.
11. Describe light chain analysis.

■ OBJECTIVES—LEVEL II

After this chapter, the student should be able to:

1. Describe myelomas in terms of treatment.
2. Describe macroglobulinemia in terms of treatment.
3. Interpret case histories with emphasis on high-risk groups and the clinical manifestations of the disease, and select and interpret appropriate clinical laboratory tests in diagnosis and evaluation of the disease.

KEY TERMS

acute leukemia

amyloidosis

chronic leukemia

heavy chain disease

Hodgkin's disease

immunofixation
    electrophoresis

immunoproliferative
    disease

leukemia

light chain deposition
    disease

lymphoid

lymphoma

monoclonal gammopathy
    of undetermined
    significance (MGUS)

multiple myeloma

myeloid

non-Hodgkin's lymphoma

plasma cell dyscrasias

Raynaud phenomena

Rituximab

Waldenström
    macroglobulinemia

▶ INTRODUCTION

The term **immunoproliferative disease** usually indicates a malignant growth of lymphocytes resulting in a lymphoma, a leukemia, or a plasma cell dyscrasia. Like all cancers, the immunoproliferative disorders arise from genetic alterations in one cell that cause the production of progeny that do not respond to normal growth signals and controls. A multistep process causes the transformation of the cell (1, 2, 3, 4).

There is no known cause of these cancers, but risk factors are related to them. Risk factors for immunoproliferative disorders include (1) acquired or congenital immunodeficiency diseases including immunosuppression resulting from transplantation, (2) autoimmune diseases, (3) certain chronic infections (*Helicobacter pylori,* hepatitis C), (4) infection with certain viruses that can be involved in the transformation process including Epstein Barr and human T-cell leukemia/lymphoma virus, (5) genetic susceptibility in patients with Down syndrome and other congenital disorders, (6) age over 60, (7) carcinogen exposure (benzene and certain pesticide or herbicide exposure), (8) previous radiation therapy, and (9) obesity (1, 2, 3, 4).

Leukemia, a disease of the cells of either myeloid or lymphoid lineage, starts in the bone marrow (Figure 13.1 ■). From the bone marrow, these cells invade the blood stream and circulate in it. These cells can then spread to the lymph nodes, liver, spleen, central nervous system, and the testicles in males. Occasionally, other cell types with tumors arising in the bone marrow are also called leukemia.

Lymphomas arise from mature lymphocytes in the organs of the lymphoid system, the lymph nodes, the spleen, the MALT, and the thymus. Lymphomas begin as solid tumors in these organs and can seed the blood and the marrow. The term dyscrasia means blood disorder. Plasma cell dyscrasias include multiple myelomas, Waldenström macroglobulinemia, **light chain deposition disease,** and heavy chain disease, which are all cancers that arise from a plasma cell. A

benign disorder called *monoclonal gammopathy of undetermined (or unknown) significance (MGUS)* is also grouped here (1, 2, 3, 4).

▶ LEUKEMIAS

Leukemias can either be myeloid or lymphoid. The myeloid leukemias (Figure 13.2(a) ■) arise from cells produced by the common **myeloid** progenitor cell, including monocytes, granulocytes, mast cells, red blood cells, and platelets. The **lymphoid** leukemias (Figure 13.2(b)) arise from B cells, T cells, NK cells, and their precursors that are progeny of the common lymphoid precursor. Leukemias are subdivided into acute or chronic; acute disease is the more aggressive disease because it grows more rapidly. Chronic leukemias grow more slowly, taking more time to progress, but are more difficult to treat. **Acute leukemia** has many immature leukocytes in the blood, and **chronic leukemia** also has excess white cells in the blood, but they are usually more mature and can be in the bone marrow (1, 2, 3, 4).

The 4 main types of leukemia are acute myeloid, chronic myeloid, acute lymphocytic, and chronic lymphocytic. Acute lymphocytic leukemia (ALL) is most often seen in children 2 to 5 years old, chronic lymphocytic leukemia is most often seen in adults over 50, and acute and chronic myeloid leukemia are most often seen in adults. Adult and childhood cases of the same disease can be very different. For example, ALL is the most common type of leukemia in children but is the most rare type in adults. Although there are twice as many cases of ALL in children as adults, 3 times as many deaths from ALL occur in adults. This is one example in which the new 2009 classification (see the next paragraph) considers these differences; ALL is now separated by cytogenetic markers (4).

Leukemias are further differentiated by the cellular characteristics of morphology, genetics, cytochemical criteria, and cell surface immunological markers detected using flow cytometry (Table 13.1 ✪). The differentiation of the leukemias is important in determining prognosis and therapy. The World Health Organization (WHO) developed a new differentiation scheme that was adapted in 2009. This new differentiation utilizes morphology, genetics, immunophenotyping, cytochemical characteristics, patient's age, site-specific lesions, and the importance of borderline cases to best categorize patients for treatment. A full description of the WHO system of classification of leukemias and lymphomas is outside the scope of an immunology class, but a brief description is included here (1, 2, 3, 4).

▶ LYMPHOMAS

Lymphomas are classified as either Hodgkin's disease or non-Hodgkin's lymphoma. **Hodgkin's disease,** also called *Hodgkin's lymphoma,* can be further subtyped to classic Hodgkin's disease (which can be further subtyped to 4 different diseases

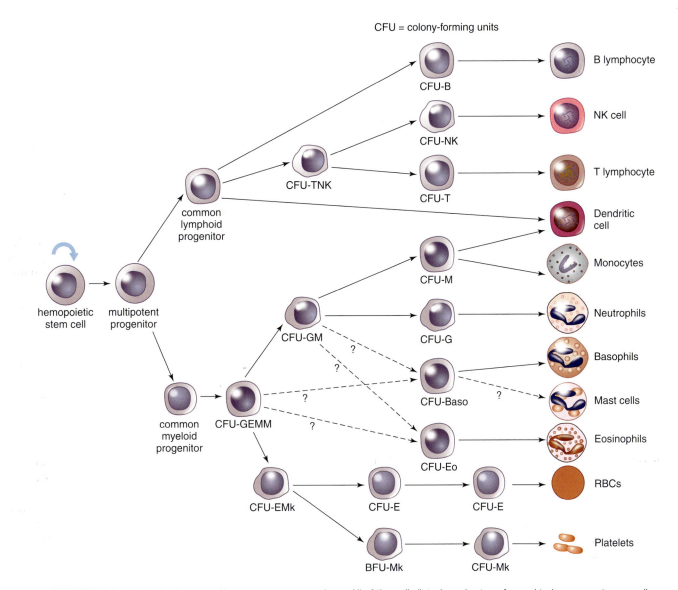

CFU = colony-forming units

■ **FIGURE 13.1**   A simple diagram of bone marrow progenitors. All of the cells listed can be transformed to become a tumor cell. These tumors are called *immunoproliferative diseases* and include leukemias, lymphomas, myelomas, and macroglobulinemias.

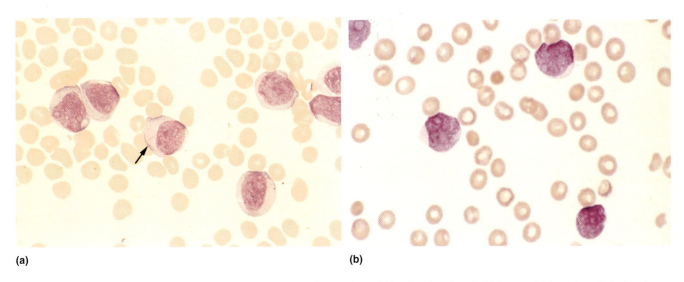

(a)   (b)

■ **FIGURE 13.2**   (a) Acute myelocytic leukemia: The tumor cells are of myeloid rather than lymphoid lineage. (b) Lymphocytic leukemia: The tumor cells are of lymphoid rather than myeloid lineage.

✪ TABLE 13.1

CD Markers Involved in Diagnosis, Monitoring, and Staging Leukemias and Plasma Cell Dyscrasias

Tumor		Antigens Used	Antigen Description
Myeloid		HLA-DR, CD34, CD33, CD11b, CD13, CD14, CD15, CD16	HLA-DR = class II CD34 = a marker for hematopoietic progenitor cells CD33, CD13 = marker on myeloid cells CD11b, CD16 = on monocytes, macrophages, granulocytes, and NK cells CD14 = monocytes, macrophage CD15 = on myeloid cells but can be on some lymphoid tumor cells as well
Lymphoid	T cells	CD2, CD3, CD5, CD7, CD34	CD2, CD3, CD5, CD7 T-cell markers CD34 hematopoietic progenitor cells
	B cells	CD10, CD19, CD20, CD21, CD34, HLA-DR	CD19, CD20, CD21 B-cell markers HLA-DR = class II CD34 = a marker for hematopoietic progenitor cells CD10 = common acute lymphocytic leukemia antigen
Myeloma		CD19, CD38, CD45, CD56	CD19 is on B cells but is lost when they mature to plasma cells CD38 is on plasma cells CD45 is on all white blood cells CD56 on 70–80% of myeloma cases and is related to prognosis
Waldenström macrogobulinemia		CD19, CD20, CD22, CD79	CD19, CD20, CD22 are B-cell surface antigens CD79 is associated with surface immunoglobulin

(Table 13.2 ✪)), and nodular lymphocytic predominant Hodgkin's disease (see Figure 13.3 ■). Identification of type and subtype of Hodgkin's disease is important in determining therapeutic choices. Hodgkin's lymphoma is seen in patients ages 15 to 35 and in those over 55. Hodgkin's disease starts in lymph nodes anywhere in the body, but most often in the chest, neck, or under the arms. It spreads from one lymph node to another in a chain, usually without skipping lymph nodes until late in the disease. Symptoms include night sweats and weight loss. In very late stage, the disease can metastasize throughout the body through circulatory spread, but this is rare (1, 2, 3, 4, 5).

✪ TABLE 13.2

CD Markers Involved in Diagnosis, Monitoring, and Staging Lymphomas

Tumor	Tumor Subtype	Subtypes	Antigens Used
Hodgkin disease	Classic	Nodular sclerosis	CD30+, CD15+
		Mixed cellularity	CD20 weak
		Lymphocyte depleted	
		Lymphocyte rich or predominant	
	Nodular lymphocytic predominant	–	usually CD30−, CD 15−, CD19+, CD20+
Non-Hodgkin lymphoma	B cell	Precursor cell	CD19+, CD20+, CD10+
		Mature cell (many subtypes of this)	Surface immunoglobulin, rearranged immunoglobulin genes
	T cell	Precursor cell	T cells: look for clonal rearrangement of T-cell receptor gene
		Mature cell (many subtypes of this)	

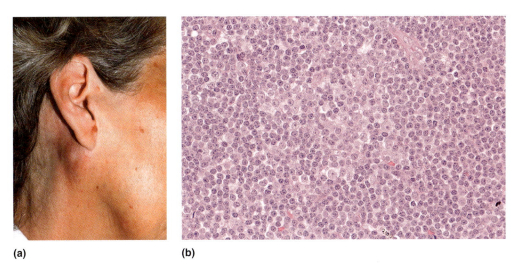

(a)   **(b)**

The cancer cells in Hodgkin's disease are called *Reed-Sternberg* cells and have a unique appearance under a microscope because the nucleus is bilobed and has 2 prominent nucleoli so that the cell is said to have an owl's eyes appearance (Figure 13.4 ■). The 5-year survival rates for persons with Hodgkin's disease is quite high: for stage I or II, about 90%; for stage III, about 80%; and for stage IV, about 65%. Hodgkin's disease is treated with chemotherapy and radiation therapy. If the disease does not respond to treatment, patients may be given a high dose of radiation or chemotherapy followed by either autologous or allogeneic stem cell transplant. A mild amount of graft versus host disease is said to be helpful in this therapy because the graft may actually help kill the lymphoma cells (1, 2, 3, 4, 5).

The many types of **non-Hodgkin's lymphoma** are classified according to morphologic appearance, genetic features, and surface CD markers. About 85% of non-Hodgkin's lymphomas are B-cell lymphomas, which include many different diseases. The remaining 15% of the non-Hodgkin's lymphomas are T-cell lymphomas, again including many different diseases. Non-Hodgkin's lymphoma is diagnosed with the general clinical symptoms of weight loss, fever, and night sweats which are found with fast growing lymphomas. Enlarged lymph nodes represent a symptom of lymphoma but can occur with response to infection; so, to determine whether the lymph nodes are enlarged because of infection or lymphoma, the patient is given antibiotics and the lymph nodes are checked again. If the nodes remain the same size or have increased, a biopsy is performed. Evidence of production of only one type of light chain in cells of the biopsy indicates that the lymphoproliferation is due to a malignant process rather than inflammation. Further testing to determine tumor spread can include a bone marrow aspiration and biopsy as well as laboratory testing (1, 2, 3, 4, 5).

Immunohistochemistry and flow cytometry are used to characterize the cells, and lactate dehydrogenase levels may be used to help determine whether the tumor is rapidly growing. Cytogenetic analysis can also characterize the tumor cells. The different types of non-Hodgkin's lymphoma can require different treatments and may have different prognoses, so characterization is important. Treatment is with chemotherapy, and the use of the monoclonal antibody may be suggested for B-cell non-Hodgkin's lymphomas. **Rituximab** is an antibody to CD20 that is on the surface of B-cell lymphomas. Radioactively labeled anti-CD20 monoclonal antibodies Bexxar and Zevalin are also used. Chronic lymphocytic leukemia and T-cell lymphomas may be treated with Campath, an antibody to the CD52 surface antigen. Interferon may shrink some lymphomas, and stem cell transplantation therapy may also be suggested as therapy for lymphomas (6).

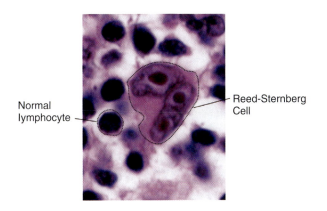

Normal lymphocyte —

Reed-Sternberg Cell

■ **FIGURE 13.4** Reed-Sternberg cells: Bilobed nucleus coupled with the prominent nucleoli gives this cell the "owl's eyes" appearance. *Source:* National Cancer Institute.

▶ PLASMA CELL DYSCRASIAS

Plasma cell dyscrasias, or plasma cell disorders, include multiple myeloma, macroglobulinemia, light chain deposition disease, heavy chain disease, and MGUS. Black patients have 3 times the incidence of plasma cell dyscrasias, and males have these diseases more often than women and in general have poorer prognosis (7, 8, 9).

MONOCLONAL GAMMOPATHY OF UNDETERMINED SIGNIFICANCE

Monoclonal gammopathy of undetermined significance (MGUS) is the most common of these dyscrasias or diseases of the plasma cells, representing 2 of every 3 cases of plasma cell dyscrasias. Monoclonal immunoglobulin is present in the sera of patients with MGUS, but neither multiple myeloma nor macroglobulinemia is present. The incidence of plasma cell dyscrasias increases with age, and the incidence of MGUS in individuals over 70 is more than 5%. The rate in which MGUS patients progress to either myeloma or macroglobulinemia is 1% a year, but this change can occur rapidly, and patients should be aware of what to look for because treatment would then be required. The serum monoclonal protein level in MGUS is less than 3 g/dL, no or only very little Bence-Jones protein is found in the urine, less than 1% of the bone marrow cells are plasma cells, there are no skeletal lesions, and there is no associated anemia, hypercalcemia, or renal failure. Patients with MGUS also have low plasma cell proliferation rate (9).

MULTIPLE MYELOMA

Multiple myeloma occurs in about 5 to 7 per 100 000 people. An uncontrolled proliferation of plasma cells occurs in multiple myeloma (Figure 13.5 ■) and results in very large increases in serum immunoglobulin levels. The immunoglobulin is monoclonal and in serum protein electrophoresis presents as a thin dark band that upon densitometry is visualized as a sharp tall peak. Multiple myeloma is usually of either the IgG or the IgA isotype, but in rare instances can be IgD or IgE. The plasma cell proliferation frequently occurs in the bone, forming areas in which it is replaced by a circular clone of tumor cells, resulting in bone lesions that on x-ray look like holes punched out of the bone. More than 30% of the cells in the bone marrow are these malignant plasma cells. The replacement of the normal cells of the bone marrow with these malignant plasma cells results in decrease in the production of normal blood cells. These patients consequently develop anemia, thrombocytopenia, and leukopenia. The bone lesions cause bone pain and hypercalcemia (7, 8).

The large increase in serum immunoglobulin results in serum hyperviscosity (increased thickness of the serum resulting from increased protein concentration) and subsequently a compensatory increase in plasma volume to reduce the

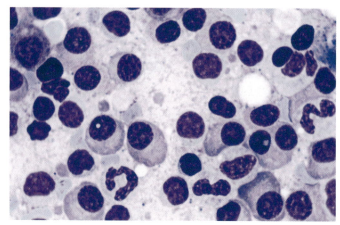

(a)

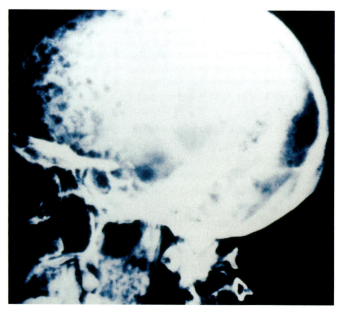

(b)

■ **FIGURE 13.5** (a) Multiple myeloma: Tumor of plasma cells. (b) Myeloma cells grow within the bone and lesions can be clearly visible on x-ray.

serum's viscosity. This increase in plasma volume results in a decrease in the number of red blood cells (RBCs), white cells, and platelets per ml of blood, thus worsening the anemia, leukopenia, and thrombocytopenia caused by the bone marrow damage. The increased plasma protein and increased calcium cause kidney damage. Spinal cord compression occurs in 20% of patients. Bone pain and fractures, increased bleeding, increased infection rate, and poor perfusion are all clinical symptoms of multiple myeloma. Serum levels of C-reactive protein and beta-2 microglobulin can be used to stage a patient with multiple myeloma (7, 8).

Treatment for myeloma includes high-dose chemotherapy and peripheral blood or bone marrow stem cell transplantation. Radiation therapy can be used to reduce tumor cell growth in areas with bone pain. Plasmapheresis to remove immunoglobulin may reduce renal failure rates. The prognosis for myeloma patients is approximately 3 years. However, it is important to note that with the advent of new therapies such as stem cell transplantation after high-dose chemotherapy, this survival time will increase (7, 8).

HEAVY CHAIN DISEASE

In **heavy chain disease,** heavy chains are made without the corresponding production and attachment to light chain. These heavy chains are not often full length because they contain deletions as a result of genetic changes. Heavy chain disease is more similar to lymphoma clinically than to myeloma because bone lesions do not occur, and the tumor cells are usually located in the mucosa of the small intestine as a lymphoma (10, 11).

IgA heavy chain disease occurs more often in the Middle East and occurs in the unexpectedly young age group of 10 to 30 years. Heavy chains may be found in the serum or the urine, or a biopsy may be necessary for diagnosis. Serum protein electrophoresis may have decreased gammaglobulins and an increase in the alpha-2 or beta peaks. The cause may be an incorrect immune response to infection; thus, the treatment can include antibiotics and corticosteroids as well as the more usual cytotoxic drugs. The prognosis is variable and can be from 1 to 2 or many years, depending on response to this therapy (10, 11).

Also more like lymphoma than myeloma, IgG heavy chain disease is found in elderly men and is associated with several autoimmune diseases. Increased infection rate, enlarged lymph nodes, liver, and spleen as well as fever occur in these patients. The prognosis is bleak with survival length commonly 1 year from diagnosis (10, 11).

IgM heavy chain disease is rare and is found in people over 50. Characteristics of this disease also include increased infection rate, enlarged lymph nodes (this time limited to the abdomen), liver, and spleen as well as fever, but bone fractures are more common in these patients. IgM heavy chain disease looks more like leukemia than lymphoma. The IgM heavy chain is not usually found in urine electrophoresis, and less than half the cases show an apparent band in serum protein electrophoresis. Kidney damage frequently occurs (10, 11).

LIGHT CHAIN DISEASE

In light chain disease, light chains called *Bence-Jones proteins* can be found in the urine, and renal damage can occur because of light chain accumulation in the kidney. These patients can also have heart, liver, and gastrointestinal involvement. Long-term survival is rare with a 1-year survival rate of about 20%. Light chain disease is also called light chain deposition disease. For light chain disease, myeloma, and macroglobulinemia, free light chain can be measured using several methods including protein electrophoresis of concentrated urine, immunofixation electrophoresis of serum or concentrated urine, and capillary zone electrophoresis, but latex enhanced immunonephelometry is an important new protocol (12, 13, 14).

WALDENSTRÖM MACROGLOBULINEMIA

In **Waldenström macroglobulinemia,** which occurs in about 7 to 10 per 100 000 people, the monoclonal production of excess amounts of IgM causes many changes in the patient's body. Waldenström macroglobulinemia was formerly classified as a myeloma but now is classified as a lymphoma because of its presence as a solid tumor in the lymphoid organs. Because the overproduced immunoglobulin has such a high molecular weight (900 000 daltons), the blood can become thick or viscous. The serum's thickness can cause circulation problems because the heart has trouble pushing this fluid through the blood vessels. Cryoglobulins, or cold precipitation of the immunoglobulin, can occur as the temperature drops and can cause pain in hands and feet due to decreased blood supply which is known as **Raynaud phenomena.** Excess light chain can cause heart and kidney damage in a process called **amyloidosis.** Amyloidosis occurs when a protein is abnormally folded and thus is insoluble and precipitates in organs and tissues causing pathology. Waldenström macroglobulinemia patients can become anemic because of the crowding out of blood-producing cells in the bone marrow by tumor cells and by the increase in fluids in the bloodstream as the body attempts to decrease the serum viscosity. Bleeding problems are seen in Waldenström macroglobulinemia patients because high levels of IgM alter platelet function. Patients can also experience weight loss and fever (15, 16, 17, 18).

✓ **Checkpoint! 13.1**

Which of the following is not found in lymphoid organs but is found in the blood stream and the bone marrow?

1. *Multiple myeloma*
2. *Heavy chain disease*
3. *Non-Hodgkin's lymphoma*
4. *Hodgkin's lymphoma*

The enlarged lymph nodes and spleen caused by tumor cell growth in Waldenström macroglobulinemia is not often seen in myeloma, and the lytic bony lesions often seen in multiple myeloma are rarely seen in Waldenström macroglobulinemia. Numbness and poor brain circulation with headache, confusion, and dizziness can also be seen in Waldenström macroglobulinemia patients. The formation of rouleaux, or stacks of red blood cells, because of the thickness of the serum can cause abnormalities in the perfusion of the eyes and result in vision problems. These patients have increased infection rates because of the feedback inhibition caused by high IgM levels. To decrease plasma IgM levels and decrease hyperviscosity problems, plasmapheresis can be performed. Waldenström macroglobulinemia is diagnosed with a complete blood count (to determine whether tumor cells are inhibiting the function of normal hematopoietic cells in the bone marrow), serum protein electrophoresis, immunofixation electrophoresis, quantitative measurements of immunoglobulins, and evidence of malignant small plasma cells in the bone marrow. Blood viscosity levels and beta-2 microglobulin levels are also important. Flow cytometry is used to analyze the tumor cells. The amount of serum IgM and the amount of serum beta-2-microglobulin are used in staging (15, 16).

Chemotherapy is given with steroid therapy to treat Waldenström macroglobulinemia. Immunotherapy with the antibody targeting either CD20 (Rituximab) (targets B cells) or CD52 (Alemtuzumab) (targets mature lymphocytes) is also used to treat these tumors. When these treatments do not work, autologous or allogeneic stem cell transplantation can be performed (15, 16).

 Checkpoint! 13.2

Name 2 things that can lead to anemia in patients with macroglobulinemia.

► LABORATORY ANALYSIS OF LYMPHOPROLIFERATIVE DISORDERS

A hematology course is better suited for a description of each type of leukemia than is an immunology course, but important classification of leukemias, lymphomas, and myelomas are based on immunological techniques. Leukemias and lymphomas are characterized via the cell surface markers that indicate cell type and degree of differentiation and whether the cells are monoclonal. This characterization is accomplished with flow cytometry (Chapter 1). Myelomas are characterized using serum protein electrophoresis, immunofixation electrophoresis, and immunoglobulin quantitation (17, 18, 19, 20, 21, 22).

ROLE OF THE FLOW CYTOMETRY LABORATORY IN DIAGNOSIS AND MONITORING

A standard operating procedure is followed in the diagnosis and differentiation of acute myeloid and acute lymphoid leukemia. Direct immunofluorescence is measured by flow cytometry. Fluorescently labeled antibody to cell type specific markers and differentiation specific markers are used to characterize the individual cell populations. The markers that were described in Chapter 2 to characterize the different cell populations are among those used to determine the phenotype of leukemias and lymphomas. The following markers used

differentiate myeloid cells (HLA-DR, CD34, CD33, CD11b, CD13, CD14, CD15, CD16) from lymphoid T cells (CD2, CD3, CD5, CD7, CD34) and B cells (CD10, CD19, CD20, CD21, CD34, and HLA-DR). Plasma cells are determined using a panel that contains CD19, CD38, CD45, and CD56 (Tables 13.1 and 13.2). Differentiation of the cell type of the tumor is important to determine the optimal therapy. After original typing, the molecules that were found on the cell surface are used as tumor markers for monitoring response to therapy and the course of the disease (17, 18, 19).

 Checkpoint! 13.3

Match the markers with the cell type

1. *HLA-DR, CD34, CD33, CD11b, CD13, CD14, CD15, CD16*
2. *CD2, CD3, CD5, CD7, CD34*
3. *CD10, CD19, CD20, CD21, CD34, and HLA-DR*

A. *B cells*
B. *T cells*
C. *myeloid cells*

LABORATORY ANALYSIS OF MYELOMA AND MACROGLOBULINEMIA

For diagnosis and prognosis of myeloma and macroglobulinemia, serum analysis for myeloma protein identification is performed for immunoglobulin by serum protein electrophoresis and immunofixation electrophoresis. It is important not to refrigerate serum prior to analysis because excess antibody, particularly IgM, can precipitate out of solution. Quantitative immunoglobulin levels are measured for each subclass. C-reactive protein and beta-2 microglobulin levels are measured for staging. X-ray skeletal studies and bone marrow biopsies are performed to determine the percentage of plasma cells. Latex-enhanced nephelometry with antibody that is specific for free light chain or urine protein electrophoresis is performed to analyze for Bence-Jones proteins (17, 18, 19).

Serum Protein Electrophoresis

Serum protein electrophoresis was important in the elucidation of the structure of immunoglobulin and was described in Chapter 1 (Figure 1.9) and Chapter 2 (Figure 2.1), but because this method is part of the laboratory analysis of a myeloma or macroglobulinemia, it is described in detail here. In serum protein electrophoresis, a small amount of serum (about 3 microliters, depending on the assay kit utilized) is placed at one end of an agarose gel. The 2 ends of the gel are placed in 2 different troughs of pH 8.6 buffer (Figure 13.6 ■). An electric current is placed with an electrode in each container of buffer, and the current moves from one container of buffer to the other by traveling through the gel. As the current travels through the

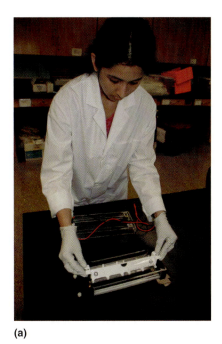
(a)

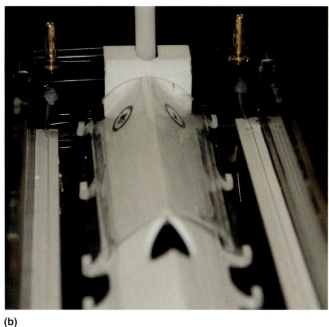
(b)

■ **FIGURE 13.6** Serum protein electrophoresis photo of gel just placed in electrophoresis apparatus showing that the 2 ends of the gel make contact between the 2 buffer baths; thus, the current goes through the gel to move the anionic (negatively charged) albumin toward the anode (positively charged).

gel, it brings with it the proteins with a negative charge at pH 8.6. Under these conditions, albumin travels most quickly toward the anode, followed by alpha-1 globulins, alpha-2 globulins, beta globulins, and finally the gamma globulins. The amount of movement of each molecule depends on:

1. The charge, size, and shape of the molecule—this can affect movement through the pores in the gel.
2. The pH of the media—this affects charge on the molecule.
3. The ionic strength of the media—high ionic strength gives better separation but more heat, which can denature the molecule.
4. The amount of current and length of time applied—an increase in either increases the distance the protein travels.
5. The temperature.
6. Electroendosmosis—movement toward the cathode because of the buffer's movement toward the cathode.

After the separation with the electric current, the gel is immediately placed in a stain that fixes the proteins in place (preventing band-width changes because of diffusion) and stains the proteins to make the bands visible. After staining, destaining is performed to remove the background staining, the gels are dried, and densitometry is performed on the gel. The gel is placed in a densitometer, and light is shown through the gel; the amount of light that is absorbed by the densely colored protein bands appears as peaks in the resultant densitometry tracing (Figure 13.7 ■) (20, 21, 22).

✔ **Checkpoint! 13.4**

1. *If you accidently made up the buffer in such a way that the proteins all had less charge, what would the electrophoresis pattern look like if you ran the gel for the same time period.*
2. *If you accidently ran the gel for half the period of time as you should have, what would the gel look like?*
3. *What would the bands on the gel look like if you increased the ionic strength of the buffer?*

The protein albumin, which is present in high amounts in serum and in which all the molecules have the same charge, appears as a dark tight band on the gel and a high and narrow peak on the densitometry tracing. Because gamma globulin is composed of many different immunoglobulin molecules with slightly different charges, it appears in normal serum as a lighter wider band that has a broader range of electrophoretic mobilities and in the densitometry tracing is a shorter broader peak. The normal amount of total serum protein is 6.4 to 8.3 g/dL, the normal amounts of albumin are 3.5 to 5.0 g/dL, of alpha-1 globulin 0.1 to 0.3 g/dL, of beta globulin 0.7 to 1.2 g/dL, and of gamma globulin is 0.7 to 1.6 g/dL (20, 21, 22).

In a patient with myeloma or macroglobulinemia, most of the immunoglobulin is made by the tumor cells and is monoclonal in origin. This antibody shows a much tighter peak, and the increased concentrations of immunoglobulin

Slit light source

The light is blocked by the stained sample. The gel is on a sliding platform which moves past the light source. The first peak is albumin which gives a sharp tall peak.

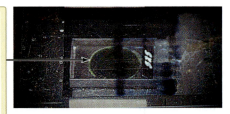

(a)

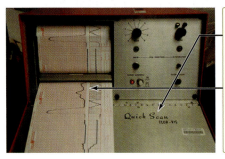

The gel is placed inside and a light shines through the gel.

Peaks are the amount of absorbance of the light as the gel moves past the light.

(b)

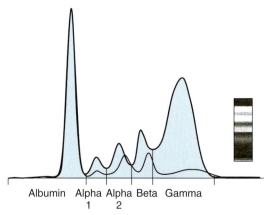

Serum protein electrophoresis

Fractions	%		Reference normal % range	Concentration	Reference normal concentration range
Albumin	28.3	<	60.0 – 71.0	2.43	43.00 – 51.00
Alpha 1	4.2	>	1.4 – 2.9	0.36	1.00 – 2.00
Alpha 2	8.2		7.0 – 11.0	0.71	5.00 – 8.00
Beta	10.5		8.0 – 13.0	0.90	6.00 – 9.00
Gamma	48.8	>	9.0 – 16.0	4.20	6.00 – 11.00

(d)

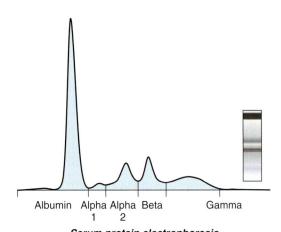

Serum protein electrophoresis

Fractions	%		Reference normal % range	Reference normal concentration range
Albumin	63.0		60.0 – 71.0	43.00 – 51.00
Alpha 1	2.1		1.4 – 2.9	1.00 – 2.00
Alpha 2	11.2	>	7.0 – 11.0	5.00 – 8.00
Beta	11.6		8.0 – 13.0	6.00 – 9.00
Gamma	12.1		9.0 – 16.0	6.00 – 11.00

(c)

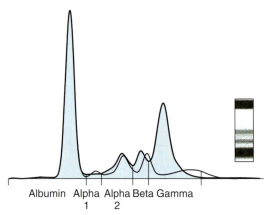

Serum protein electrophoresis

Fractions	%		Reference normal % range	Concentration	Reference normal concentration range
Albumin	50.5	<	60.0 – 71.0	4.14	43.00 – 51.00
Alpha 1	1.5		1.4 – 2.9	0.12	1.00 – 2.00
Alpha 2	10.2		7.0 – 11.0	0.84	5.00 – 8.00
Beta	7.5	<	8.0 – 13.0	0.62	6.00 – 9.00
Gamma	30.3	>	9.0 – 16.0	2.48	6.00 – 11.00

(e)

■ **FIGURE 13.7** Electrophoresis gel in a densitometer. (a) The green light from the slit light source is visible beneath the gel. (b) The densitometer showing the tracing as the scan is made. (c) SPE densitometry showing a normal pattern. (d) SPE densitometry showing polyclonal gammmopathy with a broad peak with an underlaying normal graph for comparison. (e) SPE densitometry showing an M spike in the gamma region with a shift towards the beta region with an underlaying normal graph for comparison.

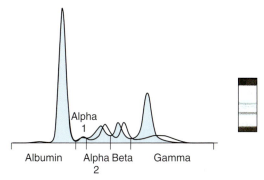

Serum protein electrophoresis

Fractions	%		Reference normal % range	Concentration	Reference normal concentration range
Albumin	59.3	<	60.0 – 71.0	4.68	43.00 – 51.00
Alpha 1	1.7		1.4 – 2.9	0.13	1.00 – 2.00
Alpha 2	9.1		7.0 – 11.0	0.72	5.00 – 8.00
Beta	8.0		8.0 – 13.0	0.63	6.00 – 9.00
Gamma	21.9	>	9.0 – 16.0	1.73	6.00 – 11.00

(f)

■ **FIGURE 13.7** *(continued)* (f) SPE densitometry showing an M spike in the gamma region.

produced by the tumor results in a high and tight peak. The serum protein electrophoresis patterns of myeloma and macroglobulinemia are very different from the patterns of hypergammaglobulinemia that can be seen with acute or chronic infection or autoimmune disease in that myeloma, and macroglobulinemia. The SPE patterns produced by tumor cells in macroglobulinemia and myeloma show a sharp peak in comparison to a broad peak of the polyclonal gammopathy caused by chronic or acute infection. The different tumor types show more subtle differences in serum protein electrophoretic pattern, generally in the mobility of the immunoglobulin peak with IgM and IgA generally showing more movement toward the anode than IgG (Figure 13.8 ■, lanes 1–10). The isotype produced by the tumor is determined by subsequent testing in immunofixation electrophoresis (20, 21, 22).

Immunofixation Electrophoresis

In **immunofixation electrophoresis,** serum is electrophoresed in serum protein electrophoresis in 6 replicates, that is, in 6 different parallel lanes on 1 agarose gel. The agarose gel is then incubated with the monospecific antiserum to IgG, IgA, IgM, and kappa and lambda light chains. The different antiserums are added so each overlays 1 lane

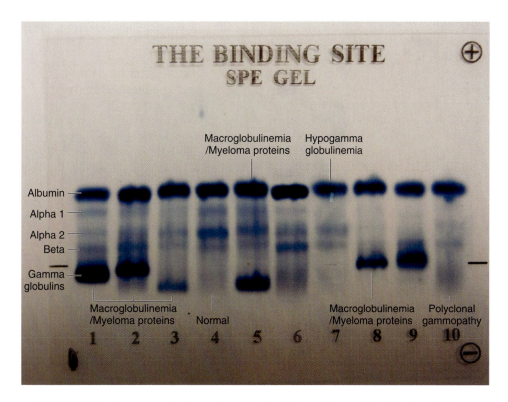

■ **FIGURE 13.8** Serum protein electrophoresis gel of 10 sera. Lanes 1, 2, 3, 5, 8, and 9 show evidence of an "M" protein, indicating either a multiple myeloma or a macroglobulinemia. IgG myeloma proteins are generally found closer to the cathode than IgM macroglobulinemia proteins, which are generally closer to the cathode than IgA myeloma proteins. However, to determine isotype for clinical use, immunofixation electrophoresis is performed.

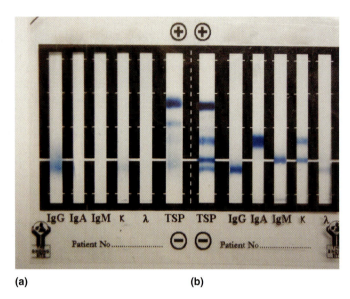

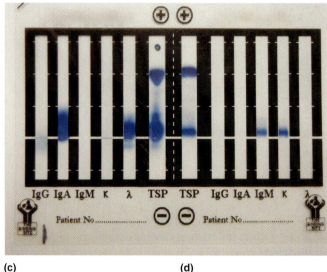

■ **FIGURE 13.9** Immunofixation electrophoresis. (a) IgG kappa myeloma, (b) Controls showing total serum protein (TSP) bands and sharp dense band in each lane, (c) IgA lambda myeloma, and (d) IgM kappa macroglobulinemia.

each. A protein fixative is added to the sixth lane to denature and precipitate the proteins for a total protein visualization. The reaction of the antibody with the immunoglobulin in the patient's sera forms a lattice immunoprecipitin reaction, thus fixing the complexes in the gel. The gels are then placed in saline and washed until unprecipitated proteins (those not fixed by lattice formation) are removed. The gel is then placed in a stain so that any precipitated proteins are stained. In normal samples, either no staining or light staining in a diffuse area in the IgG lane occurs. In polyclonal gammopathy, moderate to strong but diffuse staining occurs in all lanes. In a myeloma, sharp, dark bands are in either IgG or IgA heavy chain and 1 light chain (kappa or lambda) (Figure 13.9 ■(a) and (c)). A sharp band in the same place is also seen in the total protein lane. In macroglobulinemia, the bands will be in the IgM lane and either of the light chain lanes. The total protein lane also contains a band in the same area (Figure 13.9(d)). Figure 13.9(b) shows kit-included controls for the banding pattern that should occur in the lanes. Serum samples that show a band only in the light chain areas may indicate light chain disease or a monoclonal gammopathy of IgD or IgE, so additional testing should be performed. If a band is seen only in the heavy chain lane, the patient has heavy chain disease (20, 21, 22).

Immunoglobulin Quantitation

The percentage of total protein represented by each protein can be determined by the densitometry reading; the percentages expected are as follows: albumin 58–70%; α_1 2–5%; α_2 6–11%; β 8–14%; and γ 9–18%. The total serum protein concentration can be obtained by the biuret method or more rapidly by refractometry, nephelometry, or turbidometry. The normal total protein concentration is 6–8 g/dL.

Immunoglobulin concentrations are most often determined in the clinical laboratory by turbidometry and nephelometry. Smaller clinical laboratories quantitate immunoglobulin levels by radial immunodiffusion. The IgG concentration range in healthy adults is 0.548 to 17.68 g/dL, IgA is 0.078 to 0.322 g/dL, and IgM is 0.045 to 0.153 g/dL (20, 21, 22).

Light Chain Quantitation

A latex bead-enhanced nephelometric method that utilizes latex beads with antibody that is specific for free light chain and does not react with light chain which is in intact immunoglobulin, has become available. Free light chain is related to renal damage so quantitation is useful. In addition, levels of free light chain can be used for therapeutic monitoring and for diagnosis (20, 21, 22).

⊘ CASE STUDY 1

Mr. Grimes, an 80-year-old black male, was feeling a bit tired and weak. Among other tests, his physician ordered a serum protein electrophoresis. A sharp peak which indicated a monoclonal gammopathy was found, but this peak was not tall. The total serum protein was 8 g/dL, and the gamma globulin peak was 2.7 g/dL. Additional testing showed no protein in his urine, and no abnormalities were seen on x-ray. Immunofixation electrophoresis indicated that the monoclonal antibody being produced is an IgG kappa.

1. What do you think Mr. Grimes might have?

2. What do you think should be done at this point?

3. What risk factors for MGUS and myeloma are given in Mr. Grimes' description?

CASE STUDY 2

Christi Phillips, a 25-year-old woman, came in with a growth in the lymph node on her neck. She recently lost weight. Ms. Phillips's physician notes that the next lymph node in the chain is also enlarged. She does a biopsy and sends it to the lab for processing. The cells on the slide have a bilobed nucleus with 2 obvious and large nucleoi.

1. What is Ms. Phillips's diagnosis?
2. What is the name of the cells that were seen?
3. What is Ms. Phillips's prognosis?

SUMMARY

Malignant growth of lymphocytes causes immunoproliferative diseases, including lymphoma, leukemia, and plasma cell dyscrasias, which include multiple myeloma, Waldenström macroglobulinemia, light chain deposition disease, and heavy chain disease. Risk factors for immunoproliferative disorders are varied but include any type of immunosuppression, autoimmune diseases, certain chronic infections, viruses, genetic susceptibility, age over 60, carcinogen exposure, previous radiation therapy, and obesity (1, 2, 3, 4, 5).

Leukemia is a disease of either myeloid or lymphoid cells that begins in the bone marrow. Lymphomas begin with the aberrant proliferation of mature lymphocytes in one of the organs of the lymphoid system. Plasma cell dyscrasias are cancers that arise from a plasma cell and can include multiple myelomas, Waldenström macroglobulinemia, light chain deposition disease, heavy chain disease, and monoclonal gammopathy of undetermined significance (MGUS). The classification of the many types of leukemia begins with 4 main types of leukemia—acute myeloid, chronic myeloid, acute lymphocytic, and chronic lymphocytic—and is based on whether the cell origin is myeloid or lymphoid and whether the disease is composed of immature or mature cells (1, 2, 3, 4, 5).

Lymphomas are classified as either Hodgkin's or non-Hodgkin's lymphoma and are further subdivided after these general classifications. Hodgkin's disease has a very good prognosis and is subdivided into classical (which is subdivided to 4 diseases) and nodular lymphocytic predominant. Characteristic Reed-Sternberg cells have 2 prominent nucleoli and look like owl's eyes. Classification of the many different types of non-Hodgkin's lymphoma by morphologic appearance, genetic features, and surface CD markers is important for making therapeutic decisions and for prognostic determinations (1, 2, 3, 4, 5).

Multiple myeloma, macroglobulinemia, light chain deposition disease, heavy chain disease, and monoclonal gammopathy of unknown significance (MGUS) are plasma cell dyscrasias, or disorders. Each of these cells produces excess of either whole immunoglobulin or part of the immunoglobulin molecule. The cells in Waldenström macroglobulinemia produce IgM, but this is not the only difference between macroglobulinemia and multiple myeloma because the cells of multiple myeloma are more likely to grow in and cause lesion in the bone whereas the cells of Waldenström macroglobulinemia are more likely to grow in an organ of the lymphoid system. Waldenström macroglobulinemia is thus classed as a lymphoma. Excess immunoglobulin production in these diseases can cause a decrease in normal immunoglobulin production, serum viscosity increases that can cause platelet abnormalities, and bleeding problems. Attempts by the body to alleviate excess viscosity by adding fluid to the serum can cause anemia. In addition, the growth of myeloma cells in the marrow can crowd out normal cell production leading to anemia as well (7, 8, 9, 10, 11, 12, 13, 14, 15, 16).

Assays important in the diagnosis and monitoring of lymphoproliferative diseases include flow cytometry for the various cell surface markers, which indicate whether the cells are myeloid or lymphoid, T or B, and mature or immature. This information can be important to therapeutic decisions and prognosis. Assays important for the plasma cell dyscrasias include serum protein electrophoresis, immunofixation electrophoresis, immunoglobulin quantitation, and light chain analysis (17, 18, 19, 20, 21, 22).

REVIEW QUESTIONS

1. A cancer which produces monoclonal IgA in large amounts in a patient with skeletal lesions is a (an)
   a. acute leukemia
   b. Hodgkin's lymphoma
   c. non-Hodgkin's lymphoma
   d. multiple myeloma

2. A cancer that is diagnosed and monitored with serum protein electrophoresis, immunofixation electrophoresis, and immunoglobulin level measurements is
   a. acute leukemia
   b. macroglobulenemia
   c. multiple myeloma
   d. B and C

REVIEW QUESTIONS (continued)

3. Reed-Sternberg cells are found in
   a. acute leukemia
   b. Hodgkin's lymphoma
   c. non-Hodgkin's lymphoma
   d. multiple myeloma

4. In a monoclonal gammopathy, the gammaglobulin peak would be
   a. short and wide
   b. tall and wide
   c. short and narrow
   d. tall and narrow

5. Which disease has a monoclonal increase in the beta or gamma region of the serum protein electrophoresis but looks like a lymphoma?
   a. acute leukemia
   b. Hodgkin's lymphoma
   c. macroglobulenemia
   d. multiple myeloma

6. When a patient has a monoclonal gammopathy, the antibody response to infection should be
   a. less
   b. the same
   c. more
   d. cannot be determined

7. Rouleaux are
   a. stacks of red blood cells because of high serum protein levels
   b. stacks of red blood cells because of Reed-Sternberg cells
   c. round lesions in the kidney because of myeloma
   d. round lesions in the bone marrow because of myeloma

8. In an immunoproliferative B-cell tumor, the tumor would contain cells with
   a. gene rearrangements for either kappa or lambda chains but not both
   b. CD19 unless it is a plasma cell, and then CD38
   c. CD4 and CD3
   d. A and B

9. In immunofixation electrophoresis, the patient's serum is electrophoresed in how many lanes?
   a. 6
   b. 2
   c. 4
   d. 3

10. Risks for immunoproliferative diseases include
    a. immunosuppression
    b. Epstein-Barr virus infection
    c. radiation
    d. all of the above

REFERENCES

1. National Cancer Institute. What you need to know about cancer. http://www.cancer.gov/cancertopics/wyntk/cancer. Accessed March 17, 2012

2. National Cancer Institute. Fact sheet cancer: Questions and answers. http://www.cancer.gov/cancertopics/factsheet/Sites-Types/general. Accessed June 4, 2010.

3. American Society of Clinical Oncology (ASCO). http://www.cancer.net/patient/All+About+Cancer. Accessed March 17, 2012.

4. Jaffe ES. The 2008 WHO classification of lymphomas: Implications for clinical practice and translational research. *Hematol.* 2009; 2009:523–531.

5. National Comprehensive Cancer Network. NCCN clinical practice guidelines in oncology (NCCN Guidelines™): Non-Hodgkin's lymphoma. http://www.nccn.org/professionals/physician_gls/PDF/nhl.pdf. Accessed March 17, 2012.

6. Jacene HA, Filice R, Kasecamp W, et al. Comparison of 90Y-ibritumomab tiuxetan and 131I-tositumomab in clinical practice. *J Nucl Med.* 2007;48(11):1767–1776. Epub 2007 Oct 17.

7. National Comprehensive Cancer Network. NCCN clinical practice guidelines in oncology (NCCN Guidelines™): Multiple myeloma. http://www.nccn.org/professionals/physician_gls/PDF/myeloma.pdf. Accessed Accessed March 17, 2012.

8. Grethlein SJ, Thomas LM. Multiple myeloma: Differential diagnoses & workup. http://emedicine.medscape.com/article/204369-overview. Accessed March 17, 2012.

9. Fanning S, Hussein MA. Monoclonal gammopathies of uncertain origin. http://emedicine.medscape.com/article/204297-overview. Accessed March 17, 2012.

10. Berenson, J. Heavy Chain Disease. In: *The Merck Manual for Health Care Professionals.* http://www.merck.com/mmpe/sec11/ch144/ch144b.html. Accessed March 17, 2012.

11. Gajra A, Grethlein SJ. Heavy chain disease, Mu http://emedicine.medscape.com/article/200758-overview. Accessed March 17, 2012.

12. Bradwell AR. http://www.wikilite.com/wiki/index.php/Immunoassays_for_free_light_chain_measurement. Accessed March 17, 2012.

13. Jayamohan Y, Sacher RA, Fanning SR, et al. A light-chain deposition. http://emedicine.medscape.com/article/202585-overview. Accessed March 17, 2012.

14. Hall CL, Peat DS. Light chain deposit disease: A frequent cause of diagnostic difficulty. *Nephrol Dial Transplant.* 2001;16(9):1939–1941.

15. American Society of Clinical Oncology (ASCO). Waldenström macroglobulinemia. http://www.cancer.net/patient/Cancer+Types/Waldenstrom%27s+Macroglobulinemia. Accessed March 17, 2012.

16. Ponce D, Seiter K, Ramu V, et al. Waldenström hypergammaglobulinemia. http://emedicine.medscape.com/article/207097-overview. Accessed March 17, 2012.

17. Lab Tests Online. Triple Screen or Quad Screen. http://www.labtestsonline.org/understanding/analytes/triple_screen/glance.html. Accessed March 17, 2012.

18. National Cancer Institute. Fact sheet tumor markers: Questions and answers. http://www.cancer.gov/cancertopics/factsheet/Detection/tumor-markers/print?page=&keyword=. Accessed March 17, 2012.

19. National Academy of Clinical Biochemistry Laboratory Medicine Practice Guidelines. NACB: Tumor markers. http://www.aacc.org/EXPIRED/TumorMarkers/Pages/TumorMarkersPDF.aspx. Accessed March 17, 2012.

20. Hamilton RG. Human Immunoglobulins. In: O'Gorman MRG, Donnenberg AD, eds. *Handbook of Human Immunology.* 2nd ed. Boca Raton, FL: CRC Press; 2008: chap. 3.

21. O'Connell TX, Horita TJ, Kasravi B. Understanding and interpreting serum protein electrophoresis. *Am Fam Physician.* 2005;71(1):105–112. http://www.aafp.org/afp/2005/0101/p105.html. Accessed March 17, 2012.

22. U.S. National Library of Medicine NIH, National Institute of Health. Protein electrophoresis-serum on MedlinePlus. http://www.nlm.nih.gov/medlineplus/ency/article/003540.htm. Accessed March 17, 2012.

PEARSON
myhealthprofessionskit

Visit www.myhealthprofessionskit.com to access the interactive Companion Website for this textbook. Simply select "Clinical Laboratory Science" from the choice of disciplines. Find this book and log in by using your user name and password to access additional learning tools.

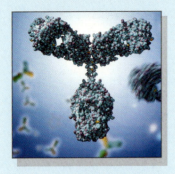

CHAPTER OUTLINE

14

Immunology of Transplantation

■ OBJECTIVES—LEVEL I

After this chapter, the student should be able to:

1. Describe the role of the ABO and Rh systems in blood transfusions.
2. Describe the ABO relationships (ie, who can give and who can receive) between blood donors and recipients.
3. Describe the different methods of blood typing and donor–recipient matching in blood transfusions.
4. List and describe the histocompatibility antigens that are involved in transplantation rejection.
5. Differentiate between autograft, isograft, allograft, and xenograft.
6. List and describe the immunologic mechanisms of graft rejection and their clinical manifestation.
7. Describe graft-versus-host disease.
8. Describe the different methods used for HLA typing.
9. Describe methods to detect anti-HLA antibodies.

■ OBJECTIVES—LEVEL II

After this chapter, the student should be able to:

1. Describe the antigen sets used in the multiplexing assay.
2. List and describe different examples of immunosuppressive agents.

KEY TERMS

acute rejection
allograft
allorecognition
autograft
chronic rejection
first-set rejection
graft

graft-versus-host disease (GVHD)
hyperacute rejection
isograft
second-set rejection
tissue typing
xenograft

▶ **INTRODUCTION**

Our body's defenses are designed to protect us from threats from our environment, whether real or perceived. To achieve this, our defense systems operate to (1) prevent a potential threat from entering our system and (2) reject and destroy such a threat should it have gained entry. Physiological barriers, such as skin, hair, mucus, and physiological reflexes such as gagging, sneezing, and coughing usually prevent entry. The immune system is very active in both actions; it can block entry by interfering with viral or bacterial adherence and preventing tissue invasion by parasites, and, of course, as has been noted in previous chapters, the body is armed with many ways to destroy a foreign entity that has already gained access to the system. The basis of discrimination of the immune system is based on the foreignness of an entity as described in Chapter 3. The immune system cannot discern what is "good" and what is "bad" for you; it simply acts against what "does not belong"; this discrimination is based on the concepts described in Chapter 3. In nature, this works well because it is a better-to-be-safe-than-sorry approach so that something that does not belong or is foreign is seen as a potential threat and, therefore, is acted against. However, modern medicine has created situations in which the entrance and establishment of a foreign entity is desired as in the case of transplantation. In this chapter, we discuss the role that the immune response plays in transplantation, the mechanisms involved in this role and their consequences, the laboratory approaches to evaluate the compatibility between a transplant donor and a transplant recipient, and the approaches that are designed to bypass immune responses to transplanted tissues.

▶ **BLOOD TRANSFUSIONS AND BLOOD GROUPS**

If transplantation refers to the transfer of cells and/or tissue from one individual to another, then the most common form of transplantation is blood transfusion. The main objective of blood transfusions is to replace a large number of red blood cells that have been lost. There are many concerns in blood transfusions, such as the potential transfer of an infectious organism from one individual to another; however, from an immunologic point of view, the major concern is the compatibility of blood groups between a donor and a recipient. More specifically, the major concern is to avoid the recipient reacting immunologically against the donor's red blood cells. Such reactivity depends on the antigens on red blood cells that define blood groups.

Hundreds of different erythrocyte antigens are assigned to numerous different blood groups. However, the clinically "relevant" antigens are limited in number; some of these belong to the ABO system of erythrocyte antigens, which are characterized by different carbohydrate moieties attached to

---

TABLE 14.1

Genotypes That Generate Different Blood Groups

Blood Group	Genotype
A	AA, AO
B	BB, BO
AB	AB
O	OO

---

certain glycoproteins and glycolipids on red blood cells. In particular, the differences in the ABO groups are determined by certain enzymes that add specific terminal sugars at the end of the carbohydrate chain of the particular glycoprotein or glycolipid. The ABO system is determined by allelic genes A, B, and O that, in turn, determine which enzymes and thus which terminal sugars will be added to the end of the carbohydrate chain. Group A transferase adds N-acetyl-galactosamine (GalNAc) to the chain, and the presence of GalNAc at the end of the chain defines the A blood group. Likewise, group B transferase adds a terminal galactose to the chain whose presence defines the B group. The AB group is defined by the presence of both A and B antigens on erythrocytes whereas the O group, lacking either enzyme, does not have either terminal sugar at the end of the chain (1, 2, 3). Refer to Table 14.1 ✪ for the different genotypes that can generate the different ABO blood groups.

The relevance of the ABO groups in blood transfusions is the fact that people have naturally occurring IgM antibodies to these antigens (although IgG antibodies against these antigens, albeit in lower concentrations, can also occur). These antibodies develop because of exposure to cross-reactive antigens from various natural sources, for example, from a wide variety of different microorganisms. People do not generate antibodies to their own blood group because of the immunological tolerance mechanisms described in Chapter 4. However, they do generate antibodies to other blood groups. See Table 14.2 ✪ for a description of the antibodies in individuals from different blood groups.

TABLE 14.2

Naturally Occurring Antibodies in Individuals of Different Blood Groups

Group	Ag on RBC	Serum Ab
A	A	Anti-B
B	B	Anti-A
AB	AB	None
O	None	Anti-A, Anti-B

✪ TABLE 14.3

Patterns of Blood Transfusions

Group	Can Give to	Can Receive from
A	A, AB	A, O
B	B, AB	B, O
AB	AB	A, B, AB, O
O	A, B, AB, O	O

The pattern of blood transfusions (ie, who can give blood to whom) is thus determined by such blood groups and corresponding antibodies. Once again, a blood transfusion gives a large amount of red blood cells; therefore, antibodies in a recipient's serum must not react with antigens on the donor's red blood cells. See Table 14.3 ✪ for different patterns of blood transfusions. Based on these patterns, someone with group O blood is considered a *universal donor* (ie, can give blood to any blood group) whereas a person with AB blood is a *universal recipient* (1, 2, 3). If the donor and recipient are not ABO compatible, transfusion reactions as described in detail in Chapter 9 will occur.

The Rh system is the other system that is relevant in blood transfusions, although its most dramatic effect is seen in the hemolytic disease of the newborn discussed in Chapter 9. The Rh system consists of numerous different antigens; the one with the most relevance because of its immunogenicity is the D antigen whose presence on red blood cells defines Rh positivity. Unlike the ABO system, there are no naturally occurring antibodies to the D antigen, so an Rh-negative recipient could be transfused with blood from an Rh-positive donor once. However, this would sensitize the recipient against the D antigen so that a subsequent blood transfusion from an Rh-positive donor could cause a dangerous hemolytic reaction in that recipient. Antibody that develops to the Rh antigen is IgG; thus, transfusing Rh-positive blood into an Rh-negative woman of childbearing years would put this woman's Rh-positive fetus in danger of hemolytic disease of the newborn because the IgG would cross the placenta and damage the newborn's red blood cells.

▶ BLOOD GROUPING

Blood grouping involves determining an individual's ABO blood group and Rh positivity. The test is a simple one that involves the collection of a small amount of blood, usually from a pricked finger, and mixing the blood with commercially available antibodies to A, B, and D (for Rh) antigens. The agglutination of the red blood cells by the antibody indicates a positive reaction. So, if anti-A antibodies agglutinate an individual's blood, that person is group A; likewise anti-B antibodies agglutinate blood from a group B individual. If both anti-A and anti-B antibodies agglutinate the sample, that individual is group AB; if neither

does, that individual is group O. In the same manner, agglutination with anti-D antibodies indicates Rh positivity while no agglutination indicates Rh negativity. Agglutination is currently determined by centrifuging the red blood cells through a gelatinous material after reaction with the specific antibodies. If the cells agglutinate, they aggregate and cannot travel through the gelatin; thus, they remain at the aqueous–gelatin interface. Conversely, if the cells do not agglutinate, they can be easily pushed through the gelatin by the centrifugation and end up at the bottom of the centrifuge tube (Figure 14.1 ■).

Another test known as *reverse grouping,* can detect the presence of anti-A or anti-B antibodies in an individual's serum. In this test, blood from an individual is centrifuged to remove all blood cells; the remaining serum is then collected, and a sample of it is mixed with red blood cells of known blood group (ie, group A or group B); then the mixture is observed for clumping. If the group A cells are clumped, the serum from that individual contains anti-A antibodies, indicating that the individual is group B blood or group O blood. Likewise, if group B cells are clumped, the serum from that individual contains anti-B antibodies and therefore that individual is group A blood or group O blood. Clumping of both group A and B cells indicates the presence of anti-A and anti-B antibodies and therefore that individual is group O. Conversely, no clumping of either A or B group cells suggests no antibodies in the serum, thus making that individual's blood group AB. This is performed in the same gelatin containing tubes and the results are shown in the last 2 tubes in Figure 14.1.

A third approach, called *cross-matching,* involves mixing red blood cells from the donor directly with serum from the recipient. Cross-matching is performed at 37° C to detect IgG antibodies; IgM antibodies are detected at room temperature. If the recipient's serum has antibodies against the donor's red blood cells, agglutination of those cells will occur, and, therefore, the donor and recipient are deemed incompatible.

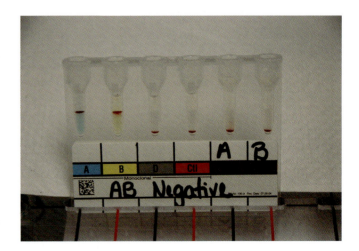

■ **FIGURE 14.1** ABO and Rh grouping using gelatin centrifugation. The blood sample above is AB negative as indicated by the agglutination of the red blood cells in the A and B tubes (on left), and the absence of agglutination in the D (Rh) tube.

✓ Checkpoint! 14.1

Why is someone with group O blood considered a universal donor but someone with AB blood is a universal recipient?

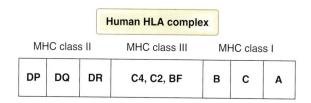

■ **FIGURE 14.2** The human HLA complex and its different regions.

▶ TISSUE AND ORGAN TRANSPLANTATION

We currently take tissue and organ transplantation for granted; these are routine procedures that have saved thousands of lives throughout the world. Tens of thousands heart, liver, pancreas, lung (often along with heart), and kidney transplants are performed every year. However, successful kidney transplants have been performed for only about 50 years. Early attempts (first in humans in 1935) led to immediate rejection because of blood group mismatch. The first successful kidney transplant was performed between identical twins in 1954.

The major barriers to organ transplantation are the lack of available organs and immune rejection of the transplanted organ because of donor–recipient immune incompatibility. A transplanted organ or tissue is known as a **graft.** There are different types of grafts: An **autograft** is a graft from the same individual (ie, the graft is obtained from one individual and transplanted in a different anatomical part of that same individual, for example, a section of skin on a burn patient). This type of graft was actually reported for repair of damaged noses back to the 6th century BC! Because an autograft is obtained from the same individual, it is genetically identical to that individual and is accepted. An **isograft,** a graft obtained from an individual who is genetically identical to the recipient, for example, from an identical twin, is also accepted. Most transplants involve an **allograft,** which is a graft from a genetically different individual of the same species (eg, human to human). Current technology is also exploring the use of **xenografts,** which are grafts from a different species (eg, from a nonhuman primate or a pig to a human) (1, 2).

▶ THE CONCEPT OF HISTOCOMPATIBILITY

The major problem in transplantation whether of cells or tissues is the recipient's reaction to components of the donor that the recipient sees as foreign. The mechanisms of the immune system that are responsible for the protection of the host are also involved in the rejection of a graft. This problem in blood transfusions can be circumvented fairly easily because the antigens of the red blood cells that are involved (ie, the ABO and Rh systems) are limited in number and because transfusion contains few cells of other types. However, when transplanting nucleated cells, tissues, or whole organs, the process becomes significantly more complex because the number of components that the recipient sees as foreign is very large. The chief players in this scenario are, not surprisingly, the

components of the major histocompatibility complex (MHC), also referred as *human leukocyte antigen (HLA)*, which are the major components that a graft recipient sees as foreign on the graft. As we discussed in Chapter 3, the MHC genes are the most polymorphic genes in the human genome; each locus has a very large number of different alleles. Because of this, matching a donor with a recipient becomes very complicated, and it is difficult to find a perfect match for a patient if no related donor is available (1, 2, 4). For a diagram of the human HLA complex, see Figure 14.2 ■.

The HLA system is inherited following a typical Mendelian inheritance pattern with an offspring inheriting 1 haplotype (a set of genes that are usually transmitted together as a single entity) from each parent. Because of the way that Mendelian inheritance of genes works, in a typical outbred (nonrelated) family, children are no more than 50% compatible with each parent, and 2 offspring from the same parents have a 25% chance of inheriting the same haplotypes. See Figure 14.3 ■ for the Mendelian patterns of inheritance of parental haplotypes. Recombinations (R) of a haplotype, although rare, also occur. Now, look at Figure 14.4 ■ and note several different alleles from parental haplotypes, including a recombination of maternal haplotypes. Considering the great polymorphism of the HLA system (ie, the different haplotypes, the different HLA loci, and the fact that each locus has dozens of different antigens and hundreds of different alleles), it becomes clear that finding an organ match with HLA compatibility is a complex and difficult task even within a related family.

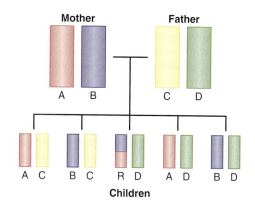

■ **FIGURE 14.3** Typical Mendelian pattern of inheritance of HLA haplotypes includes children AC, BC, AD, and BD. Child RD is unusual because a rare recombination occurs.

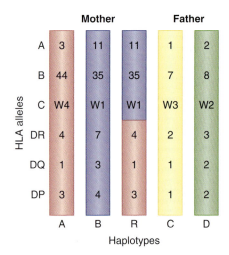

■ **FIGURE 14.4** Sample composition of maternal and paternal HLA haplotypes.

In addition, other components must be considered (1, 5). The ABO system of blood antigens also plays a role in transplant rejection. Because grafts are often highly vascularized and because ABO antigens can be found on endothelial cell (and sometimes lymphocytes to which they are absorbed from the plasma), anti-ABO antibodies in the recipient may bind to these blood antigens on the graft and initiate complement-dependent tissue damage. Also, a group of proteins called *minor histocompatibility antigens (mHA)* can play a role in graft rejection. They are not really products of the classical HLA system but can be highly polymorphic even within a species, and they can be seen as foreign even in MHC-matched transplants. An example of these is a group of proteins that are encoded by the Y chromosome in males. Because these proteins are limited to males, a female may see these proteins as foreign. An example of these proteins is a mouse protein encoded by a Y chromosome gene called *Smcy;* although females have a counterpart gene it does not match the amino acid sequence of Smcy. Therefore, this protein is unique to male mice.

▶ MECHANISMS OF REJECTION

Except when we are discussing reaction to blood antigens and to xenotransplants, the immunologic mechanisms of graft rejection are mostly mediated by cells rather than antibodies. This has been shown experimentally because transfer of serum does not transfer allograft immunity whereas transfer of lymphocytes does. In addition, T cells have been shown to mediate graft rejection (5, 6). This was shown in an experiment in nude mice, an animal model lacking a thymus and thus with no T cells. A nude mouse cannot reject allografts. T cells from a mouse that has rejected a tissue graft when transferred into another animal mediate graft rejection specifically. The subset of T cells that mediate graft rejection are both CD4+ and CD8+T cells; this is demonstrated experimentally by the fact that antibodies to either CD4 or CD8 can block or reduce rejection.

It is interesting to know that the major players in graft rejection come from both the donor and the recipient. As it may be expected, the introduction of alloantigens on a graft from a donor into a recipient causes an immune response in the recipient similar to an immune response to any foreign antigen. This process called indirect **allorecognition,** involves the uptake and processing of foreign HLA proteins from the donor graft and their presentation by the recipient's antigen-presenting cells to the recipient's T cells following the mechanisms described in Chapter 4. This results in the activation of effector mechanisms against the graft including cell-mediated cytotoxicity, delayed-type hypersensitivity, and antibody-mediated cellular responses (5, 7).

In addition, another immunological response, direct allorecognition, involves the action of donor antigen-presenting cells activating the recipient's T cells (6). Many types of grafts contain antigen-presenting cells from the donor; these "passenger" cells are able to enter the recipient's lymphatics and migrate to peripheral lymph nodes where they stimulate recipient's T cells that bear T-cell receptors against alloantigens. Some of these alloreactive T cells then migrate back to the area of the graft and attack it. The stimulation of recipient T cells by donor antigen-presenting cells may result from some similarities in HLA proteins: Although T cells usually recognize self-HLA associated with an antigenic peptide, it appears that some foreign HLA proteins may resemble a self-HLA/peptide antigen complex. It is unclear what exact contribution each mechanism provides in graft rejection, but it is clear that both mechanisms play a major role in it.

Transplant rejection follows the typical pattern of any immune response; this means that the first exposure to an allograft induces a response different than the one induced by a second or subsequent exposure to an allograft from the same individual. So, a **first-set rejection** (ie, the first encounter of an allograft) takes much longer (10–15 days) than a **second-set rejection,** which is a subsequent encounter of a graft from the same allogeneic individual (for example, when giving the recipient a second graft from the same donor) when immunological memory plays a role, and thus occurs much faster (6–8 days) (1, 2).

✓ **Checkpoint! 14.2**

Why do hematopoietic stem cells have such an important clinical significance?

► CLINICAL MANIFESTATION OF REJECTION

As stated previously, although most rejection mechanisms are cell mediated, antibodies can also play a role in graft rejection (7). Again, many grafts are highly vascularized, and the recipient may have preformed circulating antibodies against vascular endothelial cells of the donor. These antibodies may be either against the ABO blood group antigens or against HLA or other endothelial antigens of the donor. Binding of these antibodies to the endothelium causes the activation of the complement cascade as well as various clotting mechanisms, which, in turn, activate inflammatory responses and thrombus formation that block the blood vessels of the graft. Known as **hyperacute graft rejection,** this results in the deprivation of blood to the graft, causing the graft's death. Cross-matching of the donor and recipient by mixing donor cells with recipient serum to detect anti-donor antibodies in the serum can circumvent this problem. This is, indeed, performed in most transplant situations, so hyperacute rejection is very rare in modern transplantation. More commonly, a major problem in transplantation currently is **acute rejection.** This mechanism involves the activation of CD4+ and CD8+ recipient T cells attacking the graft from an allogeneic donor. This reaction can take several days to manifest; the T cells from the recipient react against the foreign HLA antigens of the transplanted tissue, causing a delayed-type hypersensitivity reaction that ultimately causes damage and inflammation of the graft. The mechanisms of tissue destruction in a delayed-type hypersensitivity reaction are described in Chapter 9. Because acute rejection takes several days to develop, it can be reduced in most cases by the administration of immunosuppressive drugs, which are discussed later.

A third mechanism by which a graft can be rejected is by **chronic rejection,** which can occur months or even years after a graft is transplanted. Chronic rejection is the major cause of long-term failure of transplanted organs and grafts. The main causes of chronic rejection are various inflammatory mechanisms, which lead to the deterioration of the vasculature of the graft, causing vascular damage, atherosclerosis, narrowing of the vessels, or decreased blood supply to the graft, leading to the graft's eventual death. Chronic rejection involves both humoral and cell-mediated mechanisms and is not usually prevented by immunosuppressive drugs. In fact, alloreactive responses may occur months or years after transplantation of a graft. Other nonimmunologic factors also contribute to chronic graft rejection. For example: injury from reperfusion and ischemia at the time of grafting may have long-term repercussions much later in the graft's life. Chronic exposure to immunosuppressive drugs, some of which exhibit some level of toxicity, may also contribute to chronic rejection. Although improvements have been made, chronic rejection has been one of the major problems in transplantation

that has not yet been ameliorated by modern technology. In fact, the mean survival time of a mismatched kidney has not changed much since the 1970s. About one-third of transplanted kidneys are rejected within 5 years, so histocompatibility matching between donor and recipient is as crucial now as it was decades ago (1, 5, 8).

► GRAFT-VERSUS-HOST DISEASE

When we think of a "graft," we may think of some inert, passive tissue that is transplanted from a donor onto an immunologically "aware" recipient, and the major obstacle to the transplant is the immune reaction of the host against the donor. However, we must remember that many grafts are live organs with all the features and characteristics of live tissue; if the graft or organ happens to be an immunocompetent tissue, a phenomenon called **graft-versus-host disease (GVHD)** can occur (9). In this situation, the *graft* is reacting immunologically against the recipient.

The most common situation in which GVHD occurs is in bone marrow transplants. Allogeneic bone marrow transplants are usually performed to replace cancerous bone marrow precursors, such as in certain leukemias or lymphomas, or to restore immune competence in some primary immunodeficiency or bone marrow diseases. Bone marrow cells from a recipient are destroyed by chemotherapy and replaced by a bone marrow transplant from an allogeneic donor. In this case, the immune cells of the donor recognize the recipient as foreign. Specifically, mature T cells in the donor's graft react to the recipient's tissues, and the incompatibility between the donor and the recipient may involve HLA components as well as minor histocompatibility antigens; therefore, GVHD can also occur between HLA-matched individuals. Symptoms of GVHD include diarrhea, skin rashes, and pneumonitis; common targets of the reaction are skin, liver, and a portion of the digestive tract. A common approach to minimize GVHD is to remove alloreactive T cells from the donor bone marrow prior to transplantation. An international database has been set up for registry of individuals who are willing to donate bone marrow or stem cells so that the best possible match can be performed (see Box 14.1 ✿)

Stem cells can also be obtained directly from the blood of a donor (10). The production of stem cells is stimulated by the administration of granulocyte colony-stimulating factor to the donor for up to 5 days; after this treatment, the cells are collected by leukapheresis and the resulting cell mixture is then subjected to selection using affinity columns containing antibodies to CD34 and CD133, which are markers for pluripotential stem cells. This selection allows the concentration of these cells so that they can be transferred to the recipient. Although this ensures a "cleaner" population of stem cells (ie, a more purified population), transplantation of

---

✪ BOX 14.1

How You Can Be a Hero

Have you ever wondered how you could become a bone marrow or stem cell donor? It is much easier than you think. Collecting your HLA profile is simple and painless and, unlike many popular myths, most peripheral blood stem cell donations do not require a surgical procedure. The first step is to join the National Marrow Donor Program (NMDP), which operates a national registry of volunteer hematopoietic cell donors and umbilical cord blood units in the United States.

To be a bone marrow or peripheral blood stem cell donor, you must be

- Between 18 and 60 years of age.
- In good health and meet certain medical guidelines.

You will be sent a kit, which contains swabs used to swab the inside of the cheeks to collect cells for analysis.

If you are chosen as a donor, you will be contacted and asked if you are still willing to donate. Before you decide, you will learn all the details of the donation procedure during an information session, and a medical examination will follow the session.

There are 2 methods of donation:

1. The first one is donation of peripheral blood stem cells (PBSC):
   - During the 5 days before donation, you will be injected with filgrastim to increase the number of blood-forming cells in your blood.
   - On the day of the donation, blood is taken the normal way, and the stem cells will be separated, and the remainder of the blood is returned to replenish the removed cells.
2. The second method is bone marrow donation:
   - This procedure will be carried out at a hospital.
   - You will be under anesthesia and feel no pain.
   - Bone marrow is taken from a bone in your pelvis.
   - Cells will be replaced in a few weeks.

Recovery time can range from 1 day to 1 week and varies from donor to donor and on the type of donation. Cells and tissues from the NMDP donors are transplanted in a wide variety of patients with different disorders of the blood, bone marrow, or immune system, ranging from leukemia to some anemias, to some metabolic disorders. To date, the NMDP has contributed to almost 40 000 transplants over the world. A patient who needs a hematopoietic transplant but has no matching donor readily available can search the registry for an unrelated matched donor. If you are interested in registering for the NMDP, you can do so directly at http://www.marrow .org/ or by writing to:

National Marrow Donor Program
3001 Broadway Street N.E., Suite 100,
Minneapolis, MN 55413-1753

---

affinity-selected CD34 and CD133 cells has also been associated with a higher incidence of HVGD. Another source of stem cells is cord blood, which has been recently used for this purpose, particularly because the incidence of GVHD using cord blood is lower. However, the number of cells obtained from this source is limited, so more than one donor source is needed.

Checkpoint! 14.3

In graft-versus-host disease, why would a graft reject a host?

▶ LABORATORY TESTING

As a first step, a general health clearance of the donor and the recipient is performed. The donor should be free of hepatitis B, hepatitis C, HIV, human T-lymphotropic virus (HTLV), and West Nile virus (WNV). In addition, the donor and the donor organ should be healthy enough for the transplantation in question. It should be clear by now that matching on the basis of histocompatibility is critical in most cases of transplantation. This matching requires several steps and depends on assessing the histocompatibility profiles of both donor and recipient. See Figure 14.5 ■ for a flowchart of testing for

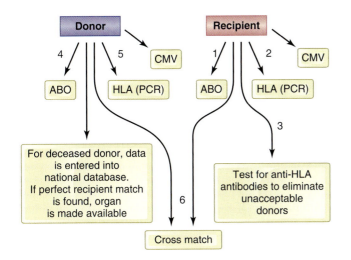

■ **FIGURE 14.5** Flowchart of typical compatibility testing for donors and recipients. Both donor and recipient are typed for ABO and HLA antigen profiles (steps 1, 2, 4, and 5). The recipient is also tested for antibodies against HLA antigens to eliminate unacceptable donors (step 3). Potentially matching individuals are then tested by cross matching (step 6), which involves mixing recipient sera with donor cells and then adding fluorescence-labeled anti-human IgG and measuring fluorescence by flow cytometry. Seropositivity to cytomegalovirus (CMV) is also assessed for both donor and recipient. When dealing with a deceased donor, results of tissue typing are entered into a national transplantation database; if a perfectly matched recipient is found, the organ is then made available for transplant.

both donor and recipient and Table 14.4 ✪ for a summary of such testing. Compatibility profiles can be derived by **tissue typing.** The first steps in tissue typing are to type for ABO and HLA antigens. We discussed ABO and Rh typing in the first part of this chapter. Matching HLA between donor and recipient requires 2 protocols: the first one is to obtain a typing of the classical HLA transplantation antigens (ie, A, B, C, DR, DQ) in both donor and recipient. The second protocol involves the detection of antibodies against these transplantation antigens. Potentially matching individuals are then tested by cross matching, which involves mixing recipient sera with donor cells, adding fluorescence-labeled anti-human IgG, and measuring fluorescence by flow cytometry.

HLA TYPING

HLA typing, in turn, can be carried out in different ways. A method that has been used historically (and is still currently used in a few labs) is the *microcytotoxicity test* (11). In this test white blood cells from donor and recipient are incubated with commercially available antibodies to various MHC alleles (both class I and class II). After a period of incubation, a source of complement is added; the cells that are positive for a particular allele are bound by the antibody specific for that allele. This, in turn, activates the complement system, which will cause the lysis of the cell. Such lysis can then be detected by the addition of a pink dye (Eosin) that can penetrate dead or damaged cells but is not taken up by undamaged cells. Thus, the turning pink of the cells that have reacted with an antibody to a particular allele indicates that those cells are positive for that allele. See Figure 14.6 ■ for the principle of the microcytotoxicity test. The advantage of this method is that it is fairly straightforward, fast, and can be used if a high level of resolution (ie, the ability to differentiate 2 closely related but still different HLA components) is not needed. This assay can be performed only on live cells; in the case of a deceased donor, tissues tend to lose the expression of their HLA antigens. Furthermore, in transplants such as bone marrow transplantation, which requires a much more precise HLA typing to distinguish even very closely related HLA antigens, the limited resolution of the assay can be a problem. This is so because the specificity repertoire of the commercially available anti-HLA antibodies, although considerably diverse, is nevertheless limited. The numbers of commercially available antibodies to class II antigens were particularly limited, so when microcytotoxicity assays were common, they had to be supplemented with an assay that helped detect differences in

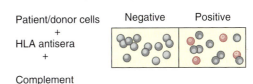

■ **FIGURE 14.6** Principle of a microcytotoxicity assay.

✪ TABLE 14.4					
Summary of Testing for Transplantation Donor and Recipient					
	Infectious Disease Testing	**ABO and Rh Blood Group**	**Molecular Testing**	**Antibody Testing**	**Cross Match**
Donor	HIV, Hepatitis B, C, HTLV, WNV, CMV	Test	HLA type by PCR	Not done	
Recipient	CMV	Test	HLA type by PCR	Test for antibody to HLA antigens by multiplex	Donors cells + recipient serum; flow cytometry

class II antigens. This assay was called the *mixed lymphocyte reaction* (1).

In the mixed lymphocyte reaction, lymphocytes from donor and recipient were mixed together and cell proliferation was detected by the uptake of radioactive thymidine. The mixed lymphocyte reaction is described in detail in Chapter 4; its advantage is that it detects incompatibility functionally (ie, it detects actual cell activation and therefore does not depend on the identification of specific HLA differences). On the other hand, MLR takes a considerable amount of time to be performed (days) and cannot be used to match donor and recipient if the donor is a cadaver. Today MLR has been primarily replaced by the more modern techniques described next. Currently, most HLA typing is accomplished by genotyping.

Genotyping involves profiling the genes that encode for the different HLA antigens rather than the antigens themselves. This is usually performed by a polymerase chain reaction (PCR), a method that amplifies a particular area of genomic DNA identified by DNA primers that are specific for that area. The principle and methodology of PCR are described in Chapter 23. The amplification of the gene, in turn, allows for analyzing whether the gene contains a particular sequence for a particular HLA antigen. This is done with the use of sequence-specific primers (or SSP) techniques. Alternatively, PCR can also be used to amplify a large number of genes at a particular HLA locus; the individual's specific gene variants can then be detected by using specific DNA probes (sequence-specific oligonucleotide probes, or SSOP) that recognize specific DNA sequences that reflect a particular gene variant. See Figure 14.7 ■ for a typical PCR machine used for genotyping and Figure 14.8 ■ for the 2 different methods of genotyping. Refer to Figure 14.9 ■ for a typical agarose gel used for genotyping. PCR-based genotyping is significantly more precise than the microcytotoxicity test and has the advantage that it needs only DNA from the donor and recipient, not live cells, and it can discriminate between closely related HLA antigens with a much higher resolution.

DETECTION OF ANTI-HLA ANTIBODIES

Patients who need transplants may have antibodies to HLA antigens that could interfere with a successful graft. These anti-HLA antibodies can develop because of stimulation by the HLA antigens present in blood transfusions; they may have developed if the recipient was pregnant and developed antibodies to the fetal HLA antigens, or they may have developed because of a previous transplanted organ or tissue.

Indirect enzyme-linked immunoassays (ELISA) can be used to detect anti-HLA antibodies; in this case, microwell plates are coated with different HLA antigens and an individual's serum is then allowed to incubate with the different HLA preparations. Antibodies from the serum can then be detected by the assay described in Chapter 7.

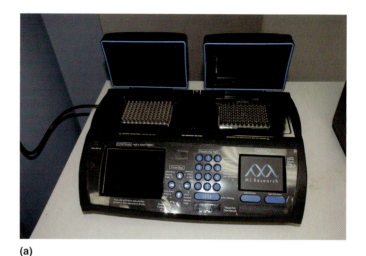

(a)

(b)

■ FIGURE 14.7   (a) Standard PCR machine used for genotyping and (b) agarose gel to detect DNA fragments.

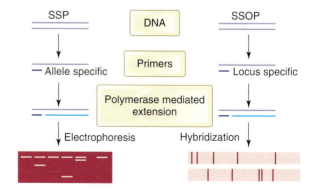

■ FIGURE 14.8   HLA genotyping by 2 different methods.

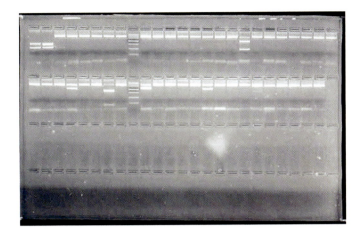

■ **FIGURE 14.9** DNA fragments visualized by gel electrophoresis on agarose gel. DNA fragments corresponding to the region amplified by PCR are separated by electrophoresis according to size. They are then stained with ethidium bromide and can be visualized under ultraviolet light. The size of the DNA fragment can then be estimated by comparing its migration pattern to fragments of DNA of known size. Because the sequence of the DNA fragment is known, its molecular size can be determined; if the size of a particular DNA fragment amplified by PCR corresponds to the size of the fragment estimated by sequencing, that DNA fragment is confirmed to be the one amplified by the PCR primers.

A relatively new assay utilizes flow cytometry to determine whether the patient has antibody to HLA antigens. This assay uses commercially available fluorescently colored beads bearing various different HLA antigens to detect anti-HLA antibodies in serum using flow cytometry (see Chapter 7). These beads, used in what is called a *multiplex system,* come in different colors that can be distinguished by flow cytometry. The manufacturer prepares the beads so that a bead set of one color is coated with a set of HLA antigens derived from one individual of known HLA type and then a bead set of another color is coated with HLA antigens of a different individual, assigning HLA antigens from many different individuals to beads of a particular color. Serum from a potential recipient is then allowed to incubate with the different sets of beads, and if the recipient has antibodies to a particular set of HLA antigens, these antibodies will bind to the bead to which those antigens are attached. After washing unbound material, the beads are allowed to incubate with an anti-human antibody that has an avidin-biotin fluorescence label on it. If this secondary antibody sticks to the bead (because it is bound to the antibody from the recipient, which in turn is bound to the HLA antigens), the bead will exhibit this additional fluorescence. Thus, by discerning such fluorescence and the color of the particular bead set, one can detect antibodies in the recipient against different sets of HLA antigens. This in turn allows for the elimination of potential donors that may have the set of HLA antigens against which the recipient is reacting. Refer to Figure 14.10 ■ for a diagram of the multiplex bead procedure. Once the antibody reactivity of a recipient to a particular set of HLA antigens is determined, more testing using bead sets with single HLA antigens can be used to narrow the specificity of such reactivity.

▶ CYTOMEGALOVIRUS

Cytomegalovirus (CMV) is a DNA herpes virus that infects humans as well as other species. In individuals with an intact immune system, CMV is kept in check and the infections it causes are usually mild and not life threatening. In immunocompetent hosts, CMV can remain latent and inactive for long periods but can be reactivated if favorable conditions occur. In general, the immune system in healthy individuals usually destroys the virus via cell-mediated immune mechanisms, so the individuals carrying the virus are usually asymptomatic. These individuals are seropositive for CMV because they have high levels of IgG to the virus. However, CMV can be transmitted from one individual to another by blood transfusions and transplantation. In the latter case, immunosuppression can make a transplant recipient particularly susceptible to CMV infection, which can result in conditions such as hepatitis, pancreatitis, pneumonitis, colitis, and even death.

The potential for infection and its timing varies from one individual to another and can differ between different organ transplants. For example, CMV disease can occur as early as 10 days after a liver transplant but months after a kidney transplant. The seropositivity of a donor and a recipient can make a difference in transplantation. Obviously, the highest risk occurs with a seropositive donor and a seronegative recipient. A better situation is a seropositive donor and a seropositive recipient, but the best scenario is having a seronegative donor. Unless aggressively treated, CMV disease can be fatal; therefore, testing for it has become a routine procedure as part of the pre-transplantation workup for both donors and recipients (12, 13).

Other testing includes organisms that are also assessed in blood transfusions, for example, hepatitis B, hepatitis C, HIV, HTLV, and WNV. CMV is tested for because these individuals are immunosuppressed. Often, testing for Epstein-Barr virus (EBV) is also done, particularly when dealing with pediatric recipients because these recipients, when immunosuppressed, may be at risk for developing post-transplant lymphoproliferative disease. In addition, the use of a questionnaire pertaining to nonmedical drug use (eg, intravenous, intramuscular, subcutaneous) and sexual practices as well as potential sexual infections (syphilis, gonorrhea) is part of donor screening.

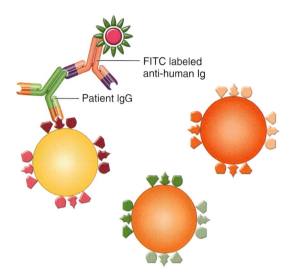

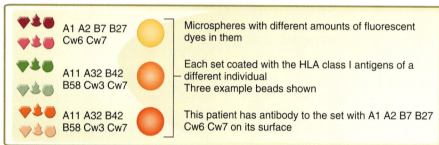

	A1 A2 B7 B27 Cw6 Cw7		Microspheres with different amounts of fluorescent dyes in them
	A11 A32 B42 B58 Cw3 Cw7		Each set coated with the HLA class I antigens of a different individual
			Three example beads shown
	A11 A32 B42 B58 Cw3 Cw7		This patient has antibody to the set with A1 A2 B7 B27 Cw6 Cw7 on its surface

■ FIGURE 14.10   Colorimetric multiplex assay to determine anti-HLA antibodies in a patient's serum.

▶ SURVIVAL AND SUCCESS

The degree of matching between donor and recipient can vary depending on the different HLA antigens that are mismatched and the organ or tissue that is being transplanted. So, in general, matching of the class II HLA antigen is more important than of class I, although mismatching of class I antigens does contribute to rejection. Tissue typing also tends to be more critical in bone marrow and kidney transplants than for liver and heart. Finally, the transplantation of tissue from an immunologically privileged site, such as corneal tissue, does not require matching (14, 15). Examples of organ transplants, specific requirements, and survival rates are shown in Table 14.5 ✪.

✪ TABLE 14.5

Five-Year Survival Rates and Requirements of Different Organ Transplants

Organ	5-Year Survival	Comments
Stem cells	80%	Stringent HLA matching required, immunosuppression required
Liver	60%	HLA matching not as critical although still needed
Heart	80%	Immunosuppression required
Kidney	80%	HLA matching very important, immunosuppression required
Pancreas	50%	Often transplanted along with kidney, immunosuppression required
Cornea	90%	Matching not critical, no immunosuppression required

► XENOTRANSPLANTATION

A major obstacle of organ transplantation is the scarcity of organs because of the low number of individuals that have committed to being organ donors. Indeed, many patients die waiting for a suitable donor. Therefore, much attention has been given to xenotransplantation, the transplantation of an organ or tissue across species. Nonhuman primates and pigs have been used as the source of organs because of their similarity in organ size and function with humans. The advantage is that successful transplants may lead to "organ farms" and to fully dedicated organ or tissue sources. Some attempts to transplant heart, liver, and bone marrow from chimps and baboons have been made but with little success. The main problem is the vigorous immune rejection among different species; in addition, the potential for spread of unrecognized pathogens (eg, viruses) has also been a major concern.

► IMMUNOSUPPRESSIVE THERAPY

Almost all transplants require immunosuppression to be successful (16). The purpose of immunosuppressive agents is to downregulate the immune responses involved in the rejection of the transplanted organ. Various immunosuppressive agents, which can be divided into 3 major classes, are used. The first one includes DNA inhibitors, such as methotrexate, cyclophosphamide, and azathioprine. These agents basically interfere with DNA synthesis, thus inhibiting cell proliferation. More selective agents such as mycophenolate mofetil tend to affect lymphocytes more specifically, reducing their effect on other proliferating cells. The second class of immunosuppressants consists of the T-cell inhibitors and includes cyclosporine A, tacrolimus (FK506), sirolimus (Rapamycin), and anti-IL-2Rα "Tac." As the name implies, their actions inhibit T-cell function, which is a necessary prelude to most immune responses. Cyclosporine A has played a major role in heart, liver, and kidney transplantation; it acts by blocking T-cell receptor signaling, thus preventing expression of IL-2 and other cytokines. Cyclosporine A binds to "immunophilins" and blocks calcineurin phosphatase, which, in turn, prevents dephosphorylation and nuclear import of NFAT, a key transcription factor for IL-2 gene expression. The third group includes corticosteroids such as prednisone and dexamethasone. Corticosteroids have multiple actions that can include interfering with the secretion of various cytokines and inhibiting the expression of adhesion molecules as well as the production of various chemoattractants and inflammatory mediators. This, in turn, results in diminished cell trafficking, diminished activation of macrophages, decreased cell-to-cell communications, and an overall downregulation of the immune response.

✓ Checkpoint! 14.4

Why do you think corneal transplants do not need immunosuppression of the recipient although the transplant is performed between 2 genetically different individuals?

► SPECIFIC IMMUNOSUPPRESSIVE THERAPIES

The immunosuppressive agents described here tend to have broad effects because they can affect different cell types. In an attempt to focus immunosuppression on specific immune cells, various antibody preparations have been used to target specific components of particular cell types. Monoclonal antibodies against T-cell components such as CD3 or IL-2R alpha have been used to deplete T cells or interfere with their function, thus reducing an immune response. Antibodies to the IL-2 receptor have been used to block T-cell activation. Even more specifically, anti-CD4 antibodies have been used to target helper T cells (17). Antibodies to adhesion molecules such as ICAM-1 and LFA-1 have also been used to interfere with cell trafficking. Because cell activations usually require reciprocal stimulation from cell to cell (a "second" signal), antibodies to cell surface molecules that are involved in this reciprocal stimulation are also used. An example of this is an antibody against B7, a protein that is necessary for secondary T-cell costimulation. Of course, antibody preparations have their own shortcomings: Because most of them are monoclonal antibodies and therefore of mouse origin, they can generate an immune response in the host. To circumvent this, current work is carried out in producing "humanized" forms of these antibodies.

► AN ALLOGRAFT WE DO NOT REJECT

Note that in Figure 14.2, an offspring carries HLA haplotypes that are from both the mother and the father; that is, they are different from the ones of each parent. In other words, each offspring has HLA haplotypes that differ from one parent because they come from the other parent. This is also true at the offspring fetal stage when the mother is carrying a fetus that has haplotypes that differ from hers (because they come from the father). Because mother and fetus are interconnected, one would expect the mother to reject the fetus as if it were an allograft from an allogeneic individual (ie, the father). But, of course, this does not happen; if it did we would have been extinct pretty quickly. Why this happens has been a long-standing puzzle in immunology and the reasons for it are still unclear. However, several hypotheses have been proposed. The simplest one is that the fetus is not considered or recognized as foreign, perhaps because the fetus is considered to be in an immunologically privileged site. However, after multiple births, women, have been shown to have circulating antibodies to the father's antigens. Other hypotheses have implicated the placenta as having an immunologically protective role for the fetus. Theories of possible mechanisms have included the fetal–maternal interface of the placenta not expressing MHC class I or class II molecules, thus making it immunologically "invisible" to maternal T cells and having certain molecules that protect it from recognition by NK cells (which recognize a lack of MHC I molecules). Secretion of cytokines that downregulate a Th1 immune response at the fetal–maternal interface (for example, TGFβ, IL-4, and IL-10) has also been suggested. This "mutual acceptance" between mother and fetus can continue to some extent after birth, perhaps because of some sort of chimerism between mother and child. This is reflected by the fact that, in general, maternal grafts have a higher survival rate than paternal grafts in recipient children.

CASE STUDY

Mr. Stearn, a patient with type I diabetes, was noncompliant for a number of years. He was in denial about his disease and as a result, he had developed proteinuria and kidney damage. His kidney damage became significant and now he is on dialysis because of kidney failure, and he needs a kidney transplant. He has 3 bothers and 1 sister who are all healthy.

1. How should you begin the testing for a possible kidney transplant?
2. What testing of Mr. Stearn's siblings should be done as possible kidney donors?

SUMMARY

Transplantation involves the transfer of cells or tissues from one individual to another. The overall purpose of this is to replace these cells or tissues, usually because they are defective (eg, a malfunctioning or damaged organ) or missing (eg, a loss of blood). Because the majority of such transfers occur between two individuals from the same species who are not genetically identical, one of the major obstacles of transplantation is an immune response from the recipient against the donor's cells or tissues. The most common form of transplantation is of blood from one individual to another. The antigens that are involved in the recipient's immune response against the donor's red blood cells are limited in number and belong to the ABO and Rh group of blood antigens; immune reactions to such antigens occur because of naturally occurring antibodies that are found in most normal individuals. Transfusion of incompatible blood can result in hemolytic transfusion reactions, which, in certain cases, can be fatal. Because of this, blood group matching between donor and recipient is of great importance before transfusion of large amounts of blood. Knowing an individual's blood group can also determine who can give to whom and who can receive from whom. Blood typing is usually performed by using commercially available antibodies against the A, B, and Rh antigens and by looking for red blood cell agglutination after incubation with these antibodies.

Tissue and organ transplantation, on the other hand, involves a much higher number of antigens that are members of the major histocompatibility complex (MHC, also referred to as HLA), which are the major components seen as foreign on the graft by a graft recipient. MHC genes are the most polymorphic genes in the human genome; each locus has a very high number of different alleles; because of this, finding an organ match with HLA compatibility is a complex and difficult task, even within a related family. There are several mechanisms of rejection, and they can involve both antibodies as well as cell-mediated responses. In addition, as in the case of the transplantation of an immunocompetent graft, the graft itself can react immunologically against the donor tissues, a phenomenon called *graft-versus-host disease*. Therefore, a successful transplant depends on the determination of HLA composition of both donor and recipient. This, in turn, is based on HLA typing. Different methods of typing are available; historically, a microcytotoxicity test had been used but although rapid and straightforward, this test had limitations and its resolution was poor. A better method is genotyping, which analyzes the actual genes coding for the different HLA types rather than the antigens themselves. Additional tests are done to determine whether the recipient has antibodies to any HLA antigens because this would cause early rejection and is used to exclude possible donors. These assays include ELISA, flow cytometry, and Luminex to detect antibodies in the recipient against different sets of the donor's HLA antigens. In most transplantation cases, however, immunosuppression of the recipient is still needed for a successful transplant because a perfect match is not often obtained. Immunosuppression is accomplished by using different pharmacological agents such as DNA inhibitors, T-cell inhibitors, and corticosteroids. Monoclonal antibodies against specific immune cells have also been used either to target those cells directly or to inhibit their functions. The exception for immunosuppression is the situation in which the transplant-involved tissue that is sequestered in an immunologically privileged site, such as the cornea. In most cases, however, the immunosuppressed individual must be carefully monitored because opportunistic organisms can become a problem.

REVIEW QUESTIONS

1. Which of the following grafts is the most likely to be accepted?
   a. autograft
   b. allograft
   c. xenograft
   d. graft-versus-host

2. Allograft rejection is mainly mediated by
   a. CD4 cells only
   b. CD4 and CD8 cells
   c. B cells
   d. neutrophils

3. The microcytotoxicity test is based on which of the following methods?
   a. using antibodies to various cytokines plus complement proteins to induce lysis of particular phenotypes and determine tissue compatibility between donor and recipient
   b. using antibodies to HLA alleles and complement to induce lysis of particular phenotypes and determine tissue compatibility between donor and recipient
   c. mixing donor and recipient white blood cells and measuring proliferation to determine tissue compatibility between donor and recipient
   d. staining cells with antibodies to HLA antigens to determine tissue type

4. Which of the following drugs is the "gold standard" for immunosuppression in organ transplantation?
   a. antibodies to the IL-4 receptor ("Tac")
   b. corticosteroids
   c. cyclosporine A
   d. monoclonal antibodies

5. Graft-versus-host disease is a major problem in which of the following situations?
   a. corneal transplants
   b. kidney and liver transplants
   c. heart transplants
   d. bone marrow transplants

6. An allograft is a transplant of
   a. tissue from a genetically identical individual
   b. tissue from a different species
   c. tissue from a haplotype-identical individual
   d. tissue from a genetically different individual from the same species

7. What is the likelihood of 2 siblings being histocompatible donors?
   a. 10%
   b. 25%
   c. 50%
   d. 75%

8. A mixed lymphocyte reaction
   a. tests the functional compatibility of a donor and recipient T cells
   b. can be performed on tissue from cadavers
   c. compares the specific MHC alleles on the host and recipient
   d. must be used before performing a transplant

9. The rejection because of already existing Ab is
   a. acute
   b. hyperacute
   c. chronic
   d. any of the above

10. Survival
   a. of bone marrow transplantation patients depends primarily on whether the donor rejects the recipient cells
   b. of bone marrow transplantation patients depends primarily on whether the recipient rejects the donor cells
   c. of an HLA mismatched kidney (mismatched at 1 loci) recipient at 6 months is 0%
   d. none of the above

11. Which of the following is *not* routinely performed today for analysis before a transplant?
   a. ABO agglutination
   b. mixed lymphocyte reaction
   c. HLA genotyping
   d. flow cytometry

REFERENCES

1. Murphy K, Travers P, Walport M. *Janeway's Immunobiology.* 8th ed. New York, NY: Garland Publishing; 8th Edition, Garland Publishing, 2012.

2. Perham P. *The Immune System.* 1st ed. New York, NY: Garland Publishing; 2005.

3. Storry JR, Olsson ML. The ABO blood group system revisited: A review and update. *Immunohematology.* 2009;25:48–59.

4. Howell WM, Carter V, Clark B. The HLA system: Immunobiology, HLA typing, antibody screening and crossmatching techniques. *J Clin Pathol.* 2010;63:387–390.

5. Chinen J, Buckley RH. Transplantation immunology: Solid organ and bone marrow. *J Allergy Clin Immunol.* 2010;125:S324–S335.

6. Issa F, Schiopu A, Wood KJ. Role of T cells in graft rejection and transplantation tolerance. *Expert Rev Clin Immunol.* 2010;6:155–169.

7. Leffell MS, Zachary AA. Antiallograft antibodies: Relevance, detection, and monitoring. *Curr Opin Organ Transplant.* 2010;15:2–7.

8. Opelz G. Factors influencing long-term graft loss. The collaborative transplant study. *Transpl. Proc.* 2000;32:647–649.

9. Flowers ME, Kansu E, Sullivan KM. Pathophysiology and treatment of graft-versus-host-disease. *Hematol. Oncol. Clin. North Am.* 1999;13:1091–1112.

10. Stern M, Ruggeri L, Mancusi A, et al. Survival after T-cell-depleted haploidentical stem cell transplantation is improved using the mother as donor. *Blood.* 2008;112:2990–2995.

11. Terasaki PI, McClelland JD. Microdroplet assay of human serum cytotoxins. *Nature.* 1964;204:998–1000.

12. Reinke P, et al. Mechanisms of human cytomegalovirus (HCMV) (re)activation and its impact on organ transplant patients. *Transpl Infect Dis.* 1999;1(3):157–164.

13. van der Bij W, Speich R. Management of cytomegalovirus infection and disease after solid-organ transplantation. *Clin Infect Dis.* 2001;33(Suppl 1):S32–S37.

14. Hong S, Van Kaer L. Immune privilege: Keeping an eye on natural killer T cells. *J Exp Med.* 1999;190(9):1197–1200.

15. Streilein, JW, Stein-Streilein, J. Anterior chamber associated immune deviation (ACAID): Regulation, biological relevance, and implications for therapy. *Int Rev Immunol* 2002;21(2–3):123–152.

16. Urschel S, Altamirano-Diaz LA, West LJ. Immunosuppression armamentarium in 2010: Mechanistic and clinical considerations. *Pediatr Clin North Am.* 2010;57:433–457.

17. Campara M, Tzvetanov IG, Oberholzer J. Interleukin-2 receptor blockade with humanized monoclonal antibody for solid organ transplantation. *Expert Opin Biol Ther.* 2010;10:959–969.

PEARSON myhealthprofessionskit™

Visit www.myhealthprofessionskit.com to access the interactive Companion Website for this textbook. Simply select "Clinical Laboratory Science" from the choice of disciplines. Find this book and log in by using your user name and password to access additional learning tools.

15

Primary Immunodeficiency Diseases

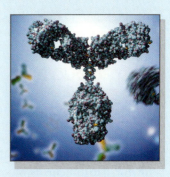

■ OBJECTIVES—LEVEL I

After this chapter, the student should be able to:

1. Describe the major arms of the immune system in which defects can lead to different immunodeficiencies.

2. Describe the mechanisms and clinical manifestation of immunodeficiencies involving antibody production.

3. Describe the mechanisms and clinical manifestation of immunodeficiencies involving T-cell defects.

4. List and describe the mechanisms of immunodeficiencies resulting from defects in the complement system.

5. Describe different mechanisms of immunodeficiency involving phagocytes, and their clinical implication.

6. Describe the pathologic mechanisms behind leukocyte adherence deficiency.

7. Describe different testing procedures to detect immunodeficiency.

8. List and describe therapeutic approaches to different forms of immunodeficiency.

■ OBJECTIVES—LEVEL II

After this chapter, the student should be able to:

1. List and describe different forms of severe combined immunodeficiencies and the mechanisms involved in them.

2. List and describe examples of immunodeficiency resulting from defects in enzymes.

KEY TERMS

adenosine deaminase deficiency
agammaglobulinemias
Bruton's disease
chronic granulomatous disease (CGD)
common variable immunodeficiency
  (CVID)
DiGeorge syndrome
hereditary angioedema (HAE)
hyper-IgM syndrome

leukocyte adherence deficiency (LAD)
purine nucleoside phosphorylase
  deficiency (PNP)
reticular dysgenesis
selective IgA deficiency
severe combined immunodeficiencies
  (SCID)
X-linked agammaglobulinemia (XLA)
X-linked immunodeficiencies

▶ INTRODUCTION

For the past 25 to 30 years, when people hear the word *immunodeficiency,* they immediately think of human immunodeficiency virus (HIV) and acquired immune deficiency syndrome (AIDS)—and justifiably so. AIDS has been one of the major epidemics in human history, affecting millions of people, spanning countries and continents, spurring countless media reports, affecting people of all walks of life, creating human and economic disasters, and generating huge amounts of both basic and clinical research as well as books and research publications. However, it must be noted that immunodeficiency spans the whole spectrum of immune responses and describes a large number of conditions in which one or more components of the immune system malfunction, resulting in either partial or total loss of immune function. In the chapters covering autoimmunity and hypersensitivity, we presented situations in which an immune response is a misdirected army and the cause of damage to the host. In this chapter, we discuss malfunctions of the immune system when one or more of its components fail to act as expected and thus prevents such system from protecting the host from a potential threat. Immunodeficiency can be either primary or secondary (ie, acquired). Primary immunodeficiencies are usually congenital defects that can affect lymphoid or myeloid lineages. The defects may be in a single gene or the result of a complex of genes, and some can affect organ development. Secondary immunodeficiencies are usually acquired (ie, caused by some external factor); the best example of a secondary or acquired immunodeficiency is AIDS, but acquired immunodeficiencies can be the result of malnutrition, radiation exposure, or immunosuppressive therapy. The scope of this chapter is not to list all the primary immunodeficiencies that have ever been described but to provide examples of different groups of primary immunodeficiencies based on the branch of the immune response they affect. If known, the underlying mechanisms will be discussed, and the clinical implications, treatments, and laboratory assays to evaluate the different conditions will be described.

▶ PRIMARY IMMUNODEFICIENCIES

Primary immunodeficiencies are genetic anomalies of various components of the immune system. They can affect a single component or multiple ones, depending on the genetic aberration involved. They can cause defects in antibody response and/or cell-mediated immunity as well as complement activation and function, phagocyte function, cell trafficking, and organ development. Interestingly, many primary immunodeficiencies are X-linked and recessive (ie, they are associated with the X chromosome) and therefore primarily affect males. Fortunately, except for specific IgA deficiency, most primary immunodeficiencies are quite rare (1, 2). Examples of primary immunodeficiencies are listed in Table 15.1 ✪, and examples of **X-linked immunodeficiencies** are listed in Table 15.2 ✪.

✪ TABLE 15.1

Examples of Primary (Congenital) Forms of Immunodeficiency

Immunodeficiency	Sample Condition
RAG1 and RAG2 deficiency	Severe combined immunodeficiency
Defective B-cell maturation	Agammaglobulinemia
Defective T-cell maturation	DiGeorge syndrome
Complement component defects	Hereditary angioedema
Defects in phagocyte functions	Defective assemble of NADPH oxidase
Defects in cell trafficking	Leukocyte adhesion deficiency

In previous chapters, we described in detail the overall complexity of the immune system, a system based on the complicated and multifaceted interactions among different cells, tissues, and a large number of diverse molecules. Most of these interactions are interdependent and pleotropic (have multiple activities); therefore, a dysfunction in even one single component of the immune system can have repercussions in several of its functions. For example, an aberration in the innate branch of the immune system can result in functional aberrations of the acquired immune system (1, 2).

▶ IMMUNOGLOBULIN DEFICIENCIES

Immunoglobulin deficiencies are usually associated with a defect in B-cell maturation or in B-cell activation (1, 3). They are collectively called **agammaglobulinemias;** they can affect the production (decrease or increase) of any immunoglobulin isotype and usually result in increased susceptibility to pyogenic infections. *Pyogenic* indicates pus-forming infections and is not to be confused with pyrogenic infections, which are fever-causing infections (Figure 15.1 ■). The defects in agammaglobulinemias can occur at any step in the development of a B cell from a stem cell to a plasma cell. The defect can also occur in signaling molecules that are necessary for B-cell function or in the mechanisms involved in isotype switch (1, 3, 4). See Table 15.3 ✪ for a few examples

✪ TABLE 15.2

Examples of X-linked Immunodeficiencies

Condition	Resulting Defect
X-SCID	Defect in the IL-2 receptor
X-linked agammaglobulinemia	Failure of B cells to mature beyond pre-B
X-linked hyper-IgM	Defective isotype switching
Chronic granulomatous disease	Failure to clear bacterial and fungal infections, development of granulomas

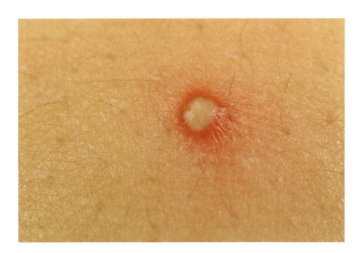

■ **FIGURE 15.1**   Pus-forming infection. Such infections occur more frequently in individuals with immunoglobulin deficiencies.
Source: Faiz Zaki/Shutterstock.

of immunoglobulin deficiencies. Except for IgA deficiencies, immunoglobulin deficiencies can be successfully treated with passive transfer of immunoglobulin.

SELECTIVE IGA DEFICIENCY

Most commonly found in individuals of European descent, **selective IgA deficiency** is the most common of the primary immunodeficiencies (1, 5). Reports in the literature on the rate of its occurrence vary from population to population from a low of 1 in 14 500 to 18 500 in Japanese individuals, to 1 in 350 to 700 Caucasian individuals, to a high of a prevalence rate of 1 in 142 persons in individuals from the Arabian peninsula. Selective IgA deficiency occurs more frequently in males than females, and, as the name implies, it results from abnormally low levels of IgA when levels of other isotypes are normal. The levels of IgA, while being abnormally low, can vary from mild to severe conditions. In general, levels of serum IgA below 5 to 7 mg/dL are considered "low" and approach the lower limits of laboratory-detectable levels of the immunoglobulin. However, levels 2 standard deviations below normal serum IgA levels (after adjusting for age) also define IgA deficiency; in this case, the condition is considered "partial deficiency." Most cases of IgA deficiency fall in this

latter category. Selective IgA deficiency does not appear to have a Mendelian distribution of transmission; in fact, patterns of transmissions have included autosomal recessive, autosomal dominant, and sporadic. This has suggested that selective IgA deficiency may actually include an assorted set of different immunologic abnormalities. For example, the genetic susceptibility to IgA deficiency is related to the genetic deficiency for common variable immunodeficiency. The idea that this is really a set of different diseases is supported by the fact that no single specific genetic defect for this disease has been identified. It is hypothesized that aberrations in B-cell differentiation to IgA-committed B cells are at its basis. This, in turn, can be attributed to different possible causes from an inherent defect in B-cell differentiation to a defect in T-cell functional help, which results in these B-cell aberration to the action of regulatory T cells (1, 5). Dysfunctions in cytokine networks have also been implicated in this disease (6) with defects in cytokines such as IL-4, IL-6, IL-7, IL-10, TGF-β, and others as being associated with the disease. It is possible that the defect may occur early in the development of B cells; this is shown by the fact that selective IgA deficiency can be transferred by the transfer of stem cells during bone marrow transplants (7). Chromosome 18 abnormalities have also been associated with IgA deficiency, and there is an increased incidence of IgA deficiency in patients who are HLA-B8, DR38.

As described in Chapter 2, IgA is the predominant isotype in extravascular secretion and the mucosal system (1, 8). The importance of this role cannot be underestimated because the mucosal system comprises an enormous surface area (~400 square meters) and is often the portal of entry for many pathogens as well as the residence of many normal commensal microorganisms. Therefore, the function of secretory IgA in the mucosal system not only serves as a method of protection against potential mucosal pathogens but also plays an important role in the maintenance of the homeostasis of commensal bacteria in the gastrointestinal tract. Because of this, one would expect that a deficiency in IgA would lead to catastrophic results in an individual, yet most people with selective IgA deficiency are asymptomatic, which suggests that other compensatory mechanisms may be involved. For example, many individuals with selective IgA deficiency have increased levels of secretory IgM. The most common symptoms in patients are mild and involve, not surprisingly, the

⊗ TABLE 15.3

Examples of B Cell and Immunoglobulin Deficiencies

Condition	Resulting Defect
Selective IgA deficiency	Increased number of infections of the respiratory and digestive tract
Hyperimmunoglobulin-M	Increased production of IgM because of defects in isotype switching; also reduced IgA, IgG, and IgE
Common variable immunodeficiency	Reduction in many different isotypes because of a combination of B-cell defects and increased T-cell inhibition
X-linked agammaglobulinemia	Reduction in all different isotypes because of a defect in B-cell differentiation

respiratory and digestive tracts. These symptoms can vary in severity from mild respiratory infections and diarrhea to severe infections leading to rare permanent damage of airway epithelia and intestines. Other conditions include increased incidences of collagen-vascular disease, allergic disorders, milk intolerance, autoimmune disease, malabsorption problems, and malignancies. Selective IgA deficiency is diagnosed by measuring levels of serum IgA; because most patients are asymptomatic, this is usually warranted by a family history of IgA deficiency or unexplained recurrent respiratory or gastrointestinal infections. In addition, because some allergic conditions and some autoimmune disorders have been associated with IgA deficiency, such testing is also indicated in patients with allergies and autoimmunity.

Of clinical importance is the fact that about 30 to 40% of patients with severe IgA deficiency produce anti-IgA antibodies, which can generate anaphylactic reactions after transfusion of blood products that contain IgA, particularly if these anti-IgA antibodies are of the IgE isotype. Because of this, testing for anti-IgA IgE antibodies is strongly indicated before blood transfusions in subjects with selective IgA deficiency. Additionally, these subjects should receive washed or deglycerolized red blood cells or blood products from IgA-deficient donors. Treatment is not necessary in asymptomatic subjects; however, because of the danger of anaphylactic reactions after transfusions in IgA-deficient subjects, it is of great value that these subjects be informed of their condition. Selective IgA deficiency should become part of their medical history and should be highlighted by having individuals wear labeled medical bracelets or medical tags. Treatment for symptomatic patients is concentrated on controlling the infections associated with the disease. This usually translates into various different antibiotic regimens. Injections of gamma globulin are not warranted because IgA is most effective at the mucosal interfaces, there is no way to replace this, and injection of IgA would likely cause development of IgE against the IgA.

As mentioned, determination of levels of serum IgA can establish the extent of selective IgA deficiency after screening for risk factors that may suggest this condition in an individual. Assays for low levels of IgA include immunonephelometry capture enzyme immunoassay.

Hyperimmunoglobulin-M Syndrome

As its name implies, hyperimmunoglobulin-M syndrome (also known as hyper-IgM syndrome) comprises different immunological malfunctions that result in elevated levels of IgM. Very low levels of IgG, IgA, and IgE characterize this syndrome. The common denominator in hyper-IgM syndrome is a defect in isotype switching in B cells (1, 9, 10). As described in Chapter 2, B cells undergo isotype switching, a process by which B-cell genes encoding for immunoglobulin heavy chains are rearranged in a unidirectional manner to switch from IgM to other isotypes. This switching and the change to different immunoglobulin classes play a major role in the immune response to infections and requires the collaboration between T and B cells described in earlier chapters. The failure in switching can be attributed either to a defect in T–B cell interactions or to defects in the actual rearrangements of isotype genes. The most common form of defect involving B–T cell interactions in hyper-IgM syndrome is a defect in the T-cell molecules CD40 ligand, which binds to CD40 receptors on B cells (11). The interaction of these costimulatory molecules is a necessary secondary stimulus for B-cell activation and isotype switch. Alternatively, molecular defects in DNA rearrangement can also play a role in hyper-IgM syndrome. Subjects with this syndrome experience severe hypogammaglobulinemia and exhibit the same symptoms as subjects with Bruton's agammaglobulinemia (to be discussed) with recurrent infections, usually in the ear, throat, and chest as well as diarrhea and osteomyelitis. Treatment is also the same with gammaglobulin replacement therapy and infection management.

Common Variable Immunodeficiency

Although many diseases derive their name from a condition that may cause different symptoms, common variable immunodeficiency (CVID) refers to the common result (most notably hypogammaglobulinemia) of a variety of immunodeficiency mechanisms (1, 12). In fact, CVID comprises a group of 20 to 30 different primary immunodeficiencies. Unlike selective IgA deficiency, CVID can result in severe clinical conditions, and patients with it are very susceptible to a variety of infections of the lungs, sinuses, ears, and bronchi and in many cases develop pneumonia. Gastrointestinal infections and shingles have also been reported for patients with CVID, and autoimmune disorders such as hemolytic anemia and thrombocytopenia can also be associated with it.

Characteristics of CVID are low levels of IgG, IgA, and/or IgM. It is a rare condition; perhaps because of its heterogeneity, its reported rate of occurrence varies in the literature, ranging from 1 in 25 000 to 1 in 100 000. However, CVID is the second most common primary immunodeficiency after selective IgA deficiency and much remains unclear about its pathogenesis. Because it comprises a variety of immunologic defects and because the symptoms are heterogeneous and the pathogenesis mostly unknown, its diagnosis is difficult and very often delayed until more and more factors point to the possibility that an individual has CVID. More often than not, some of the infections that follow CVID are treated as sporadic and incidental and in certain situations no definite diagnosis is achieved until years after its onset. In addition, other immunodeficient conditions such as hyper-IgM or X-linked agammaglobulinemia can mimic CVID, so clinical and laboratory evaluations of the CVID patient are critical for correct diagnosis. Unlike forms of agammaglobulinemias, patients with CVID initially make their own immunoglobulin. The disease can become apparent in early adulthood; unlike in the other forms of immunoglobulin deficiencies which are evident as soon as the maternal antibody is gone.

Significant decreases in serum immunoglobulin, particularly IgA and IgG, indicate CVID; however, additional tests are necessary for diagnosis. The total number of B cells appears to be normal in CVID patients; however, these cells do not seem to develop into immunoglobulin-producing plasma cells, a fact that has suggested a T-cell defect in CVID. Evaluation of the number of CD27+ switched memory B cells by flow cytometry has shown that this particular B-cell population is drastically reduced in a high percentage of CVID subjects. Because of its heterogeneity, the molecular mechanisms leading to CVID are largely unknown; however, some have been proposed as potential contributing factors. For example, it has been associated with a deficiency in a cellular signaling molecule called *CD19*. This molecule participates in B-cell receptor activation by altering the flux of calcium after the B-cell receptor has been stimulated. Mutations in the protein TACI have also been associated with CVID (13). TACI-mediated signaling plays a role in B-cell activation and regulation as well as IgA isotype switching. Treatment for CVID involves replacement of immunoglobulins by intravenous or intramuscular routes and can be quite successful. The control of the infections derived from it is imperative, particularly respiratory and gastrointestinal ones, especially considering that secretory IgA is also low in these subjects.

X-linked Agammaglobulinemia

X-linked agammaglobulinemia (XLA) (also called Bruton's agammaglobulinemia or **Bruton's disease**) is a primary immunodeficiency whose prevalence in males was first described in 1952. XLA has a frequency of about 1 case per 250 000 and is characterized by a lack of mature B cells and immunoglobulins of all isotypes (1, 3). Because of the impaired B-cell development, there is a lack of lymphoid tissue such as tonsils and lymph nodes, and individuals with XLA tend to develop infections in early life once maternal antibodies have been cleared out. Observation of the lack of tonsils is a diagnostic criterion. Infections can range from localized to systemic and can include pneumonia, otitis, gastroenteritis, osteomyelitis, urinary tract infections, meningitis, and sepsis. Cellulitis and skin abscesses can also be found, and infections from enteroviruses such as vaccine-derived poliovirus can lead to viremia and complications in the central nervous system. Individuals with XLA have pre-B in their bone marrow but lack circulating B cells and plasma cells. T cells, NK cells, and CD4/CD8 ratios are normal. The primary congenital defect in XLA is in an enzyme called *Bruton's tyrosine kinase.* This enzyme is produced in all B cells and their precursors and plays a critical role in cell signaling, particularly in functions involving the maturation of B cells from B-cell precursors. It also affects the VJ and VDJ rearrangements of the immunoglobulin variable region genes discussed in Chapter 2.

Amazingly enough, these patients, who are subjected to frequent infections, do not usually have catastrophic consequences; they usually tend to live well into their 40s, and the prognosis is better with early treatment. Children can manifest clinical symptoms of XLA at 3 to 9 months of age because this is when maternal antibodies will have diminished. If there is a family history of XLA, fetal lymphocytes can be collected in utero by amniocentesis; flow cytometry can be used to detect a decrease of CD19+ B cells and an increase of mature T cells. As with other agammaglobulinemias, a good prognosis results after treatment involving replacement of immunoglobulins by intramuscular or intravenous routes and, of course, aggressive treatment of the infections associated with this disease.

▶ T-CELL IMMUNODEFICIENCIES

In previous chapters, we discussed the critical role that T cells play in an efficient and effective immune response. It only stands to reason, then, that dysfunctions in T-cell function can have multiple effects on the immune system. Because of this and the diversity of the role of T cells, immunodeficiencies that affect T cells "only" are hard to identify. In other words, any dysfunction of T cells is likely to affect other aspects of the immune system. In fact, some of the dysfunctions in T cells have a molecular basis that also affects other cells. For example, the CD40 ligand defect described previously is a T-cell defect but, of course, it affects B cells (11). See Table 15.4 ✪ for some examples of defects in T-cell function.

DIGEORGE SYNDROME

DiGeorge Syndrome is a condition caused by a missing piece (a small deletion) of chromosome 22 (1, 3). Its occurrence is about 1 in 4000 individuals; its traits are numerous and diverse, affecting many organs and body parts, and its severity varies widely from one individual to another (14, 15, 16). Only 1 in 250 of the children with DiGeorge have complete lack of T-cell function. Transplant of fetal thymus can improve this. Thymus donors can be infants who had cardiac surgery because some thymic tissue needs to be removed to approach a fetal heart; fetal thymus from stillborn or aborted fetuses also can be used. Features of DiGeorge syndrome include heart defects, neuromuscular problems, palate defects, learning disabilities, and aberration in facial expressions. Childhood infections are also a common feature of the disease. The immunologic component of this syndrome is the dysfunctional or failed development of the thymus. The defect in thymic development varies, and some subjects with DiGeorge syndrome have very small thymic defects and an almost normal immune response. On the other hand, individuals with failed development of the third and fourth pharyngeal pouches of the thymus experience significant decrease in number of T cells and, thus, more severe immune defects. Although T cells in patients with DiGeorge syndrome tend to be functionally normal, the problem in this condition is the number of mature T cells. Because of decreased function of

❂ TABLE 15.4

Examples of T-Cell Defects and Resulting Deficiencies

Condition	Resulting Defect
DiGeorge syndrome	Faulty development of thymus and defective maturation of T cells
ZAP70 deficiency	Defective T-cell signaling
SCID (different forms)	Various T-cell defects
PNP	Decreased number of T cells because of buildup of toxic metabolites
ADA deficiencies	Decreased number of T and B cells because of buildup of toxic metabolites

T cells, subjects with DiGeorge syndrome suffer from recurrent fungal and viral infections (Figure 15.2 ■).

PURINE NUCLEOSIDE PHOSPHORYLASE DEFICIENCY

The enzyme purine nucleoside phosphorylase plays a major role in the purine salvage pathway by degrading purines and converting them into their respective metabolites. If this enzyme is defective, a buildup of excessive deoxy-GTP can occur, and this, in turn, can be toxic to T cells. **Purine nucleoside phosphorylase deficiency (PNP)** is a very rare condition in which this defect occurs, and it is characterized by a progressive reduction in the number of T cells because of the toxicity of the elevated levels of deoxy-GTP (17). Subjects with

PNP exhibit impaired cell-mediated immunity and are susceptible to various benign and opportunistic infections including recurrent or chronic infections of the lungs, skin, and urinary tract. PNP presents in infants and has been associated with autoimmune disorders such as systemic lupus erythematosus, hemolytic anemia, and idiopathic thrombocytopenia. Abnormalities of the nervous system and mental retardation have also been reported in subjects with PNP. Humoral responses in general are not affected, and antibody levels are normal or slightly elevated.

▶ SEVERE COMBINED IMMUNODEFICIENCIES

Severe combined immunodeficiencies (SCID) is a term used to describe a variety of conditions in which, as its name implies, the genetic defect affects pretty much every branch of the immune system (1) (see David Vetter, the "bubble boy," Chapter 4). SCID conditions affect the development and function of both B and T cells. **Adenosine deaminase deficiency** (ADA deficiency) is another immunodeficiency caused by a genetic defect in a gene encoding for an enzyme involved in the purine salvage pathway (1, 2, 18). Encoded in chromosome 20, adenosine deaminase (ADA) plays a major role in the breakdown of adenosine. Failure of this breakdown results in the buildup of deoxyadenosine and S-adenosylhomocysteine, products that, if at high enough levels, are toxic to both immature B and T cells. Fortunately, this condition is autosomal recessive, so 2 copies of the defective gene (ie, one from each parent) must be inherited for the disease to be expressed. Because T cells are affected even more than B cells, individuals with ADA deficiency tend to have a very small and underdeveloped thymus and a severely compromised immune system. Bone marrow transplant and gene therapy are both considered as treatment in these conditions. The first gene therapy ever utilized was used for a patient with this disorder. Those of you who have more interest in this area can read about Ashanti de Silva, the first patient treated.

Another example of SCID is **reticular dysgenesis,** a rare condition characterized by low lymphocyte counts and lack of blood monocytes and neutrophils. The most common form of SCID is X-linked severe combined immunodeficiency (X-SCID),

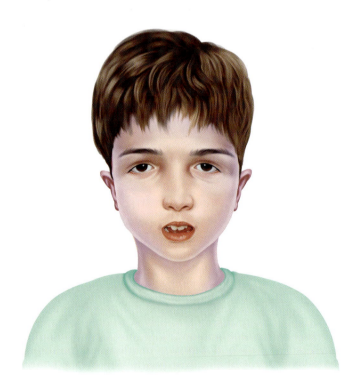

■ **FIGURE 15.2** Patient with DiGeorge syndrome. Note low set ears and wide set downward slanting eyes; often these patients also have a cleft palate.

a condition that affects lymphocytes and is characterized by a very low number of both T and B lymphocytes, severe susceptibility to numerous different infections, and profound immunodeficiency. X-SCID is the result of mutations in γc subunit of the interleukin-2 (IL-2) receptor, resulting in defects in IL-2 signaling. However, the γc subunit of the receptor for IL-2 is also shared by the receptors for several other cytokines, IL-4, IL-7, IL-9, and IL-15 (1, 19, 20, 21, 22). Thus, anomalies in the function of this γc subunit affect the function not only of IL-2 but also of numerous other cytokines, resulting in multiple functional aberrations in the immune system. See Figure 15.3 ■ for a diagram of the receptor for IL-7, showing the common γc subunit. (The critical functions of cytokines in the immune system are covered in Chapter 4.)

Subjects with X-SCID are severely susceptible to a variety of infections from early infancy; because of an essentially nonfunctioning immune system, the infections can be of many different types and occur in many locations, from lungs, to gastrointestinal, to systemic areas, and the disease is usually fatal; subjects die, at the best, in very early childhood. Treatment for X-SCID involves bone marrow transplants. Gene therapy has been attempted, and 14 patients successfully developed immune system responses, but 2 of these patients developed leukemia as a result of the movement of the inserted gene to a spot that affected cellular proliferation. The leukemia in these 2 patients was successfully treated, but these gene trials were discontinued. Those of you with further interest in this area can read about Rhys Evans, one of the patients so treated.

Another aberration of the receptor for IL-2 is the condition Janus kinase 3 (JAK-3) deficiency. JAK-3 is a signal transduction component that plays a major role in the activation and transduction of interleukin receptors (see Figure 15.3). It is commonly found in T cells and NK cells and participates in the signal transduction by cytokine receptors that utilize the γc subunit just described. Therefore, mutations in JAK-3 can also affect the function of this common γc subunit and of T cells and NK cells. Because the defect is on the JAK-3, not the γc subunit, this condition is not X-linked and can affect both males and females. The symptoms and features of the JAK-3 deficiency are similar to those of X-SCID.

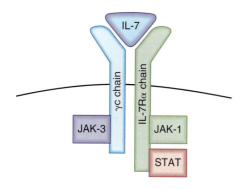

■ FIGURE 15.3   The different components of the IL-7 receptor.

Other forms of SCID are the ZAP70 deficiency, an aberration of the protein kinase ZAP70, which plays a critical role in T-cell signaling, and Omenn syndrome, a condition characterized by defects in the recombinase activating genes RAG1 and RAG2, resulting in defective lymphocyte maturation.

 Checkpoint! 15.1

Antibodies are produced by B cells. Why is it, then, that a dysfunction in T cells can result in defective antibody production?

▶ COMPLEMENT DEFICIENCIES

The critical role of the complement system in immunity is described in detail in Chapter 5. As one can imagine, because of the numerous and diverse roles of complement in an immune response, different functional aberrations in one or more of its components can result in some sort of immune dysfunction. In fact, defects in numerous different complement components have been reported for a number of different conditions. These components include early components of the classical pathway (C1q, C1r, C1s, C4, C2, and C3), late components (C5–C9), and components of the alternative pathway such as factor D or of properdin. Deficiencies have also been reported for factor H and factor I and for the mannose-binding lectin (MBL), a component of the MBL-dependent pathway (1, 2, 3, 4, 23). Depending on the component involved, deficiencies in complement components can result in either defective opsonization or defective lytic activity. Defective opsonization is usually associated with a dysfunction in C3b and C3bi, and any defect that results in diminished production of these components also causes decreased opsonization. The defect can be in either the classical pathway, the alternative pathway, or the MBL pathway because all 3 lead to C3. Defects of C3 itself have a high rate of morbidity because this complement component plays a key role in each pathway in lysis and in opsonization. Defective lytic activity is usually associated with defects in the terminal components of the complement cascade, such as those that form the membrane attack complex (MAC) (ie, C5–C9). Interestingly, subjects with these defects are more susceptible to infections from certain organisms, such as Neisseria.

Complement also plays a major role in the control of immune complexes by interfering with their aggregation and promoting their clearance. Because of this, subjects with defects in the classical complement pathway are also more susceptible to diseases that involve immune complexes, such as systemic lupus erythematosus (SLE). In particular, subjects with defects in C1qrs, C2, or C4 are at higher risk for developing SLE.

It is not in the scope of this chapter to list all possible permutations of each complement defect; however, one disease, **hereditary angioedema (HAE),** has been historically associated with complement deficiencies (25). HAE is characterized by an autosomal dominant genetic defect in the plasma component C1 inhibitor (C1INH). C1INH has different actions: It inhibits the first complement component C1, and it affects both the classical and the lectin complement pathways and thus has a "control" function on the activation of complement. In addition, it is a regulator of the coagulation pathway by inhibiting activated Hageman factor (factor XII) and inhibits plasma kallikrein. It has been suggested that failure to inhibit or control the coagulation pathway results in various kinin mediators that may cause vascular changes related to vascular permeability, vascular leakage, and edema. More specifically, kallikrein is known to cleave kininogen into bradykinin, a mediator that promotes the leakage of postcapillary venules. Failure of C1INH to inhibit the action of kallikrein allows this cascade to remain unchecked, resulting in vascular leakage and edema. It is interesting to point out that whereas the problem in most cases of immunodeficiency is a mechanism that is impaired and "fails" to function or that is turned "down" or "off," the problem in the case of HAE is a mechanism that is *not* turned off. In fact, one may argue as to whether this condition is truly an immunodeficiency (ie, a failed protection mechanism). Nevertheless, because it *is* the failure of a mechanism associated with the immune system, it has historically been considered as such. HAE has an incidence of 1 in 10 000 to 50 000 individuals in the United States and 1 in 50 000 to 150 000 individuals in the rest of the world. As the name implies, the major clinical manifestation of the disease is localized swelling, which can be mild or severe; sometimes it can be accompanied by a rash and can resolve in a few days. The areas affected vary, commonly including the hands and feet. Swelling of the gastrointestinal mucosa can cause more severe symptoms including severe pain and diarrhea. Most cases of HAE are not life threatening; however, the edema often extends to the laryngeal area and, in severe cases, can cause respiratory obstruction or blockage (1, 25). Sometimes such reactions can be caused by specific stimuli such as a local anesthetic administered during a dental procedure, but more often these reactions are spontaneous (Figure 15.4 ■).

▶ DEFECTS IN PHAGOCYTE FUNCTION

Phagocytes such as neutrophils play a major role in the clearance of infectious organisms and are essential participants of a strong immune system. Therefore, functional aberrations of phagocytes can also result in an inefficient or ineffective immune response. *Phagocytosis* is the process by which phagocytes internalize particles such as bacteria and digest them. Phagocytes are usually activated by various receptors, such as those for opsonins including immunoglobulins and complement components, or by other ligands. Once phagocytes have recognized a microorganism and have been activated, phagocytosis follows. This entails various steps from initial adherence to internalization of the microorganism into a phagolysosome where digestion occurs. Digestion is achieved by a combination of different biochemical events that include the production of various digestive and degradative enzymes as well as highly reactive and bacteriocidal metabolic intermediates of

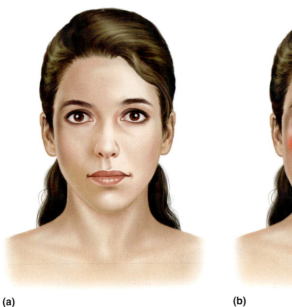
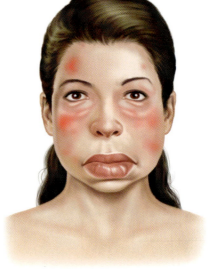

(a)   (b)

■ **FIGURE 15.4** Typical clinical manifestation of hereditary angioedema (C1 inhibitor deficiency). You can see a person having a typical edema attack (b) as compared to her normal appearance (a).

oxygen and nitrogen, such as H_2O_2 and NO. The production of these metabolic intermediates involves a process known as *oxidative burst,* an increase in oxidative metabolism of phagocytes following uptake of opsonized particles and resulting in the production of these intermediates (1, 2).

CHRONIC GRANULOMATOUS DISEASE

One of the major enzymes involved in the oxidative burst and the production of H_2O_2 is nicotinamide adenine dinucleotide phosphate (NADPH) oxidase. This enzyme transfers electrons from NADPH and combines them with molecular oxygen to generate superoxide, which in turn, after additional steps, results in the production of H_2O_2 as well as hydroxyl radical and hypochlorite, all products used to kill the ingested microorganism (1). Should this enzyme fail in its function, the phagocytic cell would be incapable of generating the reactive radicals needed for this digestive process. This is indeed the case in the condition **chronic granulomatous disease (CGD).** CGD is a term used to describe a variety of hereditary diseases characterized by an aberration of phagocytes' ability to form the reactive oxygen species needed for intracellular killing of ingested microorganisms (26). The frequency of CGD is roughly 1 in 200 000 individuals in the United States, and the common denominator is a defect in one of the 4 subunits of NADPH oxidase. In other words, phagocytes cannot assemble NADPH oxidase and produce H_2O_2 and O_2 radicals that kill bacteria.

People with CGD suffer diverse recurrent infections such as pneumonia, suppurative arthritis, various abscesses of skin or organs (such as liver), osteomyelitis, cellulitis, and impetigo. Refer to Figure 15.5 ■ for an example of cutaneous granulomatous lesions.

These individuals are also more susceptible to catalase-positive organisms, such as *Staphylococcus aureus* and species of Salmonella, Nocardia, and Klebsiella, than people with a

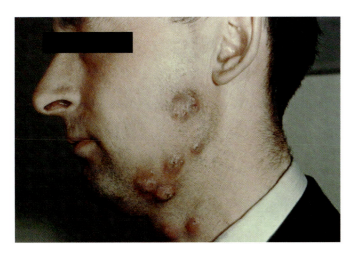

■ **FIGURE 15.5** Cutaneous granulomatous lesions on the face of a man suffering from a dermatophytic infection. *Source:* © CDC.

normal immune system. Early diagnosis is critical in CGD because the disease manifests itself in early childhood and, if uncontrolled, can be fatal.

Historically, diagnosis of CGD has relied on the nitroblue-tetrazolium (NBT) test, which measures the ability of an individual's neutrophils to reduce NBT from a colorless compound into a blue colored insoluble form that precipitates and is visible on a microscope slide. Neutrophils from a CGD subject are negative (ie, no color change) for this test. A more modern approach involves a similar mechanism but can be quantitated by flow cytometry. This test uses dihydrorhodamine-123 (DHR-123), which, when reduced, generates rhodamine, which, in turn, emits fluorescence that can be measured quantitatively. Cells, such as neutrophils, from a patient are mixed with DHR-123 and then stimulated, resulting in an oxidative burst, which, in a healthy individual, reduces DHR-123 to the fluorescent compound. In addition to being quantitative, this assay can also distinguish subjects with X-linked CGD from subjects with autosomal recessive CGD, the latter having decreased but detectable levels of this activity. An assay of similar principle measuring the activity of superoxide dismutase is the cytochrome C microplate reduction assay, which, as the name implies, measures the reduction of cytochrome C.

LEUKOCYTE ADHERENCE DEFICIENCY

Leukocyte adherence deficiency (LAD) is an autosomal recessive genetic defect in the gene that encodes for CD18, a molecule shared by the β_2-integrin, which play a critical role in the adhesion and emigration of leukocytes to extravascular sites. The movement of cells from one place to another in a directed and well-planned manner is an essential activity for an efficient and focused immune response. In fact, cells of the immune system move all the time, and their movement is not limited to a passive floating within the circulatory system. Cells of the immune system not only move but also discriminate between sites. In a way, these cells appear to "know" how to get there, and some even know how to get back. This phenomenon, often called *cell homing,* involves the preferential migration of cells and is a property common to many cells including all leukocytes (1). Cell homing is an essential phenomenon in the capacity of the immune system to protect tissues.

This brings us to the mechanism of chemotaxis, which is the directed movement of leukocytes along a concentration gradient of chemoattractants. *Chemoattractants* are substances that may be derived from the tissues or from infecting organisms, and stimulate leukocytes such as neutrophils by binding to receptors on the leukocyte surface. The movement of cells in the immune system is mediated by adhesive molecules that are present on the cells that are moving and on the surface onto which these cells move (1). Think of these molecules as some sort of chemical "Velcro" with one side of the Velcro on a cell and the corresponding other side on the surface on which these cells "walk." Adhesive molecules have many functions, not only for cell locomotion, but also for cell-to-cell interactions such as those discussed in antigen presentation. However, for this form of immunodeficiency, we will be discussing molecules associated with cell locomotion.

Neutrophils must cross 2 endothelial cell barriers to arrive at sites of infection; the interaction between surface adhesins on the neutrophils and their corresponding ligands on endothelial cells is a first step in neutrophil migration across endothelial borders. The modulation of neutrophil adhesive molecules, or adhesins, and endothelial cell attachment molecules by inflammatory mediators triggers neutrophil migration across blood vessel walls; upregulation of these ligands enhances neutrophil attachment to endothelial cells and facilitates transendothelial migration. Several adhesins are involved in these interactions.

In LAD there is an autosomal recessive genetic defect in the gene that encodes for CD18, a molecule shared by the β_2-integrins, which play a critical role in the adhesion and emigration of leukocytes to extravascular sites; this defect causes a defective expression of all 3 β_2-integrins at the cell surface. Because of this, phagocytes with defective integrin molecules cannot migrate through the vascular endothelium, and, in turn, cannot migrate from the blood stream into the tissues to the site of infection; because of this, they cannot properly destroy invading microorganisms. In addition, many other cells express the β_2-integrins, including lymphocytes, monocytes, macrophages, neutrophils, and natural killer cells and thus are also affected by this genetic defect.

The prevalence of LAD is approximately 1 in 100 000 persons. Subjects with LAD suffer from recurrent bacterial infections of the lungs, peritoneal cavity, gingiva, and often have abscesses and even infections of the stump of the umbilical cord in early infancy. These infections present in the neonatal stage and can be life threatening. As with other immunodeficiencies, diagnosis starts with unexpected recurrent infections followed by analysis of immune function, both cellular and humoral. A common finding in LAD is an extremely high number of blood neutrophils; because of this dysfunction, they are unable to leave the circulation. Specific diagnosis is straightforward, evaluating the expression of CD18 on the surface of leukocytes by flow cytometry using monoclonal antibodies to this component. Therapy is limited to bone marrow transplantation although gene replacement therapy is currently under aggressive consideration.

✓ Checkpoint! 15.2

In leukocyte adherence deficiency there is a defect in the gene that encodes for CD18, a molecule shared by the β_2-integrins, causing a defective expression of all 3 β_2-integrins at the cell surface and resulting in recurrent infections and a severe disease. Why do you think a defect in a single cellular component can have such devastating consequences?

▶ DIAGNOSTIC TESTS

Some of the diagnostics for specific immunodeficiencies have been explained in their specific sections. Fortunately, most immunodeficiencies are recessive, so disease will occur only if both chromosomes are affected; in fact, many recessive diseases are found in highly inbred populations, such as the Amish (for example, ZAP70 deficiency). Patients with immune deficiency are usually detected by a clinical history of recurrent infections that cannot otherwise be explained. The nature of the infection may suggest which branch of the immune system may be defective: for example, bacterial infections may suggest defects in antibody production and function, in the complement system, or in phagocytosis. Viral or fungal infections or infections by intracellular organisms, on the other hand, may suggest defects in T-cell function, and combined infections may suggest a hematopoietic defect or a combined deficiency. Medical history and family history are, of course, integral components of the diagnostic process; family history is critical considering the genetic nature of these immunodeficiencies. Because we are dealing with defects of the immune system, common sense dictates that clinical immunology testing of different immune functions is the basis for diagnosis of primary immunodeficiencies. Lymphopenia or drastic reduction in the number of T cells may be suggestive of a T-cell defect such as DiGeorge syndrome or a combined defect such as SCID; a decreased number of B cells and/or levels of a particular antibody or antibodies may indicate a deficiency in humoral immunity. Examples of diagnostic approaches to different immunodeficiencies are listed in Table 15.5 ✪.

Subjects with antibody deficiencies should be evaluated by taking B-cell counts (usually by measuring the expression of CD19 or CD20) and, of course, immunoglobulin levels, either total, isotype specific, or those specific to particular antigens. With infants, one must also account for the fact that maternal antibodies remain in circulation for a few months postpartum, so an antibody deficiency may not be detected because these maternal antibodies can make the infant's antibody levels appear to be normal. Antibody responses are easily evaluated against common antigens such as those received from a standard immunization, for example, diphtheria and tetanus toxoids, by measuring antibody levels to the toxoid preparations after immunization. Other antigens include various proteins and polysaccharides. A pneumococcal polysaccharide vaccine can be used to test a T-independent antibody response to polysaccharides. If, after the first immunization (ie, in an individual who has not been immunized), antibody levels are not as expected, a booster immunization should follow. If such booster administration is effective and antibody production is normal, a 4-fold increase in antibody levels should occur in healthy individuals.

One of the techniques used to evaluate changes of levels of different serum components from normal levels is serum

⊕ TABLE 15.5

Examples of Primary Immunodeficiencies, Associated Defects, and Diagnostic Testing

Condition	Defect	Test
X-SCID	Defect in the Il-2 receptor	Complete blood cell count
X-linked agammaglobulinemia	Failure of B cells to mature beyond pre-B	Serum levels of immunoglobulins and subclasses Complete blood cell counts
X-linked hyper-IgM	Defective isotype switching	Serum levels of immunoglobulins and subclasses
Complement deficiencies	Reduced opsonization and lytic activities	Levels of specific complement components
Chronic granulomatous disease	Defective phagocyte function	Function of oxidative and respiratory burst
Selective IgA deficiency	Reduction of IgA production	Serum levels of IgA
Common variable immunodeficiency	Reduction in many different antibody isotypes	Serum levels of immunoglobulins and subclasses B-cell counts
DiGeorge syndrome	Defective maturation of T cells	Complete blood cell counts
Leukocyte adherence deficiency	Defective cell chemotaxis	Surface expression of CD18 on leukocytes
PNP	Decreased number of T cells	Complete blood counts Differential T-cell counts Enzyme assays
ADA deficiencies	Decreased number of T and B cells	Complete blood counts Differential T-cell counts Enzyme assays

protein electrophoresis (SPE), which has been described earlier. In serum protein electrophoresis, C3 is in the β_2; IgA spans the beta and gamma regions, and IgG, IgM, IgE, and IgD are found in the gamma region. Normal distribution of the different areas in human serum are as follows: albumin: 58 to 70%; α_1: 2 to 5%; α_2: 6 to 11%; β: 8 to 14%; γ: 9 to 18%. Any elevation from normal levels indicates an aberration in the components belonging to a particular region. Additional evaluation of the different immunoglobulins can be done through quantitative nephelometry or enzyme immunoassays.

Evaluation of cell-mediated immunity can be conducted using a type IV or delayed hypersensitivity test (DHT), which involves the intradermal injection of a common antigen such as tetanus toxoid; the cell-mediated immunity reaction can then be observed by the localized appearance at the site of the injection of an induration and an inflammatory reaction. This is usually done during a visit to a physician; and it must be noted that a negative test (ie, no resulting inflammation) may not necessarily mean a defect in cell-mediated immunity but the possibility that the particular individual has never been exposed to the antigen used in the test.

The change in numbers of a particular cell type from normal levels is usually evaluated by flow cytometry, using specific antibodies to a variety of "cluster of differentiation" (CD) antigens. These antigens are numerous and varied and are characteristic of a particular cell type (for example, CD3 for T cells, CD19 for B cells, and CD16 for NK cells) or a particular subset, or the stage of activation or differentiation step of a cell type (eg, CD3/CD4 for helper T cells, CD3/CD8 for cytotoxic T cells). Therefore, a drastic decrease or lack of CD3+ cells may indicate DiGeorge syndrome whereas a lack of CD19+ cells may be associated with an agammaglobulinemia. The principle and details of flow cytometry are discussed in Chapter 7.

Complement deficiencies may be detected by evaluating the levels of different complement components. The total hemolytic complement (or CH50 test) analyzes total complement functionality; although the CH50 test mainly evaluates the classical pathway, it is used as an initial screening tool for complement deficiencies as well as certain autoimmune conditions such as lupus erythematosus. The CH50 test evaluates the overall activity of the complement system. The AH50 assay is used to screen for deficiencies in the alternative pathway. Decreases in such activity warrant further investigation into specific complement components, most commonly C3 and C4. As stated, aberrations in phagocytosis can be determined by measuring the oxidative ability of a phagocyte by using the NBT test, the DHR-13 test, and the cytochrome C test; subjects with LAD can be evaluated by measuring the expression of the CD18 surface marker.

With the advances in genomics and related research, more and more emphasis is now placed on identifying genetic markers that may be specific for a particular primary immunodeficiency, and much research is dedicated to studying the association between such genetic markers and immune diseases. Some genetic tests are already available for some of these conditions (for example, for the mutation in the IL-2Rγ). However, many of the tests currently available and described in this chapter are sufficient for proper diagnosis and are being used routinely and extensively.

▶ TREATMENT

As may be expected, a major component of the treatment of primary immunodeficiencies requires the control of the infections that are associated with these diseases and may involve different agents against bacterial, viral, or fungal infections. From an immunologic point of view, treatment also involves attempting to correct whatever molecular aberration causes the condition. This may include the replacement of a missing protein, a missing cell type or cell lineage, or the replacement of a missing or defective gene. In the case of agammaglobulinemia, the classic treatment is the administration of pooled or selected gamma globulins by either subcutaneous or intravenous routes. In some cases, this may be accomplished using antibodies against a particular organism from vaccinated people or "humanized" monoclonal antibodies. Unfortunately, the host may see even humanized antibodies as antigens and produce an immune response to them. For ADA deficiency, the regular intramuscular administration of ADA linked to polyethylene glycol (ADA-PEG) has been used as a treatment method. The replacement of a missing cell type or lineage is usually achieved by bone marrow transplantation or hematopoietic cell transplantation. A carefully HLA-matched donor is needed, especially to avoid graft-versus-host disease, although the risk is minimized by the use of purified stem cells. Both of these approaches are described in detail in Chapter 14. Gene replacement, on the other hand, is still under intense development.

 Checkpoint! 15.3

Why do you think certain immunodeficiencies are more common in highly inbred populations?

CASE STUDY

A friend of yours was getting an estimate from an architect to make her home more suitable for her expanding family because she has 3 children and she was about to marry a man who has 4 children. You were visiting her when the architect came. The architect was making conversation and said that it must be interesting to have so many children. The architect further said that she loved children but was not going to have any herself. The way that she said this made you ask why. She explained that she had had 2 brothers, but they had both been very ill when they were babies, were always sickly, and had died at 40. This loss of her brothers had made her afraid to have her own family. In addition, she told you that a similar thing had happened to her mother's brother who had had many infections when he was small and had died after vaccination with the live polio vaccine. The illnesses in these little boys had begun when they were all about 5 months old and had consisted of pneumonia, otitis, and meningitis. You asked her what the diagnosis had been. She replied that her family were Christian Scientists and did not go to the doctor except when it was legally mandated for most people to get a vaccine, for example.

1. What do you think was wrong with these little boys?
2. If one of these boys were still alive, is there a physical sign that would indicate he had the disease in your answer in Question 1?
3. What laboratory test would you use to determine whether the boy had the immunodeficiency you suspect?
4. If the architect were to have children, would they have this disease?
5. If the architect did have a son with the disease, how could he be treated to reduce its severity?

SUMMARY

Primary immunodeficiencies are congenital conditions that affect one or more components of the immune system. Because of its complexity, they can span the whole spectrum of the system from humoral immunity to cell-mediated immunity and from innate immunity to acquired immunity. Many immunodeficiencies are X-linked and, therefore, affect only males. Deficiencies in B-cell function and/or development and activation results in antibody deficiencies; these can include selective IgA deficiency, hyperimmunoglobulin-M, common variable immunodeficiency, and X-linked agammaglobulinemia. These are usually associated with an aberration in B-cell development, in B-cell activation and differentiation, or a defect in isotype switching. Genetic defects can also affect T cells, which in turn, result in aberrations of various different immune components. T-cell deficiencies include DiGeorge syndrome, PNP, and ADA deficiency. T cells are also affected in severe combined immunodeficiencies (SCID), which, as the name implies, affect many different components of the immune system. Of the several forms of SCID, the most severe one is X-SCID, which is caused by mutations in γc subunit of the interleukin-2 (IL-2) receptor, a subunit also shared by various other different cytokine receptors. Defect in the complement system also results in different forms of immunodeficiency; the action of complement can be either diminished or absent, rendering an individual more susceptible to infections, or, as in the case of hereditary angioedema, to uncontrolled activation of the complement components. Immunodeficiencies can also involve phagocytic cells by affecting their ability either to destroy phagocytosed organisms or to arrive at site of inflammation. The former is characterized by chronic granulomatous disease in which phagocytes cannot assemble NADPH oxidase and produce H_2O_2 and O_2 radicals that kill phagocytosed bacteria. On the other hand, cellular locomotion of phagocytes can be impaired by the lack of a common subunit (CD18) for the β_2-integrins, which are adhesive molecules used in cell locomotion. Such a situation appears in LAD.

Diagnostic approaches for primary immunodeficiencies usually start with the observation of recurrent infections that cannot otherwise be explained. The type and site of infection may implicate a particular component of a specific branch of the immune system, such as humoral immunity or cell-mediated immunity, and narrows the selection of specific tests to evaluate the functionality of that particular branch of components. These tests may include antibody levels, either total or isotype and antigen specific; evaluation of complement; cellular immunity; enzyme activity profiles; and the enumeration of a wide variety of different cell types. Treatment involves the control of the infections usually associated with these conditions; in addition, replacement of missing molecules (eg, gamma globulins), cells (eg, bone marrow or stem cell transplants), or genes (eg, gene therapy) are also direct treatment approaches to these immunologic defects. Table 15.5 summarizes examples of primary immunodeficiency conditions, associated defects, and diagnostic testing.

REVIEW QUESTIONS

1. What congenital immunodeficiency is characterized by the absence of a thymus and cardiac abnormalities?
   a. chronic granulomatous disease
   b. DiGeorge syndrome
   c. leukocyte adhesion deficiency
   d. bare lymphocyte syndrome

2. Gene therapy for X-linked SCID involves reconstitution with the gene that codes for
   a. ZAP70
   b. Phox91
   c. IL-2Rβ
   d. IL-2Rγc

3. In X-linked SCID, which immune cell populations are defective?
   a. neutrophils
   b. T cells only
   c. T and B cells
   d. macrophages and dendritic cells

4. A 6-month-old patient who presents with frequent viral infections but few bacterial infections is most likely to have a defect in
   a. B cells
   b. T cells
   c. both B and T cells
   d. complement proteins

5. Which of the following immunodeficiencies affect(s) B cells?
   a. X-linked SCID
   b. X-linked agammaglobulinemia
   c. X-linked hyper-IgM
   d. all of the above

Questions 7 and 8 refer to information in Question 6.

6. A baby was born several months ago and by the age of 2 months has developed a number of bacterial infections from which he is slow to recover. His response to viruses and fungi is not impaired. His older brother, who is 10, has this same problem, but his sister does not. On electrophoresis, we would likely see a(n)
   a. increased albumin peak
   b. increased beta globulin peak
   c. decreased gamma globulin peak
   d. increased gamma globulin peak

7. Treatment of the boy should be
   a. a bone marrow transplant
   b. gene therapy
   c. passive transfer of gamma globulin
   d. transfer of IgA to his mucosal surfaces

8. The cause of his disease is likely to be
   a. unclear
   b. a defect in maturation of pre-B cells to mature B cells
   c. a defect in lack of T-cell help
   d. AIDS virus

9. T-cell deficiency results in
   a. bacterial infections including otitis media and pneumonia
   b. increased number of fungal protozoan and viral infections
   c. increased number of infections with bacteria that are normally of low virulence
   d. none of the above

10. Complement deficiencies can result in the increased risk of
    a. allergic reactions
    b. SLE-like syndrome
    c. both of the above
    d. none of the above

REFERENCES

1. Murphy K. *Janeway's Immunobiology.* 8th ed. New York, NY: Garland Publishing; 2012.

2. Perham P. *The Immune System.* 1st ed. New York, NY: Garland Publishing; 2005.

3. Notarangelo LD. Primary Immunodeficiencies. *J Allergy Clin Immunol.* 2010;125:S182–S194.

4. Kumar A, Teuber SS, Gershwin ME. Current perspectives on primary immunodeficiency diseases. *Clin Dev Immunol.* 2006;13:223–259.

5. Yel L. Selective IgA deficiency. *J Clin Immunol.* 2010;30:10–16.

6. Borte S, Pan-Hammarström Q, Liu C, et al. Interleukin-21 restores immunoglobulin production ex vivo in patients with common variable immunodeficiency and selective IgA deficiency. *Blood.* 2009;114:4089–4098.

7. Woof JM, Kerr MA. The function of immunoglobulin A in immunity. *J Pathol.* 2006;208:270–282.

8. Hammarström L, Lönnqvist B, Ringdén O, et al. Transfer of IgA deficiency to a bone-marrow-grafted patient with aplastic anaemia. *Lancet.* 1985;1:778–781.

9. Geha RS, Hyslop N, Alami S, et al. Hyper immunoglobulin M immunodeficiency. (Dysgammaglobulinemia). Presence of immunoglobulin M-secreting plasmacytoid cells in peripheral blood and failure of immunoglobulin M-immunoglobulin G switch in B-cell differentiation. *J. Clin Invest.* 1979;64:385–391.

10. Pascual-Salcedo D, de la Concha EG, Garcia-Rodriguez MC, et al. Cellular basis of hyper IgM immunodeficiency. *J Clin Lab Immunol.* 1983;10:29–34.

11. Lougaris V, Badolato R, Ferrari S, et al. Hyper immunoglobulin M syndrome due to CD40 deficiency: Clinical, molecular, and immunological features. *Immunol. Rev.* 2005;203:48–66.

12. Deane S, Selmi C, Naguwa SM, et al. Common variable immunodeficiency: Etiological and treatment issues. *Int Arch Allergy Immunol.* 2009;150:311–324.

13. Salzer U, Neumann C, Thiel J, et al. Screening of functional and positional candidate genes in families with common variable immunodeficiency. *BMC Immunol.* 2008;9:3.

14. Tonelli AR, Kosuri K, Wei S, et al. Seizures as the first manifestation of chromosome 22q11.2 deletion syndrome in a 40-year old man: A case report. *J Med Case Reports.* 2007;1:167.

15. Restivo, A, Sarkozy A, Digilio MC, et al. 22q11 deletion syndrome: A review of some developmental biology aspects of the cardiovascular system. *Journal of Cardiovascular Medicine.* 2006;7(2):77–85.

16. Debbané M, Glaser B, David MK, et al. Psychotic symptoms in children and adolescents with 22q11.2 deletion syndrome: Neuropsychological and behavioral implications. *Schizophr. Res.* 2006;84:187–193.

17. Sasaki Y, Iseki M, Yamaguchi S, et al. Direct evidence of autosomal recessive inheritance of Arg24 to termination codon in purine nucleoside phosphorylase gene in a family with a severe combined immunodeficiency patient. *Human genetics.* 1998;103:81–85.

18. Hirschhorn R, Vawter GF, Kirkpatrick JA Jr., et al. Adenosine deaminase deficiency: Frequency and comparative pathology in autosomally recessive severe combined immunodeficiency. Clinical immunology and immunopathology. 1979;14:107–120.

19. Wang X, Rickert M, Garcia KC. Structure of the quaternary complex of interleukin-2 with its alpha, beta, and gamma receptors. *Science.* 2005;310:1159–1163.

20. Russell SM, Keegan AD, Harada N, et al. Interleukin-2 receptor gamma chain: A functional component of the interleukin-4 receptor. *Science.* 1993;262:1880–1883.

21. Noguchi M, Nakamura Y, Russell SM, et al. Interleukin-2 receptor gamma chain: A functional component of the interleukin-7 receptor. *Science.* 1994;262:1877–1880.

22. Giri JG, Kumaki S, Ahdieh M, et al. Identification and cloning of a novel IL-15 binding protein that is structurally related to the alpha chain of the IL-2 receptor. *EMBO J.* 1995;14:3654–3663.

23. Chaganti RK, Schwartz A. Complement deficiencies. E-Medicine, 2009. http://emedicine.medscape.com/article/135478-overview. Accessed March 23, 2012

25. Frank MM. Complement disorders and hereditary angioedema. *J Allergy Clin Immunol.* 2010;125:S262–S2671.

26. Heyworth P, Cross A, Curnutte J. Chronic granulomatous disease. *Curr Opin Immunol.* 2003;15:578–584.

PART 4
SEROLOGY OF INFECTIOUS CLINICAL DISORDERS

16

Acquired Immunodeficiency

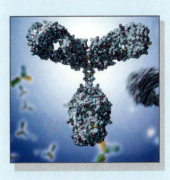

■ OBJECTIVES—LEVEL I

After this chapter, the student should be able to:

1. Describe the different forms of acquired immunodeficiency.
2. Describe the different methods of transmission of HIV.
3. Describe the different functional components of HIV and the role of each in infection and viral replication.
4. Describe the immune response of the host to HIV.
5. Describe the effect of HIV infection on the immune system and the development of AIDS.
6. Describe the different CDC and WHO classifications of AIDS.
7. Give examples of opportunistic infections commonly found in AIDS patients.
8. Describe current treatments for HIV and AIDS.
9. Describe the different diagnostic tests currently used to diagnose HIV infection and AIDS.

■ OBJECTIVES—LEVEL II

After this chapter, the student should be able to:

1. Give examples of the molecular mechanism of acquired immunodeficiencies other than HIV.
2. Describe how the immune response may both decelerate and accelerate HIV infection.

KEY TERMS

acute HIV syndrome
chemokine
clinical latency
eclipse phase
false negative
false positive
highly active antiretroviral therapy (HAART)
integrase
neutralizing antibodies
protease
provirus
reverse transcriptase
sensitivity
seroconversion
seronegative
seropositive
specificity
viremia
window period

▶ INTRODUCTION

Acquired immunodeficiencies, as the name implies, are aberrations in immune function caused by external factors. These "external" factors may include truly exogenous factors such as malnutrition, infections, certain drugs, and even trauma or environmental conditions. In addition, the external factor may be altered biological mechanisms; for example, some metabolic disorders, although not directly part of the immune system, affect its function. The interdependence of many complex cellular and molecular mechanisms in the human body is responsible for the latter situation. And although the term *acquired immunodeficiency* for the past 20 to 30 years has been associated with HIV infection and AIDS, other factors can affect immune function (1). Acquired immunodeficiencies are more common than primary immunodeficiencies; the latter are usually caused by genetic aberrations in one or more components of the immune system; the bulk of this chapter discusses HIV infection and AIDS; however, it also touches on some other causes of acquired immunodeficiencies.

▶ MALNUTRITION

Napoleon was quoted as saying, "An army marches on its stomach." Napoleon was right. No matter what the advancement and sophistication of an army's weapons and defense systems may be, its soldiers need food and energy. As banal and simplistic as it may appear, this is also true of the immune army: its soldiers (cells) need proper nutrition and efficiently functioning metabolic pathways to provide both energy for function and components of the weapon systems themselves. The cells require fuel, power, and the basic building blocks of many of their effector mechanisms. In fact, malnutrition associated with low caloric intake or protein deficiency is one of the most common causes of immunodeficiency throughout the world, particularly in areas where, for whatever reason, food is scarce. Certain chronic diseases that result in malnutrition can also be associated with immunodeficiency. Although numerous and complex molecular mechanisms tie malnutrition and immunodeficiency, it is not in the scope of this chapter to cover them all; however, the following are some examples.

Protein deficiency or protein energy malnutrition (PEM) can impact the function of cell-mediated immunity, phagocytosis, and the actions of the complement system. It can also lower the concentration of IgG, IgM, and IgA and affects cytokine function. Deficiency in vitamin C or zinc can affect mucosal barriers, thus weakening this aspect of immunity, while deficiency in vitamin D can have an effect on the ability of certain phagocytes to kill intracellular organisms. The reestablishment of proper nutrition usually reverses these effects (1, 2).

▶ METABOLIC DEFECTS, GENETIC IMPLICATIONS, AND DRUGS

Cells depend on a properly functioning metabolism, and immune cells are no different, so it is not surprising that certain aberrations of metabolic functions can affect the function of immune cells (1). An example of this is diabetes mellitus (DM); patients with DM often exhibit dysfunctions in cellular chemotaxis and phagocytosis as well as decreased T-cell proliferation and function. These effects are usually associated with the defective metabolism of glucose. Neutrophil function is often affected in patients with DM because the neutrophil depends heavily on sugar metabolism for some of its antimicrobial functions; in fact, decreased neutrophil function is directly related to the level of hyperglycemia. In addition, animal studies have shown that diabetic mice are more susceptible to staphylococcal infection than their nondiabetic littermates and that persistent hyperglycemia affects innate immunity in the diabetic animals (1, 3, 4).

In Chapter 15, we discussed several genetic defects that can directly be associated with a deficiency in one or more immune mechanism; however, this can also occur indirectly that is, a genetic aberration can affect a biological system that, although not part of the immune system, by biological connection can affect its function. A classical example of this is a chromosome abnormality called *trisomy 21*, also known as *Down syndrome,* a condition characterized by, as the name implies, the presence of an extra chromosome 21. Patients with Down syndrome are often more susceptible to various infections than healthy individuals. Although usually not life-threatening, these infections can affect the skin, the respiratory system, and the oral cavity. Phagocyte function is usually affected with decreased chemotaxis and phagocytosis (1, 5). Genetic defects in the physical barrier of innate immunity can also result in impaired immune protection. For example, patients with cystic fibrosis, which results in increased thickness of mucous secretion, are more susceptible to certain respiratory pathogens because they cannot clear them as efficiently as healthy individuals can (1).

The use of anti-inflammatory and immunosuppressive drugs such as corticosteroids, cytotoxic agents, monoclonal antibodies to TNFα, and calcineurin inhibitors can, of course, have profound effects on the immune system. The mechanism of action of these drugs is discussed in Chapter 14. Finally, although not discussed in this chapter, other factors and environmental conditions have been suggested to affect the function of the immune system, and they are actively investigated for various different purposes. These include extremes of age, ionizing radiation, high altitude, ultraviolet light, chronic hypoxia, and the effect of lack of gravity in space flights (1).

Checkpoint! 16.1

Some reports have suggested that the increased incidence of bacterial infections in patients with diabetes mellitus may be in part the result of a decreased function of neutrophils, including decreased chemotaxis and phagocytosis. What do you think would be the connection between this metabolic disease and neutrophil function?

▶ HIV INFECTION AND AIDS

Few, if any, human diseases with perhaps the exception of the medieval plague (the Black Death) have received more attention, coverage, and interest than the acquired immunodeficiency syndrome (AIDS) caused by human immunodeficiency virus (HIV) infection. AIDS has affected millions of people, and has spanned across countries throughout the world, causing enormous human suffering as well as financial burden. It has changed many social attitudes, which, in turn, have, in one way or another, affected the everyday life of many people around the globe. The Centers for Disease Control and Prevention (CDC) has estimated that in the United States, more than 1 million people may be living with HIV and that approximately 20% of them are not aware that they are infected. Although the number of new U.S. HIV infections has stayed stable annually, more than 56 000 people in the United States become infected with HIV every year and more than 18 000 individuals with AIDS die here annually (6). Some statistics on global HIV and AIDS at the end of 2008 from the Joint United Nations Program on HIV/AIDS (UNAIDS) and World Health Organization (WHO) statistics for 2010 are presented in Table 16.1 ✪ (7). The majority (more than 60%) of these individuals live in the sub-Saharan region of Africa, and approximately half of them are women and children. More than 25 million people have died of AIDS since 1981.

✪ TABLE 16.1

Global Statistics on HIV and AIDS at the End of 2010

Groups (2008 data)	Estimated Numbers
People living with HIV/AIDS	33.4 million
Adults living with HIV/AIDS	31.3 million
Women living with HIV/AIDS	15.7 million
Children living with HIV/AIDS	2.1 million
People newly infected with HIV	2.7 million
Children newly infected with HIV	430,000
AIDS deaths	2 million

Source: Data from UNAIDS, WHO, and UNICEF, published in 2010.

In the United States, men who have sex with men (MSM) is the groups most affected by HIV, accounting for more than 50% of all infections in this country each year. MSM also accounts for almost half of people living with HIV. Individuals infected by heterosexual contact comprise roughly 30% of annual HIV infections, and injection drug users account for 12%. The most common form of HIV infection/transmission is through sexual contact and exposure either through the genital track or via the rectal mucosa. The mechanism by which HIV crosses mucosal barriers is unclear, although intraepithelial dendritic cells have been implicated. In most cases, however, infection and transmission occur as repeated sexual exposure causes trauma and tissue breakdown, resulting in the breach of barriers and contact with blood. Although HIV is primarily transmitted sexually, it can also be transmitted by blood transfusions or contact with body fluids and from mothers to their infants. Contrary to some urban myths still existing today, HIV is *not* transmitted by coughing, sneezing, sharing eating or drinking utensils with an HIV infected individual, casual contact (eg, shaking hands) or by simply being around an HIV-infected individual. Nor is it transmitted through the air, water, food, or a mosquito vector. HIV is a rather fragile virus and does not survive well outside of fresh blood and other internal body fluids.

VIROLOGY

HIV is a lentivirus; it contains 2 copies of single-stranded RNA that can infect various CD4+ human cells such as T cells, monocytes, macrophages, dendritic cells, and microglial brain cells (1). Two types of HIV have been described: HIV-1 and HIV-2, both of which can result in AIDS. The HIV genome comprises 3 structural genes (gag, pol, and env) and 6 regulatory genes (tat, rev, nef, vif, vpr, and vpu). The gag gene encodes for a gag protein that is cleaved into different products: capsid (p24), matrix, nucleocapsid, p6, and p2. These products are part of the viral particle and stabilize the viral genome. The pol gene encodes for a protein that, when cleaved into different products, results in the enzymes **integrase, reverse transcriptase,** and the **protease** that cleaves the viral proteins. As with other retroviruses, the reverse transcriptase converts the viral ribonucleic acid (RNA) into DNA, and the integrase mediates the incorporation of the viral DNA into the genome of the infected cell. The infected cell's replication system is then used to generate more virions. The env gene encodes for an env protein, which, when cleaved, results in the generation of 2 viral envelope components: gp120 and gp41 (1, 8). gp120 and gp41 are the proteins that bind to cellular receptors on the cells to be infected. The role of the regulatory genes varies; the protein encoded by the tat gene upregulates the transcription of the HIV genes, and the rev protein is involved in the regulation of messenger RNA splicing. Interestingly, the product of

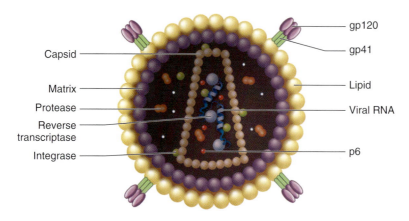

■ **FIGURE 16.1**   Basic structures of HIV.

the nef gene is a protein that inhibits the expression of MHC class I components on the surface of the infected cell, a virulence factor that allows HIV to bypass the mechanism of immune regulation of virus-infected cells described in Chapters 3 and 4 (9). Refer to Figure 16.1 ■ for some basic structures of the human immunodeficiency virus.

 Checkpoint! 16.2

Because HIV is transmitted by blood and blood products, should we worry about AIDS being acquired via the bite of a mosquito that has bitten an HIV-infected individual?

VIRAL INFECTION AND REPLICATION

In the 1980s, CD4 was shown to be a receptor for gp120; any human cell that expresses CD4 could be infected. However, the expression of CD4 alone was not sufficient for infection; cells from other species could not be infected even if they were manipulated to express human CD4. It was thus hypothesized that another "coreceptor" must be involved in the infection process. In 1995, it was shown that treating cells with certain **chemokines** (MIP-1a, RANTES) could reduce infection in culture; additionally, it was noticed that certain groups of people, while having high-risk exposure to HIV, remained **seronegative.** Seronegative refers to a negative result when a serological test is performed and **seropositive** indicates that the serological test has been performed and is positive. It was determined that these individuals were homozygous for a 32-base pair deletion in the gene for the chemokine receptor CCR5, resulting in a truncated protein. These observations led to the conclusion that 2 chemokine receptors, specifically CXCR4 and CCR5, served as coreceptors for HIV.

Infection of host cells by the virus starts with the specific binding of the virus to the host cell. This is mediated by the interaction of the gp120 viral protein with the CD4 and either the CXCR4 or the CCR5 receptors on the host cell.

These chemokine co-receptors are also involved in the fusion of the viral envelope with the cell's plasma membrane. More specifically, the interaction of the gp120 with CD4 causes a structural change in the viral envelope; this, in turn, exposes domains of the gp120 that bind to the chemokine receptor molecules. Several cell types can be infected; helper T cells, having a large number of CD4 molecules on their surface are the more commonly infected cells, but others, such as macrophages, dendritic cells, monocytes, and microglial brain cells, can also be infected.

Once the virus is attached to the cell, the gp41 protein on the virus penetrates the host cell membrane; gp41 then forms a "looplike" structure bringing the viral envelope and cell membrane together and allowing their fusion. This fusion results in the creation of a "hole" in the membrane, which allows the virus to enter the cell and release its RNA and enzymes. This process is shown in Figure 16.2 ■. The reverse transcriptase then converts this RNA into viral DNA, which is transported into the nucleus and integrates into the host cell DNA by the action of the viral integrase.

The integrated viral DNA, termed a **provirus,** can remain undisturbed in the host genome for long periods of time. Importantly, the transcription mechanisms of the reverse transcriptase are susceptible to numerous transcription errors, causing the generation of different products as a result of these "errors." These errors are believed to contribute, at least in part, to the genetic variability of HIV, which, in turn, can create viral mutations that can exhibit drug resistance and/or immune evasion. The process of reactivation and its timing is still under investigation; cellular transcription factors, however, have been implicated, the most common one being NF kappa B, a transcription factor common to various molecular pathways and heavily involved in the activation of immune cells by antigens. Upon reactivation, which can occur during antigen activation of an infected helper T cell, the viral DNA is expressed and transcribed into mRNA; translation of the mRNA results in the production of viral proteins such as tat and rev. tat encourages new virus production whereas rev stimulates the translation of the other viral proteins, gag and env. These

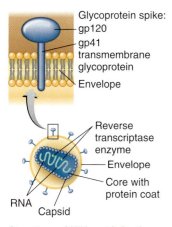

Glycoprotein spike:
gp120
gp41
transmembrane
glycoprotein
Envelope

Reverse
transcriptase
enzyme
Envelope
Core with
protein coat
RNA
Capsid

Structure of HIV and infection of a CD4⁺ T cell. The gp120 glyco-protein spike on the membrane attaches to a receptor on the CD4⁺ cell. The gp41 transmembrane glycoprotein probably facilitates fusion by attaching to a proposed fusion receptor on the CD4⁺ cell.

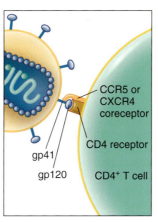

CCR5 or
CXCR4
coreceptor

CD4 receptor

gp41
gp120

CD4⁺ T cell

1 Attachment. The gp120 spike attaches to a receptor and to a CCR5 or CXCR4 coreceptor on the cell.

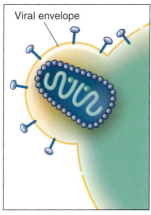

Viral envelope

2 Fusion. The gp41 participates in fusion of the HIV with the cell.

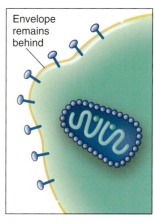

Envelope
remains
behind

3 Entry. Following fusion with the cell, an entry pore is created. After entry, the viral envelope remains behind and the HIV uncoats, releasing the RNA core for directing synthesis of the new viruses.

■ **FIGURE 16.2** Attachment and cell entry by HIV. *Source:* TORTORA, GERARD J.; FUNKE, BERDELL R.; CASE, CHRISTINE L., MICROBIOLOGY: AN INTRODUCTION, 10th, ©2010. Printed and Electronically reproduced by permission of Pearson Education, Inc., Upper Saddle River, New Jersey.

proteins promote the release of the viral RNA genome, which is packaged into new viral particles by interacting with gag.

The new virions bud out of the cell in a process somewhat reversed from the one for viral entry; the env protein is transported via the endoplasmic reticulum to the Golgi, where it is cleaved, generating new gp120 and gp41 proteins; the gp41 protein attaches the gp120 protein to the infected cell membrane, and the virion buds out of the cell; in the meantime, maturation of the new virion occurs, and the new viruses can then infect other cells repeating the process (1, 10) (Figure 16.3 ■). A scanning electron micrograph of HIV-1 budding is shown in Figure 16.4 ■.

 Checkpoint! 16.3

A salesperson from a chemical company comes to your clinic selling a new disinfectant spray, claiming that it kills 100% of HIV from environmental surfaces such as examining tables, exam room floors, and other similar surfaces. However, you show little interest in the product. Why?

HIV AND IMMUNE RESPONSES

Ironically, for a virus that can shut down the immune system, initial infection with HIV does trigger an immune response to it, and this response can be both humoral and cell mediated (1, 11). This early response is important and can delay onset of symptoms in an untreated patient group. However even more ironically, as we will see, the immune response to

HIV can also contribute to the infection and play a role in the establishment of viral reservoirs.

The immune response to HIV is the same as any immune response to a viral infection. Cytotoxic T lymphocytes are generated to kill virus-infected cells via the MHC class I, endogenous antigen epitope, CD8, and T-cell receptor mechanisms described in Chapters 3 and 4. The specificity of cytotoxic T cells is usually directed to both the envelope and internal viral proteins such as p17, p24, and p15; they can also be reactive against regulatory proteins such as nef and vif. In addition, studies have shown that virus-specific helper T cells can also be generated during an immune response against HIV and play a role in the continuous maintenance of the cytotoxic T cells against the virus.

Humoral response to HIV results in the generation of antibodies against different viral components; these antibodies are actually used for diagnosis. Some of the antibodies are directed against nonfunctional components of the virus, such as viral debris, targeting linear epitopes without much effect on viral function. Others, called **neutralizing antibodies,** target functional components such as envelope proteins involved in viral entry or that bind to the host cell's CD4 (for example, the V3 loop and the extracellular domain of gp41), and some attack conformational epitopes of different viral components that are necessary for the 3-dimensional conformation of the viral envelope.

Antibodies to HIV can be usually detected in the blood stream, mucosal surfaces, and other body fluids within 1 to 3 months after HIV infection. Depending on the isotype, these antibodies play a role in antibody-dependent cellular cytotoxicity, complement activation, and direct neutralizing or

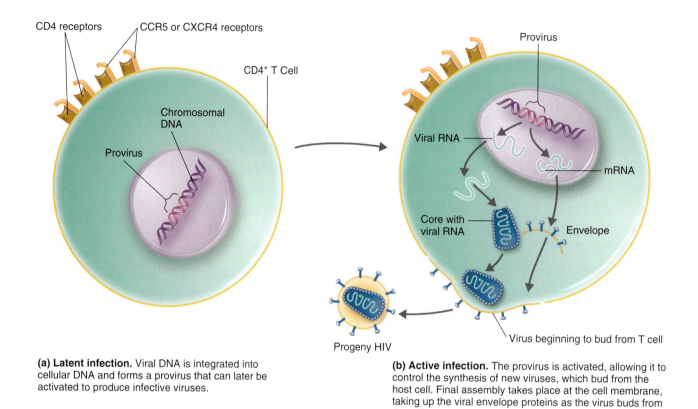

(a) Latent infection. Viral DNA is integrated into cellular DNA and forms a provirus that can later be activated to produce infective viruses.

(b) Active infection. The provirus is activated, allowing it to control the synthesis of new viruses, which bud from the host cell. Final assembly takes place at the cell membrane, taking up the viral envelope proteins as the virus buds from the cell.

■ **FIGURE 16.3**   HIV cycle in an infected cell: (a) latent infection; (b) active infection. *Source:* TORTORA, GERARD J.; FUNKE, BERDELL R.; CASE, CHRISTINE L., MICROBIOLOGY: AN INTRODUCTION, 10th, ©2010. Printed and Electronically reproduced by permission of Pearson Education, Inc., Upper Saddle River, New Jersey.

blocking responses. Early antibody responses tend to target gag proteins (eg, p24); later, antibodies to the viral envelope and some regulatory proteins become involved. These antibodies can limit viral replication by keeping the virus in check

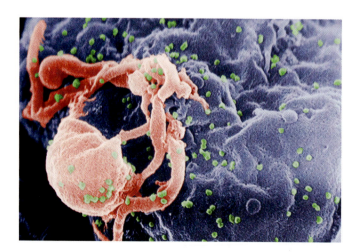

■ **FIGURE 16.4**   Scanning electron micrograph of HIV-1 budding (in green) from cultured lymphocyte. This image has been colored to highlight important features. Multiple round bumps on cell surface represent sites of assembly and budding of virions. *Source:* ©CDC/C. Goldsmith, P. Feorino, E. L. Palmer, W. R. McManus.

during the early asymptomatic stage (1). Unfortunately, the titers of these neutralizing antibodies tend to be low, and their specificity is very narrow (ie, they react with only a few selected viral epitopes); this makes them inefficient because they lack a broader cross-reactivity, as the virus mutates very rapidly and thus can escape the effect of these antibodies. In other words, early antibody responses are directed against early forms of the virus (ie, from the initial infection), but they are not effective against "newer" mutants of the virus. The product of the nef gene is a protein that inhibits the expression of MHC class I components on the surface of the infected cell; because of this, it interferes with MHC class I-dependent antigen presentation, thus downregulating the host cellular response to virally infected cells (9). So, although the initial immune response to HIV can reduce viral replication, it cannot completely eliminate the virus from the host.

PATHOGENESIS

After infection, there is a period of time called the **eclipse phase** (7–10 days), during which viral components are not easily detectable. Studies have suggested that a single virus can initiate an infection and that an established infection can arise from a single focus of infected mucosal CD4+ T cells. After the eclipse phase, virally infected cells as well as free virus arrive at the lymph nodes.

In the lymph nodes, the interaction of immune cells described in Chapters 3 and 4 takes place; activated CD4+ T cells are infected by interacting with either virally infected cells or antigen-presenting cells such as dendritic cells, which have taken up and internalized the virus. B cells can also participate in these interactions. Once into the lymphoid system, the virus can rapidly spread to the entire body through the lymphoid tissues.

The level of infection of CD4+ T cells depends on the numbers of these cells within a lymphoid area: for example, in the gut-associated lymphoid tissue, which is rich in CD4+ cells, 80% of these cells can be depleted in the first 20 days of HIV infection. And although at the highest level of viremia CD4+ T cells are low in number, they later return to normal levels. Unfortunately, viral escape from the immune system creates cellular reservoirs of the virus in many different cells, including not only CD4+ T cells but also monocytes, macrophages, dendritic cells, and microglial brain cells, which are also CD4+.

As described, the virus can remain dormant in these reservoirs for long periods of time, thus escaping immune detection. This in turn generates a situation in which the virus can cause a persistent infection that can ultimately deplete the virus-infected cells. The causes of such depletion are varied; infected cells are eliminated by cytotoxic T cells that are designed to eliminate any virally infected cell. The process of viral budding can also destroy a cell, and virally induced apoptosis contributes to cell depletion, so as depletion expands, the depleted cells cannot be replaced quickly enough.

Although different CD4+ cells are affected by the infection, the cells most affected are helper T lymphocytes; the depletion of helper T cells, in turn, creates the characteristic profound immunodeficiency associated with HIV infection. As discussed in previous chapters, the role of helper T cells in an immune response, both humoral and cell mediated, is absolutely

critical, and the depletion of this cell population can affect both branches of the immune system. Antibody production to many antigens becomes affected because of lack of T-cell help in sending signals to B cells; cell-mediated immunity is also affected by the lack of helper T cells and the cytokines they secrete in directing an immune response (1, 12, 13). The depletion of helper T cells creates an immune army depleted of all commanding and experienced officers, resulting in an immune army in complete disarray. See Figure 16.5(a) ■ for the time course of HIV infection.

SYMPTOMS AND CLINICAL CHARACTERISTICS

Early symptoms of HIV infection vary from one individual to another. Some people do not develop any symptoms when they first become infected with HIV. More commonly, however, flulike symptoms including headaches, nausea, sore throat, fever, diarrhea, and enlargement of the lymph nodes appear—Figure 16.5(b). This ailment, called **acute HIV syndrome,** can be mistaken for other simple viral infections and usually lasts from 1 week to 1 month. At this stage, **viremia** is very high—see Figure 16.5(a)—as the virus spreads throughout the lymphatic system; there is also a rapid decrease in the number of CD4+ T cells.

The host's immune response to the virus drastically reduces its numbers, and the affected individual enters the **clinical latency** stage. Unfortunately, as we have described, the virus is not totally eliminated and it remains, although in lower numbers, in both plasma and lymphoid tissues. During this period, the patient can be asymptomatic, and CD4+ T cell counts return to near normal levels; however, viral transmission from person to person still occurs during

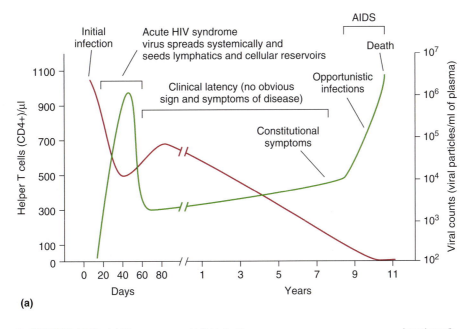

■ **FIGURE 16.5**   (a) Time course of HIV infection.   (continued)

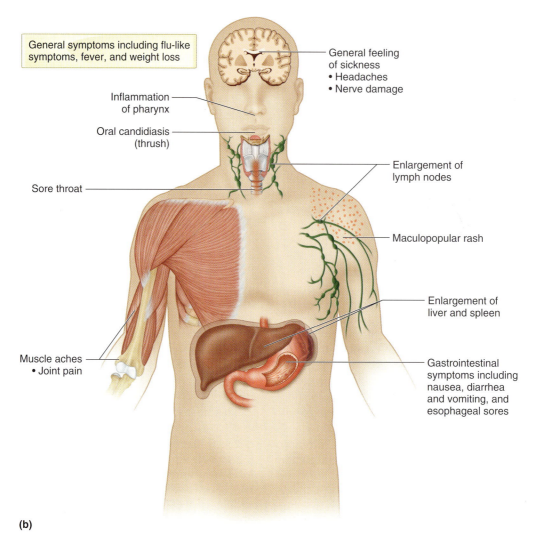

General symptoms including flu-like symptoms, fever, and weight loss

General feeling of sickness
• Headaches
• Nerve damage

Inflammation of pharynx

Oral candidiasis (thrush)

Enlargement of lymph nodes

Sore throat

Maculopopular rash

Enlargement of liver and spleen

Muscle aches
• Joint pain

Gastrointestinal symptoms including nausea, diarrhea and vomiting, and esophageal sores

(b)

■ **FIGURE 16.5**   (continued) (b) Different symptoms of acute HIV syndrome.

clinical latency, and the virus is still actively infecting host cells. Clinical latency can last for several years after initial infection; during this period, some people remain asymptomatic, while others may have mild infections or mild chronic symptoms. Eventually, as the virus continues to multiply and destroy immune cells, as in other forms of immunodeficiency, opportunistic infections occur, and the affected individual develops what has been defined as AIDS (1, 12, 13). Oral candidiasis (thrush) is a common opportunistic infection in AIDS patients (Figure 16.6 ■).

As the patient progresses from HIV infection to the clinical symptoms that define AIDS, viremia also drastically increases, as CD4+ cell counts drastically decrease; the occurrences of certain forms of cancer such as Kaposi's sarcoma (Figures 16.7 ■ and 16.8 ■) and lymphomas also increase. The immune system is not the only system affected by HIV; the virus can also infect the nervous system, particularly the brain. For example, a metabolic encephalopathy called *AIDS*

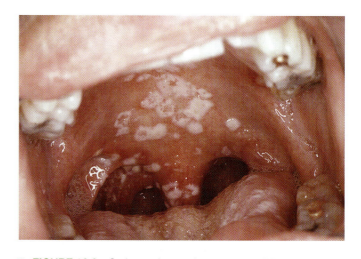

■ **FIGURE 16.6**   Oral pseudo membraneous candidiasis in a patient with AIDS. *Source:* © CDC/Sol Silverman, Jr., DDS.

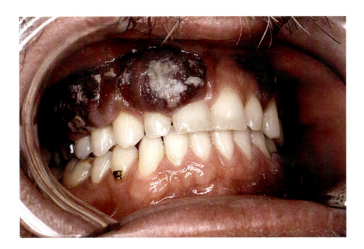

■ **FIGURE 16.7**   Intraoral Kaposi's sarcoma lesion with an overlying candidiasis infection in an HIV-positive patient. *Source:* © CDC/Sol Silverman, Jr., DDS.

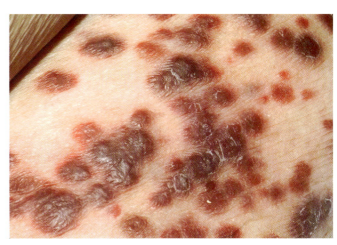

■ **FIGURE 16.8**   Kaposi's sarcoma on the skin of an AIDS patient. *Source:* © National Cancer Institute.

dementia complex can be induced by HIV infection of brain microglia and macrophages. This condition manifests itself after years of HIV infection and is characterized by various neurological disorders including impaired motor function, cognitive abnormalities, behavioral changes, forgetfulness, tiredness, confusion, disorientation, and, eventually, dementia, weakness of lower extremities, and loss of full control of body movements (1, 12, 13).

CLASSIFICATION OF AIDS

Since the discovery and early recognition of this syndrome, various attempts had been made to define the clinical and laboratory findings that can actually define the term *AIDS*. Early attempts involved the recognition of deficiencies in cell-mediated immunity with no otherwise plausible explanation. Later parameters included T cell counts and the occurrence of certain opportunistic infections. In 1993, the CDC devised guidelines for the classification of different stages of AIDS (with some guidelines on case surveillance and monitoring revised in 1999) (14, 15). The different classifications are based

on CD4 cell counts, identification of certain bacterial and fungal infections, and certain clinical conditions. Nine groups or categories (A, B, and C, and each of these divided into 3 subgroups) have been used to classify the different AIDS stages. Tables 16.2 ✪, 16.3 ✪, and 16.4 ✪ provide the details for the different classifications.

The WHO has devised 4 different levels of clinical staging for AIDS, which were revised in 2007 (16) (see Table 16.5 ✪). The advantage of this classification system is that it can be applied when resources are not available for CD4+ T cell counting or other laboratory tests. This classification is based on clinical manifestations of the disease and can be used to recognize it in a variety of different clinical settings, especially those that lack laboratory resources.

TREATMENT

As with any other immunodeficiency, one of the major components of treatment of HIV infection and AIDS is the control of ensuing opportunistic infections. Of course, antiviral treatment is also of cardinal importance. Anti-HIV therapy

✪ TABLE 16.2

CDC Classification System for HIV-Infected Adults and Adolescents

	Clinical Categories		
CD4 Cell Categories	A: Asymptomatic, Acute HIV, or PGL	B: Symptomatic Conditions, not A or C	C: AIDS-Indicator Conditions
(1) ≥ 500 cells/μL	A1	B1	C1
(2) 200–499 cells/μL	A2	B2	C2
(3) < 200 cells/μL	A3	B3	C3

Source: AIDS Education and Training Centers (AETC) National Resource Center. http://www.aidsetc.org/aidsetc?page=cm-105_disease

⊙ **TABLE 16.3**

CDC Classification System: Category B Symptomatic Conditions

Category B symptomatic conditions are defined as symptomatic conditions occurring in an HIV-infected adolescent or adult that meet at least 1 of the following criteria:

(a) They are attributed to HIV infection or indicate a defect in cell-mediated immunity.

(b) They are considered to have a clinical course or management that is complicated by HIV infection.

Examples include but are not limited to the following:

- Bacillary angiomatosis
- Oropharyngeal candidiasis (thrush)
- Vulvovaginal candidiasis, persistent or resistant
- Pelvic inflammatory disease (PID)
- Cervical dysplasia (moderate or severe)/cervical carcinoma *in situ*
- Hairy leukoplakia, oral

- Idiopathic thrombocytopenic purpura
- Constitutional symptoms, such as fever (> 38.5° C) or diarrhea lasting > 1 month
- Peripheral neuropathy
- Herpes zoster (shingles), involving ≥ 2 episodes or ≥ 1 dermatome

Source: AIDS Education and Training Centers (AETC) National Resource Center. http://www.aidsetc.org/aidsetc?page=cm-105_disease

⊙ **TABLE 16.4**

CDC Classification System: Category C AIDS-Indicator Conditions

- Bacterial pneumonia, recurrent (≥ 2 episodes in 12 months)
- Candidiasis of the bronchi, trachea, or lungs
- Candidiasis, esophageal
- Cervical carcinoma, invasive, confirmed by biopsy
- Coccidioidomycosis, disseminated or extrapulmonary
- Cryptococcosis, extrapulmonary
- Cryptosporidiosis, chronic intestinal (> 1-month duration)
- Cytomegalovirus disease (other than liver, spleen, or nodes)
- Encephalopathy, HIV-related
- Herpes simplex; chronic ulcers (> 1-month duration), or bronchitis, pneumonitis, or esophagitis
- Histoplasmosis, disseminated or extrapulmonary
- Isosporiasis, chronic intestinal (> 1-month duration)
- Kaposi sarcoma

- Lymphoma, Burkitt, immunoblastic, or primary central nervous system
- *Mycobacterium avium* complex (MAC) or *M kansasii,* disseminated or extrapulmonary
- *Mycobacterium tuberculosis,* pulmonary or extrapulmonary
- *Mycobacterium,* other species or unidentified species, disseminated or extrapulmonary
- *Pneumocystis jiroveci* (formerly *carinii*) pneumonia (PCP)
- Progressive multifocal leukoencephalopathy (PML)
- *Salmonella* septicemia, recurrent (nontyphoid)
- Toxoplasmosis of brain
- Wasting syndrome due to HIV (involuntary weight loss > 10% of baseline body weight) associated with either chronic diarrhea (≥ 2 loose stools per day ≥ 1 month) or chronic weakness and documented fever ≥ 1 month

Source: Reprinted from AIDS Education and Training Centers (AETC) National Resource Center. http://www.aidsetc.org/aidsetc?page=cm-105_disease

⊙ **TABLE 16.5**

WHO Clinical Staging of HIV/AIDS for Adults and Adolescents, Stages 1–4

Primary HIV Infection

- Asymptomatic
- Acute retroviral syndrome

Clinical Stage 1

- Asymptomatic
- Persistent generalized lymphadenopathy

⭐ **TABLE 16.5**

WHO Clinical Staging of HIV/AIDS for Adults and Adolescents, Stages 1–4 (continued)

Clinical Stage 2

- Moderate unexplained weight loss (< 10% of presumed or measured body weight)
- Recurrent respiratory infections (sinusitis, tonsillitis, otitis media, and pharyngitis)
- Herpes zoster
- Angular cheilitis

- Recurrent oral ulceration
- Papular pruritic eruptions
- Seborrheic dermatitis
- Fungal nail infections

Clinical Stage 3

- Unexplained severe weight loss (> 10% of presumed or measured body weight)
- Unexplained chronic diarrhea for > 1 month
- Unexplained persistent fever for > 1 month (> 37.6° C, intermittent or constant)
- Persistent oral candidiasis (thrush)
- Oral hairy leukoplakia

- Pulmonary tuberculosis (current)
- Severe presumed bacterial infections (eg, pneumonia, empyema, pyomyositis, bone or joint infection, meningitis, bacteremia)
- Acute necrotizing ulcerative stomatitis, gingivitis, or periodontitis
- Unexplained anemia (hemoglobin < 8 g/dL)
- Neutropenia (neutrophils < 500 cells/μL)
- Chronic thrombocytopenia (platelets < 50,000 cells/μL)

Clinical Stage 4

- HIV wasting syndrome, as defined by the CDC (see Clinical Stage 3 above)
- *Pneumocystis* pneumonia
- Recurrent severe bacterial pneumonia
- Chronic herpes simplex infection (orolabial, genital, or anorectal site for > 1 month or visceral herpes at any site)
- Esophageal candidiasis (or candidiasis of trachea, bronchionchi, or lungs)
- Extrapulmonary tuberculosis
- Kaposi sarcoma
- Cytomegalovirus infection (retinitis or infection of other organs)
- Central nervous system toxoplasmosis
- HIV encephalopathy
- Cryptococcosis, extrapulmonary (including meningitis)
- Disseminated nontuberculosis *Mycobacteria* infection

- Progressive multifocal leukoencephalopathy
- Candida of the trachea, bronchi, or lungs
- Chronic cryptosporidiosis (with diarrhea)
- Chronic isosporiasis
- Disseminated mycosis (eg, histoplasmosis, coccidioidomycosis, penicilliosis)
- Recurrent nontyphoidal *Salmoneila* bacteremia
- Lymphoma (cerebral or B-cell non-Hodgkin)
- Invasive cervical carcinoma
- Atypical disseminated leishmaniasis
- Symptomatic HIV-associated nephropathy
- Symptomatic HIV-associated cardiomyopathy
- Reactivation of American trypanosomiasis (meningoencephalitis or myocarditis)

Source: Data from the World Health Organization as cited in AIDS Education and Training Centers (AETC) National Resource Center. http://www.aidsetc.org/aidsetc?page=cm-105_disease

is usually recommended when an infected individual has a CD4+ T cell count less than 350/μl and/or the viral load is more than 100 000 copies/ml. Various anti-viral drugs are available for therapy; they are usually divided on the basis of their functional mechanisms (ie, how their actions inhibit the virus). Some are inhibitors of reverse transcriptase and are divided into nucleoside and non-nucleoside inhibitors. Others inhibit protease activity, while others interfere with cell fusion. Additional drugs inhibit the action of the viral integrase, and others inhibit the binding of the virus to CCR5, thus interfering with the mechanism of viral attachment and entry described previously. See Table 16.6 ⭐ for different examples of anti-viral drugs and their actions.

Although each of the drug categories has its own antiviral mechanism, current therapy is based on the combined use of some of these drugs. This approach, known as **highly active antiretroviral therapy (HAART)** (13, 17), involves the combination of 3 synergistic anti-HIV drugs from at least 2 of the drug categories described in Table 16.6. Recent examples of HAART include 2 nucleoside reverse transcriptase inhibitors and a protease inhibitor or 2 nucleoside reverse transcriptase inhibitors and a non-nucleoside reverse transcriptase inhibitor. The HAART approach has been quite successful in reducing viremia and restoring T cell counts; it has also drastically reduced the number of other infections and overall mortality. However, HAART has never been considered a "cure" for

⚙ **TABLE 16.6**

Examples of Antiviral Drugs and Their Actions

Drug Category	Mechanism of Action	Examples
Nucleoside reverse transcriptase inhibitors	Mimics nucleosides, incorporates into viral DNA and inhibits reverse transcriptase	azitothymidine, abacavir, lamivudine
Non-nucleoside reverse transcriptase inhibitors	Binds and deactivates reverse transcriptase directly	etravirine, efavirenz, nevirapine, delavirdine
Protease inhibitors	Prevents viral protease function resulting in failed production of cleaved products necessary for viral replication and release	nelfinavir, lopinavir, saquinavir
Inhibitors of cell fusion	Inhibits viral membrane-cell fusion, thus interfering with viral entry	enfuvirtide (Fuzeon)
Integrase inhibitors	Interferes with viral DNA integration into the host cell genome	raltegravir (Isentress), elvitegravir (under clinical trials), MK-2048 (under development)
CCR5 inhibitors	Binds to CCR5, blocking it, and thus preventing viral binding and subsequent viral entry	maraviroc (UK-427857)

HIV infections for various reasons. First, as we explained, HIV can "hide" from both the immune system and pharmacological approaches by integrating into various cellular reservoirs; second, HAART drugs never fully eradicate the virus; thus, they must be administered throughout an individual's lifetime. Third, the virus can develop resistance to the drugs, thus rendering them ineffective. In addition to antiviral therapies, recent studies have explored the administration of IL-2 and IL-7 to increase helper T cell counts, and so far, the results have been encouraging. However, HAART is still at the center of current HIV treatment modalities. Antiviral therapy has also been used as a post-exposure prophylaxis for health care workers who experience certain kinds of occupational exposures to HIV (eg, a needlestick).

As the old saying goes, every rose has its thorns, and anti-viral treatment does not come without complications. About 20% of subjects with AIDS undergoing HAART can develop what is called *immune reconstitution inflammatory syndrome* several weeks after the start of the treatment (18, 19). This syndrome is characterized by a very severe inflammatory response to various opportunistic infections. HAART has also been shown to increase the incidence of asthma 3-fold in treated HIV patients when compared to healthy controls. Drug allergies are also more prevalent in patients receiving HAART; these allergies can include severe rashes: almost 20% of patients receiving the anti-viral drug nevirapine develop some form of urticaria (rash); the use of abacavir can result in a hypersensitivity syndrome affecting many organs and resulting in fever, rash, diarrhea, myalgia (muscle aches), and arthralgia (joint aches) in almost 15% of patient treated, and, in some cases, can be fatal. In addition, antibiotics given to control infections can create problems; for example, about two-thirds of HIV-infected individuals given

trimethoprim sulfamethoxazole develop urticarial or maculopapular rashes.

To date, the best treatment for HIV infection and AIDS has been prevention. This, in turn, has been based on social and educational approaches often directed to high-risk groups such as intravenous drug users and homosexual males, although heterosexual education and the improvement of many different procedures in health care such as additional safety procedures, blood donor screening, and the prophylactic use of antiviral drugs for workers who may have been accidentally exposed to HIV have also contributed to prevention. Active programs have heavily promoted the use of condoms for sexual practices and some programs have provided free needles and syringes to intravenous drug users; the administration of antiretroviral agents to HIV-infected pregnant women and their infants has also been an approach to prevent the spread of HIV infection. However, the number of new HIV cases in the United States has not decreased since the early 1990s. Of new U.S. HIV cases, 54% are acquired from an individual who did not know that he or she was infected. The CDC has suggested a new opt-out policy for HIV screening to prevent such spread. In this policy, everyone seen at a hospital or at a physician's office would be screened regardless of the presence or absence of risk factors. This screening would be done unless the patient opted out of the test (ie, it would be done unless the patient specifically requested that it not be done).

THE HOPE FOR AN AIDS VACCINE

The ultimate battle against HIV and AIDS will be a combination of prevention, therapy, and the development of an HIV vaccine. Unfortunately, several impediments have prevented vaccine development. A vaccine usually stimulates an immune response to a pathogen and the response then eliminates it. However, as we have discussed, HIV infection does elicit an immune response, but this response is ineffective in the long run. Early trials with inactivated HIV yielded weak neutralizing antibodies that were not effective in clinical trials. Even in the presence of circulating antibodies, HIV infection can continue and develop into AIDS. The immune response to HIV may hold the virus in check initially but not permanently. Many vaccines can prevent disease but not necessarily initial infection. For example, the vaccines against influenza and poliomyelitis control the virus produced by infected cells so that it can be cleared and does not infect other cells. This approach may not be totally effective for HIV because the virus integrates into the host genome and remains latent for very long periods. Rapid mutation and variation of the HIV virus also make the development of a vaccine against a constant viral antigen difficult. This problem is not unique to HIV; for example, rhinoviruses, which cause the common cold, have this characteristic, which is why we do not have a vaccine against the common cold. The lack of an optimal animal model for HIV/AIDS has also hindered the development of a vaccine. However, higher antibody titers in the acute infection stage are related to longer lag periods before disease progression. In addition, HIV in infants who have an immature immune response progresses more rapidly. These 2 factors lead us to believe that immunity to HIV also plays a positive role, which may be increased by research efforts for a vaccine.

✓ Checkpoint! 16.4

A researcher who has developed an HIV preparation isolated off a viral strain claims that it can be used as a vaccine for AIDS because this preparation can generate a good antibody response in a laboratory animal. However, other researchers are skeptical. Why?

▶ LABORATORY TESTS FOR HIV

The tests used to identify a potential HIV infection are based on 3 different aspects of the infectious process (Table 16.7 ✪). Testing includes measuring host antibody levels against the virus, enumerating the host's CD4+ T cells, and detecting the

presence of the virus. Testing for HIV and AIDS shares a common feature with many diagnostic tests: a **window period,** which is the time between infection and the test detection of some changes that are associated with the infection. This window period varies from test to test. For example, the window period for antibody testing for HIV is about 30 days, while antigen testing has a shorter window period of approximately 15 days. Nucleic acid testing cuts it down to about 12 days. Testing is also evaluated on its sensitivity and specificity. **Sensitivity** measures the percentage of real positives that are identified as positives, that is, the proportion of positive results when HIV is present. The higher the percentage is, the more sensitive the test is. **Specificity,** on the other hand, refers to the percentage of negatives that are correctly identified as such; in other words, it is the percentage of the results that will be negative when HIV is not present.

Sensitivity and specificity affect each other; for example, an emergency Coast Guard station operating a radio signal receiver may set it to receive a wide variety of signals (low specificity) to avoid missing weak signals that may come from a true emergency call (high sensitivity). On the other hand, an amateur radio operator may set such settings on a specific strong frequency (high specificity) to talk to a fellow operator without being disturbed by other weaker signals (low sensitivity). In addition, tests can give false positives and false negatives. A **false positive** result indicates that HIV may be present in a person who is actually not infected. An example of this is the cross-reactive antibodies to antigens that may be present on another infectious organism antigenically similar to HIV. A **false negative** result, as the name implies, would miss detecting HIV (ie, the test suggests the absence of HIV in an infected person). The most common cause of false negatives is the timing of the test within the window period.

CD4+ COUNTS

Technically speaking, CD4+ T cell counting is not really a test for HIV in the true sense of the word. It is a test that measures the cells that are most affected by HIV infection, the CD4+ T cells. Their number can decrease drastically during acute HIV syndrome, recover somewhat after viremia decreases, but decline throughout the years during clinical latency and eventually drop to irrecoverable levels (1, 13)

✪ TABLE 16.7

Approaches in Testing for HIV Infection

Looking for	Test for	Techniques
Actual presence of virus	p24 (low sensitivity, no longer commonly used), viral nucleic acids	ELISA, PCR
Host antibody response to virus	IgG and IgM antibodies to viral components	ELISA, Western blot
Effect of virus on host cells	CD4+ T cell counts, either absolute or percentage	Flow cytometry

(Figure 16.5). Monitoring their count is therefore essential in monitoring both the level and course of HIV infection as well as the development of AIDS. In fact, the CDC uses CD4+ T cell counts as one of the major parameters in its classification system for HIV-infected individuals (Table 16.2). A count of less than 200 CD4+ T cells/μl defines AIDS according to the CDC (14, 15) (normal CD4+ T cell counts range between 500 and 1500 cells/μl) (13). Monitoring CD4+ counts can also be useful in checking anti-viral therapy and its efficacy and in anticipating potential opportunistic infections and designing proper antibiotic approaches. CD4+ T cell counting is classically performed by flow cytometry (see Figure 16.9 ■); the principle and procedures of flow cytometry are described in detail in Chapter 7. CD4+ T cell counts can be evaluated either as absolute counts or as a percentage of total lymphocytes. The ratio of CD4+ T cell and CD8+ T cell can also be determined. The percentage of CD4+ T cell counts is determined by dividing the number of CD4+ T cells by the total lymphocyte count (also determined by flow cytometry) and then multiplying by 100. From this, absolute counts of CD4+ T cells can be obtained by multiplying the total white blood cell counts by the percentage of lymphocytes and then by the percentage of CD4+ T cells. CD4+ T cell/CD8+ T cell ratios are also important; in AIDS patients, the number of CD4+ T cells is drastically decreased, but the number of CD8+ T cells

may increase. Care must be taken in interpreting a decrease in CD4+ T cell counts because other conditions may also lower them. These can include various different bacterial, viral, and parasitic infections, tuberculosis, sepsis, trauma, malnutrition, and stress. CD4+ T cell counts, therefore, are only a part of a comprehensive set of tests for HIV infection and AIDS.

TESTING FOR ANTIBODIES

The presence of antibodies against HIV components in a person's blood has been routinely used as a diagnostic tool for many years. For antibody testing, the window period described earlier is critical because false negatives can result from this testing if it is done too early and the patient is within such period. False negatives can also result from some immunodeficiency conditions such as hypogammaglobulinemia, and, of course, from improper collection or faulty laboratory techniques. The window period is also critical because during this period a person can transmit the virus to another individual even though no antibodies to the virus are detected. Antibody testing is fairly straightforward, relatively inexpensive, and, more importantly, very accurate. HIV-infected individuals develop anti-HIV antibodies within 30 to 60 days after exposure, and almost 100% of infected individuals show antibodies to HIV 3 months after infection. The detectable production of antibodies to HIV

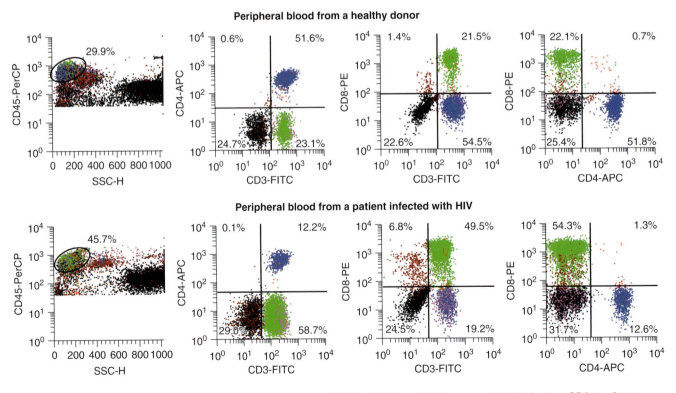

■ **FIGURE 16.9** Flow cytometry data that shows the differences in CD3+ CD4+ cells that occur with HIV infection. CD3+ cells are selected because this selects the T-cell population. CD3+ CD4+ cells decrease from 51.6% in the healthy individual (second panel top) to 12.2% in this patient with HIV (second panel bottom). This change is accompanied by an increase in the percentage of gated cells that are CD3+ and CD8+ from 21.5% in the healthy individual (third panel upper) to 49.5% (third panel lower). *Source:* Reprinted by permission of Paul Wallace and the Department of Flow Cytometry.

is called **seroconversion,** and its timing can vary from an individual to another (13). Testing for antibodies against HIV is based on 2 different approaches: screening tests, which are used for the rapid identification of potentially infected individuals, and confirmatory tests, which, as the name implies, are used to confirm infection and eliminate potentially false positive results from the screening tests.

SCREENING TESTS

The quintessential screening test for antibodies to HIV has been ELISA (the principle and procedures for ELISA techniques are described in detail in Chapter 7). ELISA has been shown to have both high sensitivity and high specificity and is still used routinely for screening for anti-HIV antibodies. Early ELISA testing involved the detection of antibodies against viral lysates from HIV-1 viruses. Because the lysates contained many different components, including contaminants from the cells used to culture the virus, they were prone to many false positive results and could not detect anti-HIV-2 antibodies. As both testing techniques and structural information on the virus developed, later assays were carried out on purified viral components or viral components created by recombinant techniques. These newer assays were more specific and could also detect antibodies to HIV-2. Modern ELISA techniques involve a "sandwich" approach (see Chapter 7) and have not only increased both the specificity and the sensitivity of the assay but also allowed the detection of anti-HIV antibodies of different isotypes.

Even modern ELISA techniques can, however, give false positive results. These can occur for a variety of reasons: from the detection of cross-reactive antigens, to the presence of certain tumors, to the administration of passive immunoglobulin, to mishandling samples or a mistake in techniques. Of course, the positive predictive value is lower when testing subjects who are a low risk for HIV infection, so to improve the positive predictive value, screening based on overall diagnosis, lifestyle, and medical history is important. However, diagnosis has the power to prevent the spread of disease, so the use of ELISA even in low-risk groups is important. Therefore, ELISA is used only as a screening test, and the use of confirmatory tests such as Western blots are necessary to confirm diagnosis. The CDC recommends that a positive ELISA test should be confirmed by a second and third identical ELISA test on the same individual. If 2 of the 3 tests results are positive, a confirmatory test must be performed.

Modern technology and the need for rapid evaluation of a potential HIV infection have resulted in the generation of rapid screening tests. These tests do not require laboratory equipment, technical staff, or complicated procedures but can be done in the field where technical resources are scarce or in clinical settings when a rapid test is required. These tests are as sensitive as the ELISA and are easy to perform without any laboratory skills. They are qualitative immune assays that use a flow-through technology and can be performed on samples of blood, plasma, or oral exudates. As with ELISA, these tests should be for initial screening only; their results must be interpreted considering history, clinical status, and whether the individual being tested belongs to a high-risk group, and should always be followed by confirmatory tests.

Several tests on the market have been approved for use in the detection of anti-HIV antibodies. Examples include OraQuick, Orasure, Uni-Gold (only for HIV-1), Clearview Complete HIV 1/2, Clearview HIV 1/2 Stat-Pak, and Reveal HIV. An FDA-approved home test, Home Access Express HIV-1 Test, requires the patient to collect a drop of blood in a proper kit and then mail it to the test facilities. OraQuick is a rapid antibody test that can provide results in about 20 minutes. The sample, whether whole blood, plasma, or oral fluids, is mixed in a vial with developing reagents, and the results are read from a testing apparatus shaped like a stick. In the case of collection of oral fluids, the stick itself can be used for this purpose (Figure 16.10 ■). Briefly, the individual being tested is asked to place the flap pad of the apparatus in the mouth above the teeth and against the outer gums and then gently swab around the outer gums, both upper and lower, using both sides of the flat pad to collect exudate, not saliva. The pad is then inserted into the reagent vial, and the results become visible from 20 to 40 minutes afterward.

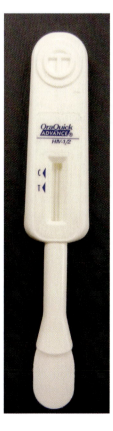

■ **FIGURE 16.10** OraQuick. A negative result would show a red line at the "C" mark, whereas a positive result would show red lines at both the "C" mark and the "T" marks. *Source:* Courtesy of OraSure Technologies, Inc.

CONFIRMATORY TESTS

All screening tests, whether ELISA or rapid, have a common caveat: A positive result does not necessarily mean that an individual is HIV infected. A false positive result can occur for various reasons, some of which have been discussed. Therefore, confirmatory tests are critical to correctly diagnose an HIV infection. The most commonly used confirmatory test for HIV is the Western blot test. Its principle and procedures are described in detail in Chapter 7. Unlike the ELISA or rapid tests, which evaluate the presence of anti-HIV antibodies as a yes-or-no approach (ie, whether there are antibodies against a mixture of viral components or not), the Western blot technique evaluates the presence of antibodies to specific viral components. Briefly, these components are separated electrophoretically by molecular size and then transferred to a solid matrix such as a nitrocellulose membrane and immobilized. The patient serum is then allowed to react with the nitrocellulose membrane. If the patient has antibodies to the different viral components that are immobilized on the membrane, these antibodies will attach to such components. As in the ELISA procedure, after washing the unbound material off the membrane, a second enzyme-labeled anti-human antibody preparation is allowed to react with the membrane, and the patient's antibodies (if any) that are attached to the viral components on the membrane will be visualized. Because the different viral components are physically separated onto the membrane, the antibody from a patient against a particular component can be identified. These enzyme labeled antibody-antigen complexes appear as stained "bands" on the nitrocellulose membrane (see Figure 16.11 ■ for a sample of a Western blot assay of HIV viral components).

Results may vary, from *no* bands to several bands. Although there is no gold standard as to how many and which bands determine a confirmatory diagnosis of HIV infection, the CDC has suggested that reactivity against *two* of the following viral components is considered a positive confirmatory test: p24, p31, gp41, and gp120/160. A test that shows less than these requirements is considered an intermediate response and should be repeated at a later date. Most HIV-infected individuals who had an intermediate test result test positive when retested later.

TESTING FOR VIRAL COMPONENTS

The most direct way to determine if an individual is infected with HIV is to detect the presence of the virus itself in that individual. However, these testing techniques are more expensive than antibody tests and are not used for screening. Early tests for viral components involved the detection of the p24 protein (a capsid or core antigen). This was a monoclonal antibody capture immunoassay (see Chapter 7) and was used in the mid- to late 1990s as a test for the virus. The rationale in choosing this component was the fact that the p24 protein increased significantly 7 to 20 days after infection and before anti-HIV antibodies could be detected. However the timeframe for the detection of p24 was very narrow, and as the

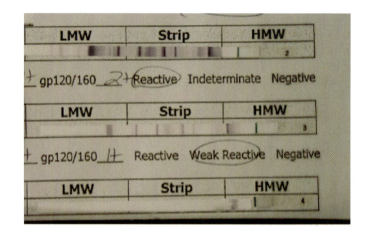

■ **FIGURE 16.11**   Western blot analysis of viral antigens. The nitrocellulose strips from the kit contain blotted viral antigens that have been separated by molecular weight using electrophoresis. (1) Strongly positive control sera. (2) Weakly positive control sera. (3) Test sera from patient. From right to left on the strips are the gp160 band, followed by the gp120 band, followed the p65, p55, p51, gp41, p40, p31, p24, and p18 bands. The patient shows a very light band at the gp160 region only. *Source:* Rittenhouse-Olson K. HIV testing and confidentiality. ASCP TechSample. Chicago, IL: ASCP; 2004.

infected individual started making antibodies to it, it became undetectable. Therefore, testing for p24 protein is no longer routinely used in the United States and Europe.

Modern tests for the presence of the virus are based on the detection of viral nucleic acids, which are obtained after the disruption of viral particles from an infected individual. Nucleic acid testing can determine the presence and the amount of virus in an infected individual and has been used in conjunction with testing for antibodies in donated blood in the United States since the mid-1990s. The principle of nucleic acid-based tests is to amplify and detect different sequences in the HIV genome. Examples of specific sequences include those encoding for HIV-I gag, HIV-II gag, HIV-env, and the HIV-pol.

Recently, genotyping has also targeted mutations in the genes of viral components that have been associated with resistance of the virus to anti-viral drugs. Examples of mutations targeted are M41L, K103N, V108I, and T215F for reverse transcriptase and Q58E, L63P, V77I, and L90M for protease. There are different forms of nucleic acid testing. In the reverse transcriptase polymerase chain reaction (RT-PCR), viral RNA is extracted from an individual's plasma and allowed to react with a preparation of reverse transcriptase; this converts the viral RNA into cDNA. The polymerase chain reaction is then used to amplify specific areas of the DNA that encode for specific viral genes. After amplification, the resulting DNA is allowed to react with specific oligonucleotides stuck to the walls of the reaction vessel and can be visualized using an enzyme-bound probe. This, in turn, can be used to quantify the amount of virus in the sample.

A more recent form of RT-PCR is the real-time RT-PCR. This test follows the same principle of the conventional RT-PCR; however, the resulting products are analyzed as they are produced (ie, in real time). This test incorporates a fluorescent label into the amplified products, and the amount of fluorescence detected is a reflection of the amount of product produced, which, in turn, can be quantitated. Another sensitive method is the branched DNA test (bDNA) on Quantiplex bDNA test. After viral particle disruption and the release of viral RNA, special oligonucleotides (label extenders and capture extenders) that bind to viral RNA and to certain oligonucleotides bound to the wall of a microtiter plate or vessel are added. A different set of oligonucleotides that bind at several locations to this RNA is added; then, other oligonucleotides that bind at several locations to those previous oligonucleotides are added. This creates a large complex (i.e. "branches") that amplifies the signal. Finally, enzyme-labeled oligonucleotides that bind to the last set of oligonucleotides are added; the presence and amount of the enzyme can be detected by a color reaction, which allows quantification of the viral RNA in the original sample. This method is very sensitive and can detect all known subtypes of HIV. Another method of amplifying RNA sequences is the nucleic acid sequence based amplification (NASBA). The NASBA can amplify RNA like PCR, and it has the advantage that it can be done at a constant temperature (41° C), thus not necessitating a thermocycler (20). The principle and methodology of different nucleic acid tests are discussed in detail in Chapter 23. See Box 16.1 ○

○ BOX 16.1

What to Do if You Are Stuck by a Syringe Needle from a Potentially HIV-Infected Sample?

Needlestick injuries are quite common in health care and the laboratory. These can occur when drawing blood, administering an intravenous or intramuscular medication, or performing tasks that involve the use of sharps. The most common injuries occur while recapping a needle or by failing to place used needles in approved sharps containers. Needlestick injuries can transmit diseases even in the absence of bleeding. In general, the chances of becoming HIV infected from a needlestick are relatively small, at an estimated rate of only 1 in 300 occurrences. However, in spite of the low probability of infection, a needlestick from a potentially HIV-infected sample should be treated as a medical emergency. If a needlestick injury occurs, the injury area should be cleaned with soap and water followed by disinfection with 70% alcohol. "Milking" the wound to increase blood flow is not recommended because this procedure may push infected cells more deeply into the tissue. Any rubbing or scraping of the wound should also be avoided because this creates a localized inflammatory condition that recruits white blood cells at the site, increasing the chance that they will be infected. The same is true for using bleach to clean the wound, so it should be avoided. Reporting the incident immediately is also very important; this allows the recording of the incident and the subsequent management following appropriate procedures. Most clinical and laboratory settings have well-defined protocols and procedures for these incidents. Health care workers who experience certain kinds of occupational exposures such as needlesticks are offered anti-viral therapy as a form of postexposure prophylaxis. This has cut the probability of HIV infection from such exposure by 80 to 20% of 1 in 300 or 1 in 1500.

TESTING ALGORITHMS

We have discussed the different tests for HIV infection, including screening and confirmatory tests. In 2009, the CDC published a status report describing a series of HIV testing algorithms recommended for clinical laboratories. This report can be found at http://www.aphl.org/aphlprograms/infectious/hiv/Documents/StatusReportFINAL.pdf.

○ CASE STUDY

A drug dealer from New York City was tested and found to be HIV positive and was counseled on precautions that he should take in his relationships to avoid infecting others. He moved to a small city and often traded drugs for sex. Over the course of several years, he had unprotected sex with 48 young women. His HIV status became known, and the man was found guilty of reckless endangerment and statutory rape and was sentenced to years in prison.

1. What tests should be done to determine whether these young women are infected?
2. The first screening test results were positive for 39 of the 48 women. What additional testing should be done first for them?
3. Of the 9 women who tested negative, 3 had had sex with the infected man more than 6 months earlier, 3 had had sex with him between 3 and 6 months earlier, 2 had sex with him about 1 and 3 months earlier, and one had sex with him this morning for the first time. What should be done with these women?
4. What confirmatory test should be performed after the positive ELISA results? What would indicate a positive result in this test?
5. What tests indicate how much HIV has affected the patient's immune system?
6. What tests can be used during therapy to determine whether the anti-virals are working?
7. What tests can be used to determine whether the HIV-infected person is resistant to a certain therapy?

SUMMARY

Acquired immunodeficiencies are abnormalities in immune function caused by various nonimmune factors; these include malnutrition, infections, certain drugs, trauma, environmental conditions, altered biological mechanisms, and some metabolic disorders. In recent years, the most prevalent form of acquired immunodeficiency has been acquired immunodeficiency disease (AIDS) caused by human immunodeficiency virus (HIV) infection. The number of infected people has been staggering, and AIDS has been a major human epidemic as well as a clinical and social challenge for the past 30 years.

HIV infections are transmitted in a variety of ways, most commonly through sexual exposure but also by blood transfusion, intravenous drug use, and mother-to-fetus transmission. HIV is a retrovirus and has been subdivided into 2 types, HIV-1 and HIV-2.

Both can result in AIDS, but HIV-1 is more common; HIV-2 is found mainly in West Africa. HIV infects human cells by binding to 2 different host cell surface receptors: CD4 as well as CXCR4 and CCR5, which serve as coreceptors. Several cell types can be infected; helper T cells, which have a large number of CD4 molecules on their surface, are the more commonly infected cells, but others, such as macrophages, dendritic cells, monocytes, and microglial brain cells, which also express CD4, can be infected. Once the virus is attached to the cell, the viral envelope and cell membrane fuse together, resulting in viral entry. The viral reverse transcriptase then converts this RNA into viral DNA, which is transported into the nucleus and integrated into the host cell DNA by the action of the viral integrase. The viral DNA can remain undisturbed into the host genome for long periods of time. Upon reactivation, the viral DNA is expressed and transcribed into mRNA; translation of the mRNA results in the production of viral proteins. These proteins promote the release of the viral RNA genome, which is packaged into new viral particles. New virions bud out of the cell in a protease-dependent process somewhat reversed from the one for viral entry; new viruses can then infect other cells, repeating the process.

The host immune response to the virus can be both humoral and cell mediated. Humoral response results in the generation of antibodies against different viral components. Antibodies to HIV can be usually detected in the blood stream, mucosal surfaces, and other body fluids within 1 to 3 months after HIV infection; these antibodies can limit viral replication by keeping the virus in check during the early asymptomatic stage; however, whereas the initial immune response to HIV can reduce viral replication, it cannot completely eliminate the virus from the host.

The major targets of the virus are CD4+ T cells; they are infected by interacting with either virally infected cells or antigen-presenting cells such as dendritic cells that have taken up and internalized the virus. Once in the lymphoid system, the virus can rapidly spread to the entire body through the lymphoid tissues; viral escape from the immune system creates cellular reservoirs of the virus in many different cells, including monocytes,

macrophages, dendritic cells, and microglial brain cells. This generates a situation in which the virus can cause a persistent infection that can ultimately deplete the virus-infected cells.

The clinical scenario in HIV infection and AIDS is the ultimate depletion of CD4+ T cells, a total breakdown of immune function, and the subsequent appearance of opportunistic infections and certain malignancies. The clinical classification of AIDS is based on several different parameters including CD4+ T cell counts, various clinical symptoms, and the nature of the opportunistic infections and malignancies.

Treatment involves the combination of various different antiviral drugs, each with different and specific antiviral actions. Highly active antiretroviral therapy (HAART) involves the combination of 3 synergistic anti-HIV drugs from at least 2 functional drug categories, for example, 2 nucleoside reverse transcriptase inhibitors and a protease inhibitor or 2 nucleoside reverse transcriptase inhibitors and a non-nucleoside reverse transcriptase inhibitor. Drug treatment comes at a price because side effects from the treatments are common. Laboratory diagnostic tests for HIV infection and AIDS include CD4+ T cell counts, the detection of anti-viral antibodies in the infected individual, and the detection of viral components. CD4+ T cell counts are usually performed using flow cytometry. Antibody testing regimens include screening tests such as ELISA or rapid tests, and confirmatory tests such as Western blots. Viral components such as p24 can be detected directly, but modern approaches involve viral nucleic acid testing that analyzes specific viral genes that encode for specific viral components. These tests include reverse transcriptase polymerase chain reaction (RT-PCR), real-time RT-PCR, nucleic acid sequence based amplification (NASBA), and branched DNA tests. A vaccine for HIV has so far been elusive; several obstacles have been encountered, the major ones being the antigenic variability of the virus and its ability to integrate into the host genome for long periods of time, thus evading immune detection. See Table 16.8 ✪ for a summary of different acquired immunodeficiencies.

✪ TABLE 16.8

Summary of Acquired Immunodeficiencies

Cause	Sample Condition	Effect
Malnutrition	Protein deficiency	Impaired cell-mediated immunity, phagocytosis, and actions of the complement
Metabolic disorders	Diabetes mellitus	Impaired chemotaxis and phagocytosis; decreased T-cell proliferation and function
Genetic defects	Down syndrome	Decreased phagocyte functions such as chemotaxis and phagocytosis
Alterations of physical barriers	Cystic fibrosis	Decreased clearance of pathogens from mucosal surfaces
Pharmacological agents	Use of anti-inflammatory drugs, corticosteroids, TNFα, or calcineurin inhibitors	Multiple effects
Environmental conditions	Exposure to ionizing radiation, high altitude, exposure to ultraviolet light, chronic hypoxia, lack of gravity	Multiple effects
Viral Infection	HIV infection	Long-term infection and/or depletion of various cells including CD4+ T cells leading to AIDS

REVIEW QUESTIONS

1. The reverse transcriptase of HIV
   a. transcribes viral DNA to cell DNA
   b. transcribes viral RNA to DNA
   c. transcribes cellular DNA to viral RNA
   d. is attached to the viral DNA

2. The current therapy for HIV consists of the use of
   a. reverse transcriptase inhibitor and a protease inhibitor
   b. 2 reverse transcriptase inhibitors and a protease inhibitor
   c. 2 reverse transcriptase inhibitors, a protease inhibitor, and a decoy CD4 molecule
   d. none of the above

3. During the latent phase of HIV infection,
   a. viral replication is held in check by the immune response
   b. viral replication occurs primarily in macrophages
   c. virus alone kills infected cells
   d. viral RNA is integrated into the host DNA

4. A window period is the amount of time
   a. between infection and a positive HIV test
   b. between a positive HIV test and AIDS
   c. between infection and clinical AIDS
   d. between the sample and the result

5. For what reason(s) do protease inhibitors slow the course of HIV infection?
   a. The genome is made of protein.
   b. Proteolytic processing is required for viral protein function.
   c. Serum proteases made by the infected host attack the virus.
   d. All of the above.

6. A student came to the health center with a malaise, fever, fatigue, and a complaint of being sick all the time. Her medical history for the previous 6 years has been uneventful, but 6 years before her visit to the clinic (1983), she had received open-heart surgery to repair a congenital defect. The operation required that many units of blood be transfused. Physical exam reveals a frail, thin young woman who is obviously ill. Her temperature is 102° F. Her white blood count shows a dramatic decrease in lymphocyte number. She has a *Pneumocystis carinii* infection. What laboratory tests make sense for this case?
   a. HIV enzyme immunoassays (EIA)
   b. HIV Western blot
   c. CD4+/CD8+ ratio
   d. all of the above

7. A van was set up outside of a local bar so that couples would get an EIA for HIV before they went home with each other for the evening. A young entrepreneur had this idea as a way to help couples be sure that their new partner is not HIV infected and as a way to make money; the price tag for his assay was high. Would you buy stock in his company?
   a. yes, because the EIA has no false positives or negatives
   b. yes, because everyone knows that Western blot is not needed
   c. no, because of the window period, this service would not be very useful and the false positives would be a problem
   d. no, because the CD4 to CD8 ratio is the only way to know for sure

8. Strategies to block which cellular receptor are being tried to prevent HIV infection?
   a. CCR5
   b. gp120
   c. CD4
   d. MHC

9. Opportunistic infections associated with HIV infection are due primarily to a
   a. declining number of CD4+ T cells
   b. declining number of CD8+ T cells
   c. failure to produce anti-HIV antibodies
   d. failure to activate a potent dendritic cell response

REFERENCES

1. Chinen J, Shearer WT. Secondary immunodeficiencies, including HIV infection. *J Allergy Clin Immunol.* 2010;125:S195–S203.

2. Cunningham-Rundles S, McNeeley DF, Moon A. Mechanisms of nutrient modulation of the immune response. *J Allergy Clin Immunol.* 2005;115:1119–1128.

3. Daoud AK, Tayyar MA, Fouda IM, et al. Effects of diabetes mellitus vs. in vitro hyperglycemia on select immune cell functions. *J Immunotoxicol.* 2009;6:36–41.

4. Alba-Loureiro TC, Munhoz CD, Martins JO, et al. Neutrophil function and metabolism in individuals with diabetes mellitus. *Braz. J. Med. Biol. Res.* 2007;40:1037–1044.

5. Douglas SD. Down syndrome: Immunologic and epidemiologic association enigmas remain. *J Pediatr.* 2005;147:723–725.

6. Hall HI, Song R, Rhodes P, et al. Estimation of HIV incidence in the Unites States. *JAMA.* 2008;300:520–529.

7. United Nations Programme on HIV/AIDS (UNAIDS) and World Health Organization (WHO). AIDS Epidemic Update. 2009. http://data.unaids.org/pub/report/2009/jc1700_epi_update_2009_en.pdf. Accessed March 27, 2012

8. Chan, DC, Fass, D, Berger, JM, et al. Core structure of gp41 from the HIV envelope glycoprotein. *Cell.* 1997;89:263–273.

9. Stumptner-Cuvelette P, Morchoisne S, Dugast M, et al. HIV-1 Nef impairs MHC class II antigen presentation and surface expression. *Proc Natl Acad Sci. U.S.A.* 2001;98:12144–12149.

10. Zheng YH, Lovsin N, Peterlin BM. Newly identified host factors modulate HIV replication. *Immunol. Lett.* 2005;97(2):225–234.

11. McMichael AJ, Borrow P, Tomaras GD, et al. The immune response during acute HIV-1 infection: Clues for vaccine. *Nature Rev Immunol.* 2010;10:11–23.

12. Baliga CS, Paul ME, Chine J, et al. HIV infection and the acquired immunodeficiency syndrome. In: Rich RR, ed. *Clinical Immunology: Principles and Practice.* 3rd. ed. Philadelphia, PA: Elsevier Saunders; 2008: 553–560.

13. Murphy K, Travers P, Walport M. *Janeway's Immunobiology.* 8th ed. New York, NY: Garland Publishing, 2012.

14. Centers for Disease Control and Prevention. 1993 revised classification system for HIV infection and expanded surveillance case definition for AIDS among adolescents and adults. *MMWR Recomm Rep.* 1992;18 (41)(RR-17):1–19.

15. Centers for Disease Control and Prevention. Guidelines for national human immunodeficiency virus case surveillance, including monitoring for human immunodeficiency virus infection and acquired immunodeficiency syndrome. *MMWR Recomm Rep.* 1999;48(RR-13):1–27, 29–31.

16. World Health Organization. WHO Case Definitions of HIV for Surveillance and Revised Clinical Staging and Immunological Classification of HIV-Related Disease In Adults and Children. 2007. http://www.who.int/hiv/pub/guidelines/HIVstaging150307.pdf. Accessed March 28, 2012

17. Burgoyne RW, Tan DH. Prolongation and quality of life for HIV-infected adults treated with highly active antiretroviral therapy (HAART): A balancing act. *J Antimicrob Chemother.* 2008;61:469–473.

18. Camargo JF, Kulkarni H, Agan BK, et al. Responsiveness of T cells to interleukin-7 is associated with higher CD4 1 T cell counts in HIV-1-positive individuals with highly active antiretroviral therapy-induced viral load suppression. *J Infect Dis.* 2009;199:1872–1882.

19. French MA. HIV/AIDS: Immune reconstitution inflammatory syndrome: A reappraisal. *Clin Infect Dis.* 2009;48:101–107.

20. Weber B. Screening of HIV infection: Role of molecular and immunological assays. *Expert Rev Mol Diagn.* 2006;6:399–411.

17

Hepatitis

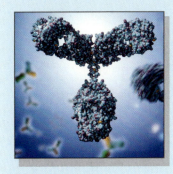

■ OBJECTIVES—LEVEL I

After this chapter, the student should be able to:

1. Describe the symptoms of hepatitis.
2. Compare and contrast the possible viral agents in terms of epidemiology, risk factors, and laboratory diagnosis in the assessment of a patient with acute viral hepatitis.
3. Describe the hepatitis A and B vaccines.
4. Explain the effect of vaccination for hepatitis B and hepatitis A on subsequent assays for antibodies to hepatitis and assays for the hepatitis antigens.
5. Understand the infection risks associated with patients who have the various hepatitis viruses for laboratory and personal safety. Describe what these are for each type of hepatitis.
6. Describe indicators that suggest that a patient may have a delta infection.
7. Describe the assays that would allow for the differentiation of a chronic carrier of hepatitis B from a patient with an acute hepatitis B infection.
8. Explain which antibody indicates hepatitis B virus infection resolution.
9. Describe what assays should be performed if hepatitis C is suspected.
10. Describe the course that should be taken in the reporting of hepatitis A, and when, if ever, hepatitis E should be suspected.
11. Indicate what assays should be done when a patient's liver enzymes are elevated.

■ OBJECTIVES—LEVEL II

After this chapter, the student should be able to:

1. Use your understanding of the Ab and Ag tests for hepatitis to describe the effect of advanced HIV on the use of these diagnostic tests.
2. Evaluate laboratory results to determine the cause of liver disease and whether the patient has an acute or chronic infection or whether their infection has resolved.
3. Compare and contrast the treatment methodologies of the different types of hepatitis.
4. Evaluate case studies in terms of risk factors and symptoms to determine the likely cause of the liver disease.

KEY TERMS

alanine aminotransferase (ALT)	hepatitis A
	hepatitis B
aspartate aminotransferase (AST)	hepatitis C
	hepatitis D
bilirubin	hepatitis E
HBc	hepatotropic viruses
HBeAg	recombinant immunoblot
HBsAg	assay (RIBA)
hepatitis	

▶ INTRODUCTION

The definition of **hepatitis** is any inflammation of the liver (Figure 17.1 ■); the disease can be caused by viruses, alcohol, drugs, toxins, and autoimmunity. Inflammation of the liver is accompanied by certain changes regardless of its cause. **Alanine aminotransferase (ALT)** and **aspartate aminotransferase (AST)** levels are elevated in hepatitis because they leak from damaged and dying liver cells. Unless there is increased production of bilirubin because of increased red blood cell lysis, hyperbilirubinemia, also indicates liver injury. **Bilirubin** is a breakdown product of heme, usually from red blood cells, and is a water insoluble pigment in bile. For bilirubin to be excreted in the stool, it must be conjugated to glucuronic acid by the liver. However, liver damage and bile duct blockage prevent this, resulting in elevated serum bilirubin. Elevated bilirubin is responsible for the yellowing of the skin and the whites of the eyes seen in the jaundice associated with hepatitis. Hepatitis with jaundice is called

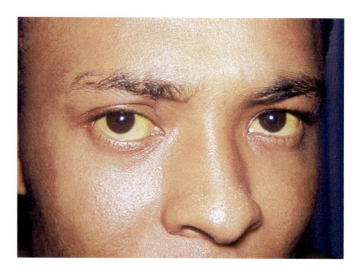

■ **FIGURE 17.2** Jaundice seen in the eyes and the skin of a patient with hepatitis A. *Source:* ©CDC/Dr. Thomas F. Sellers/ Emory University.

icteric (Figure 17.2 ■), and without jaundice is called *anicteric*. Alkaline phosphatase may also be elevated in hepatitis when there is obstruction of the bile duct. Hepatitis also affects clotting time, so the prothrombin time (PT) or the adjusted PT, known as the international normalized ratio (INR), are increased in severe hepatic disease. The physical symptoms of hepatitis can include nausea, abdominal pain, fever, malaise, anorexia, dark urine, clay-colored stool, and jaundice (1, 2, 3, 4, 5, 6, 7).

If, on a general chemistry screen, the AST/ALT levels are elevated or if physical signs and symptoms of liver

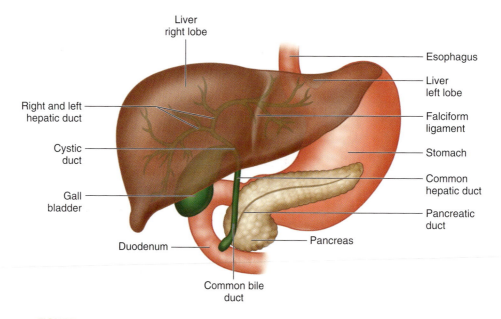

■ **FIGURE 17.1** Anatomy of the biliary tree, liver, and gall bladder.

abnormalities are identified during the annual physical, additional tests for the possible cause of the liver abnormalities are performed, which, depending on the history and physical of the patient, may include testing for hepatitis viruses. The viruses that cause hepatitis include **hepatotrophic viruses** (those that are liver cell seeking) and nonhepatotropic viruses. The hepatotrophic viruses include hepatitis viruses A, B, C, D (also called *delta*), and E. The nonhepatotropic viruses, which primarily infect other cells but can infect liver cells and cause hepatitis, include several viruses in the herpetoviridae family including Epstein-Barr virus (infectious mononucleosis), varicella zoster (chicken pox), and cytomegalovirus. Only the hepatotrophic viruses hepatitis A, B, C, D, and E will be discussed in this chapter. The term *non-A, non-B hepatitis* was used to refer to a hepatitis caused by a virus that tested negative in the only assays for viral agents of hepatitis available at the time, assays for hepatitis A and hepatitis B. Non-A, non-B hepatitis referred to are what we now call *hepatitis C and E*. Because hepatitis A and E are most often spread by a fecal-oral route and hepatitis B, D (delta), and C are most often bloodborne infections, the viruses are discussed in the order listed rather than alphabetical order (1, 2, 3, 4, 5, 6, 7).

✓ Checkpoint! 17.1

A patient had elevated ALT and AST and hyperbilirubinemia but tested negative for hepatitis A, B, C, D, and E. What could be a reason for the hepatitis that this patient is experiencing?

▶ FECAL-ORAL HEPATITIS: HEPATITIS A AND E

HEPATITIS A

Epidemiology

Hepatitis A is a single-stranded positive strand RNA virus in an icosahedral capsid belonging to the Picornaviridae viral family. Hepatitis A causes acute hepatitis after an incubation period of about 28 days. It is shed in high concentrations in the patient's feces from 2 weeks before symptoms occur until 1 week after the symptoms appear. In the United States, about half of the cases of hepatitis A occur without any known source or risk factor. In 2007, 2979 cases of acute symptomatic hepatitis A were reported, with about 25 000 total cases estimated as the result of underreporting and asymptomatic cases. This is about 1 case per 100 000 people in the United States. This number of cases represents a 92% drop since the 1995 introduction of the hepatitis A vaccine (7, 8, 9, 10, 11, 12, 13).

Risk groups for hepatitis A are men who have sex with men, international travelers (especially in Mexico and South and Central America), illegal drug users, and children living in communities with high rates of disease. Each of these risk groups is related to fecal-oral contact, the first group the result

of anal sex and international travelers through contaminated food and water. International travelers to regions with a high hepatitis A risk (Figure 17.3 ■) should be aware that all water should be bottled, all ice ingested should be prepared from bottled water, and all shellfish, fruits, and vegetables should be consumed only if they are cooked or peeled. Melons can contain hepatitis A virus and so should not be consumed. Heating thoroughly for 1 minute at 185° C destroys hepatitis A in food. In some areas, plastic water bottles are reused and filled with local tap water that may be infectious, so water should be consumed only from bottles that are unsealed in your presence. In addition, in some regions, the reuse of water bottles can involve resealing with superglue to give the appearance of factory-bottled water. If in doubt, drink carbonated water, which is alternatively called "water with gas" (7, 8, 9, 10, 11, 12).

The risk of hepatitis A for drug users requires some explanation. Some drugs travel across borders in condoms that have been ingested, and because these condoms travel through the body to their final destination, they are exposed to fecal material. Intravenous drugs users have been found to become exposed to hepatitis A this way. In addition, marijuana users also have been found to be exposed to hepatitis A because in some places, crops are fertilized with human fecal material (13).

Diagnosis

Hepatitis A does not become chronic, and people cannot be re-infected with it, although rarely (less than1%) a relapsing form of hepatitis in which symptoms recur can happen. Antibodies formed to the virus protect from re-infection. Thirty-five percent of hepatitis A cases require hospitalization, and 0.8% of these cases die. The rare fatality occurs mainly in people over 50 and is associated with previous alcoholic or other viral damage to the liver. There is no extra risk for pregnant women. The probability of a cure is nearly 100%. Young children are frequently asymptomatic. The physical signs and symptoms of hepatitis—yellowing of the skin, fatigue, loss of appetite, and muscle and joint aches—are quite similar regardless of which virus caused the inflammation of the liver, making laboratory diagnosis very important for treatment and prognosis. Additionally, hepatitis A is a reportable infection for which there is national surveillance, so proper diagnosis is important. The diagnosis for hepatitis A, initially involves screening for IgM antibodies to the hepatitis A virus (HAV), while total anti-HAV antibodies can be used diagnostically later (Figure 17.4 ■). Total anti-HAV antibodies can be assessed to determine immune status of the patient. Several assays are available for analysis of anti-HAV levels; these assays are either (1) indirect enzyme immunoassays, (2) competitive direct enzyme immunoassays in which enzyme labeled anti-HAV competes with patient anti-HAV for binding to the HAV antigen coated well, or (3) capture immunoassays in which the patient's IgM is captured by an anti-human IgM, and hepatitis A viral particles are added and then enzyme labeled antihepatitis A antibody is added (7, 8, 9, 10, 11, 12).

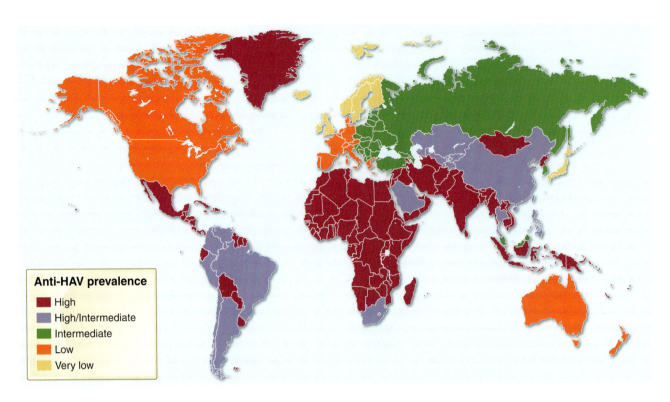

■ **FIGURE 17.3**   Geographic distribution of hepatitis A prevalence (anti-HAV-antibody), 2005.

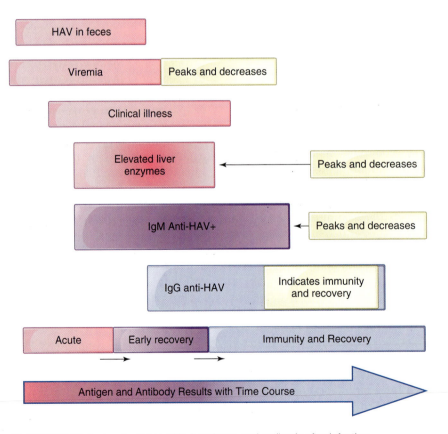

■ **FIGURE 17.4**   Levels of hepatitis A antigens and antibody after infection.

Vaccine and Postexposure Prophylaxis

The vaccine for hepatitis A is recommended by the CDC's Advisory Committee on Immunization Practices for children at their first birthday, for children ages 2 to 18 who did not receive the vaccine at their first birthday, adults traveling to or working in countries with a high or intermediate risk of hepatitis A, men who have sex with men, users of illegal drugs whether injectable or not, people at occupational risk for hepatitis A, individuals with clotting factor disorders, and individuals with chronic liver disease. The only people thought to be at occupational risk for hepatitis A are those doing research on the virus and studying live virus in their research laboratories. GlaxoSmithKline (GSK) and Merck & Co., Inc. produce hepatitis A vaccines. The vaccines are killed or inactivated viruses. Three different vaccines are made: 2 single antigen vaccines, VAQTA (Merck) and HAVRIX (GSK), and a combination vaccine called Twinrix (GSK), which contains both hepatitis A antigens and hepatitis B antigens. The vaccine protection lasts ≥ 14 to 20 years in children and ≥ 25 years in adults. No postvaccination testing is needed because of the high degree of protection conferred to the hepatitis A virus (7, 8, 9, 10, 11, 12).

Individuals with known exposure to hepatitis A virus can receive either an injection of immune globulin or, for exposed individuals 1 to 40 years old, the hepatitis A vaccine. The vaccine is the preferred choice because it also protects the individual from infection due to any subsequent exposure. The groups who should receive the postexposure prophylaxis include people who have household, sexual, or close personal contact with individuals who have confirmed cases of hepatitis A, such as child care workers and physical attendants. In a day care setting, all individuals in the classroom should be vaccinated. Restaurant patrons that consumed food served by infected food handlers who had bad hygiene and handled foods that are served uncooked or handled food after cooking should be vaccinated within 2 weeks. Patrons of institutional cafeterias who are likely to have been exposed multiple times should be vaccinated. Postexposure prophylaxis when there is a single case in a dormitory or school is not suggested, but if there are multiple cases indicating spread, the population in that setting should receive the vaccine as postexposure prophylaxis (7, 8, 9, 10, 11, 12).

HEPATITIS E

Epidemiology

Like hepatitis A, **hepatitis E** is a fecal-oral form of hepatitis caused by a single positive strand RNA virus with an icosahedral capsid belonging to its own family, Hepeviridae. Contaminated water causes epidemic infections whereas contaminated food and animals cause sporadic cases. Hepatitis E is not usually spread from person to person, nor does it appear to be spread sexually. It is found most often in Southeast and Central Asia and India and has been found in Mexico (Figure 17.5 ■). Serological evidence shows that 40% of 16- to 25-year-olds in India had been infected. It is second only to hepatitis B as a cause of viral hepatitis in the Middle East and Africa, and it is also frequently

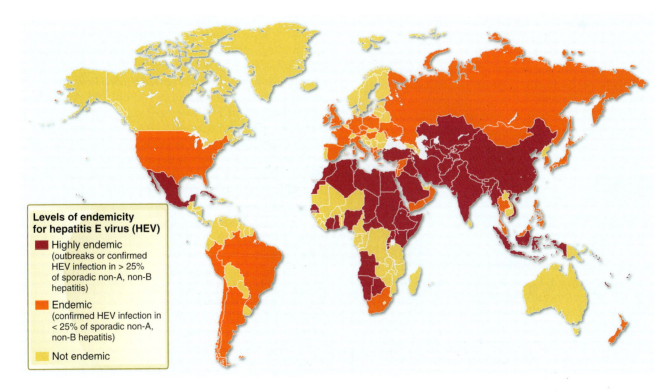

■ FIGURE 17.5 Hepatitis epidemiology.

found in refugee camps (14, 15). Hepatitis E is rare in the United States, and its cause is usually travel associated.

Hepatitis E causes an acute form of hepatitis from 2 weeks to 2 months after infection. Clinically, it appears like the other forms of hepatitis and is not usually severe, and only 40% of people who are infected become ill. Young children are often asymptomatic. Most patients recover within a few weeks, and hepatitis E does not become chronic. The concern is that 1% of the cases become fulminant and in these cases, the disease is fatal. Of particular concern is the fact that when pregnant women become infected, the mortality rate for these women is as high as 30% in the third trimester. The fetus is commonly infected when a pregnant woman is infected and fetal demise may occur. Hepatitis E is also of special concern in individuals who already have chronic hepatitis or other liver damage and for whom the mortality rate can be as high as 70%. Travelers to endemic areas should take the precautions concerning water, ice, and uncooked fruit and vegetables discussed in the hepatitis A section (14, 15).

Diagnosis and Vaccines

Because hepatitis E is rare in the United States, diagnostic tests for this virus are not commonly performed here, but hepatitis E blood tests are available in other countries. When available, testing includes serology for IgM and IgG to hepatitis E specific antigens and RT-PCR (polymerase chain reaction) for viral RNA. Because there is no treatment for hepatitis E, sufferers should rest, drink fluids, and not take any medicines toxic to the liver or drink alcohol. No vaccine is currently available for hepatitis E, although a promising candidate has recently received press after very successful phase III trials. This candidate vaccine developed by GlaxoSmithKline had 96% efficacy when tested in Nepal (see Box 17.1 ✪). This vaccine would be particularly important for pregnant women and individuals who already have chronic liver disease. Unfortunately, further development of the vaccine is questionable because of the lack of commercial viability of protecting against a disease that is predominantly seen in undeveloped countries (16, 17, 18, 19).

✪ BOX 17.1

The story of the first visualization of the hepatitis E virus is too interesting not to share. Dr. Balayan, after studying an outbreak of non-A, non-B hepatitis in the Soviet Union, wanted to isolate the virus that caused the outbreak. However, he had no refrigeration and was afraid that without refrigeration, he would not be able to get live virus back to his laboratory. To ensure arrival of the live virus to his lab in Moscow, he drank a milkshake made of yogurt and stool from an infected patient. He went to his lab in Moscow and when he became ill, he isolated the virus from his own stool and visualized it under an electron microscope! And to keep the interesting story going, a collaborator of Dr. Balayan, Dr. Tsarev, emigrated to the United States and became a scientist at the National Institute of Allergy and Infectious Diseases. Dr. Tsarev was one of the key investigators in the development of the new hepatitis E vaccine.

▶ BLOODBORNE HEPATITIS: HEPATITIS B, D, AND C

HEPATITIS B

Epidemiology

Hepatitis B is a virus with partially double-stranded circular DNA that is attached to a polymerase protein and surrounded by a nucleocapsid. That in turn is surrounded by a lipoprotein envelope of the cell from which the virus budded. The nucleocapsid is composed of the core protein **HBc.** The hepatitis B surface antigen **(HBsAg)** is in the lipoprotein envelope. The **HBeAg** is between the nucleocapsid and the lipoprotein envelope. Excess HBsAg is produced and exists in particles called *Australian antigens* (Figure 17.6 ■) (20, 21, 22, 23, 24).

Hepatitis B causes acute hepatitis approximately 90 days after infection (60–150 days). Infection is through contact with infectious blood or body fluids via mucosal contact or through breaks through the skin (percutaneous). Even dried blood can spread the disease, and hepatitis B can be transmitted in dried blood for 7 days after it was shed. Persons at risk for a hepatitis B infection are those who have sex with an infected person, men who have sex with men, people who had multiple sex partners in the previous 90 days, health care workers who are occupationally exposed to blood, hemodialysis patients, travelers to countries with high prevalence, household contacts of infected persons, residents and staff of facilities for developmentally disabled people, injection drug users, and infants born from an infected mother. Males are diagnosed with hepatitis B at a rate 1.6 times higher than that of females (20, 21, 22, 23, 24).

Many infected people are asymptomatic, including most children under 5, newly infected immunosuppressed people, and 50 to 70% of infected people of ages over 5. Symptoms of acute hepatitis B are those described under general hepatitis symptoms with the addition of joint pain and rash. Of people reported with acute hepatitis B, 40% need hospitalization. Fulminant hepatitis and death can result in 0.5 to 1% of hepatitis B cases. People over 60 suffer more severe illnesses (20, 21, 22, 23, 24).

Unlike hepatitis A or E, a hepatitis B infection can become chronic; that is, the virus remains in the person's body after the acute infection has ended. Chronic hepatitis develops in about 5% of the adults with an increased risk in the elderly, 25 to 50% of the children, and about 90% of the infants who are infected with hepatitis B. Patients with anicteric hepatitis B are more likely to develop chronic hepatitis than are people with icteric hepatitis. During the acute phase, an increased immune response kills liver cells and thus is more likely both to cause an icteric infection and to clear the virus. In some people with chronic hepatitis B, the symptoms of acute hepatitis remain; however, most people with chronic hepatitis remain symptom free for 20 to 30 years. Liver scarring (cirrhosis) or liver cancer (hepatoma) can occur in 15 to 25% of patients with chronic hepatitis B. The cirrhosis can cause liver failure and death, and in countries without advanced medical care, hepatoma leads to death usually within a year (20, 21, 22, 23, 24).

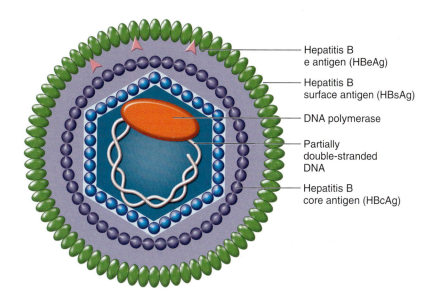

■ **FIGURE 17.6**   Structure of the hepatitis B virus.

In 2007, the CDC reported 4519 cases of acute hepatitis B in the United States (Figure 17.7 ■) and noted that because so many cases of hepatitis B are asymptomatic, these reported cases are about a tenth of the actual number. The overall U.S. incidence is 1.5 cases per 100 000. This number is a significant decrease (82%) from the levels before the vaccine was routinely recommended. The decrease has allowed recognition of previously unrecognized risk factors: 157 cases of hepatitis B were found to have resulted from shared use of glucose monitoring equipment by diabetics in nursing homes. About 1.25 million people in the United States have chronic hepatitis B, (20, 21, 22, 23, 24).

Two billion people have been infected worldwide with hepatitis B with 350 million chronic hepatitis cases. Hepatitis B is most common in China and other parts of Asia; other areas of high incidence include the Amazon, southeast and south-central Europe, the Middle East, and India. In developing countries, almost all children are infected with hepatitis B. Liver cancer caused by hepatitis B is in the top 3 causes of death for men in these countries. Hepatitis B is tenth in the list of major causes of worldwide mortality (20, 21, 22, 23, 24) (Figure 17.8 ■).

Diagnosis

Diagnosis of hepatitis B is determined by measuring levels of antigen and antibody against different viral antigens (Figure 17.9 ■). The levels of the antigen and antibodies are different in acute resolving infections and those acute infections which become chronic (Figure 17.10 ■). The presence of hepatitis B surface Ag (HBsAg) is one of the first measurable signs of infection; it disappears within 4 to 6 months if the patient is recovering but remains elevated if the patient develops chronic hepatitis B. Antihepatitis B core (anti-HBc) antibody develops at the same time as symptoms, but because it lasts for a lifetime, isotyping is needed to determine present versus past infection. IgM anti-HBc indicates a recent infection and is positive when HBsAg has just disappeared, so it can be important in diagnosis. Anti-HBcAg is the same in acute and chronic hepatitis B. HBsAg and HBeAg positivity indicates that the patient is infectious because these are part of the virion. HBeAg becomes positive shortly after HBsAg and indicates that the patient is highly infectious (20, 21, 22, 23, 24).

When anti-HBcAg IgM is negative with anti-HBcAg IgG positive and HBsAg is positive, the patient is chronically infected because the virus antigen should have disappeared prior to the development of IgG anti-HBcAg. Positive measurements 6 months apart for either HBV antigen or HBV DNA also indicate a chronic infection. Anti-hepatitis D antigen (anti-HDV) indicates a co-infection with hepatitis D virus. IgM anti HBcAg and HBsAg measurements are used in screening donor blood.

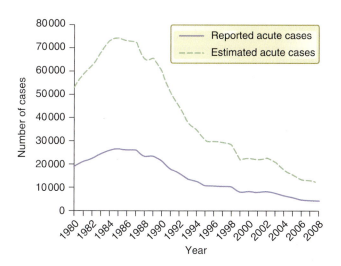

■ **FIGURE 17.7**   Incidence of acute hepatitis B in the United States, 1980–2008.

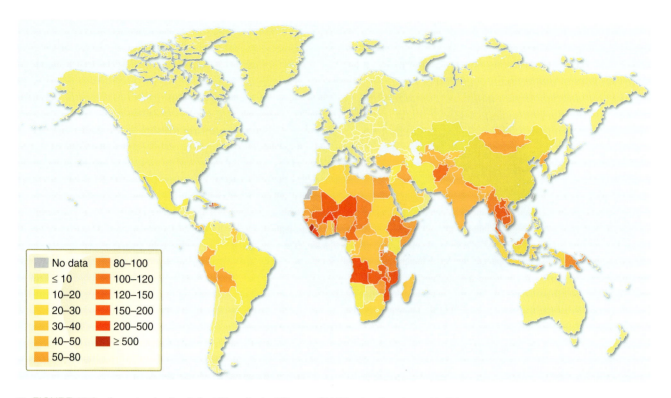

■ **FIGURE 17.8** Age-standardized disability-adjusted life year (DALY) rates from hepatitis B by country (per 100 000 inhabitants).

Legend:
- No data
- ≤ 10
- 10–20
- 20–30
- 30–40
- 40–50
- 50–80
- 80–100
- 100–120
- 120–150
- 150–200
- 200–500
- ≥ 500

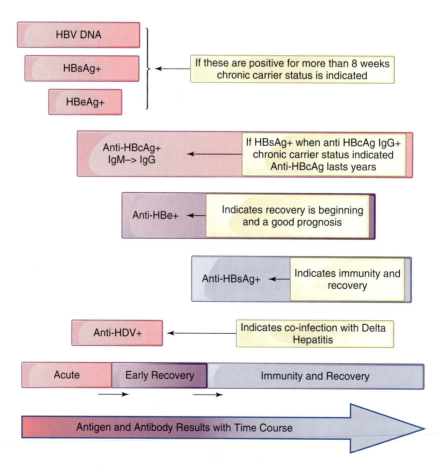

HBV DNA

HBsAg+

HBeAg+

If these are positive for more than 8 weeks chronic carrier status is indicated

Anti-HBcAg+ IgM–> IgG

If HBsAg+ when anti HBcAg IgG+ chronic carrier status indicated Anti-HBcAg lasts years

Anti-HBe+

Indicates recovery is beginning and a good prognosis

Anti-HBsAg+

Indicates immunity and recovery

Anti-HDV+

Indicates co-infection with Delta Hepatitis

Acute   Early Recovery   Immunity and Recovery

Antigen and Antibody Results with Time Course

■ **FIGURE 17.9** Hepatitis B antigens and antibody in an acutely infected patient with recovery. Note the indicators of recovery and conversely those of chronic infection.

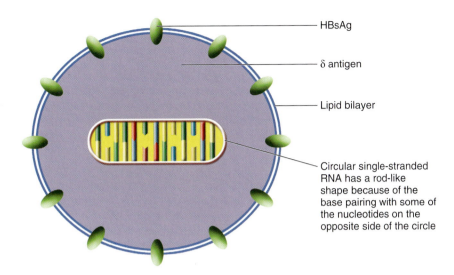

HBsAg

δ antigen

Lipid bilayer

Circular single-stranded RNA has a rod-like shape because of the base pairing with some of the nucleotides on the opposite side of the circle

■ **FIGURE 17.10**   The hepatitis D virion.

Antibody to HBeAg indicates that the patient is recovering from the infection. Antibody to HBsAg can be measured after the disappearance of HBsAg and indicates recovery because this antibody provides protective immunity. Anti-HBsAg is present without any of the other markers in vaccinated individuals. These antibodies are not produced in individuals who become chronically infected (20, 21, 22, 23, 24).

A chronic hepatitis B infection can become reactivated when a patient takes corticosteroids or chemotherapy; in this case, the IgM anti-HBcAg may reappear in the serum. In chronic hepatitis B, the presence of either HBcAg, and HBV DNA indicates active viral replication, and serum that is negative for these indicates a low replicative state. The antigens are generally detected by capture enzyme immunoassays. The IgM antibodies may be detected either by an isotype-specific indirect assay or by a capture assay in which the IgM antibody is captured onto a surface coated with anti-human IgM, followed by addition of the hepatitis antigen, and then by addition of alkaline phosphatase–labeled antibody to the antigen and finally followed by addition of substrate. The antibodies can also be detected by a competitive direct assay in which the antigen is coated on a plate and the patient's antibody is added and alkaline phosphatase–labeled antibody to the antigen is added so that the patient antibody competes with the kit antibody for binding to the antigen in the well. Both acute hepatitis B and chronic hepatitis B are nationally reportable diseases (20, 21, 22, 23, 24).

Testing for chronic infection is recommended for persons from countries with high prevalence of hepatitis B, unvaccinated people born in the United States whose parents came from regions of high prevalence, men who have sex with men, immunosuppressed individuals, pregnant women, infants of HBsAg+, mothers, injection drug users, persons with elevated AST/ALT, household and sexual contacts of hepatitis B virus-infected people, people with HIV, and source patients whose blood was involved in an occupational exposure (20, 21, 22, 23, 24).

Treatment

There is no treatment for acute hepatitis B because of the high spontaneous recovery rate. Antiviral therapy may be given for severely ill patients, but no controlled case studies have been conducted. Chronic hepatitis B with active viral replication is treated with interferon-alpha, pegylated interferon-alpha 2a, lamivudine, adefovir dipivoxil, entecavir, and telbivudine. Interferon-alpha is a cytokine named for its ability to interfere with viral replication, and pegylation (adding a polyethylene glycol) increases the time it remains in the body. Lamivudine (3TC) (also used for HIV) is a reverse transcriptase inhibitor, and hepatitis B has a step in its life cycle in which viral RNA, which has been produced by a cellular RNA polymerase from the viral DNA, is replicated to DNA via a viral reverse transcriptase. Adefovir dipivoxil, telbivudine, and entecavir are also reverse transcriptase inhibitors used for hepatitis B, but they do not work for HIV. These treatments do not cure chronic hepatitis, but they do decrease viral replication. These patients should be monitored to evaluate whether the disease is progressing to liver cirrhosis or liver cancer (hepatocellular carcinoma). Fulminant acute HBV infection can be treated with a liver transplant along with high dose passive transfer of human anti-hepatitis B immunoglobulin and antivirals (20, 21, 22, 23, 24).

Vaccine

The first vaccine developed to protect against hepatitis B was composed of hepatitis B surface antigen isolated from the plasma of people infected with hepatitis B and then heat inactivated. This vaccine was discontinued, and now 5 different vaccines for hepatitis B are licensed in the United States. Two of them, Engerix-B and Recombivax, contain recombinant HBsAg only. The 3 remaining vaccines contain recombinant HBsAg with other antigens: Comvax contains recombinant HBsAg + Haemophilus influenza type b conjugate; Pediarix contains recombinant HBsAg, diphtheria, tetanus, acellular pertussis, and inactivated poliovirus; and Twinrix contains hepatitis A and recombinant HBsAg (20, 21, 22, 23, 24).

The recombinant HBsAg is produced in yeasts, so individuals who are allergic to yeast cannot receive any of these vaccines. The protection lasts at least 20 years after vaccination if the individuals were older than 6 months when they received their vaccine. Studies are still underway to determine how long protection lasts if the individual vaccinated was under 6 months. Postvaccination testing to ensure that protective titers developed to vaccination should be performed on certain individuals for whom immunity to hepatitis B is of particular importance. This includes infants born to HBsAg+ mothers, health care workers at high risk of exposure to hepatitis B, sex partners of people with hepatitis B, hemodialysis patients, HIV-infected persons, and other immunocompromised people. The postvaccination testing should be done 1 to 2 months after the third dose of the vaccine. Booster doses are recommended when antibody levels go lower than 10 mIU/ml for hemodialysis patients and for immunocompromised people. Currently, boosters are not recommended for healthy individuals. A mutation has been found in which the 3-D conformation of the HBsAg has changed so that it is not neutralized by the antibodies developed after vaccination; what effect this will have in the future is unknown (20, 21, 22, 23, 24).

A strategy was developed in 1991 to decrease the number of hepatitis B cases in the United States which includes vaccination of (1) all infants at birth, (2) children and adolescents who were not previously vaccinated, and (3) adults at increased risk. The strategy also includes screening of all pregnant women prior to delivery and immunoprophylaxis with anti-HBV immunoglobulin (HBIG) of all babies born to HBV positive women. In the case of exposure of a health care worker who was not previously vaccinated with HBsAg, they should receive multiple doses of HBIG. A new protocol using a dose of HBIG followed by the hepatitis B vaccine series is being considered (20, 21, 22, 23, 24).

 Checkpoint! 17.2

An IV drug user had elevated ALT and AST and hyperbilirubinemia. Assays for IgM anti-HAV, IgM anti-HBcAg, HBsAg, and anti-HCV were performed and IgM anti-HBcAg was found. What diagnostic result(s) would show that the disease was resolving?

HEPATITIS D

Epidemiology

Hepatitis D virus, also called *hepatitis delta virus,* is a virus with small circular single-stranded RNA and is the only known animal virus with circular RNA. Hepatitis D virus requires co-infection with the hepatitis B virus to replicate. It uses the envelope proteins of hepatitis B virus to assemble into new particles and to attach and enter into new cells. The genome of the hepatitis D virus codes for only 2 proteins, a long delta antigen and a small one. These are RNA-binding proteins. The host cell supplies the rest of the proteins that are needed for its replication. Because of the dependence of hepatitis D virus on hepatitis B virus, the hepatitis D virus is called a subviral satellite of hepatitis B virus. It is transmitted like hepatitis B with percutaneous (through the skin) or mucosal exposure. Hepatitis D acquired with hepatitis B is called a *co-infection;* the infection of a patient already infected with hepatitis B who becomes infected with hepatitis D is called a *superinfection.* Like hepatitis B virus, hepatitis D virus is very stable and can infect after drying (25, 26).

About 20 million people who have chronic hepatitis B also have hepatitis D, a little less than 5% of the people infected with chronic hepatitis B. Both acute and chronic hepatitis B infections have a worse prognosis if the patient also has hepatitis D. The mortality rate for hepatitis B virus with hepatitis D virus is 10 times higher than hepatitis B virus alone with fatality of 2% of the acute dual infections and 20% of the chronic dual infections. Prevalence rates of hepatitis D are highest in Russia, Romania, southern Italy, Africa, South America, and the Mediterranean countries (25, 26).

Diagnosis

Hepatitis D can be diagnosed by looking for antibodies to HDV antigens in hepatitis B virus infected patients. RT-PCR is also used to detect hepatitis B virus. There is no separate vaccine for hepatitis D virus, but it can be prevented with the vaccine for hepatitis B (25, 26).

HEPATITIS C

Epidemiology

Hepatitis C virus is a single-stranded RNA virus that is spherical, enveloped, and a member of the Flaviviridae family (Figure 17.11 ■). Six main genotypes of hepatitis C virus exist with more than 50 subgroups. In viral multiplication, a number of mutant viruses develop with enough mutations to be called a quasispecies. The genetic variability results in difficulty for the patient in eliminating the virus, difficulty for vaccinologists in the development of a vaccine, and difficulty in treatment of the virus as resistant mutants develop (27, 28, 29, 30).

Hepatitis C causes an acute infection 6–7 weeks after infection; however, most people are not symptomatic with the acute infection. In 2007, only 849 cases of acute hepatitis C were reported in the United States, but because of the effects of both underreporting and the asymptomatic nature of the disease, 17 000 new cases are estimated to have occurred in 2007. The number of new cases of hepatitis C reached a peak in 1992, when the number of new cases began to decrease as the result of the implementation of blood supply screening for hepatitis C virus in the United States. The number of new cases fell until 2003 when a plateau was reached (27, 28, 29, 30).

Prior to 1992, many of the cases came from blood transfusions because no established test for the presence of hepatitis C existed. Prior to diagnostic tests for hepatitis C, individuals who had hepatitis but tested negative by the assays for hepatitis

Envelope

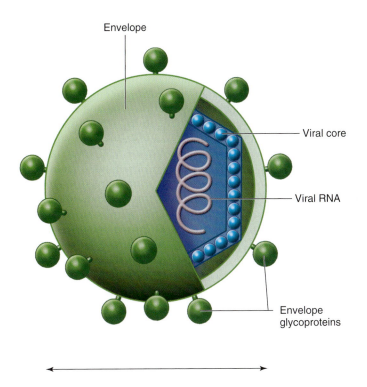

Viral core

Viral RNA

Envelope glycoproteins

■ **FIGURE 17.11**   Hepatitis C virion structure.

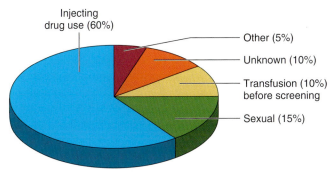

Injecting drug use (60%)

Other (5%)

Unknown (10%)

Transfusion (10%) before screening

Sexual (15%)

■ **FIGURE 17.12**   Sources of hepatitis C infection.

A and B were said to have non-A, non-B hepatitis. This term was used to refer to both hepatitis C and E. Since blood testing became widely used in 1992, most of the new cases of hepatitis C have been associated with injection drug use. The risk factors for hepatitis C are injectable drug use, having multiple sexual partners during the incubation period, men who have sex with men, surgery with a transfusion especially before 1992, occupational exposure to blood, receipt of a tattoo, and sharing a toothbrush or a razor with a hepatitis C virus–infected person as well as maternal-neonatal transmission from a hepatitis C+ mother (27, 28, 29, 30) (Figure 17.12 ■).

Transmission of hepatitis C by transfusion is now rare as the result of blood screening. Individuals who test positive for hepatitis C but do not fall into a risk group should be investigated because an unsafe practice in which the person engages may be discovered in a health care setting. Outbreaks have been found associated with unsafe practices at an endoscopy clinic as well as other nonhospital health care facilities. The risk of acquiring hepatitis C after a needle stick from a hepatitis C+ patient is about 1.8%, and the risk to an infant born to a hepatitis C positive mother is about 4%. People who have sex with people who have chronic hepatitis C have a low but present risk of infection. In a monogamous relationship with a hepatitis C positive partner, 1% of the partners become infected. Re-infection of the patient with the same strain of hepatitis C or with different strains is possible after the patient has cleared the acute infection because antibody to hepatitis C virus is not protective (27, 28, 29, 30).

The symptoms of acute hepatitis C are the general symptoms of hepatitis; however, 70% of the people with hepatitis C are asymptomatic in the acute phase. If symptoms do occur they do so 6 to 7 weeks after exposure. Like symptomatic acute hepatitis B, symptomatic acute hepatitis C is less likely to develop into chronic hepatitis than is an asymptomatic acute phase. The impact of hepatitis C is seen in the number of chronically infected individuals with more than 4 million chronically infected people living in the United States. This is an astonishing 1.6% of the U.S. population. Imagine 1.6 people of every 100 friends that you have on Facebook! Of people infected with hepatitis C virus, 75 to 85% develop a chronic infection. In addition, 60 to 70% of the people infected with hepatitis C will progress to chronic liver disease, 5 to 20% will slowly (~20 years) develop liver cirrhosis, and 1 to 5% will die of either liver cirrhosis or hepatoma. The number of deaths from chronic hepatitis C is estimated to be about 8 000 to 10 000 cases in the United States per year (27, 28, 29, 30).

Most people with chronic hepatitis C do not have symptoms, but as the liver damage progresses, symptoms can occur. Fatigue is the primary symptom of chronic hepatitis, and upper right quadrant abdominal tenderness, nausea, poor appetite, bruising, and joint and muscle pain can also occur. As the disease progresses and liver cirrhosis occurs, all of these symptoms can occur with enlarged liver and spleen, jaundice, muscle wasting, and ascites (fluid in the peritoneal cavity). In addition, hepatitis C is the most common cause of mixed essential cryoglobulinemia, which occurs in 1 to 2% of patients with hepatitis C. In mixed essential cryoglobulinemia immune complexes are formed that contain the virus, antibody to the virus, complement, and rheumatoid factor. These complexes, which form in the cold and dissolve upon warming, deposit throughout the body causing symptoms of type III hypersensitivity including rashes and joint pain. Raynaud's phenomena, which causes pain, numbness, paleness, and/or tingling of the fingers and toes when exposed to the cold, can develop as the result of the cryoglobulinemia (30, 31, 32, 33).

Diagnosis

Hepatitis C is diagnosed by using a group of tests utilizing immunological and molecular biology techniques. The immunologic assays measure anti-hepatitis C antibodies in 2 different ways. The screening test involves a third-generation indirect enzyme immunoassay that uses a mixture of viral antigens in a microtiter well or on microbeads. This assay measures antibody to structural and nonstructural proteins of the hepatitis C virus as a collective yes or no answer. That is, the assay will be positive if the patient has antibodies to any of the antigens in the hepatitis C virus. This assay is inexpensive and is used for screening. False positive results can occur, so a positive result must be repeated to see whether it is repeatedly reactive. After repeated reactive anti-HCV EIA results, a more specific confirmatory test is done (30, 31, 32, 33).

A **recombinant immunoblot assay (RIBA)** that shares similarities with the Western blot has been developed (see Chapter 7). In brief, recombinant antigens or synthetic peptides are manufactured and placed in separate areas on a nitrocellulose strip; then an indirect enzyme immunoassay is performed on the strip with the patient's antibody binding the antigens and enzyme-labeled secondary antibody binding to the patient's antibody; the enzyme causes substrate to change color and precipitate. The currently used RIBA includes recombinant c33c and NS5 antigens and synthetic 5-1-1, c100, and c22 peptides (33).

The molecular techniques test for the presence of viral RNA. They can be qualitative (yes or no for viral presence) or quantitative and yield information about the viral load. Qualitative tests include PCR assays or a transcription-mediated assay. Quantitative assays available include a branched chain DNA assay and a variety of quantitative PCR assays. After a positive molecular result, genotype testing is performed because the

different genotypes of hepatitis C respond differently to treatment. Liver biopsy is performed because people with liver cirrhosis will not respond to therapy. Patients with liver cirrhosis should be screened with alpha 1-fetoprotein (AFP) (Chapter 12) and ultrasound for hepatoma annually (30, 31, 32, 33).

In general, screening begins with the EIA-3; a positive result requires it to be repeated in duplicate, and if these are positive (the serum is repeatedly reactive), 1 of 2 protocols can be used. The protocols differ in the value placed on how high above background the signal in the enzyme immunoassay is. In a protocol that does not use this value, the serum is tested after a repeatedly reactive EIA result as in the flow chart in Figure 17.13 ■. Negatives are, of course, reported and positive results are tested either by RIBA for antibody confirmation or by a molecular technique for viral RNA (30, 31, 32, 33).

If the molecular test is performed next, a positive result is reported and indicates that the patient is currently infected and a negative molecular result is reflexed to the RIBA. If the antibody tests are positive but the molecular tests are negative this patient may be one of the 25% of the hepatitis C patients who cleared the infection; however, the molecular test should be repeated because the patient can be transiently negative for viremia. If the RIBA was performed after the EIA-3 and is positive, a molecular assay is performed. If the molecular assay is positive, the patient is currently infected (30, 31, 32, 33).

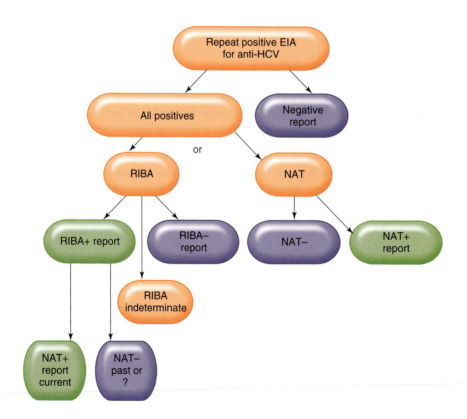

■ **FIGURE 17.13** Flow chart for the diagnosis of hepatitis C. Hepatitis C reporting not using the signal-to-cutoff ratio values from the EIA analysis.

If the signal-to-cutoff ratio is used and the signal from the EIA is high (with the cutoff value being the reading at which a patient's sample would be considered negative), the sample can be confirmed with a molecular test for hepatitis C RNA without a RIBA. A positive EIA that had a low signal-to-cutoff ratio would be followed by a RIBA; if positive, it would be followed by a molecular assay. Figure 17.14 ■. See Table 17.1 ✪ for a summary of CDC recommendations for hepatitis C testing (30, 31, 32, 33).

As in all serological testing for antibody, in hepatitis C testing, the antibody assays of a patient who is immunosuppressed may be negative, so the only way to determine whether the patient is infected is to run the molecular assays.

Treatment

No postexposure prophylaxis is available for hepatitis C because immune globulin is ineffective because antibodies are not protective. For this reason, no vaccine has been developed. Pegylated alpha interferon is combined with ribavirin for treatment. Interferon interferes with viral replication and although ribavirin alone has no effect, adding it to the interferon increases the response rate 2- or 3-fold. About 55% of the patients become negative by molecular assays using this treatment. Genotypes 2 and 3 respond best to therapy (70–80%) and allow a shorter course of drug treatment. Patients who already have cirrhosis do not respond to treatment. Patients who do not have any symptoms with normal liver enzymes may wait to be treated; however, response rates are better when viral load is low. Pegylated interferon has multiple side effects, including those on mood that can cause severe personality changes, aggravation of any autoimmune disease present, and bone marrow suppression whereas ribivirin can cause anemia, so drug treatment is not a trivial choice. Transplantation can be used when liver failure is eminent (33).

✔ **Checkpoint! 17.3**

A man who had been tattooed in prison in 1988 came to the hospital with elevated AST and ALT and hyperbilirubinemia. In prison, tattooing is often done without sterile equipment. He is fatigued and has joint pain. Assays for IgM anti-HAV, IgM anti-HBcAg, HBsAg, and anti-HCV were performed. He was found to have a positive result for anti-HCV in the EIA-3. What should be done?

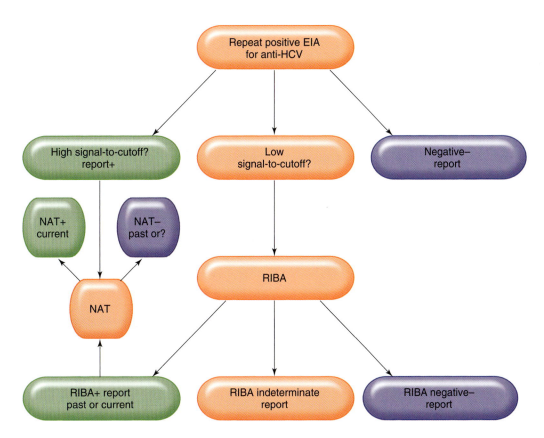

■ **FIGURE 17.14** Flow chart for the diagnosis of hepatitis C. Hepatitis C reporting using the signal-to-cutoff ratio.

✪ TABLE 17.1

Centers for Disease Control and Prevention. Flowchart for Hepatitis C Testing

Reference for Interpretation of Hepatitis C Virus (HCV) Test Results

If Your HCV EIA Test Result Is:			Interpretation		Action
Anti-HCV Screening Test*	Anti-HCV Supplemental Test		Anti-HCV	HCV Infection	Additional Testing or Evaluation
	RIBA	HCV RNA			
Negative	Not Needed	Not Needed	Negative	None	No
Positive	Not Done	Not Done	Not Known	Not Known	Supplemental anti-HCV (RIBA) or HCV RNA
Positive	Not Done	Negative	Not Known	Not Known†	Supplemental anti-HCV (RIBA)
Positive (high s/co ratio§)	Not Done	Not Done	Positive	Past/Current	Evaluate for chronic infection and liver disease
Positive	Negative	Not Needed	Negative	None	No
Positive	Positive	Not Done	Positive	Past/Current	Evaluate for chronic infection and liver disease
Positive	Positive	Negative	Positive	Past/Current†	Report HCV RNA; Evaluate for chronic infection and liver disease
Positive	Positive/Not Done	Positive	Positve	Current	Evaluate for chronic infection and liver disease
Positive	Indeterminate	Not Done	Indeterminate	Not Known	Test for HCV RNA or repeat anti-HVI testing
Positive	Indeterminate	Positive	Positive	Current	Evaluate for chronic infection and live disease
Positive	Indeterminate	Negative	Indeterminate	Not Known†	Test for HVC RNA or repeat anti-HCV testing

* EIA (enzyme immunoassay) or CIA (enhanced chemiluminescence immunoassay).

† Single negative HCV RNA result cannot determine infection status, as persons might have intermittent viremia.

§ Samples with high signal-to-cutoff ratios usually (>95%) confirm positive, but supplemental serologic testing was not performed. Less than 5 of every 100 might represent false positives; more specific testing should be requested, if indicated.

ⓔ CASE STUDY

You live with your friend Meghan who is also in the clinical laboratory scientist program. You have both been vaccinated to prevent hepatitis B. You had all 3 of the shots that you were supposed to, but Meghan received only the first shot. She has an appointment for the next shot in the series right after spring break. During spring break, she went to Mexico and had a great time. Meghan loved the seafood, the music, and the tequila. She mentions to you that although the food was great, she felt that the seafood at the resort she was staying at could have been cooked a bit more. The shrimp and fish still had that kind of transparent look, and the clams were supposed to be steamed but she had to pry them open.

Two weeks later, school is back in session, and you are about to take the fourth immunology exam. Meghan feels tired, her muscles ache, and her eyes look a bit yellow. Hmm, hepatitis is in this section of the immunology exam—or are you just seeing things?

1. What are Meghan's risk factors for viral hepatitis?

2. What should the initial testing be?

3. Meghan's IgM anti-HAV was positive, but all the other assays were negative. What should be done now?

SUMMARY

Hepatitis A and E are spread through fecal-oral contamination, whereas hepatitis B, D, and C are spread through exposure to blood. Hepatitis A and E do not become chronic, but hepatitis B, D, and C can. More than half of the chronic liver disease in the United States results from the effects of hepatitis B and C (Figure 17.15 ■). When a patient with the clinical signs and symptoms of hepatitis with elevated liver enzymes presents, several assays are performed to distinguish among the types of hepatitis viruses seen in the United States (1, 2, 3, 4, 5, 6). Assays for IgM anti-HAV, IgM anti-HBcAg, HBsAg, and anti-HCV are performed. Patients who are positive for hepatitis C should receive the hepatitis B and hepatitis A vaccines to protect their livers from any further damage; similarly, a patient with hepatitis B should receive the vaccine for hepatitis A if he or she has any of the risk factors (33). Although rashes and joint pain are seen in hepatitis B and C but not in hepatitis A or E, an anti-HAV assay may be performed even with these additional symptoms. Hepatitis E is rarely seen in the United States but can be considered in travelers who return and then have symptoms of hepatitis. Rapid diagnosis of any of the hepatitis viruses is important to prevent spread of disease (33).

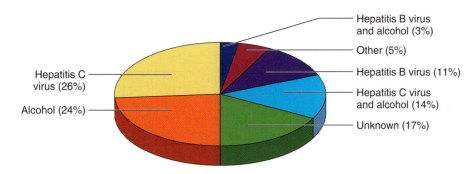

■ **FIGURE 17.15**   Primary causes of chronic liver disease in the United States.

REVIEW QUESTIONS

1. Hepatitis A
   a. spreads through the use of shared needles
   b. spreads through the fecal-oral route
   c. is prevented by the hepatitis vaccine that is required for admission to clinical laboratory science programs
   d. is a DNA virus

2. Hepatitis B
   a. spreads most commonly through blood and sexual transmission
   b. never becomes chronic
   c. is never found in Asia
   d. is not in the saliva of patients

3. Delta hepatitis
   a. is very infectious without any other cofactors or viruses required
   b. coinfects with hepatitis A only
   c. coinfects with hepatitis B only
   d. coinfects with hepatitis C only

4. I ate raw clams that came from South America and later I began to feel ill with a tender right upper abdominal quadrant and the yellowing of the whites of my eyes. I developed elevated liver enzymes. A laboratory scientist who analyzed my test results said that I did not have type A or B hepatitis. Which type of hepatitis did I probably have?
   a. hepatitis A
   b. hepatitis B
   c. hepatitis D
   d. hepatitis E

5. Between the time that I ate the raw clams and the time I began to feel ill, I decided to take a part-time job on the weekends because my kids wanted a pool in the backyard. I had a job in a local restaurant as a waitress. Considering how this virus spreads will this be a problem?
   a. yes
   b. no

6. Etiologic agents of viral hepatitis are all of the following except:
   a. Epstein-Barr virus
   b. hepatitis C virus
   c. hepatitis B virus
   d. hepatitis A virus

7. Hepatitis E
   a. spreads through the use of shared needles
   b. spreads through the fecal-oral route
   c. is prevented by the hepatitis vaccine
   d. is a DNA virus

8. Hepatitis C
   a. spreads most commonly through blood
   b. never becomes chronic
   c. is never found in Asia
   d. always causes a mild disease

9. Which type of hepatitis virus cannot infect by itself?
   a. hepatitis A
   b. hepatitis B
   c. hepatitis C
   d. hepatitis D

10. A 16-year-old female IV drug user comes to the hospital with yellow skin and yellowing in the whites of her eyes. Chemical analysis shows elevated liver enzymes. She has a rash on her skin and has arthritis in multiple joints in her body. She has protein in her urine. Of the following, which is probably the causative agent of her disease?
    a. hepatitis A
    b. hepatitis B
    c. hepatitis D
    d. hepatitis E

REVIEW QUESTIONS *(Continued)*

11. Referring to Question 10, which of the girl's contacts should be tested?
    a. those who are needle sharers
    b. those who are in the same classroom
    c. those who are sexual contacts
    d. A and C

12. Fred tests positive for anti-HBsAg, and his test for HBeAg is now negative. This indicates that he is
    a. a chronic carrier
    b. acutely infected
    c. in recovery with good prognosis
    d. coinfected with delta hepatitis

REFERENCES

1. Daniels D, Grytdal S, Wasley A. Surveillance for acute viral hepatitis—United States, 2007 *MMWR*. Surveillance summaries: /CDC. 05/22/2009; 58(SS03):1–27. http://www.cdc.gov/mmwr/preview/mmwrhtml/ss5803a1.htm. Accessed March 18, 2012.

2. http://www.who.int/mediacentre/factsheets/fs280/en/. Accessed May 21, 2012.

3. http://www.webmd.com/hepatitis/understanding-hepatitis-basics. Accessed May 21, 2012.

4. Hepatic and biliary disorders: Testing for hepatic and biliary disorders: Laboratory tests. *Merck Manual for Health Care Professionals*. http://www.merck.com/mmpe/sec03/ch023/ch023b.html#CEGCJEFJ. Accessed March 19, 2012.

5. Acute hepatitis. *Merck Manual for Health Care Professionals*. http://www.merck.com/mmpe/sec03/ch027/ch027b.html#sec03-ch027-ch027b-438. Accessed March 19, 2012.

6. Teo C-G. Other Infectious Diseases Related to Travel. *CDC Travelers Health* (Yellow Book). 2011: chap 5. http://wwwnc.cdc.gov/travel/yellowbook/2010/chapter-5/hepatitis-e.aspx. Accessed March 19, 2012

7. Kalia H, Martin P. Acute viral hepatitis. In: Schlosssberg D, ed. *Clinical Infectious Disease*. New York, NY: Cambridge University Press; 2008: chap 42.

8. Abbott AXSYM System HAVAB 2.0 product manual. Abbott Park, IL: Abbott Laboratories Diagnostic Division.

9. Hepatitis A information for health professionals. http://www.cdc.gov/hepatitis/HAV/index.htm. Accessed March 19, 2012.

10. Hepatitis A FAQs for health professionals. http://www.cdc.gov/hepatitis/HAV/index.htm. Accessed March 19, 2012.

11. Yao JDC. Laboratory Testing for Hepatitis A and E. http://www.mayomedicallaboratories.com/mediax/articles/hottopics/2008-09-hav/2008-09-hav-handout.pdf. Accessed March 19, 2012.

12. Lemon SM. Type A viral hepatitis: Epidemiology, diagnosis, and prevention. *Clin Chem*. 1997;43:1494–1499. http://www.clinchem.org/cgi/content/full/43/8/1494 . Accessed March 19, 2012.

13. Epidemiologic notes and reports hepatitis A among drug abusers. *MMWR Weekly*. 1988;37(19);297–300, 305. http://www.cdc.gov/mmwr/preview/mmwrhtml/00000024.htm. Accessed March 19, 2012.

14. World Health Organization. Hepatitis E. http://www.who.int/mediacentre/factsheets/fs280/en/. Accessed May 21, 2012.

15. Centers for Disease Control and Prevention. Hepatitis E FAQs for health professionals. http://www.cdc.gov/hepatitis/HEV/HEVfaq.htm#section1. Accessed March 19, 2012.

16. Hepatitis E Vaccine: A time of testing. http://www.niaid.nih.gov/topics/hepatitis/hepatitisE/Pages/nepalHepEVaccine.aspx. Accessed May 21, 2012.

17. Hepatitis E Vaccine: The story of the hepatitis E Vaccine. National Institute of Allergy and Infectious Disease. http://www.niaid.nih.gov/topics/hepatitis/hepatitisE/Pages/storyHepatitisEVaccine.aspx. Accessed March 19, 2012.

18. Zhu F-C, Zhang J, Zhang X-F, et al. Efficacy and safety of a recombinant hepatitis E vaccine in healthy adults: A large-scale, randomised, double-blind placebo-controlled, phase 3 trial. *Lancet*. 2010;376(9744): 895–902. doi: 10.1016/S0140-6736(10)61030-6.

19. Hepatitis E vaccine: Why wait? *Lancet*. 2010;376:845. http://www.thelancet.com/journals/lancet/article/PIIS0140-6736%2810%2961393-1/fulltext. Accessed June 1,2012.

20. Hepatitis B National Institute of Allergy and Infectious Disease. http://www.niaid.nih.gov/topics/hepatitis/hepatitisB/Pages/Default.aspx. Accessed March 19, 2012.

21. Centers for Disease Control and Prevention. Hepatitis B FAQs for health professionals. http://www.cdc.gov/hepatitis/HBV/HBVfaq.htm. Accessed March 19, 2012.

22. Centers for Disease Control and Prevention. Testing and Public Health Management of Persons with Chronic Hepatitis B Virus Infection. http://www.cdc.gov/hepatitis/HBV/TestingChronic.htm. Accessed March 19, 2012.

23. World Health Organization. Hepatitis B. http://www.who.int/mediacentre/factsheets/fs204/en/. Accessed March 19, 2012.

24. Biomerieux Clinical Diagnostics Hepatitis Fact Sheet: Hepatitis B. http://www.biomerieux-diagnostics.com/servlet/srt/bio/clinical-diagnostics/dynPage?node=viral_hepatitis. Accessed March 19, 2012.

25. Taylor JM. Hepatitis delta virus. *Review Article Virology*. 2006;344(1):71–76.

26. Previsani N, Lavanchy D. World Health Organization hepatitis delta. http://www.who.int/csr/disease/hepatitis/HepatitisD_whocdscsrncs2001_1.pdf. Accessed March 19, 2012.

27. Centers for Disease Control and Prevention. Hepatitis C FAQs for health professionals. http://www.cdc.gov/hepatitis/HCV/HCVfaq.htm#section1. Accessed March 19, 2012.

28. Hepatitis C: The test on lab tests online. http://www.labtestsonline.org/understanding/analytes/hepatitis_c/test.html#. Accessed March 19, 2012.

29. Cryoglobulin: On lab tests online. http://www.labtestsonline.org/understanding/analytes/cryoglobulin/test.html#. Accessed March 19, 2012.

30. Pascual M, Perrin L, Giostra E, et al. Hepatitis C virus in patients with cryoglobulinemia type II. *J Infect Dis*. 1990;162(2):569–570.

31. National Digestive Diseases Information Clearinghouse, Hepatitis C: Current Disease Management. http://consensus.nih.gov/2002/2002Hepatitisc2002116html.htm/. Accessed March 19, 2012.

32. Chiron Hepatitis C Virus Encoded Antigen (Recombinant c33c and NS5 antigens; Synthesis 5-1-1, c100 and c22 peptides) Chiron*RIBA*HCV 30 SIA Product insert. Date issue February 1999.

33. New York State Department of Health Clinical Guidelines for the Medical Management of Hepatitis C. http://www.health.ny.gov/publications/1840/. Accessed March 19, 2012.

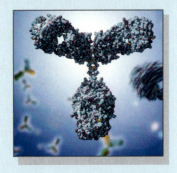

18

Herpesviridae Family and Other Serologically Diagnosed Viruses

■ OBJECTIVES—LEVEL I

After this chapter, the student should be able to:

1. Describe the similarities of the viruses of the Herpesviridae family.
2. Discuss Epstein-Barr virus (EBV) in terms of virus type, infection course, immunity, and population affected.
3. Describe the following viral antigens in terms of when antibodies form and when the antigens are present: viral capsid antigen (VCA), EBV early antigen diffuse (EA-D), early antigen restricted (EA-R), EBV early antigen, and EBV nuclear antigen (EBNA).
4. Describe the incubation period of EBV.
5. Describe a heterophile Ag and differentiate between the Davidsohn differential tests of infectious mononucleosis, Forssman Ab, and serum sickness.
6. Describe how an infectious mononucleosis diagnosis is made.
7. Describe the etiology of cytomegalovirus (CMV) in terms of viral family.
8. Describe the different routes of CMV infection and delineate the fluids that contain CMV.
9. Discuss the effects of a congenital CMV infection.
10. Compare and contrast the clinical signs and symptoms of CMV in a healthy individual, a pregnant woman, a newborn, and an immunocompromised individual.
11. Describe herpes simplex 1 and 2 disease and diagnosis.
12. Describe varicella zoster virus disease and diagnosis.
13. Describe rubeola (measles) in terms of disease and diagnosis.
14. Evaluate the significance of serologic and molecular biology laboratory results.
15. Describe the etiology and epidemiology of rubella infection.
16. Explain the signs and symptoms of acquired and congenital rubella infection.
17. Compare the immunologic manifestations of acquired and congenital rubella infections.
18. Describe the use of the enzyme immunoassay for rubella.
19. Describe laboratory diagnosis of varicella.
20. Describe the difference between a primary infection with varicella zoster and a reactivation.
21. Define toxoplasmosis, other infections, rubella, cytomegalovirus, and herpes simplex virus (TORCH).
22. Describe the signs and symptoms of mumps.
23. Describe the signs and symptoms of influenza.
24. Describe the signs and symptoms of West Nile virus infection.

After this chapter, the student should be able to:

1. Interpret case histories with emphasis on the clinical symptoms and pathogenesis of the disease and the role of the clinical laboratory tests in diagnosis and evaluation.

2. Analyze the clinical significance of 1 positive serological test for CMV in a pregnant woman. Compare this with the significance of an increase in a paired titer. What tests are performed to analyze for this infection?

3. Compare and contrast how a CMV infection should be treated in a healthy individual, a pregnant woman, a newborn, and an immunocompromised individual such as a tranplant recipient.

4. Describe the varicella zoster vaccine.

5. Describe the reason that 1 case of mumps brought into this country could result in ~2000 cases.

KEY TERMS

congenital rubella syndrome
cytomegalovirus (CMV)
Davidsohn differential
Epstein-Barr virus (EBV)
Forssman antigen
herpes simplex virus 1 (HSV1)
herpes simplex virus 2 (HSV2)
Herpesviridae family
heterophile antibody
infectious mononucleosis
influenza
measles
Mono-Diff test
monospot test

mumps
Paramyxoviridae family
Paul-Bunnell antigen
Reyes syndrome
rubella
serology
seropositive
serum sickness antigen
toxoplasmosis, other infections, rubella, cytomegalovirus, and herpes simplex virus (TORCH)
varicella zoster virus (VZV)
West Nile virus (WNV)

▶ INTRODUCTION

In the previous chapter, the hepatitis viruses were grouped together because they all cause a disease of the liver. Viruses are placed in this chapter because an important part of their diagnosis involves **serology,** which is defined as the study of serum or other bodily fluids for the detection of antibodies or antigens. This chapter discusses many of the viruses that are diagnosed by serological techniques with the exception of human immunodeficiency virus, which is covered in a chapter by itself because of its worldwide importance.

More than one system is used to classify viruses, and although classification can be based on many different criteria, most classification schemes include stratification based on the genetic material in the virus. Classification of viruses is based in part on whether the genetic material is DNA or RNA, double-stranded or single-stranded, a positive or negative strand, segmented or not segmented, linear or circular. Many other characteristics can be involved in classifications

including whether the virus is enveloped or non-enveloped and what proteins or enzymes are produced (1).

Many viruses are diagnosed either by using molecular techniques or by incubation with cells followed by analysis of the cytopathic (cellular changes) effect produced by the viral infection. The viruses discussed first in this chapter are all members of the **Herpesviridae family,** which are viruses that contain double-stranded DNA (ds DNA) and have a latency period. Rubella, a Togavirus, is described after the Herpesviridae family and is important because infection during pregnancy has severe consequences. Measles (rubeola) and mumps are paramyxoviruses that caused common childhood diseases in this country until a successful vaccine was developed. Both measles and mumps are still prevalent in countries with low immunization rates and can still be brought into the United States by travelers. West Nile virus (WNV) is an emerging infection in the United States; although many cases of WNV can be subclinical, infection can lead to severe consequences. The final virus to be discussed in this chapter is influenza, which is included because of the seasonal surge in cases every year with risks of influenza pandemics never far from mind (1).

▶ THE HERPESVIRIDAE FAMILY

The Herpesviridae family includes Epstein-Barr virus (EBV), cytomegalovirus (CMV), herpes simplex virus 1 (HSV1), herpes simplex virus 2 (HSV2), and varicella zoster virus (VZV). These are all DNA viruses that contain linear double-stranded DNA, are enveloped, and have an icosahedral capsid (Figure 18.1 ■). An important feature of this family is that all of the viruses exhibit latency and cause lifelong infections.

✓ **Checkpoint! 18.1**

What viruses are in the Herpesviridae family?

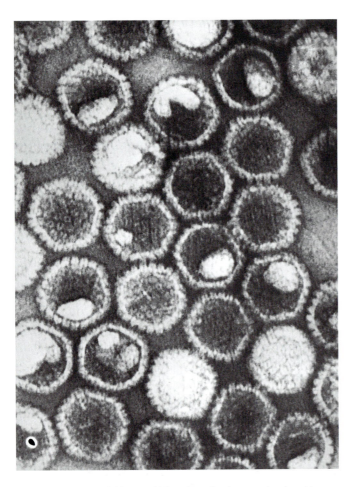

■ **FIGURE 18.1**   A Herpesviridae virus, the herpes simplex virion. It has an icosahedral capsid with double-stranded DNA. *Source:* © CDC/Dr. Fred Murphy; Sylvia Whitfield.

EPSTEIN-BARR VIRUS

Epidemiology

Epstein-Barr virus (EBV) is the causative agent for infectious mononucleosis and is associated with Burkitt's lymphoma and nasopharyngeal carcinoma. Infection results from direct contact with saliva of an infected person, not through air or blood. It is spread through shared drinking glasses and straws and through kissing, hence the common name the "kissing disease." The symptoms of the disease begin 30 to 50 days after infection (2, 3).

Throughout the world, half the children have EBV infections by the time they are 5 years old and have mild unremarkable or asymptomatic disease. Approximately 95% of adults worldwide are **seropositive** for EBV. In developed countries, the age of acquiring the infection is later, but this percentage of adults is still seropositive. Many children in the United States have relatively mild EBV infections early in life. However, when people are infected with EBV during the teenage years and early adulthood, infectious mononucleosis, instead of mild or asymptomatic disease, develops in 35 to 50% of the cases. **Infectious mononucleosis** involves the familiar clinical symptoms of malaise, sore throat, enlarged tonsils, fever, and swollen glands. Enlarged spleen and liver damage (hepatitis) can occur, and care must be taken not to rupture the spleen (Figures 18.2 ■ and 18.3 ■) (2, 3).

The symptoms can last for 1 to 2 months, but the virus remains in a latent form for the patient's lifetime. Reactivations occur during which saliva contains active virus, but symptoms rarely return. In a very small number of people with latent EBV infections, Burkitt's lymphoma or nasopharyngeal cancer can develop. Although associated with these cancers, EBV alone does not cause these malignancies. Burkitt's lymphoma (Figure 18.4 ■) is seen primarily in Africa and New Guinea. Nasopharyngeal carcinoma is seen primarily in southern China and Greenland and among Eskimos (2, 3, 4).

Diagnosis and Treatment

Patients with infectious mononucleosis exhibit an elevated white blood cell count and produce reactive lymphocytes (Figure 18.5 ■). These symptoms, the age of the patients, and the results of the serologic tests **monospot test** and **Mono-Diff test** are used to diagnose infectious mononucleosis. Patients with infectious mononucleosis have heterophile antibodies.

Heterophile antibody (Chapter 2) is defined as an antibody that reacts with antigens from 2 or more species in a pattern without evolutionary relatedness. Heterophile antibodies are usually IgM antibodies and are often found to react with carbohydrate antigens. Paul and Bunnell found that people with infectious mononucleosis make heterophile antibodies that agglutinate sheep red blood cells. The antigen on the sheep red blood cells that reacts with the infectious mononucleosis serum is the **Paul-Bunnell antigen.** This property led to the development of an inexpensive assay for infectious mononucleosis called the monospot test (2, 3).

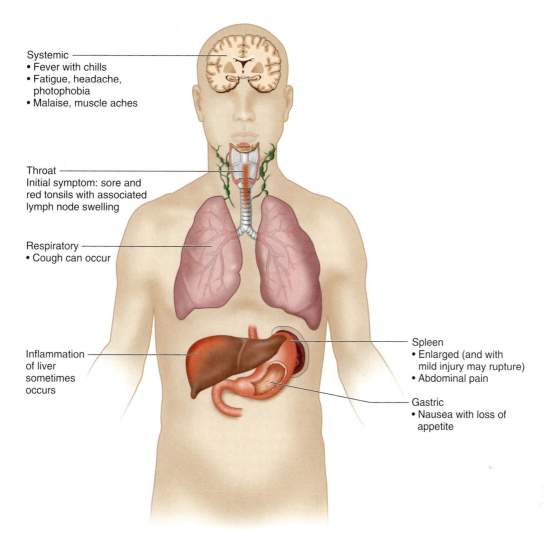

Systemic
• Fever with chills
• Fatigue, headache, photophobia
• Malaise, muscle aches

Throat
Initial symptom: sore and red tonsils with associated lymph node swelling

Respiratory
• Cough can occur

Inflammation of liver sometimes occurs

Spleen
• Enlarged (and with mild injury may rupture)
• Abdominal pain

Gastric
• Nausea with loss of appetite

■ **FIGURE 18.2**   The symptoms of infectious mononucleosis.

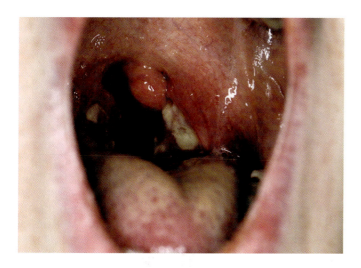

■ **FIGURE 18.3**   Diffuse pharyngeal erythema seen with infectious mononucleosis. *Source:* © Hercules/Robinson/Alamy.

The monospot test, also called the *presumptive test,* mixes patient serum with sheep red blood cells. If the cells agglutinate, this is a presumptive positive result for infectious mononucleosis. However, this is complicated by the fact that 2 other types of serum can cause agglutination of sheep red blood cells: normal patients with antibody to **Forssman antigen** and people who have had serum sickness and react with an antigen on the sheep red blood cells because of previous stimulation with animal serum. Serum sickness and Forssman antibodies also react with guinea pig kidney, but infectious mononucleosis antibodies do not. Serum sickness and infectious mononucleosis antibodies react with bovine erythrocyte stroma, but Forssman antibodies do not (2, 3).

The Mono-Diff (or Davidsohn differential) test exploits these differences to differentially diagnose patients with infectious mononucleosis. In the Mono-Diff test (Figures 18.6 ■, 18.7 ■, 18.8 ■, and Table 18.1 ✪) the patient serum is placed

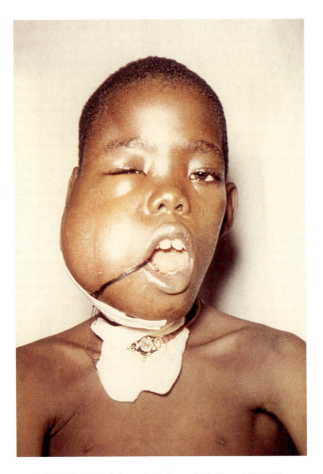

■ **FIGURE 18.4** A large facial manifestation of Burkitt's lymphoma, a non-Hodgkin's lymphoma, in a Nigerian boy. *Source:* © CDC/Rober S. Craig.

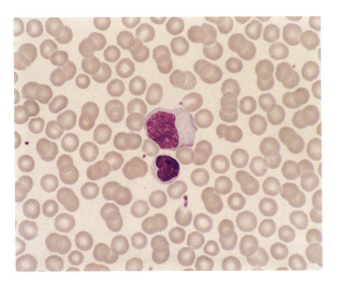

■ **FIGURE 18.5** Two lymphocytes that are reactive in a 19-year-old college student with infectious mononucleosis. Note large amount of cytoplasm but no nucleolus. *Source:* Joaquin Carrillo-Farga/Photo Researchers, Inc.

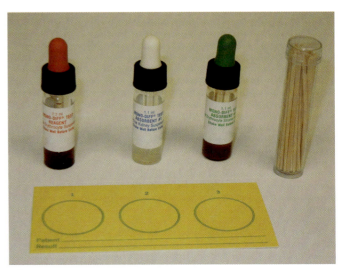

(a)

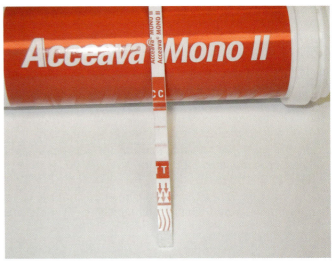

(b)

■ **FIGURE 18.6** (a) A Mono-Diff test. This test contains the indicator cells for the presumptive test and for absorptions, a kidney extract and a suspension of bovine erythrocyte stroma. (b) The Acceava mono immunochromotograaphy rapid test. *Source:* Alere Inc.—Acceava Monoll is an Alere product. All nghts reserved.

in the first circle on the card and is mixed with the indicator sheep or horse red blood cells, and after three minutes the cells are observed for agglutination. If these cells agglutinate, the next 2 steps are performed. In the next circle, the patient serum is mixed first with a guinea pig kidney cell suspension and then the indicator red blood cells are added. In the last circle, first the serum is mixed with bovine erythrocyte stroma and then with the indicator red blood cells. If agglutination is observed in the first circle (the presumptive) and the second circle (kidney absorption) but not in the third circle, the

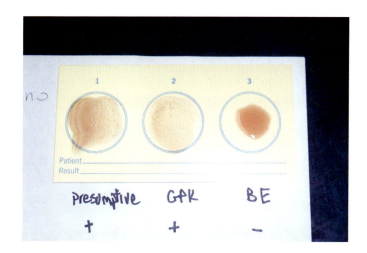

■ **FIGURE 18.7**   A Mono-Diff test in which the presumptive well contains the patient's serum mixed with indicator red blood cells (1) (agglutination+); in the GPK circle, the serum was mixed first with guinea pig kidney (2) (agglutination+) and then the indicator red blood cells were added; in the BE circle, the serum was premixed with bovine erythrocyte stroma; and then the indicator red blood cells were added (3) (agglutination−). This differential shows that the patient has infectious mononucleosis.

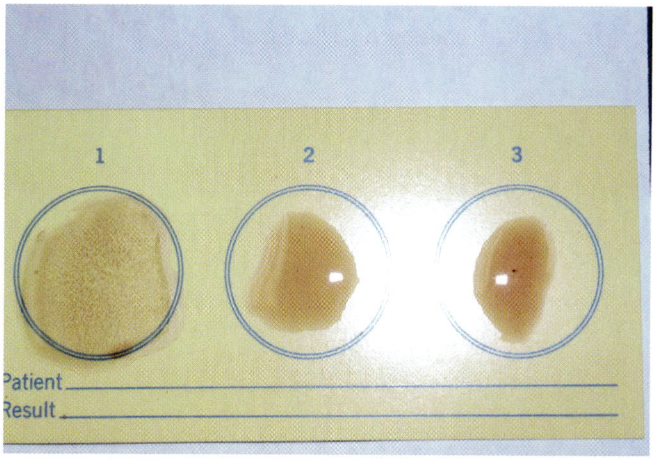

■ **FIGURE 18.8**   A Mono-Diff test in which the presumptive well contains the patient's serum mixed with indicator red blood cells (1) (agglutination+); in the GPK circle, the serum was mixed first with guinea pig kidney (2) (agglutination−), and then the indicator red blood cells were added; in the BE circle, the serum was premixed with bovine erythrocyte stroma, and then the indicator red blood cells were added (3) (agglutination−). This differential shows that the patient has serum sickness.

patient has infectious mononucleosis (Figure 18.7). A patient who has agglutination in the first circle but not in either of the other circles has serum sickness. A patient whose serum causes agglutination in the first and last circles has Forssman antibodies (2, 3).

The **Davidsohn differential** can be explained with the help of Figure 18.9 ■. This figure depicts the Paul-Bunnell antigen of infectious mononucleosis as a circle, the Forssman antigen as a square, and the **serum sickness antigen** as a triangle. The sheep red blood cells have all 3 of these antigens on their surface, which is why all 3 of these sera agglutinate sheep red blood cells. The guinea pig kidney has on its surface the antigen of serum sickness as indicated by a triangle and the Forssman antigen by a square. Thus, an antibody from

✪ **TABLE 18.1**

Results Seen in Mono-Diff Tests

Heterophile Antibody Type	Agglutination of Sheep Red Blood Cells 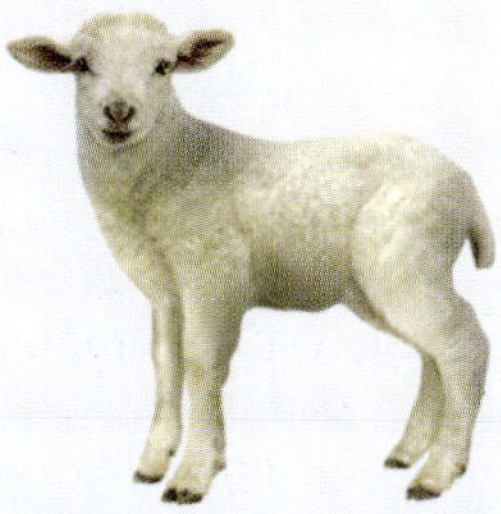	Agglutination of Sheep Red Blood Cells (after absorption with guinea pig or horse kidney) 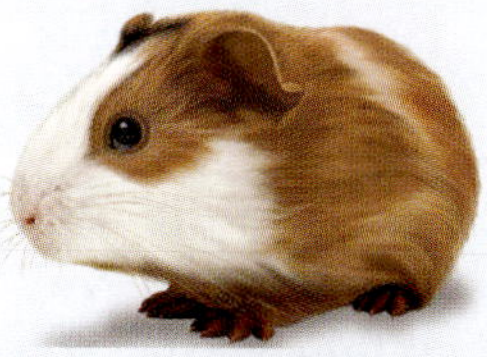	Agglutination of Sheep Red Blood Cells (after absorption with bovine erythrocyte stroma) 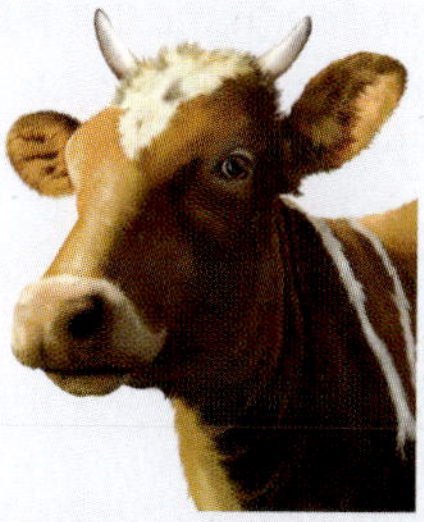
Infectious mononucleosis	+	+	−
Forssman	+	−	+
Serum sickness	+	−	−

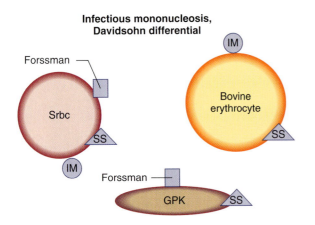

Infectious mononucleosis, Davidsohn differential

■ **FIGURE 18.9**   A schematic showing how the Davidsohn differential works.

a patient with either Forssman antibody or serum sickness antibody will bind to the guinea pig kidney and none will be left to agglutinate the sheep red blood cells. Finally, the bovine erythrocytes contain the infectious mononucleosis antigen depicted by the circle and the serum sickness antigen depicted by the triangle; thus, when preincubated with the bovine erythrocytes, both of these antibodies will bind and will not be available for agglutination of the red blood cells (2, 3).

Serum sickness, which was discussed in Chapter 9, is a type III hypersensitivity reaction that develops when a patient with a disease such as diphtheria or tetanus receives an antitoxin developed by immunizing an animal with the toxin. The patient develops antibodies to the serum proteins and antibody of the species that produced the protective antibodies. The patient antibody would react with the animal antigens and, if in high enough concentrations, immune complexes would form in the patient, causing damage. Since the advent of vaccines to these pathogens, passive transfer of immunoglobulin is not often used in this way, and few patients have serum sickness antibodies. The result of this is that the monospot can be simplified because there is no longer concern about the serum sickness antibody. Take a moment before you read further to look at Figure 18.9. By looking at this figure and realizing that you do not need to worry about false positive reactions from people with serum sickness, could you invent a new test?

We hope you took a moment and that you realize that you have wonderful problem-solving skills because you would develop an assay using bovine erythrocytes. If you came to this conclusion, congratulations! That is the basis of the new assays, which involve a yes or no reaction with the bovine erythrocyte antigen. A common type of this assay is similar to the human chorionic gonadotropin (hCG) immunochromatographic pregnancy test described in Chapter 7.

In the hCG sandwich assay test strip, colloid-labeled antibody to hCG binds the hCG, and they travel together up the strip and bind to another hCG antibody "painted" on a line farther up the strip. The hCG pregnancy test is an antibody-antigen-antibody sandwich. In the immunochromatographic assay for infectious mononucleosis using a related heterophile antigen, colored bovine erythrocyte antigen binds to the heterophile infectious mononucleosis antibody, and they travel together up the strip until they bind to an antigen-coated area on the strip and form a line. This is an antigen-antibody-antigen sandwich. Remember that heterophile antibodies are usually IgM antibodies, and the multiple binding sites facilitate this type of sandwich assay (2, 3). A possible problem for this assay is that patients now can be treated with humanized mouse monoclonal antibodies for autoimmune disease and for cancer, and may develop antibodies to the humanized mouse antibody, called human anti-mouse antibodies (HAMA). The effects of HAMA on this new assay for infectious mononucleosis must be determined. However, the age groups who receive the monoclonal antibody therapy are in general older than the age group that will be screened for mononucleosis so this should minimize any problems.

With the modification, the diagnostic assay is now easier, requiring one step instead of three for most patients; however, 10 to 15% of the infectious mononucleosis patients do not have a positive test for antibody to these heterophile antigens. A different assay must be done for patients with the signs and symptoms of infectious mononucleosis who have negative heterophile tests to differentiate whether this is a false negative infectious mononucleosis case or a cytomegalovirus infection, an adenovirus infection, or a *Toxoplasma gondii* infection. The additional testing is viral-specific antigen testing. Like diagnosis of hepatitis B, diagnosis of a presumptive antibody negative infectious mononucleosis patient utilizes several different antigens and antibodies. The assays used are IgM and IgG to the Epstein-Barr viral capsid antigen (VCA), IgM to the EBV early antigen (EA-D), and antibody to the EBV nuclear antigen (EBNA) (2, 3).

IgM antibody to the viral capsid antigen appears first and then IgG to this antigen, which lasts a lifetime, occurs. IgG to the viral capsid antigen indicates that the patient is not susceptible to infection because they have recovered from a past infection. IgG to EA-D occurs in about a week but disappears quickly. Antibody to EBNA is slow to occur but then lasts a lifetime. Current infectious mononucleosis is indicated by a positive anti-VCA and a negative anti-EBNA. The presence of antibody to EBNA and VCA indicates past infection. Antibodies to early antigen and antibodies to EBNA indicate reactivation. See Figure 18.10 ■ for the time course of the appearance and disappearance of these antibodies. The symptoms of infectious mononucleosis are treated with no attempts to decrease viral load because this is a self-resolving disease (2, 3).

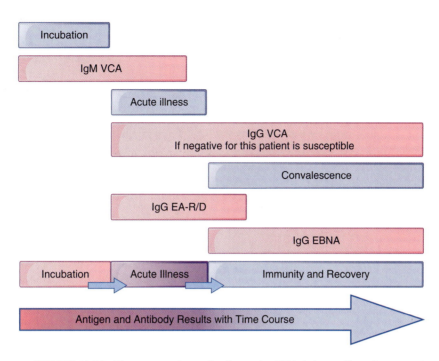

■ **FIGURE 18.10**   Time course for antibodies to the EBV viral–specific antigens.

CYTOMEGALOVIRUS

Epidemiology

Cytomegalovirus (CMV), another member of the Herpesviridae family, was briefly introduced in the transplantation section in Chapter 14. CMV is spread by close contact through saliva, urine, or other body fluids. In the United States, 50 to 80% of adults have been infected with cytomegalovirus by the time they are 40. Most people are asymptomatic, but some may experience sore throat, fatigue, fever, or swollen glands, all of which are symptoms similar to those seen in infectious mononucleosis (5).

CMV is important clinically because it can cause serious disease in immunocompromised people including transplant recipients and can cause birth defects. Of babies born with congenital exposure to CMV, 80% are asymptomatic at birth and remain so. Ten percent of the babies are symptomatic at birth, may be born prematurely, and may have liver, spleen, and/or lung problems. These infants may have a small head size, small overall size, and may have seizures at birth. They also may have hearing loss and/or vision loss, lack of coordination, and may die soon after birth. The remaining 10% of newborns who are infected *in utero,* although asymptomatic at birth, develop vision and hearing problems up to 2 years after birth. Cytomegalovirus is also a major problem in immunocompromised people including transplant recipients and people with HIV infections or lymphoproliferative diseases and those taking immunosuppressant drugs. The manifestations of CMV seen in these individuals include pneumonia, retinitis, and gastrointestinal disease. CMV infections in immunocompromised individuals can result in death (5).

Diagnosis and Treatment

CMV can be diagnosed by PCR, viral culture, or by Ab tests for IgM or IgG to CMV. For IgG diagnosis, paired samples of serum obtained in the acute and the convalescent phase should be analyzed for IgG to CMV with a 4-fold rise indicating a current infection. An alternative to paired serum analysis that allows earlier diagnosis involves tests to analyze for low affinity IgG, which indicates an acute infection prior to affinity maturation. IgM levels are positive in an initial infection and in reactivation of the infection. It is important to note that false negative serological tests can result when the tested patient is immunocompromised (5).

CMV is one of a group of infectious agents that cause congenital infections and birth defects. The acronym for this group is TORCH and it includes **toxoplasmosis, other infections, rubella, cytomegalovirus, and herpes simplex virus.** Infants are tested for these infections at birth (5).

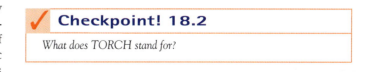

✓ Checkpoint! 18.2

What does TORCH stand for?

HERPES SIMPLEX 1 AND 2

Epidemiology

Herpes simplex viruses are also in the Herpesviridae family and like all members of this family, have an icosahedral capsid with double-stranded DNA. **Herpes simplex virus 1 (HSV1)**

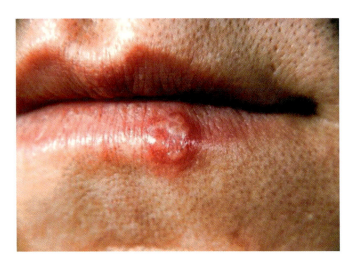

and **herpes simplex virus 2 (HSV2)** can cause a "cold sore" at the mouth or can cause genital herpes, depending upon the site of infection. HSV1 is most often associated with the oral cold sore (Figure 18.11 ■) whereas HSV2 is most often associated with sexually transmitted genital lesions (Figure 18.12 ■). Most people infected with these viruses have minimal or no symptoms. The symptom of infection that occurs at either the mouth or genitals is the appearance of painful blisters in the region. These blisters burst and create sores, which can last 2 to 4 weeks. The blister often reappears more than once, often 4 or 5 times the first year after infection. As time goes on, each successive occurrence is usually less severe (6, 7, 8, 9).

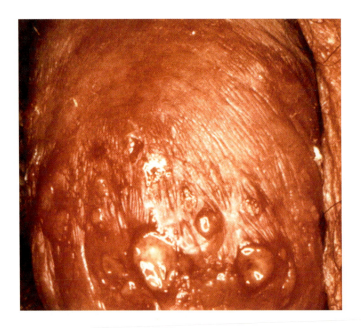

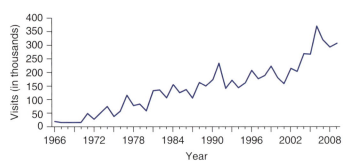

■ **FIGURE 18.13**   Genital herpes—U.S. initial visits to physicians' offices, 1866–2009.

Symptoms of HSV can be very severe in the immunosuppressed and can require hospitalization as the result of disseminated infection, hepatitis, or central nervous system (CNS) effects. The genital infection is quite common; a recent survey showed a slight decrease to ~17% of the population (or 1 of every 6 people!) between 14 and 49 years of age (Figure 18.13 ■). Genital herpes is transmitted from an infected person when the sore or symptoms are present, so those infected should abstain from sex with an uninfected partner during this time. Abstinence at these times, while helpful, will not stop all transmission because the virus can be spread when the infected partner shows no signs or symptoms of it. The open sores of herpes viral infections can increase the risk of HIV transmission. People with genital herpes should use condoms, which can reduce transmission, but condoms do not cover all areas that can transmit or be infected by the virus (6, 7, 8, 9).

As mentioned, HSV is in the group of agents that can cause TORCH congenital infections. If a woman has an obvious herpes infection with sores at the time of delivery, the child is delivered by caesarean section rather than vaginally to reduce the risk of transmission. A primary infection with herpes virus in late pregnancy increases the risk of transmission to the baby. The risk of transmission from a mother to her infant is low, but infection in the infant if left untreated often progresses to serious disseminated disease. Babies can have skin lesions, which are blisters with a red base that burst and crust over (Figure 18.14 ■). Of infected infants, 35% have developmental abnormalities because of a HSV infection of their central nervous system, and 25% progress to disseminated infection affecting the liver and respiratory system. The prognosis of disseminated disease in infants is very poor with more than 50% dying of the disease and the rest developing long-term developmental problems (6, 7, 8, 9).

Diagnosis and Treatment

Viral culture of HSV1 and 2 from genital lesions is not very sensitive, and PCR assays are not yet FDA approved for diagnosis. Assays that look for virus may be negative because viral shedding is mainly present when lesions are evident, which is intermittent.

Serological evidence of infection is an FDA-approved testing method for HSV and is used to type the infection. For

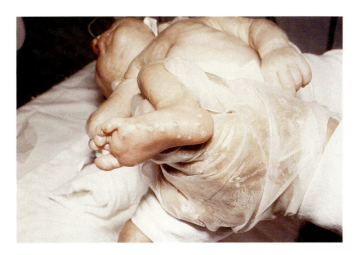

■ **FIGURE 18.14** Congenital herpes simplex infection. *Source:* © CDC/Judith Faulk.

the most accurate typing of whether the patient has HSV1 or HSV2, serotype specific glycoprotein G (gG)-based assays should be performed. Point-of-care tests are available for HSV2 diagnosis (Figure 18.15 ■). False positive tests may be obtained and is a particularly important possibility when testing people who are of low risk. Testing is important because proper education should reduce the risk of spread. It is important to note that false negative serological tests can result when the tested patient is immunocompromised (6, 7, 8, 9).

Antiviral therapy is used in symptomatic patients to decrease symptoms, and proper condom use and abstinence during outbreaks can reduce the risk of spread. The antivirals that are useful include oral therapy with acyclovir, valacyclovir, and famciclovir. Topical therapy has not been found to be effective. Intravenous therapy with acyclovir is recommended in severe infections and in infections of infants.

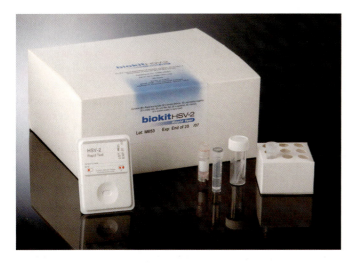

■ **FIGURE 18.15** Herpes simplex 2 rapid test. *Source:* Hardy Diagnostics, www.hardydiagnostics.com

VARICELLA ZOSTER

Epidemiology

Chicken pox and shingles are caused by another member of the Herpesviridae family, the **varicella zoster virus (VZV).** On primary infection, this virus causes a blistering rash (with ~250–500 blistery lesions common) on the body with the lesions found mostly on the head and trunk (Figure 18.16 ■). This is accompanied by a fever in most individuals. Headache, photophobia, fever, and diarrhea may also occur. VZV is highly contagious and is spread by aerosols produced by coughing and sneezing and by the skin lesions both by aerosols and

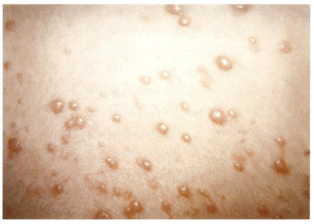

(a)

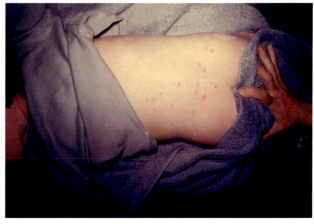

(b)

■ **FIGURE 18.16** (a) Chicken pox vesicles. *Source:* © CDC/ Joe Miller. (b) Chicken pox on back of young patient. *Source:* © CDC/Dr. Heinz F. Eichenwald.

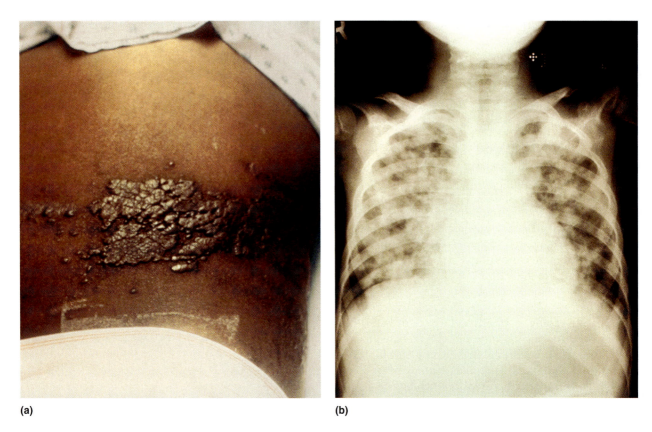

(a)   (b)

■ **FIGURE 18.17** (a) Varicella zoster virus recurring as shingles, a painful rash limited to an area enervated by 1 or 2 nerves. This occurs in 20% of all people living in the United States. The virus, latent since the original chicken pox infection, is reactivated by age, stress, or being immunocompromised. *Source:* CDC. (b) Chest x-ray of a child showing pulmonary manifestations of a chicken pox infection. This child was immunocompromised because of leukemia. *Source:* © CDC/Dr. Joel D. Meyers.

direct contact. The patient is infectious 1 to 2 days before the rash appears and remains infectious until every blister has formed a scab. The symptoms appear 2 to 3 weeks after exposure. Complications include bacterial skin infections that occur when the patient scratches the itchy blisters and also the more serious pneumonia and encephalitis (Figure 18.7(b)). About 10% of patients develop complications severe enough to see their health care provider, and 2% are hospitalized. This is an important consideration for those who are "on the fence" about vaccination. The secondary bacterial infections—pneumonia and the encephalitis—can be life threatening, so vaccination is important (10, 11, 12, 13).

Chicken pox in a pregnant woman during the first trimester can cause miscarriages and birth defects including mental retardation, blindness, and shortened limbs. Chicken pox infections in a woman in her third trimester can cause the child to have early shingles infections (10, 11, 12, 13).

After the chicken pox infection has resolved, VZV becomes latent in a nerve dorsal root ganglia until reactivation. The secondary illness caused by reactivation of this virus is called *shingles*. It occurs most often in individuals older than 50 but can appear in younger people, especially if they are immunocompromised. The shingles blisters are painful and occur in a limited area enervated by 1 or 2 nerves (Figure 18.17 ■). The blisters are usually only on 1 side of the body, and, like chicken pox, are usually found on the head and trunk. Pneumonia, blindness, and encephalitis can occur as complications. A persistent pain can develop in some individuals, which does not resolve when the lesions do. Shingles is contagious but not nearly as contagious as the primary chicken pox infection (10, 11, 12, 13).

Diagnosis and Treatment

Diagnosis of VZV can be made on clinical appearance, especially when there has been an increase in the number of cases. Severe disease, atypical disease, and disease that may have exposed a high-risk individual all warrant laboratory testing. To identify the virus, direct immunofluorescence with fluorescently labeled antibody to the viral antigens can be performed on swabs from the lesions, or PCR can be done with the same material. Viral culture takes more than 1 week and is not sensitive. When using antibody testing by EIA, a significant increase in paired titers or a high titer IgM is diagnostic for acute infection. Immunity to VZV can be determined by comparing IgG titers to a standard serum from a reference facility (10, 11, 12, 13).

Symptomatic treatment to reduce the itching of VZV infections includes the use of oatmeal baths and calamine lotion. Aspirin should be avoided because the combination of aspirin and chicken pox has been associated with **Reyes syndrome,** a very severe disease of children affecting the brain and the liver (10, 11, 12, 13).

Severely ill people can receive acyclovir as anti-viral therapy. Preventative therapy in the form of varicella zoster immune globulin (VZIG) can be administered to people who are exposed to chicken pox and are likely to have a severe case. Individuals who are immunocompromised (people with leukemia or lymphoma and those with cellular immune defects, premature babies, and people receiving immunosuppressant therapy) and pregnant women are all candidates for the immune globulin therapy. A live attenuated vaccine is available to prevent chicken pox, and a more concentrated form of this vaccine is available to prevent shingles (10, 11, 12, 13).

 Checkpoint! 18.4

What vaccine protects an individual from rubella?

▶ OTHER SEROLOGICALLY DIAGNOSED VIRUSES

RUBELLA

Epidemiology

Rubella or *3-day* or *German measles* is in the Togaviridae, not the Herpesviridae, family. Rubella is an enveloped virus that contains single-stranded positive sense RNA in an icosahedral capsid within a lipid bilayer membrane that was obtained from the cell from which it budded. It replicates quickly. Rubella most commonly occurs in young children as a fever and sore throat followed by a rash (Figure 18.18 ■). Adults exhibit similar symptoms with the addition of joint pain. A global pandemic of rubella occurred from 1962 to 1965 during which the United States reported 12 million cases of rubella, 2100 neonatal deaths, 20 000 births with congenital rubella syndrome, and more than 11 000 spontaneous or therapeutic abortions caused by rubella. **Congenital rubella syndrome** includes mental retardation, cataracts, deafness, heart malformations, spleen, and liver damage (Figure 18.19 ■). While the most devastating impact of this disease was on neonates infected *in utero,* 2000 cases of encephalitis developed in infected children and adults during the 1965 to 1972 period. In 1969, a live attenuated rubella vaccine was licensed in the United States, and in 1989 an improved 2-dose vaccine schedule was developed and its use encouraged (Figure 18.20 ■). In 2004, the end to endemic rubella in the United States was documented. The less than 25 cases annually reported in the United States are associated with people who bring the cases from abroad (14, 15, 16, 17, 18, 19).

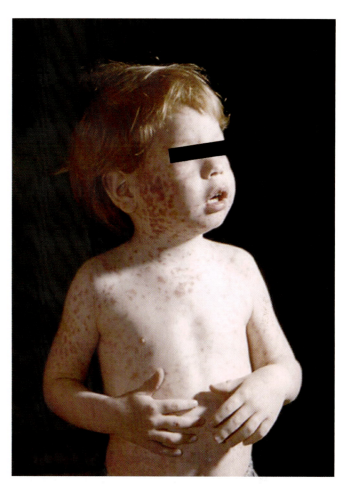

■ **FIGURE 18.18**   Rubella rash in a young child. Rubella is also called *3-day measles* or *German measles. Source:* © CDC.

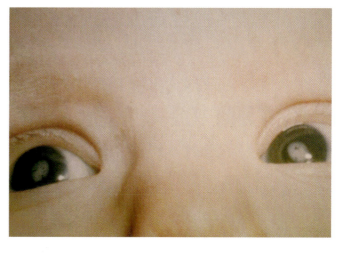

■ **FIGURE 18.19**   Cataracts seen in a child with congenital rubella syndrome. *Source:* © CDC.

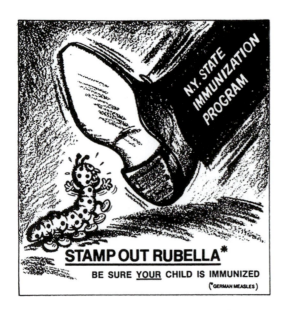

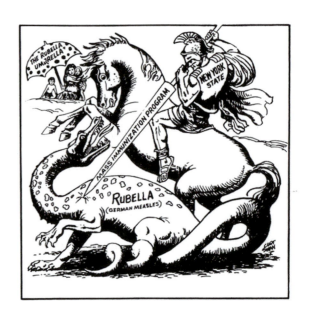

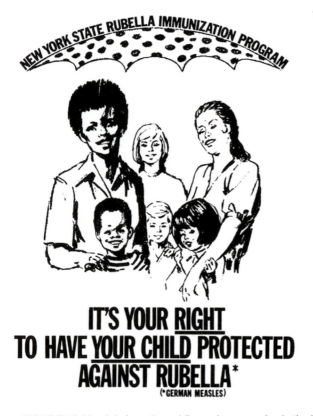

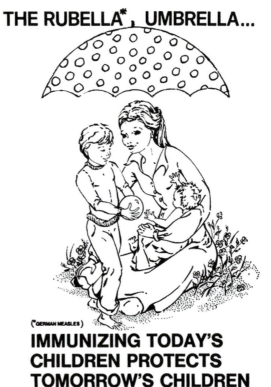

■ FIGURE 18.20 Ads from the public service campaign in the late 1960s and early 1970s that encouraged people to get vaccinated. Vaccination has reduced and nearly eliminated the devastating effects that rubella had on infants infected *in utero. Source:* © CDC

Diagnosis and Treatment

An enzyme immunoassay is available to measure antibody to rubella and can be used to diagnose rubella, but in the United States it is used primarily as a way to determine whether a woman of child-bearing age is immune to or susceptible to rubella. If the woman is not immune, she will be vaccinated before she attempts to become pregnant. The vaccine is a live attenuated virus and is part of the measles, mumps, and rubella (MMR) vaccine. The MMR vaccine is not recommended for women who are already pregnant. A cutoff of 15 IU/ml indicates that the patient can be considered immune. A standard is included in the EIA kit and the patient's sample is compared to the standard to determine immune status. Because most women in the United States at time of childbirth have high titers of antibody to rubella, infants born to these women also have high titers received through placental passive transfer. These antibody levels are high enough that it is advisable to wait until 12 to 15 months to vaccinate the newborn with MMR (14, 15, 16, 17, 18, 19).

Treatment of rubella involves alleviating the symptoms. Treatment of congenital rubella is done to repair the heart, remove cataracts, and decrease any symptoms that can be treated. Vaccination remains important even though rubella is no longer endemic in the United States because this disease can be easily brought into the country, from the many other countries that have not reached this level of disease elimination (14, 15, 16, 17, 18, 19).

MEASLES (RUBEOLA)

Epidemiology

Measles is a member of the **Paramyxoviridae family** of viruses as are mumps and respiratory syncytial virus. These viruses are single-stranded negative strand RNA viruses. Very few people in the United States get measles (131 cases from January 1, 2008, to July 31, 2008), but worldwide it is still a leading cause of death of children (164 000 deaths worldwide in 2008). This disease and these deaths are preventable by the MMR vaccination, and The Measles Initiative was launched to decrease deaths from measles. The Measles Initiative was formed by a partnership of the American Red Cross, the United Nations Foundation, the U.S. Centers for Disease Control and Prevention, UNICEF, and the World Health Organization. The effort began in 2001 because of the 733 000 worldwide deaths from measles that year, and this initiative had produced a 78% drop in the number of deaths by 2008 (20, 21, 22, 23, 24, 25).

In the midst of this effort to decrease deaths due to measles in the United States, the number of unvaccinated children has increased, and although 131 cases may seem to be a small number of cases of measles, this was a significant increase from 37 in 2004, 66 in 2005, and 55 in 2006. Of these 131 cases, 112 were not vaccinated and of these, 63 were not vaccinated because of their parent's beliefs. In 1998, a *Lancet* article linked the MMR vaccine to the development of autism and inflammatory bowel disease. This article had a profound effect on vaccination rates, dropping them from 92% to less than 80% in the United Kingdom and causing about 125 000 children in the United States to remain unvaccinated. Later, 10 of the 13 authors of the paper renounced it, and *Lancet* retracted the article amid proof that the data had been doctored. The trust that people had in the safety of vaccines was severely affected by this paper now proven to have been falsified. It is extremely sad to realize that lives were lost from the lack of vaccination caused by misled parents (20, 21, 22, 23, 24, 25).

In an unvaccinated population, 1 case of measles spreads to an average of 12 to 18 people. It is so contagious that an unvaccinated person who lives in an area that is not protected by herd immunity will probably contract measles. *Herd immunity* occurs when a significant percentage of the population is immunized. When an infection arrives in a herd immunity from an outside source, it will not spread because most people are immune. To prevent the spread of measles, 83 to 94% of the population must be vaccinated (20, 21, 22, 23, 24, 25).

Measles virus is spread through respiratory secretions from coughs and sneezes and can survive on surfaces such as door handles and stair handrails for up to 2 hours. Measles causes a characteristic dense rash on the face, trunk, arms, and legs (Figure 18.21 ■) as well as sore throat, high fever (up to 105° F), cough, runny nose, red eyes, and light sensitivity. The signs and symptoms occur 7 to 18 days after infection. Red spots with bluish white centers called *Koplik spots* are seen in the mouth (Figure 18.22 ■) (20, 21, 22, 23, 24, 25).

Diagnosis and Treatment

Testing for anti-measles antibodies is primarily done to determine immune status. The rash and fever are characteristic enough that diagnosis was formerly made clinically because every physician was very familiar with the symptoms. However, today it is so rare that a physician who suspects measles should have the enzyme immunoassay for antibodies performed. IgM antibodies indicate a current infection as does a 4-fold increase in IgG titers between the acute and

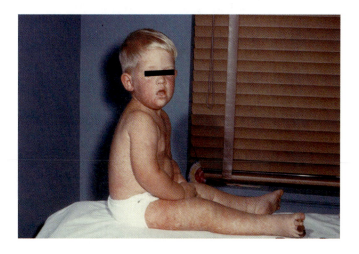

■ **FIGURE 18.21** The characteristic dense maculopapular rash of measles on the face of a child. Macules are small flat spots; papule are small raised spots. *Source:* © CDC.

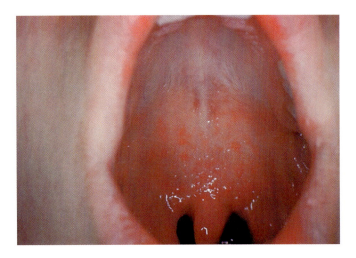

■ **FIGURE 18.22** Koplik spots in the mouth of a patient with measles. *Source:* © CDC/Dr. Heinz F. Eichenwald.

convalescent illness. Although there is only 1 antigenic strain of measles, several strains can be differentiated genetically. A nasal or throat swab may be taken for viral culturing followed by PCR to identify a vaccine strain or a wild-type strain. For epidemiologic purposes, genotyping to determine which wild-type strain was involved may also be done by PCR. There is no treatment to decrease the viral load; the treatment is to treat the symptoms only and involves the use

of acetaminophen or ibuprophen to reduce the fever (20, 21, 22, 23, 24, 25).

MUMPS

Epidemiology

Mumps, like measles is a Paramyxovirus, having single-stranded negative strand RNA as its nucleic acid. The protection against mumps provided by the MMR vaccine is not as robust as the protection against measles and rubella, and cases of mumps are seen in vaccinated individuals. The protection after 1 vaccination is estimated to be 61 to 91% and after 2 injections is 76 to 95%. Different strains of mumps have slight antigenic variations, and although all are antigenically similar and protection usually occurs, slight differences may yield this less than complete vaccine efficacy. In 2010, an outbreak occured in New York and New Jersey that resulted in more than 2000 cases. This outbreak arose from one boy who became infected in the United Kingdom and then attended a summer camp in the United States. The symptoms of mumps are swollen parotid salivary glands, and the submaxillary and sublingual salivary glands may also be enlarged (Figure 18.23 ■). In addition, fever, headache, muscle aches, loss of appetite, and fatigue usually occur. It is spread through direct contact with secretions or through items contaminated by secretions (fomites). Patients are contagious 1 to 2 days before the swelling begins and up to 5 days after the swelling is apparent. Of

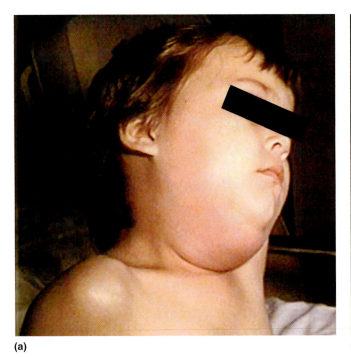
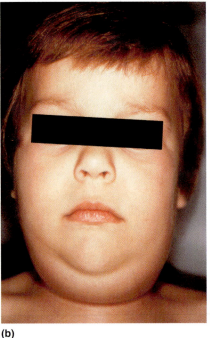

(a)   (b)

■ **FIGURE 18.23** Mumps swelling of the salivary glands. *Source:* (a) © CDC/NIP/Barbara Rice and (b) © CDC/ Patricia Smith; Barbara Rice.

patients, 15 to 20% are asymptomatic. The disease can cause bilateral orchitis in postpubertal males in 30 to 40% of the cases. Mastitis can occur in a similar percentage of girls over 15. Rare more serious complications include sterility, paralysis, and even death (25, 26, 27).

Diagnosis and Treatment

Like rubella and measles, mumps is a reportable disease. The laboratory analyses for a case definition of mumps by the Council of State and Territorial Epidemiologists (CSTE) includes detection of the virus by (1) isolation of mumps virus from the patient (viral culture) or (2) detection of mumps RNA by RT-PCR or (3) detection of an acute immune response to mumps virus by detection of anti-mumps IgM, detection of a 4-fold rise in titer of IgG against mumps, or a seroconversation from negative to positive for IgG to the mumps antigens (25, 26, 27).

WEST NILE VIRUS

Epidemiology

West Nile virus (WNV) is a Flavivirus and as such has single-stranded positive sense RNA that is enveloped and icosahedral. WNV is transmitted by mosquitoes and normally infects birds (Figure 18.24 ■ and 18.25 ■). Many different species of birds are infected, but crows are often linked with the disease. Birds sometimes die after infection, and care should be taken when handling dead birds. People become infected when an infected mosquito bites them. Handling infected animals, blood, or tissues can also transmit the virus. In 2010, every state except New Hampshire had at least 1 case of reported WNV infection with 981 total cases and 45 deaths. Of these cases, 601 were neuroinvasive causing severe illness (Figure 18.26 ■). Most WNV cases are asymptomatic or develop a mild disease called *West Nile fever*. About 1 of 100 infected individuals develop meningitis or encephalitis. The symptoms of these severe

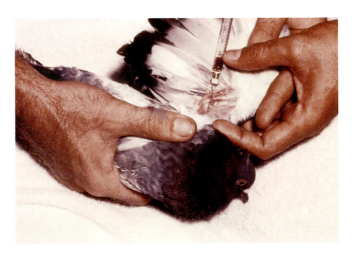

■ **FIGURE 18.25** Bird being tested for West Nile virus. *Source:* © CDC.

diseases are high fever, headache, rash on the back or chest, confusion, and weakness and can progress to convulsions, paralysis, and coma. WNV has also been found to be transmitted through blood transfusion, organ transplantation, transplacental transfer, and breast feeding, but these are rare. The evidence of this type of transmission necessitates testing blood and tissue for WNV prior to transfusions and transplantation (28, 29).

> ✔ **Checkpoint! 18.5**
>
> *Including what you have learned in this and other chapters, name viruses for which testing is done prior to the use of blood for blood transfusion.*

Diagnosis and Treatment

IgM and IgG testing is done on the blood of a patient with symptoms to determine the presence of antibodies to WNV. IgG testing on the cerebral spinal fluid is done when symptoms of encephalitis or meningitis are present. Nucleic acid testing is performed on blood prior to its use for transfusions and to check mosquitos and birds for infection. A vaccine is available for dogs but none is available for people. To avoid infection, prevent mosquito bites by draining areas with stagnant water and using mosquito repellent. Supportive care with treatment of symptoms is the only therapy that is currently available (28, 29).

INFLUENZA VIRUS

Epidemiology

Influenza is an Orthomyxoviridae virus and as such has single-stranded negative sense RNA that is segmented into 8 segments. *Myxo* in the name means that it interacts with mucins on the cell surface for infection. The surface of the

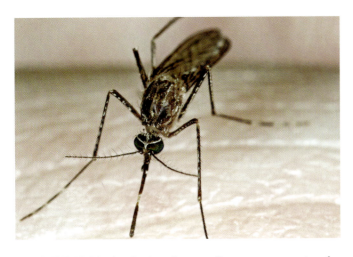

■ **FIGURE 18.24** A culex tarsalis mosquito, a common vector of the spread of West Nile virus. *Source:* © CDC/James Gathany.

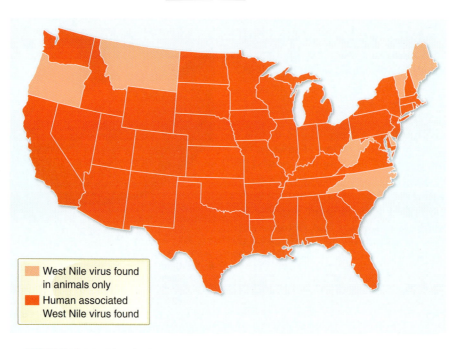

West Nile virus found
in animals only

Human associated
West Nile virus found

■ **FIGURE 18.26**   Map depicting the 2010 West Nile virus infections.

virion contains a hemagglutinin (H), which binds to surface sialic acid, and neuraminidase (N), which cleaves sialic acid for virus exit from the cell (Figure 18.27 ■). There are 3 groups of influenza viruses based on the internal nucleoprotein: Influenza A, B, and C. Influenza A causes the most widespread disease called *pandemics,* influenza B causes less widespread disease, and influenza C causes more mild disease that does not become widespread (30, 31, 32).

The reasons for the repeat waves of influenza infection are the changes in the surface hemagglutinin and neuraminidase antigens caused by 2 different factors: antigenic drift and antigenic shift. *Antigenic drift* is the result of minor changes caused by mutations in the genome of the virus, and *antigenic shift* is the result of a reassortment in a doubly infected cell in which a virion is packed with a segment of RNA from a different virus, creating a new virus. This reassortment can occur in a cell that is doubly infected with a bird (avian) or an animal (for example, swine) influenza virus and a human influenza virus. If the human virus picks up the alternative viruses RNA, the new virus will no longer have the H antigen to which humans have some immunity, and the virus will cause a pandemic. Only influenza A can infect animal strains, so only it can recombine with animal viruses to cause pandemics (30, 31, 32). Influenza A has 3 subtypes of the hemagglutinin that bind to human cells H1, H2, and H3. Two different neuraminidases, N1 and N2, have been found in humans for influenza A. Influenza virus causes an acute respiratory disease that can be mild to severe. Patients have a runny nose, muscle or body aches, sore throat, cough, fatigue, and sometimes fever, vomiting, and diarrhea. Complications of flu can include ear infections, sinusitis, bronchitis, and pneumonia. Flu can make chronic problems such as asthma and congestive heart disease worse. People who have asthma, diabetes, heart disease, or are older than 65 or very young are more likely to have severe disease. About 90% of the cases of deaths resulting from influenza occur in people 65 or older. The number of influenza-caused deaths per year range from a low of 3349 in 1986 to a high of 48 614 in 2003–2004 (30, 31, 32).

When someone with the flu coughs, sneezes, or talks, it can spread to people up to 6 feet away as they inhale the droplets into their lungs. People can also contract the flu if they touch a contaminated article and then touch their own nose or mouth. People can spread the flu 1 day before they show signs or symptoms of it. Adults can spread the virus 5 to 7 days after their symptoms start, and children may be able to spread the disease longer. Patients are contagious until 24 hours after the fever (if present) has ended (30, 31, 32).

Diagnosis and Treatment

Rapid influenza diagnostic tests detect the presence of the viral influenza antigens in respiratory specimens, yielding a positive or negative test result. These tests are not very sensitive, so a person with signs and symptoms of disease with a negative rapid test will undergo additional testing using RT-PCR or viral culture with a direct immunofluorescence assay. Anti-viral treatment for influenza utilizes Tamiflu (oseltamivir) or zanamivir (inhaled), neuraminidase inhibitors that are most helpful if used within 48 hours of the appearance of symptoms. The treatment reduces the extent and duration of the illness (30, 31, 32).

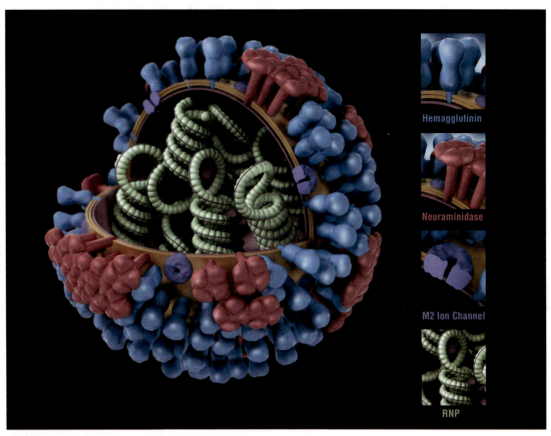

(a)

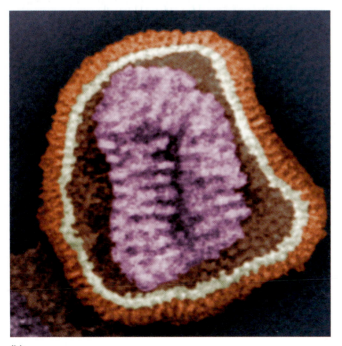

(b)

■ **FIGURE 18.27** (a) Drawing of influenza virion showing the hemagglutinin (H) and the neuraminidase (N) surface antigens. Differences in these antigens leads to subgrouping the viruses (such as H1N1). Source: © CDC/Douglas Jordan. (b) A negative stained scanning electron micrograph of the influenza virion. Source: © CDC/Erskine L. Palmer, Ph.D.; M. L. Martin.

⊘ CASE STUDY 1

You are so tired and are worried that your immunology professor will notice you sleeping in class. Even though immunology is your favorite class, you were up all night studying biochemistry and you are tired! It was worth it, though; you think that you aced the biochemistry test because you totally understand amino acid titrations now. But now, how to stay awake? Ahh, there is your best friend JoAnn with the latte with a double shot of espresso that she has every morning. JoAnn does not even take biochemistry because she had it last year. You ask her whether just this once you can have her latte, and she says sure; she has only had a few sips but it is yours now. You finish the latte and go to immunology class where you learn about viruses. The following Wednesday, JoAnn is not in class and she still is not in class on Friday. You call her and find that she has a really bad sore throat, high fever, and is really tired. Her left side hurts. She had just dragged herself to the health center and she was waiting for her results.

Her monospot looked like this:

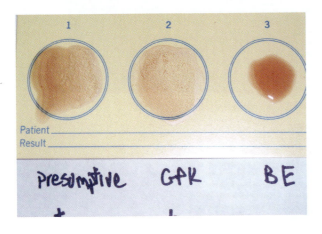

The first well contained the presumptive reaction (her serum with sheep red blood cells), the second well was the reaction after absorption with guinea pig kidney, and the third well was after absorption with bovine erythrocytes.

1. Does JoAnn have infectious mononucleosis?
2. Is it a sure thing that you are going to get infectious mononucleosis?

⊘ CASE STUDY 2

You were enjoying a break from all the activities at the Sunny Days camp for children with disabilities where you were a volunteer counselor. Your best friend Sally came out of the kitchen eating an ice cream sundae. On a hot day like this, it looked really good to you,

and she gave the rest to you because she did not have much of an appetite. Two days later, Sally's parotid salivary glands were huge and she had a fever, a headache, and muscle aches.

1. What disease do you think Sally has?
2. Should you be worried that you will have it too?

SUMMARY

No single chapter could contain a description of all viruses of medical importance for which serology is important, and this chapter has covered only a selection of them (Table 18.2 ⊘). Additional viruses for which serology is important include the respiratory viruses parainfluenza, respiratory syncytial virus and adenoviruses, the gastrointestinal rotavirus, and the vector-transmitted arboviruses, which cause encephalitis. In adenoviruses, parainfluenza, respiratory syncytial, and rotavirus, serological tests displaying a 4-fold rise in IgG titer or the presence of IgM can be diagnostic. Antigen detection can also be used to diagnose all of these infections.

Many characteristics can be used in classification of viruses, but classification is based in part on whether the genetic material is DNA or RNA, is double-stranded or single-stranded, is the positive or negative strand, and is segmented or not segmented and whether it is linear or circular.

The Herpesviridae family contains Epstein-Barr virus (EBV), cytomegalovirus (CMV), herpes simplex 1 (HSV1) and 2 viruses (HSV2), and varicella zoster virus (VZV). These viruses contain double-stranded DNA and have a latency period. EBV causes infectious mononucleosis and Burkitt's lymphoma and is related to nasopharyngeal carcinoma. It is diagnosed by measuring antibody to the Paul-Bunnell antigen that is on sheep red blood cells and bovine red blood cells but not on guinea pig kidney cells. Because antibody to sheep red blood cells is also found in patients with serum sickness and normal people with Forssman antibody, differential absorption is performed with guinea pig kidney and bovine erythrocytes to differentiate the diagnosis. Of people with infectious mononucleosis, 10 to 15% test false negative for the Paul-Bunnell antigen. In these cases, the assays used for diagnosis are IgM and IgG to the Epstein-Barr viral capsid antigen, IgM to the Epstein Barr virus early antigen, and antibody to the Epstein-Barr virus nuclear antigen (1, 2, 3, 4).

Cytomegalovirus infections can look clinically like a mild case of infectious mononucleosis. CMV becomes clinically important because of the dramatic effects that it can have for a woman who is infected while pregnant and for an immunocompromised patient. Eighty percent of babies infected *in utero* show no effects. Ten percent will be symptomatic at birth and may be born prematurely, have liver, spleen, and/or lung problems, have a small head size and small overall size, and have seizures at birth. They also may have hearing loss and/or vision loss and lack of coordination and may die soon after birth. Ten percent of newborns infected *in utero*, although asymptomatic at birth, develop vision and hearing problems that appear up to 2 years after birth. CMV infections in

⊙ TABLE 18.2

Chapter Summary Table

	Type of Virus	Antigen or Nucleic Acid Testing	Antibody Testing	Disease
Epstein-Barr	Herpesviridae	No	Heterophile antibodies Presumptive test (monospot), Davidsohn differential (Mono-Diff) Immunochromatography Viral antigen tests IgM, IgG to VCA, EBNA IgM to EA-D	Infectious mononucleosis
Cytomegalovirus (CMV)	Herpesviridae	PCR viral culture	IgM or IgG to CMV Paired titers	Mild disease in healthy people Severe disease in immunocompromised, babies infected *in utero*
Herpes simplex 1 and 2	Herpesviridae	PCR and viral culture not approved by FDA	Serology for diagnosis serotype specific glycoprotein G (gG)-based assays to differentiate type 1 and type 2	Oral or genital "cold sores" Severe in immunocompromised
Varicella zoster	Herpesviridae	Clinical appearance direct immuno-fluorescence or PCR on swabs	Antibody look for paired titers or high titer IgM For immunity to VSV compare titers to reference	Chicken pox, shingles Complications can include encephalitis, pneumonia Birth defects in babies *infected in utero*
Rubella	Togaviridae	No	EIA for antibody to rubella Antibody levels compared to reference to determine immunity	German measles, rubella Fever, sore throat, rash Congenital rubella syndrome
Measles (rubeola)	Paramyxoviridae	Viral culture/PCR for vaccine vs wild-type strain and which wild-type strain	EIA to determine immune status Paired titer for diagnosis	Measles—leading cause of death in children worldwide
Mumps	Paramyxoviridae	Viral culture PCR	IgM anti-mumps 4-fold rise in titer of IgG anti-mumps	Mumps—swollen parotid salivary gland, fever, headache, muscle aches Orchitis, mastitis possible in post-puberty
West Nile virus	Flavivirus	Nucleic acid testing on blood prior to use	IgG testing on symptomatic individual	West Nile fever mild disease 1% get encephalitis, meningitis
Influenza virus	Orthomyxoviridae	Rapid test for viral antigens RT-PCR Viral culture	No	Flu

transplant patients and other immunocompromised people can result in pneumonia, retinitis, gastrointestinal disease, and even death (1, 2, 3, 4).

Herpes simplex virus infections cause either oral or genital cold sores. Genital herpes infections are sexually transmitted. Antivirals, abstinence during outbreaks, and condom use can all reduce transmission. Of babies infected with HSV infection *in utero,* 35% have severe disease (6, 7, 8, 9).

Varicella zoster causes chicken pox and shingles. Two vaccines are available to prevent these disease manifestations. Babies infected *in utero* can be miscarried or have birth defects including mental retardation, blindness, and shortened limbs (10, 11, 12, 13).

Rubella, a Togavirus, causes a rash and a fever in children with the addition of joint pain in adults. Most of the serological testing for antibody to this virus is done to ensure that women of child-bearing years are immune. This is done to reduce the number of cases of congenital rubella syndrome. Congenital rubella syndrome includes mental retardation, cataracts, deafness, heart malformations, and spleen and liver damage (see Box 18.1 ⊙) (14, 15, 16, 17, 18, 19).

Measles (rubeola) and mumps are paramyxoviruses that caused common childhood diseases in this country until a successful vaccine was available. Both are still prevalent in countries with low immunization rates and can still be brought into the United

⊕ BOX 18.1

Congenital Rubella

Rubella had lasting impact on our country in two ways, the first much more controversial than the second. Prior to the 1960s, abortions were thought to be desired only by people that were social deviants, but the huge number of rubella related congenital defects which occurred during these years changed that. During this time, many families thought about the "what if" question. What if the woman became infected with rubella while she was pregnant? How would this affect their families and other children? The fact that this question, whatever its answer, came into the minds of mainstream individuals altered perceptions about abortion and this may have had an impact on the subsequent 1973 *Roe v. Wade* decision.

The second lasting impact of rubella was due to the fact that many children were born in 1964 and 1965 with congenital rubella caused disabilities. The sheer number of children with disabilities placed a spotlight on the lack of services for individuals with disabilities. In 1965 Federal grants were provided to states to educate children with disabilities, and in 1968 and 1972 early childhood and headstart programs for children with disabilities were enacted. Finally, in 1975 the public law "Education for all Handicapped Children" was enacted.

States by travelers. West Nile virus is an emerging mosquito-borne infection in the United States. Its infection is usually subclinical, but infection can lead to death. Influenza virus has segmented RNA as its nucleic acid, and this property allows for trade of genetic information with another virus in a process called *antigenic shift,* which can result in pandemics (20, 21, 22, 23, 24, 25, 26, 27, 28, 29, 30, 31, 32).

For diagnosis, antigens can be detected in direct analysis from the patient or after viral culture in tissue culture. Antibodies can also be measured, which requires looking either for IgM or a 4-fold rise in titer of IgG. Although there are cytopathic methods and new molecular methods for viral diagnosis, serology remains very important in diagnosing viral diseases.

REVIEW QUESTIONS

1. Rubella
   a. in an adult causes severe arthritis-like symptoms
   b. in an infant infected *in utero* can cause deafness
   c. is in the herpes virus group
   d. all of the above

2. In the United States, why is rubella vaccination not given until 12 to 15 months after birth?
   a. Children younger than 2 do not make good antibody to capsular polysaccharides.
   b. Children receive many other vaccinations earlier in their lives, so we do not want competition to occur.
   c. Attenuated organisms are not given to such young children.
   d. Maternal antibody would interfere with infant Ab development.

3. Viral capsid antigen of Epstein-Barr virus
   a. is found only in a few of the people who are infected
   b. causes the production of an IgM antibody early in the infection
   c. causes the production of aberrant macrophages
   d. is not on Epstein-Barr virus

4. Epstein-Barr nuclear antigen
   a. causes the production of a late but long lasting antibody
   b. stimulates the production of IgG antibody in the acute phase of the infection
   c. causes the production of an antibody that disappears quickly
   d. is found in the cytoplasm and in the nucleus of infected B cells

5. What kind of red blood cells are used in infectious mononucleosis absorption?
   a. guinea pig red blood cells
   b. human red blood cells and bovine red blood cells
   c. horse red blood cells and sheep red blood cells
   d. bovine red blood cells

6. What 3 types of antibody can cause a positive presumptive test for infectious mononucleosis?
   a. infectious mononucleosis, malaria, serum sickness
   b. infectious mononucleosis, serum sickness, pregnancy
   c. infectious mononucleosis, healthy humans with Forssman Ab, serum sickness
   d. infectious mononucleosis, leprosy, healthy human

7. With what diseases is Epstein-Barr virus associated?
   a. infectious mononucleosis, leprosy, Burkitt's lymphoma
   b. infectious mononucleosis, Burkitt's lymphoma, hepatoma
   c. infectious mononucleosis, Hodgkin's lymphoma, nasal pharyngeal adenocarcinoma
   d. infectious mononucleosis, Burkitt's lymphoma, nasal pharyngeal adenocarcinoma

8. Chicken pox and shingles both are caused by the same virus,
   a. cytomegalovirus
   b. rubeola
   c. varicella zoster virus
   d. Togaviridae

9. In the Davidsohn differential assay after absorption with guinea pig kidney, infectious mononucleosis antibody will
   a. be absorbed, not agglutinate the sheep red blood cells
   b. be absorbed and agglutinate the sheep red blood cells
   c. not be absorbed and not agglutinate the sheep red blood cells
   d. not be absorbed and agglutinate the sheep red blood cells

10. In immunodeficient people, cytomegalovirus infections
    a. are asymptomatic
    b. cause gumma formation
    c. can cause pneumonia or vision loss
    d. can cause a vesicular skin lesion like that seen in HSV

11. *In utero*, a cytomegalovirus infection can cause the baby to experience
    a. hearing loss and mental retardation
    b. a vesicular skin lesion like that seen in HSV
    c. blue baby syndrome
    d. autoimmune anemia because of cross-reacting antigens

12. Which of the following viruses is not in the herpes virus group
    a. rubella
    b. chicken pox
    c. cytomegalovirus
    d. Epstein-Barr virus

13. CMV
    a. in babies can cause hearing loss, visual impairment, and mental retardation
    b. in the immunodeficient can cause ocular disease, pneumonia, and hepatitis
    c. In HIV patients can cause interstitial pneumonia
    d. All of the above

14. Which antibody to Epstein-Barr virus related antigens may last a lifetime?
    a. anti-EA-D
    b. anti-EA-R
    c. anti-EBNA
    d. anti-pol

15. CMV is in which of the following fluids?
    a. blood
    b. urine
    c. breast milk
    d. all of the above

16. To prevent spread of a herpes simplex 2 genital infection,
    a. condoms should be worn
    b. abstinence during outbreaks should be practiced
    c. antivirals should be used
    d. all of the above

17. A particularly important reason to be sure that a child is vaccinated for measles is
    a. that measles is one of the most common causes of death for children
    b. that measles is still prevalent in other countries and can be brought to the United States
    c. that measles can cause orchitis and sterility
    d. A and B

18. The reason that a vaccinated child could get mumps is
    a. that mumps is resistant to vaccine protection
    b. that the protection that the child received from vaccination was not strong enough
    c. that the vaccine causes Th1 cell activation only
    d. all of the above

19. The influenza rapid test
    a. detects the anti-flu antibody in the patient's serum
    b. detects the anti-flu antibody in nasal secretions
    c. detects the flu antigen in the patient's serum
    d. detects the flu antigen in nasal secretions

20. To diagnose a viral infection that is so common that a historical infection in the patient would not be uncommon, one should look for
    a. IgM to the virus
    b. paired titers of IgG that show a 4-fold rise in titer
    c. paired titers of IgG that show a 10-fold rise in titer
    d. A and B

REFERENCES

1. Wong D. http://virology-online.com/questions/89-1.htm. Accessed March 24, 2012

2. Luzuriaga K, Sullivan JL. Infectious mononucleosis. *N Engl J Med.* 2010;362:1993–2000.

3. Centers for Disease Control and Prevention, National Center for Infectious Diseases. Epstein-Barr virus and infectious mononucleosis. http://www.cdc.gov/ncidod/diseases/ebv.htm. Accessed March 24, 2012.

4. Armed Forces Institute of Pathology Electronic Fascicles Version of the Atlas of Tumor Pathology. [CD-ROM]

5. Centers for Disease Control and Prevention. Cytomegalovirus (CMV) and Congenital CMV infection. http://www.cdc.gov/cmv/testing-diagnosis.html. Accessed March 24, 2012.

6. Centers for Disease Control and Prevention. Fact sheet. Genital herpes. http://www.cdc.gov/std/Herpes/Herpes-Fact-Sheet-lowres-2010.pdf. Accessed March 24, 2012.

7. Centers for Disease Control and Prevention. Sexually transmitted disease treatment guidelines. 2006. http://www.cdc.gov/std/treatment/2006/genital-ulcers.htm. Accessed March 24, 2012.

8. Centers for Disease Control and Prevention. Sexually transmitted disease treatment guidelines. Diseases characterized by genital ulcers http://www.cdc.gov/std/treatment/2006/genital-ulcers.htm#genulc3. Accessed March 24, 2012.

9. Taeusch HW, Ballard RA, Gleason CA, et al. Avery's diseases of the newborn. Philadelphia, Pa: Elsevier, Saunders; 2005.

10. Centers for Disease Control and Prevention. Vaccines and preventable diseases: Varicella disease questions & answers. http://www.cdc.gov/chickenpox/about/index.html. Accessed May 25, 2012.

11. Centers for Disease Control and Prevention. Vaccines and immunizations: Shingles (herpes zoster) vaccination. http://www.cdc.gov/chickenpox/vaccination.html. Accessed March 24, 2012.

12. Harpaz R, Ortega-Sanchez IR, Seward JF. MBBS, prevention of herpes zoster recommendations of the advisory committee on immunization practice. *MMWR.* 2008;57:1–30. http://www.cdc.gov/mmwr/preview/mmwrhtml/rr57e0515a1.htm. Accessed March 24, 2012.

13. Arup Consult. The Physician's Guide to Laboratory Test Selection and Interpretation Varicella Zoster Virus. http://www.arupconsult.com/Topics/VZV.html#tabs=1. Accesssed March 25, 2012.

14. Reef SE, Cochi SL. The evidence for the elimination of rubella and congenital rubella syndrome in the United States: A public health achievement. *Clinical Infectious Diseases.* 2006;43:S123–S125.

15. Centers for Disease Control and Prevention. Vaccines and preventable diseases: Rubella (German measles) vaccination. http://www.cdc.gov/vaccines/vpd-vac/rubella/default.htm. Accessed March 23, 2012.

16. Chamberlain, C. Epidemic played large role in shift of attitudes on abortion. http://news.illinois.edu/news/10/0623abortion.html. Accessed June 23, 2010.

17. Schein JD, Shein EG. Brief history of Deafblind people in the United States. http://www.deafblind.ufl.edu/PDF_attachments/PepNetCh1.pdf. Accessed June 3, 2012.

18. U.S. Department of Education. History: Twenty-five years of progress in educating children with disabilities through IDEA. 2007. http://www2.ed.gov/policy/speced/leg/idea/history.html. Accessed March 23, 2012.

19. Plotkin SA. Correlates of protection induced by vaccination. *Clin Vaccine Immunol.* 2010;7:1055–1065. http://cdli.asm.org/content/17/7/1055.full.pdf+html. Accessed June 3, 2012.

20. WHO/UNICEF. Joint annual measles report 2009. Strengthening immunization services through measles control. http://www.measlesinitiative.org/mi-files/Reports/Measles%20Initiative/Annual%20Reports/Annual%20measles%20report%20Final%2029Mar2010_compressed.pdf. Accessed March 24, 2012.

21. Centers for Disease Control and Prevention. Most U.S Measles cases reported since 1996. Many do not vaccinate because of philosophical beliefs [online newsroom press release]. http://www.cdc.gov/media/pressrel/2008/r080821.htm. Accessed March 24, 2012.

22. American National Red Cross. Measles initiative. http://www.measlesinitiative.org/. Accessed March 24, 2012.

23. Centers for Disease Control and Prevention. Bam! Body and mind. Immune platoon disease database. http://www.cdc.gov/measles/downloads/bam-measles-508.pdf. Accessed March 24, 2012.

24. Center for Infectious Disease Preparedness—UC Berkeley School of Public Health. Concepts for the prevention and control of microbial threats—2. http://www.idready.org/slides/01epiconceptsII-slides.pdf. Accessed March 24, 2012.

25. Lab Tests Online. A public resource on clinical lab testing from the laboratory professional who do the testing. Measles and mumps. http://www.labtestsonline.org/understanding/analytes/measles/test.html. Accessed March 24, 2012.

26. Update: Mumps outbreak—New York and New Jersey, June 2009–January 2010. *MMWR.* http://www.cdc.gov/mmwr/preview/mmwrhtml/mm5905a1.htm. Accessed March 24, 2012.

27. Center for Disease Control and Prevention. Mumps vaccination. http://www.cdc.gov/mumps/vaccination.html. Accessed March 24, 2012.

28. Centers for Disease Control and Prevention. Epidemic/Epizootic West Nile virus in the United States: Guidelines for surveillance, prevention, and control. http://www.cdc.gov/ncidod/dvbid/westnile/resources/wnv-guidelines-aug-2003.pdf. Accessed March 24, 2012.

29. Lab Tests Online. A public resource on clinical lab testing from the laboratory professionals who do the testing: West Nile virus. http://www.labtestsonline.org/understanding/analytes/west_nile/test.html. Accessed March 24, 2012.

30. Centers for Disease Control and Prevention. Seasonal influenza (flu): The influenza viruses. http://www.cdc.gov/flu/about/viruses/. Accessed March 24, 2012.

31. Estimates of deaths associated with seasonal influenza—United States 1976–2007. *MMWR.* 2010;33: 1057–1062. http://www.cdc.gov/mmwr/preview/mmwrhtml/mm5933a1.htm. Accessed March 24, 2012.

32. Levinson W. *Review of Medical Microbiology and Immunology.* Chap 39 RNA Enveloped Viruses. San Francisco, CA; McGraw-Hill Professional, 2006.

PEARSON
myhealthprofessionskit™

Visit www.myhealthprofessionskit.com to access the interactive Companion Website for this textbook. Simply select "Clinical Laboratory Science" from the choice of disciplines. Find this book and log in by using your user name and password to access additional learning tools.

19

Bacterial Serology

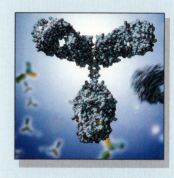

■ OBJECTIVES—LEVEL I

After this chapter, the student should be able to:

1. Describe various mechanisms of immune response to bacteria and their antigens.
2. Discuss different approaches by which bacteria evade or downregulate the host immune responses against them.
3. Describe the classification of hemolytic streptococci and the different patterns of hemolysis.
4. List and describe different clinical conditions associated with *Streptococcus pyogenes,* including clinical presentation, diagnosis, and treatment.
5. List and describe different laboratory approaches for the detection of streptococci.
6. Describe the pathological effects of *Helicobacter pylori* and laboratory tests used to detect it.
7. Describe different laboratory tests to detect *Mycoplasma pneumoniae.*
8. List and discuss the different rickettsial diseases and the life cycle of their infectious agents.
9. Discuss different serology and diagnostic tests for the detection and diagnosis of rickettsial diseases.
10. Describe clinical situations that favor the overgrowth of *Clostridium difficile,* and discuss the clinical implications associated with its overgrowth.
11. List and describe laboratory tests for the detection of *Clostridium difficile.*
12. Describe microbiological features of spirochetes.
13. Discuss the host immune response to *Treponema pallidum.*
14. List and describe the different clinical stages of syphilis.
15. List and describe diagnostic tests for syphilis.
16. List methods of prevention and treatment for syphilis.
17. Describe clinical features and immunopathology of Lyme disease.
18. Describe the tick that transmits Borrelia burgdorferi that causes Lyme disease, and the mode of disease transmission.
19. List and describe clinical diagnostic methods for Lyme disease.
20. List and describe different laboratory tests for Lyme disease.

■ OBJECTIVES—LEVEL II

After this chapter, the student should be able to:

1. Describe how *Helicobacter pylori* can survive in the low pH of the stomach.
2. Describe the life cycle of the tick that transmits Lyme disease.

KEY TERMS

adhesins	gumma
agglutination	hemolysis
aneurysm	hypervolemia
chancre	Jarisch-Herxheimer
circumoral pallor	reaction
cold agglutinins	Lancefield serotyping
cytopathic effect	M protein
ecthyma	myalgia
exudate	porins
flocculation	superantigen
granuloma	transplacental passage

▶ INTRODUCTION

We previously used the analogy of a military defense structure to describe the immune system. We discussed its organization, different interrelated components, systems of communication and control, and specific weapons. We also described the recognition mechanisms that this system uses to recognize a potential enemy, the features that allow recognition to occur, and the characteristics of a potential enemy that make it recognizable. We explained that a potential enemy is basically anything that is molecularly foreign or different from the host. Realistically, however, what are the actual enemies in a host's everyday life? The major ones, as you can imagine, are microorganisms that can cause and transmit an infectious disease. Thus, immune responses designed to protect us from such an enemy are directed to the microorganisms themselves, their components, or their products (for example, a toxin). As in any "war," the enemy is not a passive or inert entity and often has the ability to either fight back or evade both recognition as well as attack; in this chapter, we discuss the immune response to certain specific microorganisms, their mode of counteraction, the disease with which they are associated, and the methodology involved in their detection.

▶ HOST DEFENSE MECHANISMS

The first and most basic defensive approach against microorganisms is the prevention of entry; this is usually achieved by physical barriers. The skin is the best defensive wall of the host. Mucus surfaces in the respiratory and digestive tracts also prevent entry. Nose hairs may not be the most attractive things on a first date, but they are important tools of defense by interfering with entry; cilia and their outward movement can also push foreign particles toward the outside. All in all, these barriers prevent the entrance of potential pathogens, thus preventing colonization and infection. Furthermore, these barriers not only act as physical obstacles to entry but also have dynamic mechanisms of defense. For example, mucus from mucosal surfaces contains antimicrobial enzymes such as lysozyme (Figure 19.1 ■). Should any of these barriers

be breached, broken, or bypassed, the next line of defense is performed by the components of the innate immune system (Chapter 1). Major frontline soldiers of the immune system involved in first bacterial encounters are phagocytic cells such as macrophages and neutrophils. The latter can be seen as the marines of the immune army, arriving at the site of bacterial insult via chemotaxis and through diapedesis (squeezing between cells to cross blood vessel walls), processes that are described in Chapter 1. See Figure 19.2 ■ for an artist's depiction of a neutrophil's journey to reach the site of infection and its subsequent phagocytic activity. Chemotaxis, transedothelial migration, and phagocytosis are described in detail in previous chapters (1). The rationale for showing this figure is that many microorganisms can interfere at any step of such processes. For example, some microorganisms such as *Neisseria* species can interfere with chemotaxis by affecting the release of specific neutrophil chemoattractants. Some microorganisms can interfere with the binding of the phagocyte to the microorganisms; additional defensive methods of bacteria include resisting the degradation (digestion) process of phagocytes by either interfering with the emptying of digestive and reactive chemicals into the phagosomes, or, more drastically, by redirecting the process so that these reactive chemicals are released inside the cell, thus killing the phagocyte and sparing the microorganism. Additional host weapons include the acute phase response, the production of pyrogenic (fever-producing) substances such as leukotrienes and prostaglandins, and the activation of the complement system. Some of

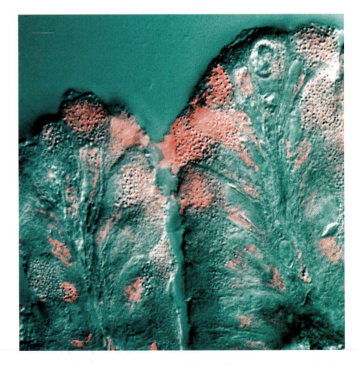

■ **FIGURE 19.1**   A surface mucous cell bordering on the stomach lumen secretes mucus (pink stain). *Source:* Underwood J (2006) The Path to Digestion Is Paved with Repair. PLoS Biol 4(9): e307. doi:10.1371/journal.pbio.0040307.

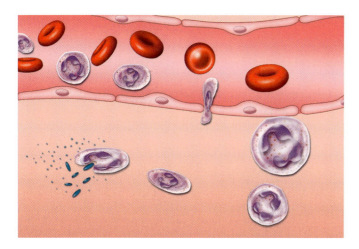

the acute-phase proteins coordinate their action with complement; opsonization of the microorganism is a major mechanism making it more susceptible to phagocytosis. All these molecules and mechanisms are described in detail in previous chapters. Once again, several microorganisms have the ability to interfere with the activation of the complement system, thus evading its effects.

Of course, once the innate immune system is engaged, acquired or specific responses follow, including the production of antibodies and the generation of cell-mediated immune responses. Some microorganisms can evade an immune response even at these levels. Some microorganisms can produce proteases that degrade antibody molecules: For example, *Streptococcus sanguis* produces a protease that can cleave molecules of IgA.

▶ SPECIFIC MICROORGANISMS

It would be very difficult to cover in a chapter all the possible microorganisms that cause disease and for which serologic testing is performed. Therefore, in this chapter, we discuss representative microorganisms that are of importance in human health and disease and that are a major target of diagnostic/serologic testing.

▶ STREPTOCOCCI

Streptococci are round gram-positive, oxidase and catalase negative, facultative anaerobic bacteria from the Firmicutes phylum (2). The name comes from the Greek, describing something that can be easily twisted (*coccus* indicates a circular shape), like a string or a chain, due to the fact that this bacterium divides along only one cell axis and thus is usually seen in pairs or characteristic chains of single organisms. Refer to Figure 19.3 ■ for a photomicrograph of *Streptococcus*

pyogenes from a specimen of pus. Streptococcal infections are associated with a variety of conditions including strep throat, endocarditis, meningitis, pneumonia, skin infections (eg, erysipelas), dental caries, and necrotizing fasciitis, more commonly known as "flesh-eating" disease. Many species are harmless, are part of the normal flora in both the respiratory and digestive tracts in humans, and are also found in other species such as cows, monkeys, and dogs (2). Some even have industrial applications, for example, in the making of certain forms of Swiss cheese.

Streptococci species are differentiated based on the way they break down blood (**hemolysis**) in a blood agar plate. Streptococci that can oxidize iron in hemoglobin are classified as α-hemolytic and can be recognized by a green-colored halo around them on blood agar. Species that can completely destroy red blood cells are defined as β-hemolytic and can be recognized by a completely clear halo around them on blood agar (2). Paradoxically, species that do not hemolyze blood are called γ-*hemolytic,* even though no hemolysis actually occurs. Different patterns of alpha and beta hemolysis are shown in Figure 19.4 ■, and a basic classification of streptococci is shown in Figure 19.5 ■.

β-hemolytic streptococci are further classified by **Lancefield serotyping,** a system developed by Rebecca Lancefield. This subdivision comprises 20 different groups labeled A through H and K through V and is based on differences in the carbohydrate composition of the components of the cell wall. These bacteria are also classified by phylogenetic analysis based on different 16S rRNA sequences. Although there are

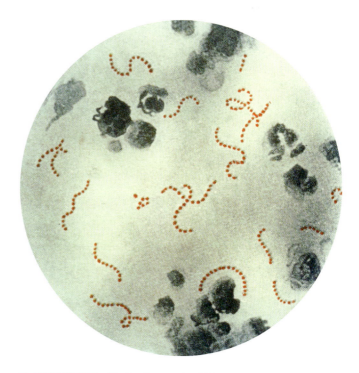

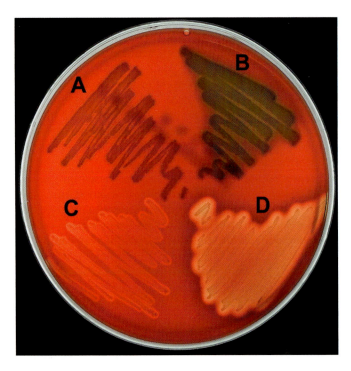

■ **FIGURE 19.4** Different patterns of α- and β-hemolysis on a blood agar plate: (a) α-hemolysis—viridian streptococci, (b) α-hemolysis—*S. pneumoniae*, (c) β-hemolysis—Group B streptococci, and (d) β-hemolysis—Group A streptococci. *Source:* Contributed by Dr. Elaine Haase and Carol Golyski. Photo by Eric Haase.

many kinds of streptococci, the main ones that have clinical relevance include *Streptococcus pneumoniae,* (α-hemolytic) and the Lancefield A and B groups of the β-hemolytic streptococci (2).

GROUP A STREP

Streptococcus pyogenes is the β-hemolytic Group A streptococcus that is responsible for most streptococcal infections (although other groups can also cause infections). These infections include acute pharyngitis, impetigo, scarlet fever (Figure 19.6 ■), acute rheumatic fever, acute glomerulonephritis, sepsis, pneumonia, and meningitis. Some of these infections, such as necrotizing fasciitis (Figure 19.7 ■), can be quite severe and some can even result in death (3). Jim Henson, the well-known creator of the Muppets, died in 1990 of a *S. pyogenes* infection.

The cell wall components of *S. pyogenes* include proteins, group specific carbohydrates, peptidoglycan, and lipoteichoic acid (LTA). A major virulence factor of *S. pyogenes* is a component called **M protein,** which is associated with colonization and the ability of the organism to evade phagocytosis. More than 50 types of M protein have been identified on the basis of antigenic specificity, and, in fact, it is a major source of antigenic shift or drift. Functionally, the M protein can bind fibrinogen and can block the binding of complement components to the underlying peptidoglycan, thus inhibiting phagocytosis (4). In addition, the M protein contains immunogenic epitopes that mimic those found in mammalian muscle and connective tissues. This can lead to cross-reactive autoimmune responses leading to conditions such as autoimmune rheumatic carditis (rheumatic heart disease) and rheumatic fever (5, 6). Furthermore, *S. pyogenes* produces an exotoxin known as Streptococcal pyrogenic exotoxin A1 (SpeA1), which acts as a **superantigen** (7). A superantigen activates T cells nonspecifically, resulting in their polyclonal activation and an enormous release of different cytokines. This happens because the superantigen can bind simultaneously to

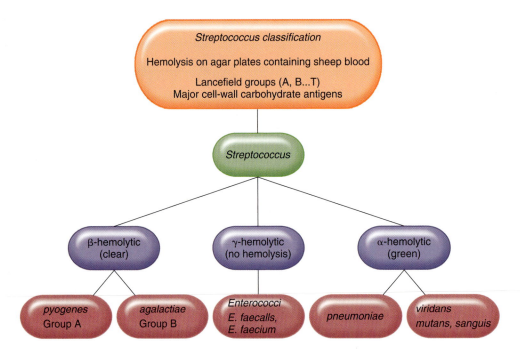

■ **FIGURE 19.5** Basic classification of streptococci-based on hemolysis.

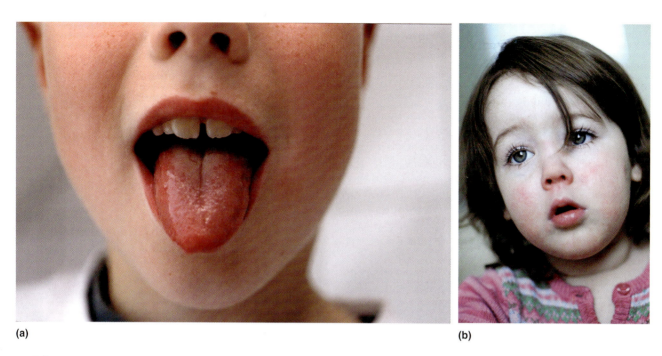

(a)   **(b)**

■ **FIGURE 19.6**   "Strawberry tongue" and circumoral pallor in scarlet fever. *Source:* (a) © imagebroker / Alamy (b) CDC/Donald Kopanoff.

MHC class II components and T-cell receptors but bypasses the antigen-specific presentation mechanism described in Chapter 4. Superantigens bind to MHC class II components first and then to a set of T-cell receptors with a particular variable beta motif. Refer to Figure 19.8 ■ for a diagram of this and the differences between a "regular" antigen and a superantigen. By bypassing the unique specificity of the antigen-binding pockets of the MHC and TCR, superantigens can activate a large number of different (in terms of antigen specificity) T cells, thus resulting in their massive response (1). Different toxins in the streptococcal family have high-affinity binding to a particular subset of MHC class II molecules. The SpeA1 toxin binds to HLA-DQ type with high affinity, and

binding occurs at one of 2 binding sites. On the T-cell receptor side, SpeA1 binds T cells expressing the Vβ subset of T-cell receptor proteins Vβ 2.1, 12.2, 14.1, and 15.1. The polyclonal activation of T cells results in a massive and detrimental release of cytokines such as IL-1, IL-2, and TNFα. This causes strong and often harmful inflammatory responses both at the local and systemic levels (7).

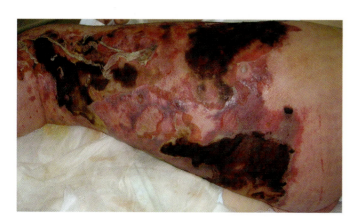

■ **FIGURE 19.7**   Preoperative photograph of a 43-year-old Caucasian male with necrotizing fasciitis on the day of admission; extensive erythema and necrosis of the left leg. *Source:* Piotr Smuszkiewicz, MD, PhD.

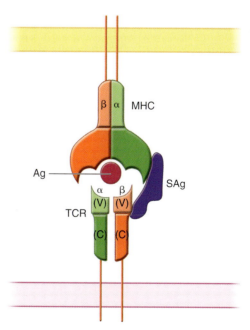

■ **FIGURE 19.8**   Differences between an antigen (Ag, in red) and a superantigen (SAg, in purple) and their interactions with MHC and T-cell receptors.

CLINICAL IMPLICATIONS OF *S. PYOGENES* INFECTIONS

Impetigo

Impetigo (also known as "school sores") is a contagious bacterial infection that is more commonly found in young, particularly preschool, children (although it does rarely occur in adults). The simpler form of impetigo is called *bullous impetigo* because of its characteristic fluid-filled blisters (bullae) that are usually located on the legs, arms, and trunk. The blisters are usually not painful although they may itch and can break, resulting in the formation of a yellowish crust (Figure 19.9 ■). The condition is not life threatening; it is transmitted by direct contact, by nasal carrier, or by scratching the lesions. It is usually treated with local antiseptic and local antibiotic ointments and, in more severe cases, with oral antibiotics such as diclozacillin or erythromycin. If the infection goes deeper and penetrates the dermis, a condition called **ecthyma** results. This is a more serious condition, which is characterized by painful pus-filled sores and ulcers and swelling of nearby lymph glands. Even after healing, the ulcers can leave some scarring. Untreated impetigo can be self-limiting, but in rare cases, it can lead to glomerulonephritis as well as sepsis. Again, treatment involves local debridement and treatment with antibacterial agents (hexachlorophene and systemic ampicillin, cefdinir, imipenem, erythromycin, or vancomycin).

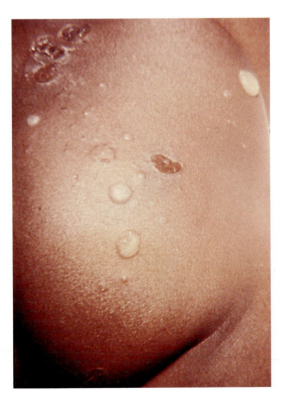

■ **FIGURE 19.9** Gluteal lesions of impetigo. *Source:* © CDC.

✓ **Checkpoint! 19.1**

The M protein is a major virulence factor of S. pyogenes. *Why is this component so important in* S. pyogenes *infections?*

Pharyngitis (Strep Throat)

Group A streptococci is the most common bacterial cause of pharyngitis in children 5 to 15 years of age. Pharyngitis is characterized by fever, chills, and, as expected, sore throat, headaches, and a red pharynx with **exudate** and anterior cervical lymphadenitis (8, 9). See Figure 19.10 ■ for a classical clinical picture of strep throat. Sometimes these symptoms can mimic those of *Mycoplasma pneumoniae* in high school students. Interestingly, strains that cause pharyngitis tend not to cause skin infections and vice versa. M types 1, 3, 5, 6, 14, 18, 19, and 24 primarily cause streptococcal pharyngitis. An important and serious sequelae to pharyngitis is rheumatic fever, which can occur in about 3% of victims of epidemics of pharyngitis. Delayed sequelae can include arthritis, endocarditis, CNS symptoms, skin lesions, and subcutaneous nodules. In addition, antibodies against streptococci can cross-react with host tissues resulting in autoimmune reactions (10, 11).

Scarlet Fever

An exotoxin produced by *Streptococcus pyogenes* is the main cause of scarlet fever (3). This condition was a major cause of death, especially in the late 19th century, when it took a particularly virulent form. It is now effectively treated with the use of antibiotics; it is a disease typical of childhood, and most adults have lasting immunity. Its incidence has declined drastically since the 1950s, and its clinical form is much milder than that seen in the late 1800. Scarlet fever is characterized by (of course) fever, sore throat, and a characteristic rash, which appears on the chest, armpits, skin folds, groin,

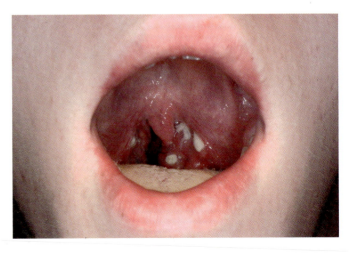

■ **FIGURE 19.10** Inflammation of the oropharynx and petechiae (small red spots) on the soft palate caused by strep throat. *Source:* CDC/Dr. Heinz F. Eichenwald.

and ears. Somehow it spares the face, creating a white mask-like pattern around the mouth called **circumoral pallor** (Figure 19.6). It also causes the tongue to become bright red, resembling a strawberry (Figure 19.6). The rash peels off after a few days (11).

Rheumatic Fever

Another sequelae of a Group A streptococcal infection such as pharyngitis can be an inflammatory disease called rheumatic fever (3). Unlike the infection itself, the culprits in rheumatic fever appear to be cross-reacting antibodies to bacterial antigens, which mimic host components immunologically and generate a type II hypersensitivity reaction to self-antigens. Common cross-reactive antigens in the host involve the heart, joints, skin, and brain tissues (5, 6). It has been suggested that some components of the M protein can cross-react with cardiac myosin, glycogen from muscles, and components of smooth muscle cells in arteries. Once again, acute rheumatic fever occurs more commonly in children (although adults can be affected too), and symptoms appear 2–3 weeks after a streptococcal infection. There is a 1% risk of developing rheumatic fever following untreated pharyngitis in the civilian population. The causal strain adheres to the oral and pharyngeal cells and then releases its degradation products (12). These, in turn, present antigenic determinants that cross-react with human tissues, particularly in cardiac valves and tissues of the myocardium, causing extensive tissue damage (13) (Figure 19.11 ■). Rheumatic fever can occur when bacteria are no longer present.

Glomerulonephritis

S. pyogenes can also cause acute proliferative glomerulonephritis (AGN), a disorder involving damage to the small blood vessels of the kidney (3, 14). AGN can occur as sequelae of streptococcal infections, and it follows more commonly a skin infection such as impetigo rather than strep throat (although the latter can also cause it). The tissue damage seen in AGN has been attributed to a type III hypersensitivity reaction caused by the deposition of immune complexes following infection. These immune complexes adhere to the basal membrane of the glomeruli, where the activation of the complement system results in glomerular destruction. Clinical symptoms can vary in type and severity and can include hematuria (blood in the urine), decreased urine flow, **hypervolemia,** edema, hypertension, fever, headache, malaise, anorexia, nausea, vomiting, renal necrosis, and renal failure. Because the kidneys are affected, edema is caused by an increase in hydrostatic pressure and an overload of fluids associated with the inflammatory damage. The urinary sediment shows dysmorphic red blood cells, red cell casts, leukocytes, and occasionally leukocyte casts.

Toxic Shock Syndrome

Toxic shock syndrome (TSS), also called toxic shock-like syndrome (TSLS), or streptococcal toxic shock syndrome (STSS), is a very serious and potentially fatal condition caused by toxins produced by bacteria such as *Streptococcus pyogenes* (it can also be caused by toxins from *Staphylococcus aureus*). Symptoms

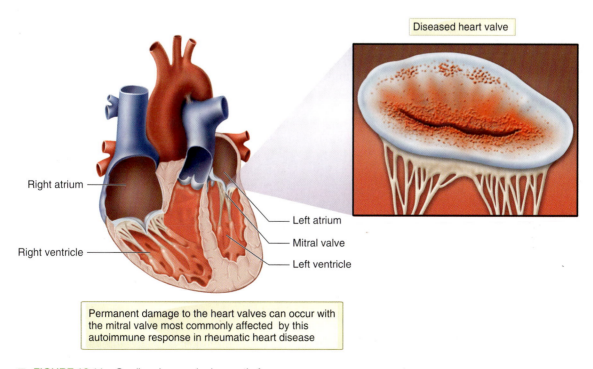

Diseased heart valve

Right atrium

Right ventricle

Left atrium

Mitral valve

Left ventricle

Permanent damage to the heart valves can occur with the mitral valve most commonly affected by this autoimmune response in rheumatic heart disease

■ **FIGURE 19.11** Cardiac damage in rheumatic fever.

and signs of TSS vary depending on the causative organism. In the case of *S. pyogenes,* TSS is usually seen in people who also have skin infections by that organism; it is characterized by high fever, malaise, hypotension, and cognitive problems such as confusion, and can lead to stupor, coma, and the failure of multiple organs. The pathophysiology of TSS is caused by a toxin that acts as a superantigen (see earlier discussion and Figure 19.8), resulting in the polyclonal activation of many different T cells and a subsequent massive release of cytokines ultimately leading to the catastrophic organ and system failures seen in the syndrome. This condition requires attention on an emergency basis with hospitalization, often in intensive care units; treatment involves stabilization and vital support, removal of the source of infection, and aggressive antibacterial treatment (3). With proper medical intervention, recovery can be achieved in 2 weeks to a month, but in extreme cases TSS can cause death within a few hours.

DETECTION AND DIAGNOSTICS FOR STREPTOCOCCI

Detection and identification of streptococci relies on different approaches: the culture of the organism itself, the detection of the organism based on immunological assays or DNA testing, and the detection of antibodies in an infected individual. Obviously, culture approaches require the ability to reach and sample a locus of infection where the organism may be found, so this is more often done in cases of strep throat, because the infected site can be reached. Culture involves the use of sheep blood agar plates and can take up to 48 hours; a halo of beta-hemolysis (see Figure 19.4) around the colonies is suggestive of Group A streptococcus. Additional testing includes sensitivity to antibiotics such as bacitracin. *S. pyogenes* also produces the enzyme L-pyrrolidonyl arylamidase; this enzyme can hydrolyze a substrate called L-pyrrolidonyl-β-naphthylamide, and in doing so, it releases L-pyrrolidone and β-naphthylamine. Addition of a particular developing reagent (p-dimethylaminocinnamaldehyde) produces a reddish-yellow color, which is a positive indication for the presence of *S. pyogenes.*

A rapid immunoassay test called the rapid strep test (RST) has been developed; this test involves the detection of certain antigens that are unique to Group A streptococci (15). The test is simple and fast and can be easily performed in a doctor's office: a patient's throat is swabbed and the swab is then placed into a commercially available kit that detects such antigens immunologically by immunochromatography within minutes. The test is highly specific (more than 95%); however, its sensitivity is only about 80%. Contamination of the swabbed area by gargling, liquids, or food can affect the results of the test. A negative RST should be followed by culture testing. Some streptococcal antigens can also be used for serotyping; for example, different antigens of the M protein have been associated with different serotypes of the organism; this may help in identifying the source, magnitude, or directional spread of an epidemic. However, this approach has

limitations because it depends on the availability of specific antibodies against a particular serotype, and new serotypes may go undetected. Molecular biology approaches have helped in identifying particular bacterial strains. In particular, a gene encoding the cell surface M protein (the emm gene) has an area that encodes for more than 100 different serotypes of *S. pyogenes.* By using PCR, this area can be amplified, and sequence analysis of a hypervariable area of this gene can then determine the serotype of a particular isolate. This approach bypasses the problems of antibody serotyping, such as the lack of availability of specific antibodies and cross-reactivity.

Antibodies to Streptococcal Products

Culture of *Streptococci* or direct detection of their components relies on the ability to obtain clinical bacterial isolates, something that is reasonably easy in a condition such as strep throat. However, when bacterial colonization is not directly accessible, for example, in rheumatic fever, the host antibody response to the infection can be of diagnostic value. The most common antigens against which antibodies are produced are various bacterial exotoxins, such as DNAses A through D, streptolysin O (a toxin that plays a role in the organism's β-hemolytic property) and streptolysin S (a cardiotoxic exotoxin also involved in beta-hemolysis), hyaluronidase (which is thought to facilitate the spread of the bacteria through tissues by breaking down components of connective tissues such as hyaluronic acid), streptokinase (which converts plasminogen into plasmin, which, in turn digests fibrin and other proteins), NADase, and different pyogenic toxins, which act as superantigens (16). The detection of antibodies against some of these components suggests a strep A infection. Most commonly tested are antibodies to streptolysin O, DNAse B, and hyaluronidase. Streptolysin O is called "O" because it is oxygen liable; it participates in the hemolysis characteristic of strep A, and although the presence of antibodies to streptolysin O indicates exposure to bacteria, it does not necessarily indicate active infection. A significant rise in titers from what are termed "acceptable values" (less than 200 units in adults and less than 300 units in children where no clinical symptoms are evident) suggests disease. Titers of anti-streptolysin antibodies start to increase 1 to 3 weeks post-strep infection, can peak in 3 to 5 weeks, and then decrease to original levels in a few months. These increases in titers must be correlated with clinical diagnosis. Testing for anti-streptolysin O antibodies was one of the earlier methods to test for strep A infections and remains a significant diagnostic approach to this day. Classically, the test was performed by measuring the ability of the antibodies to interfere with the lysis of red blood cells by streptolysin O. That is, if antibodies against streptolysin O were present, they would prevent it from lysing test red blood cells resulting in no lysis, therefore indicating a positive antibody test. Results were based on titers from the dilution of a patient's blood. Values are reported as the reciprocal of the highest dilution that still prevents hemolysis. As indicated, what are considered "normal" titers vary with the age of the individual and can be different in different populations. A more modern approach to the detection of anti-streptolysin O antibody is nephelometry. In the case of the anti-streptolysin antibodies, serum is mixed with purified streptolysin; If antibodies are present in the serum, immune complexes form, increasing the light scattering of the sample, which is measured by a nephelometer, and extrapolated to the amount of antibody present.

Anti-DNAse B

Another antigen produced by Group A strep is DNAse B, which is highly specific for these organisms; antibodies to DNAse B are elevated in patients with rheumatic fever and post-streptococcal glomerulonephritis, so testing for anti-DNAse B antibodies is often performed in concurrence with testing for anti-streptolysin O antibodies (16). This combination ensures the detection of almost 95% of previous strep infections. Because DNAse B can degrade DNA, one of the classical methods used to detect antibodies to DNAse B (similar in concept to the neutralization approach used for the detection of antibodies to streptolysin O) is to measure a *decrease* in the ability of DNAse B to depolymerize DNA because of interference of antibodies. In other words, anti-DNAse B antibodies can interfere with the ability of the DNase to degrade DNA. Therefore, failure of the enzyme to degrade DNA *in vitro* is a positive test for the presence of anti-DNAse B antibodies. The test is usually performed in a solution of a DNA-methyl green conjugate. Under normal conditions, that is, when the DNA is intact, the color of the solution is green. Upon addition of DNAse, the breakdown of the DNA causes the color to decrease and eventually disappear into a clear solution. If anti-DNAse B antibodies from an individual are present in the serum, addition of the latter to the solution prevents the DNAse from hydrolyzing the DNA; therefore, if the solution does *not* change color or if the color change is different from a negative control, the results are positive (ie, antibodies are present in the sample). The colors of the tubes are graded according to color changes, from zero indicating total color disappearance (ie, clear) to +4, indicating no loss of color. Again, the results are based on titers, using the reciprocal of the highest dilution that decreases color change with a score between 2 and 4. Because of the differences in epidemiology of Group A streptococci between populations, normal levels can vary, so it is recommended that the upper limit for normal streptococcal serology be determined for individual populations. Levels of anti-DNAse B antibodies are also detected using ELISA as well as nephelometry, where, in a similar manner to streptolysin O antibodies, immune complexes scattering light in a solution can reflect the levels of anti-DNAse B antibodies present in a sample.

Streptozyme Test

If one wishes to use the "shotgun approach" as the popular colloquialism goes, the streptozyme test is available for such purpose. This is a screening test for antibodies against streptokinase, streptolysin O, DNAse, NADase, and hyaluronidase. The streptozyme test is commonly used to detect suspected poststreptococcal conditions such as rheumatic fever. The major advantage of the streptozyme test is that it can detect a number of different antibodies at the same time; it is also not susceptible to some of the false positive results that can occur in the streptolysin O test. However, it cannot determine which of the antibodies has been detected and is not as sensitive in children as it is in adults. In fact, in children, it can give false negative results. The test is a classical hemagglutination test, using sheep red blood cells coated with the different streptococcal antigens; antibodies in a patient's sample will react with one or more of the antigens and cause the red cells to agglutinate, indicating the presence of antibodies to one or more of the antigens in the patient's sample. The test is quick and simple and can be easily carried out, but because of its shortcomings, it should be used only as an initial screening test and followed by the more specific tests already described.

Treatment of *S. pyogenes* infections involves the use of penicillin; in the case of penicillin allergies, erythromycin may be used. Some strains that are resistant to erythromycin have developed, so cephalosporins can be used in people with mild allergy to penicillin.

▶ *HELICOBACTER PYLORI*

Helicobacter pylori is a microaerophilic gram-negative bacterium shaped like a helix; its name comes from the Greek, meaning something that's twisted, like a coil, and the *pylori* refers to the pyloric valve of the stomach, the upper area of which this organism tends to inhabit. It is a very common resident of the stomach and is found in half of the world's population. It is more prevalent in developing countries and more than three-quarters of the people infected with this organism are asymptomatic. This bacterium is a causative agent of duodenal and gastric ulcers, and, in more severe cases, it has been associated with cancer of the stomach (2, 17).

H. pylori has the ability to penetrate the mucosal lining of the stomach, and its coil-like shape is thought to enable it to do so. *H. pylori* has several outer membrane proteins that serve different functions. Some act as **adhesins,** others are part of the bacterium's flagellum, others are **porins,** and others have biochemical properties such as iron transport. As a gram-negative organism, *H. pylori's* membrane contains phospholipids and lipopolysaccharide (LPS). Flagella allow for bacterial motility; the major components of the flagella are 2 flagellins: FlaA and FlaB (18). See Figure 19.12 ■ for a diagram of *H. pylori* and its virulence factors.

H. pylori has the ability to survive the harsh environment of the stomach by producing the enzyme urease. This enzyme can cleave the stomach urea to produce ammonia and carbon dioxide, which then go through chemical reactions, ultimately producing bicarbonate, which neutralizes the stomach

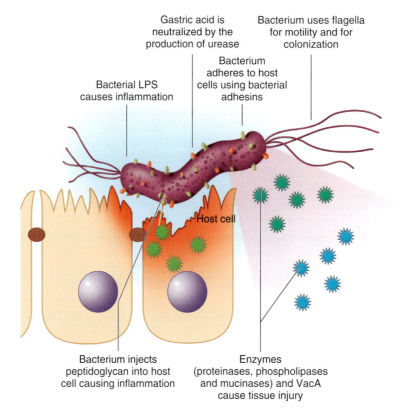

■ **FIGURE 19.12**   Schematic diagram of virulence factors of *Helicobacter pylori*.

acids. The ammonia can also damage the epithelial cells, as can other substances produced by the bacterium, such as different enzymes (mucinases, proteases, phospholipases) and vacuolating cytotoxin A (VacA) (see Figure 19.12). *H. pylori* can burrow into the mucosal layer of the stomach and can sense pH gradients, thus moving into areas that are more neutral (pH-wise); it does so by chemotaxis, using its flagella; the coil shape is thought to aid in this movement, perhaps through screwlike motion. Its adhesins bind to various components (lipids, carbohydrates) of the epithelial cells and allow the bacterium to adhere to them. *H. pylori* can also inject the protein CagA into the epithelial cells; this, in turn, disrupts the cell cytoskeleton and interferes with the cell's intracellular signaling mechanisms and the expression of different cell genes. CagA can also contribute to the immune and inflammatory response to the organism because it is highly immunogenic. So, in addition to the damage done by the bacterium itself, the presence of *H. pylori* also causes a strong inflammatory reaction at the site where it colonizes; in some cases, it also causes the increased production of the gastrin hormone, which increases acid production in the stomach. Damage to the stomach is the result of a combination of bacterial products, inflammatory responses, and fluctuations of gastric acid levels (2, 17, 18, 19). Refer to Figure 19.13 ■ for a diagram of gastric ulceration.

The great majority of people infected with *H. pylori* are asymptomatic (17) even though they may have chronic gastritis. Ulcers ultimately develop in roughly 15% of infected individuals. Treatment involves the use of proton pump inhibitors and antibiotic regimens until the organism is eradicated.

DIAGNOSIS AND TESTING

The diagnosis for *H. pylori* infections starts with symptomology that can include an upset stomach, indigestion, a sense of fullness not relative to the amount of food eaten, stomach pain, and heartburn, although these symptoms can be caused by other conditions such as gastroesophageal reflux and cancer. Testing for *H. pylori* includes the use of noninvasive tests such as testing for antibodies against the organism, testing for microbial antigens, stool testing, and the carbon-urea test. More reliable tests tend to be invasive and include performing a biopsy check during endoscopy and a rapid urease test. In this test, urease produced by the organism breaks down urea, and this reaction can be detected by colorimetric methods that detect a pH change due to the production of ammonia and bicarbonate. Histology examination and bacterial culture are also used to detect the presence of *H. pylori*. More recently, an ELISA test using urine samples has been developed. The carbon-urea test relies on the bacterial urease,

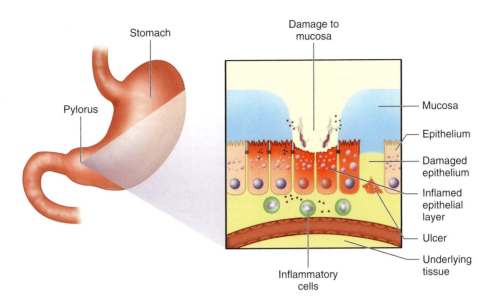

■ **FIGURE 19.13**   Diagram of gastric ulceration by *H. pylori*. *H. pylori* travels through the stomach's mucus layer and adheres to mucosal epithelial cells. The production of ammonia neutralizes the stomach acids allowing the organism to proliferate. The gastric ulceration is the result of bacterial products, inflammation, and gastric acids.

which breaks down urea releasing carbon dioxide. In the carbon-urea test, radioactively labeled urea is ingested and if the organism is present, its urease breaks it down, releasing radioactively labeled carbon dioxide, which can be detected in the patient's breath. Some drugs can result in false negatives because they can interfere with the activity of *H. pylori* urease.

The most reliable method of detection is biopsy with histological examination and bacterial culture. Unfortunately, even this method has its shortcoming because the organism is not usually widespread throughout the infected tissues, so the location of the biopsy is critical in its success to detect the organism. Stool testing is usually performed to monitor the elimination of the organisms through feces and involves an enzyme-labeled immunoassay to test for bacterial antigens in the stool. Serologic testing involves the detection of antibodies against *H. pylori* in an infected individual. Antibodies to *H. pylori* can include different isotypes; however, most serologic screening involves the detection of antibodies of the IgG class. This is because by the time the symptoms of infection become evident, the organism is well established in the infected individual whose antibody response by then tends to be of the IgG class. Assessing antibodies against *H. pylori* in an infected individual can be performed by different immunological methods, including ELISA, latex bead agglutination, immuno-dot blot, or quick tests using flow-through ImmunoMembrane technology. However, the most common method is ELISA. Because *H. pylori* is antigenically variable, several antigens from a wide variety of different *H. pylori* strains are used as targets. Common antigens against which infected individuals produce antibodies are the vacuolating cytotoxin A (VacA) and the CagA protein described earlier (19, 20).

One important point to remember is that an infected individual will have elevated antibodies to *H. pylori* for quite some time, even for years in untreated cases. It takes months for these antibodies to decrease in titers after treatment so if antibody levels are used to monitor treatment and elimination of the organism, it is imperative that antibody testing be done at different points during and after treatment and earlier samples be stored so that a decrease in antibody titers can be demonstrated. Several rapid in-office tests for *H. pylori* are available from different companies; these tests are also immunoassays, testing for antibodies against the organism in a potentially infected individual. Most of the immunoassays use whole blood as the source sample although some use urine or saliva. The best serological method for detection of anti-*H. pylori* antibodies is still the clinical laboratory ELISA. The approximate sensitivity and specificity of different tests are described in Table 19.1 ✪. Molecular biology tests using PCR amplification of specific *H. pylori* DNA are also available in the market (21); however, they only detect the possible presence of the organism but cannot distinguish a live versus dead one, nor can they confirm active infection because residual DNA may remain even after the organism has been killed.

✓ **Checkpoint! 19.2**

The environment of the stomach is chemically very harsh with very low pH and the presence of various other strong chemicals. In this environment, organic matter is usually digested or broken down. How, then, can H. pylori *survive and even thrive in this environment?*

✪ TABLE 19.1

Approximate Sensitivity and Specificity of Different Tests for *H. pylori*

Test	Sensitivity (%)	Specificity (%)
Reference lab serology (IgG)	90–93	More than 95
Office-based serology (IgG)	50–85	75–100
Urine ELISA (IgG)	70–96	77–85
Saliva ELISA (IgG)	82–91	71–85
Stool test (antigen)	~90	More than 95
Urea breath test	More than 95	95
Gastric biopsy with Steiner's stain	95	More than 95
Rapid UREASE test	93–97	More than 95
H. pylori culture	70–80	100
Stool PCR test	63	93

▶ *MYCOPLASMA PNEUMONIAE*

Mycoplasma pneumoniae is a bacterium belonging to the class of Mollicutes, a group of microorganisms that lack a peptidoglycan cell wall. Its cell membrane is similar to that of eukaryotic cells because it does not have a cell wall. It is therefore not affected by antibiotics such as the beta-lactams, which carry out their action by affecting bacterial cell walls. It is, however, susceptible to other antibiotics such as erythromycin, fluoroquinolones, and tetracyclines (2). *Mycoplasma pneumoniae* is the causative agent of a form of bacterial pneumonia called, appropriately, mycoplasma pneumonia. This condition is common and affects all ages; it is contagious and usually spreads by transmission of respiratory droplets, spreading quickly through families, households, areas in which people tend to concentrate, and hospital settings.

Mycoplasma pneumoniae can attach to the respiratory mucosa, and once there, it can extract nutrients from the host's tissues and reproduce. It usually colonizes both upper and lower respiratory tracts, causing the inflammation of the pharynx, bronchi, and lungs, and it can remain there for months. Symptoms including bronchitis, sore throat, headaches, and chills usually progress slowly compared to other forms of pneumonia (22). Mycoplasma pneumonia is also called "atypical pneumonia" because symptoms can also be extrapulmonary. These can include anemias, rashes, meningeal inflammation, and arthritis. Inflammation is the usual culprit in all these symptoms. Techniques for the detection of *M. pneumoniae* are limited; it is a "fussy" organism; it dries quickly and is difficult to transport, so culture is often a limited choice and impractical (2).

DIAGNOSIS AND TESTING

Historically, the detection of *M. pneumoniae* was performed by testing for **cold agglutinins,** which are autoantibodies thought to be generated from cross-reactive antigens on the microorganism. The antibodies are called this because of their ability to agglutinate red blood cells at lower than body temperatures (thus the name "cold"). Only about half of infected individuals exhibit cold agglutinins, so the method is not reliable for diagnosis, especially when considering that other microorganisms including some viruses can also cause cold agglutinins. Therefore, the cold agglutinin test now has more of a historical significance than a practical one.

More modern methods involve the detection of antibodies against *M. pneumoniae*. These immunological methods include ELISA, latex agglutination, and immunofluorescence. The most commonly used and reliable method is ELISA; it requires a minimal amount of sample and can detect antibodies of the IgG and IgM isotype separately. The indirect immunofluorescence test also can detect anti-*M. pneumoniae* antibodies of both IgG and IgM classes. This test involves placing a sample of an individual's serum on a slide to which antigens from *M. pneumoniae* are bound. After the reaction time and the removal of unbound material, fluorescence-labeled anti-human IgG or anti-human IgM are added to the plate, and after a second wash, the amount of fluorescence can be evaluated and results can be extrapolated from a serial dilution of the patient's original sample. The use of molecular biology techniques for the detection of *M. pneumoniae* is still under active development. Although several PCR techniques to detect *M. pneumoniae* DNA, including real-time PCR and RNA amplification, are available, the molecular approach to detection is still being improved and a recent study suggested that a combination of different testing methods, both molecular and serological, is the best approach for the detection of *M. pneumoniae* (23).

▶ *RICKETTSIA*

The organisms belonging to the genus *Rickettsia* represent diverse microorganisms that exhibit different shapes (threads, cocci, rods); the name of the genus derives from Howard Taylor Ricketts, who studied Rocky Mountain spotted fever and eventually died of typhus in 1910. Rickettsiae are gram-negative obligate intracellular parasites, meaning that they can survive and replicate only within the host's cell. They are nonmotile and nonspore-forming, and their intracellular growth requirements make their study complicated because they cannot be grown in classical microbiological growth media but must be cultured in tissues such as chicken embryos (2, 24). However, they are susceptible to antibiotics. They can cause different human diseases including typhus, Rocky Mountain spotted fever, African tick bite fever, and other forms of tick fevers. Rickettsiae are transmitted by various insects such as ticks, lice, and fleas and usually infect humans via these vectors. More recent vectors, including arthropods, leeches, and protists, have been identified (24, 25). Based on clinical outcomes, they have been divided into (1) the typhus group, (2) the scrub typhus, and (3) the spotted fever group (although the scrub typhus group, (eg, *R. tsutsugamushi*) has recently been reclassified as a new genus). The typhus group includes *R. typhi* and *R. prowazekii,* whereas the spotted fever groups include *R. rickettsii, R. akari, R. japonica,* and *R. felis*. Different groups of rickettsiae are shown in Table 19.2 ✪.

The diseases caused by rickettsiae in the United States are mainly Rocky Mountain spotted fever and typhus (either epidemic or endemic). Rocky Mountain spotted fever is a very serious disease and can be fatal; its causative agent, *Rickettsia rickettsii* is transmitted by the Dermacentor tick. Although treatable with modern antibiotics such as tetracycline, Rocky Mountain spotted fever is still a cause of death of almost 5% of infected individuals, particularly because it is often difficult to diagnose. Symptoms include fever, headache, loss of appetite, vomiting, significant muscle and joint pains, and a rash (Figure 19.14 ■). Hospitalization is usually required, and complications can include severe disease manifestations in the central nervous system and respiratory, gastrointestinal, and renal systems. Immediate treatment is absolutely critical.

Epidemic typhus is caused by *Rickettsia prowazekii,* which is transmitted by human body lice. The lice feed on an infected human, then transmit the organism, which goes through the lice's digestive system, and ends up in the feces. When the louse bites another person, the bite causes an area of itching, and the scratching pushes the feces into the bite wound. Epidemic typhus is called so because it often presents itself after natural or humanmade disasters such as wars or other catastrophic events. The disease is characterized by high fever, chills, muscle pain, rashes, severe cough, severe headaches, and hypotension as well as neurological complications such as confusion, stupor, and delirium (24, 25). During World War II, soldiers were routinely

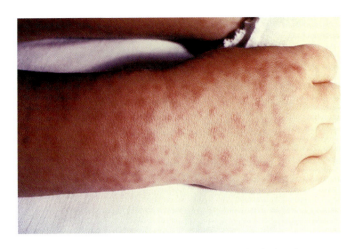

■ **FIGURE 19.14** Child's right hand and wrist displaying the characteristic spotted rash of Rocky Mountain spotted fever. *Source:* © CDC.

sprayed with DDT to kill the lice vector. Treatment involves the use of antibiotics, particularly those that act intracellularly such as tetracycline. A vaccine is also available and is highly effective.

Rickettsia typhi is the causative agent of endemic typhus (also known as Murine typhus); unlike epidemic typhus, endemic typhus is transmitted by fleas (24). Fleas from rats are the most common vectors, and common symptoms include muscle pain, chills, fever, headache, cough, nausea, and vomiting. The disease is easily treated with antibiotics such as tetracyclines and chloramphenicol, and death is rare.

SEROLOGY AND DIAGNOSTICS

As with other organisms described in this chapter, immunological techniques play a major role in the detection of rickettsiae. These include immunofluorescence, immuno-dot blot, agglutination, and ELISA. The indirect immunofluorescence

✪ TABLE 19.2

Different Rickettsial Groups, Diseases, and Geographical Locations

Disease	Location	Organism
Rocky mountain spotted fever	Western Hemisphere	*Rickettsia rickettsii*
Rickettsialpox	United States, former USSR	*Rickettsia akari*
Boutonneuse fever	Mediterranean area, Asia, Africa, India	*Rickettsia conorii*
Siberian tick typhus	Siberia, Mongolia, China	*Rickettsia sibirica*
Australian tick typhus	Australia	*Rickettsia australis*
Oriental spotted fever	Japan	*Rickettsia japonica*
African tick bite fever	South Africa	*Rickettsia africae*
Epidemic and sporadic typhus	Worldwide	*Rickettsia prowazekii*
Murine (endemic) typhus	Worldwide	*Rickettsia typhi*

test is the most commonly used and accepted test, and it can target different species and different antibodies depending on the kit specifications. For example, one kit tests for IgG (or IgM) utilizing inactivated *R. rickettsii* antigen and *R. typhi* antigen. This kit consists of slides with 8 wells each with each well containing 2 individual antigen spots. The kit is intended for the semi-quantitation of antibodies to spotted fever and typhus fever group *rickettsiae*. Micro-immunofluorescence assay kits for antibodies to various *Rickettsiae* species are also available. ELISA kits using *R. rickettsii* rOmpB, an immunodominant protein antigen, are also available to detect IgG and IgM antibodies against different *Rickettsiae* species. Rapid rickettsia IgG/IgM combo test, a flow-through membrane technology test is also available.

Historically, an agglutination assay called the Weil-Felix test was used to test the serum of patients with epidemic typhus. The test is based on the fact that *Rickettsia* species exhibit antigenic cross-reactivity with certain *Proteus* species. Thus, serum containing anti-rickettsial antibodies would also cross-react with a bacterium called *Proteus vulgaris*. The cross-reacting antigens turned out to be different polysaccharide antigens of the *Proteus* species, each of which could cross-react with different *rickettsiae*. Thus, according to which strains of *Proteus vulgaris* the patient's serum would agglutinate, some conclusions could be made concerning the strain of *rickettsia* with which the patient was infected. Unfortunately, the test lacked both sensitivity and specificity and, although still used in some cases, it has now pretty much been replaced by more modern and accurate methods. As with other organisms, molecular biology methods are available to detect and differentiate different *rickettsiae* groups such as the spotted fever, the scrub typhus, or the typhus groups. Various components are tested for, such as the 47 kDa, gltA, and ompB gene targets (26).

 Checkpoint! 19.3

The study of many microorganisms depends on culturing the organisms in growth media, thus generating enough organisms in vitro for biological, biochemical, and diagnostic studies. Unfortunately, this approach does not apply to rickettsiae. Why?

▶ CLOSTRIDIUM DIFFICILE

There are some situations in which human manipulation to improve a clinical condition can actually result in the development of another one. An example of this is an infection caused by *Clostridium difficile*, a gram-positive, spore-forming bacterium that belongs to the *Clostridia* genus and that is a normal human commensal intestinal organism in 3 to 5% of the population (2). Overabundance of *Clostridium difficile* in the intestines can cause severe diarrhea and can lead to pseudomembranous colitis, a serious inflammation of the colon. Overpopulation of *Clostridium difficile* can be caused by the

administration of antibiotics, which can wipe out the normal flora of the intestine, facilitating the thriving of *Clostridium difficile* in the affected areas. Certain antibiotics such as fluoroquinolones are particularly associated with *C. difficile* infections (27). Under those conditions, bacteria that normally compete for space and nutrients with *C. difficile* are eradicated, and *C. difficile* basically takes over, resulting in what is called *antibiotic-associated diarrhea (ADD)*. Refer to Figure 19.15 ■ for *C. difficile* colonies on blood agar and a photomicrograph of the organism. The clinical manifestations of a *C. difficile* infection are due to certain toxins produced by the organism (2, 28), particularly enterotoxin (toxin A) and cytotoxin (toxin B), which are glucosyltransferases that can disrupt the function of some cells, leading to inflammation, bloating, and diarrhea (although their specific roles are still under discussion). Symptoms can be confused with those of other conditions such as inflammatory bowel disease, and can range from mild to severe and even life threatening in some cases, particularly in older patients. In simpler cases, the infection can be eliminated spontaneously by stopping the particular antibiotic regimens that are causing the problem; more serious cases require the administration of metronidazole or vancomycin. Symptoms and findings in adults include significant diarrhea (with 3 or more loose and watery stools per 24 hour period, a condition called *C. difficile*-associated diarrhea, or CDAD), high fever, abdominal pain, and stools with unusual or particularly fetid odor. Often the source of infection is a hospital or a nursing home, but it can also be an outpatient setting or the community at large. Transmission is usually through the fecal-oral route, and the production of spores makes the organism particularly resilient because it can remain in hospital settings for long periods.

TESTING

Because *C. difficile* produces toxins for this pathogenic action, their detection and/or their effect offers a major approach in testing for *C. difficile*. The classical testing for *C. difficile* is toxigenic culture. In this assay, *C. difficile* is isolated from a stool sample and selected by culturing it in selective culture media; the organisms are then added to a culture of a fibroblast cell line, and the cytopathic effect of these toxins on the fibroblasts is observed. Once there is evidence of cytopathic effects, antiserum against the toxin is added, and the neutralization of the **cytopathic effect** confirms the identification of *C. difficile* (29). This test is the most sensitive and specific for *C. difficile*, but it is time consuming and labor intensive and requires significant experience in microbiology by the operator.

Enzyme-linked assays are now available for the detection of both toxin A and toxin B from *C. difficile*. The ELISA methods have a sensitivity of 70 to 100% and a specificity of more than 90%. ELISA testing is also used to monitor the elimination of the toxins from the stools in order to evaluate the treatment effectiveness. Rapid immunochromatography assays are also available for these toxins.

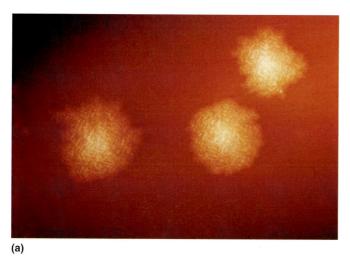

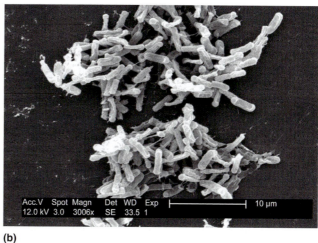

(a) **(b)**

■ **FIGURE 19.15** *Clostridium difficile:* (a) on blood agar and (b) scanning electron microscopy. *Source:* (a) © CDC/Dr. Holdeman and (b) © CDC/ Lois S. Wiggs.

Different tests using real-time PCR are also available; in fact, the FDA approved 3 of them for use in 2009. Although they use somewhat different extraction methods and vary in cost and length of procedure, all have sensitivity and specificity of more than 95%. The methods and principles of different forms of PCR are described in Chapter 23. More recently, the FDA approved a novel PCR technique, called *loop-mediated isothermal DNA amplification (LAMP)* for the detection of *C. difficile*. The illumigene *C. difficile* assay, unlike conventional PCR assays that amplify a single piece of DNA, uses a series of different primers at a constant temperature that allow for the identification of a highly conserved region of the toxin A sequence of the PaLoc pathogenicity locus of the organism. The test takes less than an hour and does not require sophisticated RT-PCR equipment.

▶ SPIROCHETES

Spirochetes are a group of motile bacteria that exhibit a characteristic coil or screw shape; they are mostly anaerobic (with some exceptions), and they have a central protoplasmic cylinder surrounded by a cytoplasmic membrane (2). Traditionally classified as gram-negative because of the similarities of their cell wall with that of gram-negative organisms, such classification has recently been under question because of differences in staining among different spirochete species, the weakness of the staining for those species that do retain the stain, and because of the marginal use of gram-staining due to their very small size (some of the smaller ones cannot be visually identified by light microscopy and require dark-field microscopy). Unique to spirochetes is also the position of their flagella or axial filaments; they run along the length of the organism between the cell wall and the outer membrane and are anchored at the extremities of the organism. In fact, contraction of the filaments distorts the bacteria to give it

its helical shape. The shape of spirochetes is also involved in their movement, allowing the organism to move using a screw-like motion. See Figure 19.16 ■ for a diagram of a representative spirochete. Spirochetes can cause a variety of different conditions, including syphilis, Lyme disease, yaws, pinta, leptospirosis, relapsing fever, necrotizing ulcerative gingivitis, and chronic periodontitis. The Order Spirochetales includes three families; the *Brachyspiraceae,* the *Leptospiraceae,* and the *Spirochaetaceae.* Examples of disease-causing spirochetes are *Treponema pallidum* pallidum, *Treponema pallidum* pertenue, *Borrelia burgdorferi, Borrelia recurrentis,* and the *Leptospira* species. It is not in the scope of this chapter to cover all spirochetes and the diseases they cause; rather, we discuss the 2 most representative diseases from Spirochete*s*, which also involve serological testing: syphilis and Lyme disease.

TREPONEMA PALLIDUM PALLIDUM

Treponema pallidum has 4 subspecies: pallidum, endemicum, carateum, and pertenue, each causing a different disease. *Treponema pallidum* subspecies pallidum (in this chapter simply referred as *T. pallidum*) is the infectious agent that causes

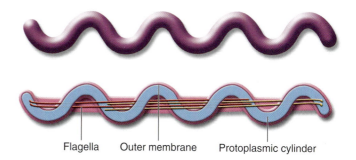

Flagella   Outer membrane   Protoplasmic cylinder

■ **FIGURE 19.16** Drawing of spirochete's mobility system (with internal flagellae).

syphilis. It is a motile spirochete that is usually transmitted by sexual contact, although it can also be transmitted from mother to child through the placenta, which usually results in congenital syphilis (30, 31). Typical to spirochetes, its corkscrewlike motility allows the organism to move through mucosal tissues and gain access to an individual's bloodstream. *T. pallidum* is an obligate parasite, that is, it depends completely on the host for survival and cannot live without it. Its nutritional requirements are complex and poorly understood, so the organism cannot be cultured solely *in vitro*. In addition, *T. pallidum* lacks many surface proteins found in many other microorganisms, although some called treponema rare outer membrane proteins (TROMPs) have been identified. This lack of surface proteins has made the production of a vaccine very difficult so far and is thought to play a role in the ability of the organism to either escape or survive an immune response. The most effective protection against the organisms comes from physical barriers such as skin and mucosal membranes. Once breeched, the organism can enter the host tissues where both innate and acquired immunity play a role in defense. However, antibody responses to *T. pallidum* are often ineffective and incapable of destroying the organism. Activation of T cells, secretion of cytokines, and subsequent phagocytosis by macrophages play a role in the elimination of the organism from lesions; however, *T. pallidum* can survive in the host for many years. See Figure 19.17 ■ for a photomicrograph of *T. pallidum*.

SYPHILIS

Syphilis is a disease that is almost always transmitted by sexual contact, although its mode of transmission can include **transplacental passage** from mother to fetus (30, 31). Although of obscure origin, the name is thought to come from a fictional tale of a legendary shepherd named Syphilus who was given the disease by the god Apollo because of Syphilus's

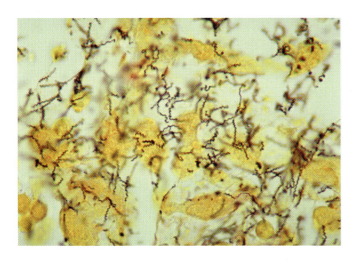

■ **FIGURE 19.17** *Treponema pallidum* using a modified Steiner silver stain. *Source:* © CDC/ Dr. Edwin P. Ewing, Jr.

BOX 19.1

It is YOUR Fault...

The word *syphilis* is thought to have originated with the legend of the shepherd Syphilus. However, several other names have been given to the disease in a wonderful form of collegiality and friendship among nations. Names used in Europe in the past included the *French disease* in Italy, Poland, and Germany; the French, somewhat disturbed by the whole thing, called it the *Italian disease*. Of course, in Holland it was known as the *Spanish disease,* and the Russians happily gave the blame to the Poles, calling it the *Polish disease.* For the Turks, it was the *Christian disease* (of course); not to be outdone, Tahitians called it the *British disease* (I mean, hello!!). All this was due to travelers (sailors, soldiers, merchants) going from country to country, spreading the disease, usually by frequenting the host country's prostitutes. The Scots, on the other hand, were a bit more politically diplomatic and simply called it the *Grandgore.* Smart move....

defiance of him (Box 19.1 ✪). The symptomology of syphilis is complex and can be confusing. Before serological testing, its diagnosis was difficult, and the disease was often confused with other conditions. Modern antibiotic treatments are successful in treating the disease but without proper treatment, it can progress and cause widespread damage to many organs and tissues, including brain, heart, major arteries, eyes, and bones, and in some cases, it can cause death. Common manifestations involve the genitals (Figure 19.18 ■), although it also causes dermatological manifestations (Figure 19.19 ■), as well as other extragenital lesions (Figure 19.20 ■). Once declining in its rate in developing countries due to the use of antibiotics and more conservative sexual practice because of the AIDS epidemic, syphilis has been on the increase in recent years (2000 and after), mainly in the homosexual male population. It appears that risky sexual practices and increased promiscuity may be important factors for this increase.

Stages of Syphilis

Syphilis can be divided into 4 stages: primary, secondary, latent, and tertiary; each stage has its own clinical manifestation and/or features. In primary syphilis, 1 week to 3 months after initial exposure, almost always via sexual contact, the point of infection develops a lesion called **chancre.** It is a painless ulceration that most often appears on the genitalia; see Figure 19.18(b); it also can involve other areas; see Figure 19.20(a). The lesion is usually at the site of entry of the organism and after 4 to 6 weeks, it heals by itself without any other symptoms. Because it is painless and goes away spontaneously, many individuals tend to ignore it and do not seek medical treatment. If untreated, after 1 to 6 months, roughly one-fourth of the primary cases develop into the secondary stage, which is the most contagious. Secondary syphilis presents with a variety of different symptoms including enlarged lymph nodes, fever, loss of weight, sore throat,

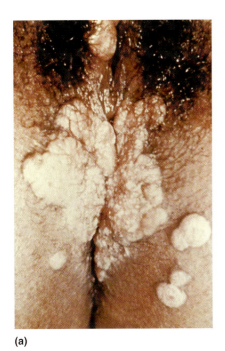

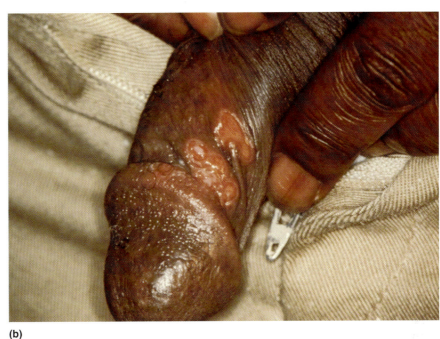

(a)   (b)

■ **FIGURE 19.18** Genital manifestations of syphilis: (a) Vaginal syphilis. Secondary syphilis manifested as perineal wartlike growths. *Source:* © CDC. (b) Chancres on the penile shaft due to a primary syphilitic infection. *Source:* © CDC/M. Rein, VD.

headache, stiffness of head and neck, light sensitivity, and an overall general feeling of discomfort or illness. Widespread rashes and lesions can involve the trunk (Figure 19.19) and limbs, including the palm of the hands and the soles of the feet. Wart-like growths called *condyloma latum* can be found in the genital areas; Figure 19.18(a). All of these lesions contain live organisms, and they are highly infective. In more severe (although rare) cases, secondary syphilis can lead to

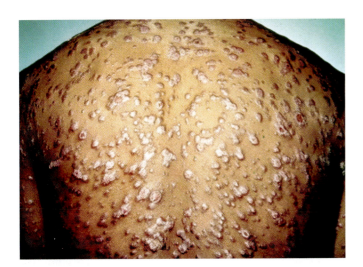

■ **FIGURE 19.19** Dermatologic manifestations of secondary syphilis on an old man with AIDS. On dark field examination, the lesions were teeming with spirochetes. *Source:* Herbert L. Fred, MD and Hendrik A. van Dijk. "Images of Memorable Cases—50 years at the bedside"

meningitis, kidney and liver disease, arthritic disease, connective tissue inflammation, especially around the bones, and inflammation of the eyes (32).

Secondary syphilis is followed by a period of latency lacking any signs or symptoms of disease. This is appropriately named the latent stage of syphilis; it is divided into early and late phases based on the time elapsed from initial exposure. By definition, the latent stage has serological evidence of disease but no symptomology. The definitions of early and late are somewhat vague because in most cases, the initial timing of infection is not known. In general, the early phase is defined as suffering from syphilis for less than 2 years, and the late phase is having had syphilis for more than 2 years without clinical symptoms. Patients in the early phase tend to be more infectious than in the late phase although the latent stage is not nearly as infectious as the secondary stage. However, when considering treatment, it is important to assume a late phase when the time of initial infection is not known; the early phase can be treated with a single administration of long-acting penicillin whereas the late phase requires 3 weekly administrations. In the both the secondary stage and the early latent stage, transplacental transmission of syphilis from mother to fetus can occur. If untreated, the fetal infection, called congenital syphilis, can create serious problems including miscarriages, stillbirths, premature births, or the death of the newborn. Untreated babies can develop a wide variety of clinical problems including seizures, developmental delays, deformities, problems in dentition, enlargement of liver and spleen, jaundice, and anemia. They can also develop rashes and lesions that can be infectious. In very rare and extreme cases, the infants

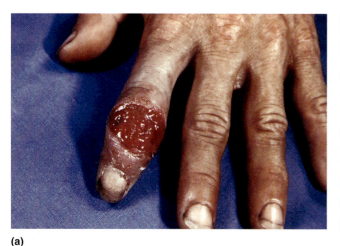

(a)

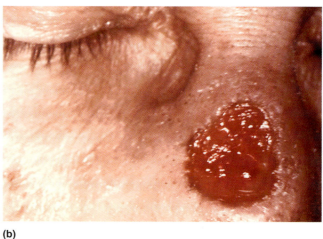

(b)

■ **FIGURE 19.20** Chancre of the hand from syphilis. (a) The chancre is usually firm, round, small, and painless, appearing at the spot where syphilis entered the body, and lasts 3 to 6 weeks, healing on its own. If adequate treatment is not administered, the infection progresses to the secondary stage. The primary lesion can be smaller than that shown. *Source:* © CDC. (b) Gumma of nose due to a long-standing tertiary syphilitic *Treponema pallidum* infection. *Source:* © CDC/ J. Pledger.

can develop tertiary syphilis. Fortunately, congenital syphilis is easily treated by prevention, which involves treatment of the mother, a treatment which is most effective if administered before 16 weeks of pregnancy but can be effective even before the last month of pregnancy. Because of an effective and aggressive treatment plan developed by the Centers for Disease Control and Prevention, the number of cases of congenital syphilis has dropped drastically in the last decade (33, 34).

Following untreated latent stage syphilis, about half of the patients can develop tertiary syphilis (31, 35). This can occur as early as a year after initial exposure, but typically it manifests decades after that. Typical of this stage are granulomas called **gummas;** see Figure 16.20(b). **Granulomas** are chronic festering balls or pockets of inflammatory molecules and cells constantly, and unsuccessfully, trying to clear the infecting organism. They can occur pretty much everywhere in the body from bones, to tissues, to skin. They cause a constant state of inflammation, can affect a patient's anatomy, and in some cases can cause grotesque deformities. A model of the head of a patient suffering from tertiary syphilis is shown in Figure 19.21 ■. Other complications include cardiac abnormalities, particularly affecting the ascending aorta, causing inflammation and **aneurysms,** aortic valve dilation, and subsequent regurgitation (which is detected as a heart murmur). This, in turn, results in insufficiency and massive left ventricular hypertrophy. There is a *huge* enlargement of the heart; in fact, the heart can grow to such a size that this condition is called *cor bovinum* (Latin for "cow's heart") because of its size. The coronary arteries can also be affected, resulting in their narrowing. The increase in heart size can cause secondary effects such as difficulty in breathing and swallowing, rib cage damage, and persistent cough because of the pressure on the laryngeal nerve that controls the cough reflex. Ruptured aneurysms and heart failure are common causes of death. Neurological complications of tertiary syphilis include

neurosyphilis (although this condition can occur at earlier stages too). The manifestations of neurosyphilis are numerous and diverse and include paresis of the insane characterized by

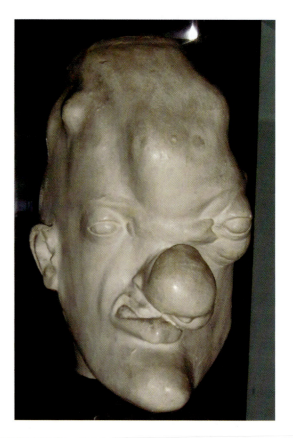

■ **FIGURE 19.21** Head of a patient with tertiary syphilis. *Source:* Axel Boldt.

changes in behavior and personality, changes in emotional reactions, and psychotic symptoms of abrupt and dramatic onset; manifestations also include hyperreactive reflexes and irregularities in the function of the pupils, a condition called *Argyll-Robinson pupil*. Additional complications of neurosyphilis include a gradual degeneration of sensory neurons called *tabes dorsalis;* this affects the nerves that help maintain a person's sense of position, direction, and standing as well as vibration and touch. Symptoms include locomotor ataxia, which results in a characteristic walking gait; other complications of neurosyphilis include weakness, tingling, burning and painful sensations without any apparent cause, visual problems, loss of coordination, deafness, and dementia (31). Neurosyphilis is commonly found in patients with HIV infections, although the reasons for this are unclear. Again, the advent of antibiotic therapy has kept the number of cases of neurosyphilis under control.

Prevention

Because syphilis is most commonly transmitted by sexual contact, common sense dictates that patient education, sexual abstinence, and avoidance of any sexual contact with an unknown or potentially infected person are the best preventive methods. *T. pallidum* can infect through the mucosa (both intact or damaged) and through minor breaks in skin, even in those areas that cannot be protected by a condom (although condoms do reduce transmission). A person who has a sexual contact with an individual suffering from any stage of the disease must be assumed as potentially infected and so tested and treated accordingly.

Treatment

Although this is a serious disease, syphilis can be well controlled if properly and promptly treated. The standard approach for treatment is the use of antibiotics, particularly penicillin G, administered intramuscularly. People allergic to penicillin can be desensitized and administered penicillin although tetracyclines and doxyclycline may be useful as a treatment (although this is still under investigation). Pregnant women allergic to penicillin should be desensitized and then treated with penicillin. The treatment modalities and doses vary with the stage of the disease. Early stages may be treated with a single dose, but later stages may require multiple subsequent administrations. A reaction called **Jarisch-Herxheimer reaction** may occur in certain patients after penicillin treatment. This condition, characterized by fever, tiredness, and worsening of any skin and mucosal symptoms, usually lasts no longer than 24 hours (31, 36).

Diagnostic Tests and Serology

The most direct way to detect *T. pallidum* is to actually see the organism, which can be done using microscopy. Although this may seem straightforward and simple, it has its disadvantages. First, it requires access to active lesions from which the organism can be isolated; thus, it cannot be used in stages when the lesions are not present. Second, an experienced technician

and microscopist are key factors because the organisms can be confused with other nonpathogenic spirochetes. Darkfield microscopy whose lens condensers allow light to go through only a particular specimen (ie, organism) also requires live organisms because recognition is based not only on bacterial morphology but also characteristic bacterial mobility. This, in turn, requires expeditious and careful specimen processing because the organism is relatively fragile and can dry quickly. Improper specimen handling may result in false negative results, so additional tests are always recommended to follow microscopy. Also because other *Treponemas* may be identified, the correlation of microscopic findings with clinical findings (signs and symptoms) is imperative for proper identification and diagnosis. A more forgiving microscopic technique involves fluorescence microscopy, either direct or indirect. In the direct method, fluorescence-labeled antibodies to *T. pallidum* are used for detection; in the indirect method, antibodies to *T. pallidum* are allowed to react with the organism, then fluorescence labeled anti-immunoglobulin antibodies are allowed to bind to the antibodies bound to the organism. This second method somewhat amplifies the sensitivity of the technique, but both methods require washes, so some of the organisms may be lost in the procedure. The major advantage of the fluorescence methods is that it does not require live organisms; a disadvantage of it is potential cross-reactivity of the antibodies with other organisms even when using commercially available monoclonal antibody preparations. Modern detections involve several other laboratory approaches (32).

Some of the laboratory tests for *T. pallidum* involve the detection of various antibodies in a patient's blood. These antibodies can be directed either to the organism itself (treponemal tests) or against components of cells that arise as a consequence of cellular damage by the organism (nontreponemal tests) (32). Examples of nontreponemal tests are the Venereal Disease Research Laboratory (VDRL) test, and the rapid plasma reagin (RPR) test. These tests are based on the detection of antibodies to cardiolipin, a lipid generated from damaged cells, and are inexpensive and fairly rapid; however, their specificity is not the best because other conditions can cause false positive results. These can include some viral infections such as hepatitis, measles, and varicella as well as diseases such as tuberculosis, malaria, Chagas disease, and endocarditis. Intravenous drug use and sample contamination can also result in false positives. Therefore, nontreponemal tests are usually considered screening tests and are followed by more precise treponemal tests. In addition, they are still routinely used for screening donated blood, although the transmission of syphilis through blood donors is almost negligible because *T. pallidum* does not usually survive blood storage conditions. In fact, recent controversy has surfaced over the rationality of including testing for syphilis in blood donations.

The VDRL test in different forms has been around for a while; it was developed before World War I by August von Wasserman. Its current form was developed right after World

War II (37). The principle of the test, as mentioned, is to detect anticardiolipin antibodies in a patient's serum. It is a **flocculation** test using extracts of bovine heart as the antigen; the antigen preparation is mixed with cholesterol and lecithin and the test is performed on a slide with several rings to contain the suspension. After inactivating complement by heating the test serum sample at 56° C, the sera to be tested are added to the slide. Along with the test samples, standard sera (controls), ranging from negative to mildly reactive to strongly reactive, are added in different circles on the slide. The antigen suspension is then added and flocculation is observed. The presence and amount of flocculation of the test samples are then compared to the control samples, and an initial semiquantitative level of reactivity can then be determined. "Positive" samples are then retested using serial dilutions. This test is also used with samples from spinal fluids in the detection of neurosyphilis.

The RPR test also measures antibodies to cardiolipin, but it is based on the **agglutination** technique. In the RPR, charcoal particles are coated with the antigen preparation; EDTA, thimerosal, and choline chloride are added to the particle suspension to preserve the antigen and to deactivate complement in the test samples. Antigen and samples are mixed within a circle on a plastic card; the use of the charcoal particles makes the detection of a positive reaction easier. If antibodies are present, the reaction causes the charcoal particles to agglutinate and clump up in a visible dark clump. The amount of both antigen and test sera is carefully measured, and results are then compared to standardized control sera (38). Once again, "positive" test samples are then retested using serial dilutions. And as mentioned, both VDRL and RPR tests are best used as screening methods to be followed by more specific ones.

Tests that follow nontreponemal tests can detect antibodies directed to *T. pallidum* itself and are thus called *treponemal tests* (32). Techniques that can detect antibodies to *T. pallidum* include agglutination and fluorescence tests. A classical agglutination test for *T. pallidum* is the *Treponema pallidum* hemagglutination assay (TPHA). This test uses red blood cells coated with *T. pallidum* antigens placed in a microtiter plate. Serum samples as well as controls are then allowed to react with the red blood cells in the plate. If antibodies to *T. pallidum* are present in the sample, agglutination of the red blood cells occurs and it is seen as an even "halolike" distribution of red blood cells in the well. If no antibodies are present, no agglutination occurs, and the red blood cells sink to the bottom of the well, forming a well-defined, small "button." Because cross-reactivity with other treponemas can occur, test samples are usually absorbed with those potentially cross-reacting antigens using a species of nonpathogenic Treponemes called the Reiter's strain. The TPHA has been pretty much replaced by an agglutination assay using gel particles instead of red blood cells, but the principle is the same. The *Treponema pallidum* particle agglutination (TP-PA) test uses gel particles sensitized with *T. pallidum* of the Nichols strain, a pathogenic serotype. Once again, agglutination appears as a uniform halo in the well, and negative results are indicated by a well-defined button of gel particles at the bottom of the well. Recent studies have suggested that the agglutination tests may not be as sensitive as other immunoassays such as ELISA (38). Antibodies to *T. pallidum* can also be detected by immunofluorescence using the fluorescent treponemal antibody absorption (FTA-ABS) test. For this test, patient sera is first heat inactivated and then absorbed with nonpathogenic strains of treponemas to remove any cross-reacting antibodies (which is why the test has the word *absorption* in its name). The serum is then allowed to react with the Nichols strain of *T. pallidum*, which has been fixed onto appropriate test slides. If antibodies to *T. pallidum* are present in the serum, they will bind to the antigen fixed on the slide. After appropriate washes, a second, anti-human immunoglobulin antibody conjugated to fluorescein is added; the latter then binds to the human antibody bound to the antigen and after a second wash, and fluorescence can be semiquantitated under a fluorescence microscope. None to weak to strong fluorescence (rated from 0 to +4) can give a semiquantitative measure of the amount of antibody against *T. pallidum* present in the patient's serum. Enzyme immunoassays have also been developed for syphilis. As in other approaches, these tests detect either antibodies to cardiolipin or to the organism itself. An example of nontreponemal ELISA tests is the Reagin II, which detects antibodies to a cardiolipin antigen in a similar principle as the VDRL and RPR tests (39). Several companies also offer treponemal specific ELISA kits to detect antibodies of different isotypes against recombinant *T. pallidum* antigens. The ELISA method allows for automation of detection better than other methods and is used in the detection of antibodies from spinal fluids. ELISA tests have high specificity and sensitivity, both surpassing 95%. In fact, because of the ease and automation of ELISA testing and because of its high specificity and sensitivity, it has recently been proposed that ELISA tests should precede more conventional tests (ie, carry out an ELISA test first and, if positive, follow by more conventional test such as VDRL and RPR tests). Molecular biology techniques are also available, and others are under development: Some include reverse transcriptase PCR targeting a 366 base pair region of the S rRNA of *T. pallidum*. Others are highly specific for the *polA* gene of *Treponema pallidum*. Another, undergoing further testing, is a TaqMan real-time PCR assay that allegedly detects *T. pallidum* from swabs and biopsy specimens from genital and mucosal ulcers, placental specimens, and cerebrospinal fluid (40). Finally, the FDA is also currently evaluating different Western blot assay kits against specific treponemal antigens.

✓ **Checkpoint! 19.4**

What has been a major impediment in the development of a vaccine for T. pallidum?

LYME DISEASE

Lyme disease, also called Lyme borreliosis, is a very common tick-borne disease caused by several microorganisms belonging to the *Borrelia* genus. Different species within the genus cause disease in different geographical areas of the world (41, 42). The disease is transmitted to humans by a deer tick of the *Ixodes* genus (Figure 19.22 ■), which received their name because they travel on and feed on deer; however, they do not acquire the infection from deer, although the deer play a role in their life cycle. The tick acquires the organisms by feeding on other animals that act as natural reservoirs, most commonly mice and sometimes rats (43). In the eastern parts of North America, the ticks causing the disease are *Ixodes scapularis;* in the west, they are *Ixodes pacificus*. Most of the U.S. cases of Lyme disease are in Maine, Vermont, New Hampshire, Rhode Island, Massachusetts, Connecticut, New York (eastern), New Jersey, Pennsylvania, Delaware, Maryland, Virginia (northern), Minnesota (eastern), and Wisconsin. This disease is also common in Europe, Asia, and Australia. The name of the disease comes from two adjacent towns in the New London County in Connecticut: Lyme and Old Lyme. The disease was first observed and described in 1975 in these towns as a cluster of cases of people with unusual rashes, malaise, fever, and arthritic symptoms. By the late 1970s, the deer tick had been recognized as a carrier of the disease, and in 1981, the causative organism was identified by Willy Burgdorfer and named *Borrelia burgdorferi* after its discoverer. The most infectious step in the life cycle of the tick is the nymphal stage at which the ticks are very small and can go undetected; they also feed for a long time, which is a critical factor in the success of the infection. In fact, the transmission rate of the infection is very low: it is estimated that only 1% of tick bites result in Lyme disease because transmission of

the organism requires the tick to remain attached to the host and feed for a long time, in general at least 24 hours (43). See Figure 19.23 ■ for the typical life cycle of ticks. Interestingly, the host of certain species of ticks can influence whether a particular species of tick can spread the *Borrelia burgdorferi* bacteria. Ticks that feed on certain lizards in the western part of North America do not spread the disease as efficiently because the lizards appear to have an innate resistance to the microorganism.

Stages and Clinical Manifestations

Individuals with Lyme disease exhibit multiple and diverse signs and symptoms. Symptoms can differ from one infected individual to another and can even be different in different geographical areas. The disease itself can be divided into 3 different stages, and symptomology varies from one stage to another. Because the tick is most likely to spread the B. *burgdorferi* during the nymph stage, symptoms tend to be more frequent during the period of such stage, which is usually during the summer months. Initial infection starts with the tick bite; anywhere from a few days to almost a month after the bite, a very characteristic, painless "bull's-eye rash" called erythema migrans (EM) appears at the site of the bite (Figure 19.24 ■). This early localized infection represents the first stage of the disease. The rash is not seen in about 20% of the cases. Early infections can also present with headaches, fever, **myalgia,** and an overall sense of sickness. This stage can last from a few days to several weeks and is followed by an early disseminated infection associated with the spread of the organism into the bloodstream and throughout the body. At this stage, a patient may experience myalgia that varies in location, joint and bone pain, irregular heartbeats and palpitation, and dizziness.

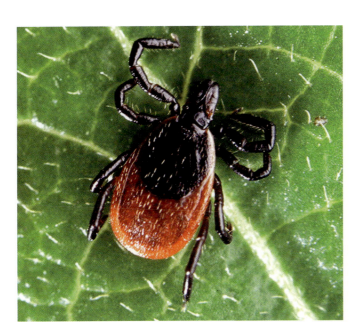

■ **FIGURE 19.22** Adult deer tick (*Ixodes scapularis*). *Source:* Scott Bauer/USDA/ARS.

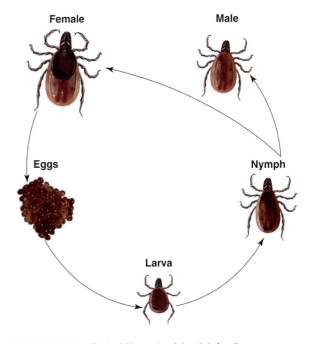

■ **FIGURE 19.23** Typical life cycle of the tick family.

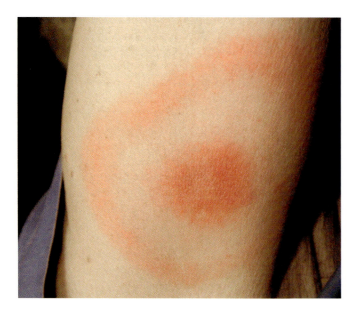

■ **FIGURE 19.24** Erythematous rash in Lyme disease in the pattern of a "bull's-eye" at the site of a tick bite on a woman's posterior right upper arm that caused Lyme disease. *Source:* © CDC/ James Gathany.

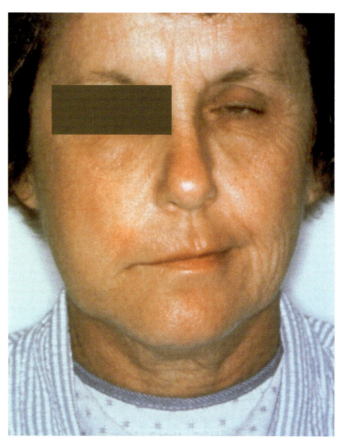

■ **FIGURE 19.25** This patient presented with a case of facial palsy caused by an infection by the bacterial spirochete *Borrelia burgdorferi* and was subsequently diagnosed with Lyme disease. *Source:* © CDC.

In more severe cases (about 10% of untreated individuals), more severe symptoms can occur. These include a set of neurological problems called *neuroborreliosis* and may include partial facial paralysis (facial palsy; Figure 19.25 ■) and meningitis. Other symptoms include memory loss, sensitivity to light, lack of sleep, and unusual mood swings. At this stage of the disease, rashes can also appear at various sites other than the site of the initial bite. After a few months, if a patient remains untreated or if treatment is not successful, the disease can develop into a late infection stage. This stage of the disease can be a serious condition, affecting different tissues and organs, including the heart, the brain, muscles, joints, and nerves. Numerous and quite diverse symptoms can occur; they can include extreme tiredness, arthritis (usually of the knees), cognitive difficulties, shooting pains, tingling, delusional behavior, some forms of psychosis, and loss of sense of reality. In some cases, these symptoms can result in permanent damage causing, for example, paralysis of lower body (paraplegia) (44, 45, 46).

Immunopathology

Much of the pathology seen in Lyme disease is actually a consequence of the immune response of the host to *B. burgdorferi*. At the initial bite site, the bacterium is actually protected by substances from the saliva of the tick that inhibit initial localized immune responses to the microorganism. Neutrophil migration to the site appears inhibited; this, in turn, prevents the organisms from being eliminated by these cells and allows the organism to colonize the site. Once *B. burgdorferi* is established in the dermis, a subsequent inflammatory response to the organism is responsible for the characteristic EM rash. The host immune system produces a strong immune response, both humoral and cellular, against *B. burgdorferi*. This, however,

turns out to be a double-edged sword because it not only is ineffective in eliminating the organism but also is responsible for many of the clinical manifestations of the disease. Once disseminated throughout the body, *B. burgdorferi* can remain in the host from months to years, evading the immune response by various means, including downregulating the expression of certain bacterial proteins that are immunogenic, by antigenic variations of some of these proteins, or by interfering with the action of complement. The disseminated secretion of inflammatory cytokines such as IL-6 and TNF-α in response to the microorganism can result in many of the symptoms seen in the disease, including both inflammatory as well as neurological ones. It has been proposed that the production of stress hormones and inflammatory responses in response to an infection by *B. burgdorferi* may interfere with the function of various neurotransmitters and their receptors, possibly contributing to the neuropathology of the disease (47, 48, 49).

Treatment

The obvious preventive approach is to avoid areas where ticks are likely to be. Early tick removal from people who have been bitten can also be effective because infection depends on the tick's ability to feed for a long time, usually at least 24 hours. It is important to remove the tick as close to the skin as possible without crushing it or severing its head from its body. For infected individuals, early treatment usually results in curing the disease. Standard treatment for Lyme disease is based on the administration of antibiotics. Different treatment regimens are required at different stages; antibiotics of choice include doxycycline, erythromycin, amoxicillin, and ceftriaxone, and treatment times can vary from 10 days to a month. In neuroborreliosis, *B. burgdorferi* may cross the blood-brain barrier; in this case, antibiotics that can act across the barrier, such as minocycline, should be prescribed (3, 50).

Diagnosis and Laboratory Testing

Lyme disease is diagnosed on the basis of clinical signs and symptoms, such as the characteristic EM, facial paralysis, and arthritic symptoms, as well as a history of tick bite or exposure to areas in which the disease is endemic. Diagnosis can be difficult at times because not all infected individuals exhibit the EM or other physical manifestations, and symptoms may be similar to other diseases. In fact, Lyme disease can be confused with many different inflammatory/autoimmune diseases such as SLE, rheumatoid arthritis, Crohn's disease, and multiple sclerosis. In cases of suspected diagnosis, laboratory testing is then performed to confirm it. Culture of *B. burgdorferi* in the laboratory is very difficult, so it is not used as a diagnostic tool. Instead, several forms of laboratory testing are employed; most of them are serological and involve the detection of the host's antibodies to *B. burgdorferi*. Unfortunately, these tests can be ineffective in the early stages of the disease because antibody responses to the infecting organism take a while to develop (up to 6 weeks after initial tick bite), so early treatment is recommended when the disease is suspected for reasons already stated. The most common symptom associated with the disease and that justifies early treatment is the characteristic EM rash although, as mentioned, not all infected individuals develop it. Again, careful early diagnosis to avoid confusion with other diseases is very important in the choice of early treatment (44, 45, 46, 47).

Serology of Lyme Disease

Testing for antibodies against Borrelia antigens can be performed using different techniques. It must be pointed out, however, that the presence of antibodies does not necessarily indicate active disease because both IgM and IgG, especially at lower titers, may remain in the host for quite some time after initial infection. Complicating the issue, cross-reactivity to different antigens must also be considered because the presence of other organisms such as cytomegalovirus, herpes virus, and Epstein-Barr virus can lead to false positive results. Because of the time it takes for a host to produce antibodies to Borrelia antigens, serology testing is most effective in the later stages of the disease. However, false negatives tend to be much more common (more than 30%) than false positives (up to 3%). Historically, immunofluorescence has been used to detect antibodies to Borrelia. Commercially available slides to which Borrelia antigens have been bound are allowed to react with serial dilutions of a patient's sera. After washing the unbound material, fluorescence-labeled anti-human immunoglobulin antibodies are allowed to react with the slides, and after a second wash, fluorescence is evaluated as a reflection of the presence of anti-Borrelia antibodies in the patient's sample. Although useful, this technique is subject to false positive results, particularly because of cross-reactivity with similar microorganisms (eg, other spirochetes such as *T. pallidum*). Although there are variations in defining a sample as "positive," a titer of about 1:256 is usually necessary to define a sample as positive. The advantage of the immunofluorescence technique is that patterns of immunofluorescence staining can give a clue to a true versus a false positive (some false positive results have distinctive bead or droplet-like patterns); however, distinguishing different patterns requires a highly experienced technician, and the results are not always reliable. Other immunological techniques, including ELISA and Western blotting, are now commonly used. The Centers for Disease Control and Prevention has recommended a 2-tier protocol that includes initial testing by ELISA, followed by a more specific Western blot assay. To repeat, these tests are only secondary to clinical suspicion of Lyme disease and are performed as confirmatory tests for the disease. Both ELISA and Western blot testing can be complicated because different microbial antigens used by various manufacturers can lead to different results. In fact, some antigens used may be specific to a certain geographical region where a particular species of *Borrelia* is found; because of this, a false negative result may be obtained when an individual who has been infected in a certain region is tested for an organism present in a different region. The advantage of the ELISA method over immunofluorescence is that antibody concentrations can be evaluated beyond just serial dilutions. In general, ELISA kits also come with calibrating positive controls (ie, positive sera), which can be used to obtain a semiquantitative evaluation of antibody concentrations in a patient's sample. The principle and methods of ELISA procedures are described in Chapter 7. Briefly, microtiter plates or strip wells are coated with different Borrelia antigens, and the patient's sample is added to the wells and allowed to react with the antigens. After washing the unbound material, an enzyme-conjugated anti-human immunoglobulin preparation is added to the wells, and after a second wash, an enzyme substrate is added and the resulting color development is measured using a spectrophotometer. Antibody concentrations in the samples can then be calculated by comparing the readings obtained from the sample with the readings from the calibrated positive control supplied with the ELISA kit. As with immunofluorescence, timing of testing and cross-reactivity are also issues affecting ELISA results. At early stages, ELISA has a sensitivity of about 70%, which increases to almost 100% in people with disseminated symptoms (47, 50, 51).

According to CDC guidelines, once a sample has been deemed positive by ELISA, it must then be tested by Western blotting (described in Chapter 7) against a battery of different Borrelia antigens. The assay manufacturer supplies nitrocellulose strips to which Borrelia antigens separated by electrophoresis have been bound. The patient's samples are then tested against these antigens by allowing them to react with the strips. After washing, anti-human immunoglobulin preparations labeled with an enzyme are allowed to react with the strips and after a second wash, the enzyme's substrate is added, resulting in the development of color at the site to which the human immunoglobulin preparations are bound. This, in turn, indicates the presence of antibodies to the particular antigen that is bound to that particular site on the strip. The different antigens are usually identified by their molecular weight, which, in turn, determines their specific position on the nitrocellulose strip (43). See Figure 19.26 ■ for a typical Western blot for Lyme disease with IgG to Lyme antigens measured in A and IgM to Lyme antigens measured in B.

The difference between the ELISA and Western blotting methods is that although the ELISA method detects antibodies to a mixture of bacterial antigens (ie, does the patient have antibodies to *Borrelia burgdorferi?*), the Western blot techniques assesses an individual's antibodies to specific Borrelia antigens (ie, which ones and how many?). As mentioned, choice of different bacterial antigens makes this analysis complicated. In addition, different individuals may develop antibodies to different antigens, so it is not clear what rule of thumb is commonly accepted to identify a "positive" subject. The CDC defines a subject as being positive who has IgM against 2 of the following 3 bands: OspC (22-25), 39, and 41. In the case of IgG antibodies, *positivity* is defined by reactivity against 5

of the following ten bands: 18, OspC (22-25), 28, 30, 39, 41, 45, 58, 66, and 93. However, this approach also has interpretation problems; antibodies to a specific antigen are visualized by observing "bands" of stain on the blot (Figure 19.26). If the band is well defined and clear, there are no problems, but one that is faint or "fuzzy" may complicate the interpretation of the results. In addition, although some bacterial antigens such as the OspC and the 39kDa bands are very specific for *Borrelia burgdorferi,* others (eg, the 41kDa band, which represents the bacterial flagella and which is a band that also commonly appears in control sera) are not. Moreover, one must remember that the identity of these bacterial antigens are derived from their molecular weight; this, in turn, complicates the interpretation of the results further because other cross-reactive bacterial components may also have similar molecular weights. This happens to be true for the 60 and/or 66 kDa, which are components commonly found in bacteria other than *Borrelia burgdorferi.* Furthermore, the reactivity of a patient's serum with certain bacterial components may vary at different times of an individual's immune response to the antigens, so certain bands may not appear at the same time after infection in different individuals. Finally, one must remember that immunofluorescence, ELISA, and Western blotting all measure a subject's antibodies to *Borrelia burgdorferi.*

More recently, a new ELISA whose accuracy rivals that of the Western blot has been developed; it has a reported specificity of 99% (and almost twice the sensitivity of a standard Western blot in early infections). This ELISA method employs a peptide as antigen (called *C6*) that mimics a highly conserved and highly immunogenic portion of a protein from *Borrelia burgdorferi.* The advantage of C6 ELISA method is its increased accuracy when compared to the whole-cell sonicate ELISA and its simplicity over the Western blot and thus it may become a "stand-alone" alternative to the 2-tiered method recommended by the CDC (52).

Polymerase Chain Reaction

Although serology measures antibodies against *Borrelia burgdorferi,* another diagnostic approach is to detect the presence of the organism itself in a potentially infected individual. Because isolation and culture of *Borrelia burgdorferi* is difficult, PCR can be used to detect genetic material from *Borrelia burgdorferi,* and different PCR kits have been developed to detect the presence of bacterial DNA in a particular sample are available. The principle and methodology of the PCR technique are described in Chapter 23. Unlike the serology approaches, PCR can be very specific because it can target very specific stretches of bacterial DNA, such as DNA encoding for some of the Osp components; because specific DNA probes can identify discrete and unique sequences of bacterial DNA, cross-reactivity is not as much of a problem as in the serology approaches. Specificity of PCR can approach 100%. However, the problem with it is sensitivity. False negative results are common, especially when testing blood or cerebrospinal fluids (CFS)

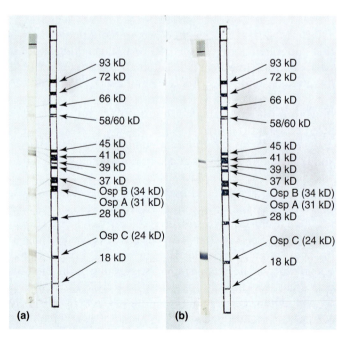

■ **FIGURE 19.26** Western blot patterns for different *Borrelia* antigens: (a) IgG Western and (b) IgM Western.

for which sensitivity can drop to 15% and 40%, respectively. Therefore, PCR is used only as an adjunct technique when diagnosis is very difficult and, in the majority of cases, is limited to testing CSF and synovial fluids. In addition, PCR can also be used to detect *Borrelia burgdorferi* in ticks that have been removed from an individual who has been bitten.

✓ Checkpoint! 19.5

Lyme disease is transmitted by tick bites. The rate of infection is usually very low, but it increases if the infected tick is at the nymphal stage. Why?

 CASE STUDY 1

While away at college, a young woman named Anna had a sore throat (acute pharyngitis), a headache, fever, and chills. Because she was going to take the Graduate Record Exam (GREs) in 2 weeks, she felt that she did not have time to go to the student health office. She decided that she would just tough it out and the sore throat would go away. She explained this decision to her mother when they talked on the phone. Her mother was rather upset by her decision and told Anna that with these symptoms, she should go to the health clinic right away because avoiding treatment could have serious consequences.

1. What did her mother think Anna had?
2. What did Anna's mother think could happen if this infection was not treated?
3. What samples would be taken at the health clinic, and what laboratory tests would be performed for diagnosis?
4. Anna tested positive for *Streptococcus pyogenes* by the rapid test. She is severely allergic to penicillin. What should be prescribed?

 CASE STUDY 2

Your dad didn't eat much at Thanksgiving dinner. This is very unlike him, so you asked him why. He said that he has not been feeling that well for the last few months. He is not very hungry and always has the sensation of being full. When he does eat, he has indigestion, heartburn, and stomach pain. You were studying your immunology notes while you were home on break, and you really think that your dad has a stomach ulcer and the associated bacterial infection.

1. What organism do you think is causing your dad's ulcer?
2. What do you think is causing problems in your dad's stomach?
3. What serologic methods could be used to diagnose this problem?
4. What treatment should be used to make your dad feel better?

CASE STUDY 3

An elderly woman was admitted to the hospital with aspiration pneumonia. After antibiotic therapy, her pneumonia resolved, but she had a high fever and developed severe and very smelly diarrhea.

1. What do you think she has?
2. What testing should be done to determine whether your diagnosis is indeed the cause of her diarrhea?

CASE STUDY 4

Your best friend Lily loves to hike, and she always seems to be telling you of her wild adventures running around in some park or another. A few months before school started, she was hiking on Bear Mountain in Connecticut, which is part of the Appalachian Trail. She said it was really cool because full blueberry bushes surrounded the trail. She also saw lots of deer while hiking. She tells you that the twin lakes near the mountain were refreshing to swim in. She is trying to talk you into going next year and shows you photos. In a photo of Lily on the mountain, you notice a rash on her leg. It has a red center, a blanched circular white area, and a red irregular circle around it. You ask her about it and she says that she did have a headache and muscle aches during the trip at the same time that she had the rash, but it all went away.

1. What do you think the rash was?
2. Lily needs to be tested for Lyme disease. How is this test performed?

SUMMARY

The immune system is designed to protect the host from biologically foreign entities that may cause it harm. The most common entities able to do this are microorganisms that can cause and/or transmit an infectious disease. Immune responses to achieve such protection are usually directed to the microorganisms themselves, their components, or their products. The immune responses to such microorganisms can also be used to detect their presence or to evaluate the disease or damage they can cause to the host. Many microorganisms in turn have the ability to downregulate or evade the immune responses mounted by the host. This chapter discussed selected microorganisms that cause human diseases and for which serological approaches are used to identify and monitor the disease they cause. Group A *streptococci* (*Streptococcus pyogenes*) cause a variety of clinical conditions including pharyngitis, impetigo, scarlet fever, rheumatic fever, glomerulonephritis, necrotizing fasciitis, sepsis, pneumonia, toxic shock syndrome, and meningitis. Detection and identification of streptococci rely on different approaches:

the culture of the organism itself, the detection of the organism based on immunological assays or DNA testing, and the detection of antibodies in an infected individual. Culture of blood agar can identify the organism based on the pattern of hemolysis and susceptibility to certain antibiotics. Immunoassays such as the rapid strep test are also used in diagnostics. Other diagnostic approaches include PCR and serological evaluation of antistreptococcal antibodies. *Helicobacter pylori* is a common resident of the stomach and a causative agent of duodenal and gastric ulcers, and, in more severe cases, cancer of the stomach. Testing for *H. pylori* includes noninvasive tests such as those for antibodies against the organism, microbial antigens, stools, and the carbon urea. More reliable tests tend to be invasive and include a biopsy during endoscopy and a rapid urease test. *Mycoplasma pneumoniae* is the causative agent of mycoplasma pneumonia, a common contagious condition affecting all ages and usually spread by transmission of respiratory droplets. Modern diagnostic methods involve the detection of antibodies against *M. pneumoniae*. These include ELISA, latex agglutination, and immunofluorescence; ELISA is the most commonly used and reliable method. The genus *Rickettsiae* represent diverse microorganisms that can cause different human diseases including typhus, Rocky Mountain spotted fever, African tick bite fever, and other forms of tick fevers. Rickettsia are transmitted by various insects such as ticks, lice, and fleas and usually infect humans via these vectors. They are classified under different types and can vary within different geographical areas. As with other organisms described in this chapter, immunological techniques play a major role in the detection of rickettsia, including immunofluorescence, immuno-dot blot, agglutination, and ELISA. The indirect immunofluorescence test is the most commonly used and accepted test for the detection of rickettsia; it can target different species and different antibodies depending on the kit specifications. *Clostridium difficile* is a normal human commensal intestinal organism in 3 to 5% of the population. Overabundance of *C. difficile* in the intestines can cause severe diarrhea and can lead to a serious inflammation of the colon. Overpopulation of *C. difficile* can be caused by the administration of antibiotics, which can destroy the normal flora of the intestine, facilitating the thriving of *C. difficile* in the affected areas. The clinical manifestations of a *C. difficile* infection are due to certain toxins produced by the organism; these toxins are also the targets of diagnostic tests for the organism. The classical testing for *C. difficile* is toxigenic culture, although different ELISA and PCR methods for their detection are also available. Spirochetes are a group of motile bacteria traditionally classified as gram-negative organisms that exhibit a characteristic coil or screw shape; 2 major human diseases caused by spirochetes are syphilis and Lyme disease. Syphilis, a disease caused by the *Treponema pallidum* subspecies pallidum, is almost always transmitted by sexual contact, although its mode of transmission can include transplacental passage from mother to fetus. The disease is divided into 4 stages: primary, secondary, latent, and tertiary; each stage has its own clinical manifestation and/or features. Because syphilis is most commonly transmitted by sexual contact, the best preventive methods are patient education, sexual abstinence, or avoidance of any sexual contact with an unknown or potentially infected person. Syphilis can be well controlled if properly and promptly treated; the standard treatment is the use of antibiotics. Diagnostic approaches include visual identification of the organism by microscopy, either directly or indirectly, and the detection of antibodies in an infected individual, either against the organism itself (treponemal tests), or against components of cells that arise as a consequence of cellular damage by the organism (nontreponemal tests). Examples of nontreponemal tests are the Venereal Disease Research Laboratory (VDRL) test and the rapid plasma reagin (RPR) test. These tests are based on the detection of antibodies to cardiolipin, a lipid generated from damaged cells. Treponemal tests include agglutination tests and fluorescence tests. A classical agglutination test for *T. pallidum* is the *Treponema pallidum* hemagglutination assay (TPHA). Enzyme immunoassays have also been developed for syphilis. A nontreponemal ELISA test is Reagin II, which detects antibodies to a cardiolipin antigen using the principle similar to that of VDRL and RPR tests. Several companies also offer ELISA kits to detect antibodies of different isotypes against recombinant *T. pallidum* antigens, and novel, Western blot-based diagnostic kits are under evaluation by the FDA at the time of this writing. PCR approaches are also available to detect genetic material from *T. pallidum*. Lyme disease is a common tick-borne disease cause by several microorganisms belonging to the *Borrelia* genus. The disease is transmitted to humans by deer ticks, which, in turn, acquire the organisms by feeding on mice and other animals that act as natural reservoirs. Individuals with Lyme disease exhibit multiple and diverse signs and symptoms. Symptoms can differ from one infected individual to another and can even be different in different geographical areas. The disease itself can be divided into 3 different stages, and symptomology varies from one stage to another. The pathology seen in Lyme disease is actually a consequence of the immune response of the host to its causative organism, *B. burgdorferi*. Diagnosis of Lyme disease is based on clinical signs and symptoms, such as the characteristic EM, facial paralysis, and arthritic symptoms as well as a history of tick bite or exposure to areas in which the disease is endemic. Lyme disease can be confused with many different inflammatory/autoimmune diseases such as SLE, rheumatoid arthritis, Crohn's disease, and multiple sclerosis. Therefore, proper diagnosis is critical in the choice of treatment modalities. Serological tests are usually secondary to clinical diagnosis and are used as confirmatory approaches. These include immunological approaches such as immunofluorescence, ELISA, and, subsequently, Western blotting. PCR approaches to detect genetic material from *Borrelia burgdorferi* are also available. Early treatment usually results in the cure of the disease. Standard treatment for Lyme disease is based on the administration of antibiotics.

REVIEW QUESTIONS

1. Ticks that harbor the disease-causing organism acquired the organism from the white-footed mouse.
   a. True
   b. False

2. The Lyme disease-causing organism is similar to the organism that causes syphilis in appearance, and indeed, the diseases share some similarities.
   a. True
   b. False

3. Lyme disease is a multisymptom disease that can involve skin, nervous system, heart, and joints.
   a. True
   b. False

4. Antibodies to the Lyme disease-causing organism are used diagnostically
   a. True
   b. False

5. The Western blot for Lyme antibody never shows any positive bands for individuals who do not have Lyme disease.
   a. True
   b. False

6. In congenital syphilis,
   a. the baby is never asymptomatic at birth
   b. the baby can show a rash, neurosyphilis, and/or anemia
   c. the baby can show hypogammaglobulinemia
   d. all of the above

7. Syphilis is
   a. not sensitive to heat, cold, and drying outside the body
   b. usually treatable with penicillin
   c. analyzed for by a laboratory test using phosphatidylinositol
   d. easy to culture in a serum supplemented media

8. The primary stage of syphilis
   a. occurs after sexual contact with a person with primary or secondary lesions
   b. occurs after the organism enters through a small break in the skin
   c. usually presents with a lesion called a chancre
   d. all of the above

9. Which of the following is *not* a major symptom of tertiary syphilis?
   a. gummas
   b. cardiovascular disease
   c. tabes dorsalis
   d. respiratory disease

10. Specific treponemal Ags used to detect Ab against *T. pallidum* are in which of the following assays
    a. VDRL
    b. RPR
    c. Davidsohn differential
    d. TPHA

11. M protein is a virulence factor because
    a. it has a net negative charge that repulses the phagocytic cells
    b. it limits C3 deposition by limiting C activation on its surface
    c. it has a protease activity that cleaves antibody
    d. both A and B

12. Suppurative infections caused by *Streptococcus pyogenes* include
    a. otitis media, scarlet fever, erysipelas, cellulitis, puerperal sepsis, abscess formation
    b. rheumatic fever
    c. glomerulonephritis
    d. B and C

13. The antistreptolysin O assay uses antibody to
    a. neutralize the lytic activity of streptolysin O
    b. add to the lytic activity of streptolysin O
    c. opsonize *Streptococcus pyogenes* for phagocytosis
    d. neutralize the DNAse activity of streptolysin O

14. The anti-streptolysin O assay can be negative even if the patient has strep throat because
    a. Ab titers do not increase until 1 to 2 weeks after infection
    b. Ab response in only 75 to 80% of acute rheumatic fever patients
    c. ASO titers do not increase in people with skin infections
    d. all of the above

15. In a streptococcal infections, the groups strep A through H were grouped by Rebecca Lancefield based on
    a. surface carbohydrates
    b. the antigenic structures of the M and T protein antigens
    c. the animal they infected
    d. the enzymes the bacteria contained

16. The VDRL reagin antibody test for syphilis
    a. is positive only for primary syphilis
    b. involves the use of heat-inactivated serum
    c. involves complement fixation
    d. involves the Reiter organism

REVIEW QUESTIONS (continued)

17. The secondary stage of syphilis is characterized by
    a. lesions called gumma
    b. a primary chancre
    c. a papule
    d. a rash

18. Your brother was bitten by a tick carrying *Borrelia burgdorferi*. After the tick was on your brother for 30 hours, it jumped off walked around under your kitchen table and found your ankle and latched on. After 15 minutes, you noticed the tick and removed it.
    a. You and your brother will get Lyme disease.
    b. Neither of you will get Lyme disease.
    c. You will get Lyme disease, but you brother will not.
    d. Your brother might get Lyme disease, but you will not.

19. Nonsuppurative infections caused by *Streptococcus pyogenes* include
    a. otitis media, erysipelas, cellulitis, puerperal sepsis, abscess formation
    b. rheumatic fever
    c. glomerulonephritis
    d. B and C

20. *Helicobacter pylori* can survive in the stomach with its low pH because
    a. it produces an enzyme called *urease*, which can cleave the stomach urea to produce ammonia and carbon dioxide, which ultimately produce bicarbonate that neutralizes the stomach acids
    b. *H. pylori* can burrow into the mucosal layer of the stomach and can sense pH gradients, thus moving into areas that are more neutral in pH
    c. it produces low pH products of its own, so it is accustomed to surviving in low pH
    d. A and B

REFERENCES

1. Janeway CA, Travers P, Walport M, Shlomchik MJ. *Immunobiology*. 5th ed. New York, NY: Garland Publishing; 2001.

2. Ryan KJ, Ray CG, eds. *Sherris Medical Microbiology*. 4th ed. New York, NY: McGraw Hill; 2004.

3. Bisno AL, Stevens DL. *Streptococcus pyogenes*. In: Mandell GL, Bennett JE, Dolin R, eds. *Principles and Practice of Infectious Diseases*. 7th ed. Philadelphia, PA: Elsevier Churchill Livingstone; 2009.

4. Bisno AL, Brito MO, Collins CM. Molecular basis of group A streptococcal virulence. *Lancet Infect Dis*. 2003;3(4):191–200.

5. Bencivenga JF, Johnson DR, Kaplan EL. Determination of group A streptococcal anti-M type-specific antibody in sera of rheumatic fever patients after 45 years. *Clin Infect Dis*. 2009 Oct 15;49(8):1237-9

6. Faé KC, da Silva DD, Oshiro SE, et al. Mimicry in recognition of cardiac myosin peptides by heart-intralesional T cell clones from rheumatic heart disease. *J. Immunol*. 2006;176(9):5662–5670.

7. Papageorgiou A, Collins CM, Gutman DM, et al. Structural basis for the recognition of superantigen streptococcal pyrogenic exotoxin A (SpeA1) by MHC class II molecules and T-cell receptors. *The EMBO Journal*. 1999;18:9–21.

8. Choby BA. Diagnosis and treatment of streptococcal pharyngitis. *Am Fam Physician*. 2009;79(5):383–390.

9. Marx, J. *Rosen's Emergency Medicine: Concepts and Clinical Practice*. 7th ed. Philadelphia, PA: Mosby/Elsevier; 2010: chap. 30.

10. Johnson DR, Kurlan R, Leckman J, et al. The human immune response to streptococcal extracellular antigens: Clinical, diagnostic, and potential pathogenetic implications. *Clin Infect Dis*. 2010;50:481–490.

11. Shulman ST, Tanz RR. Group A streptococcal pharyngitis and immune-mediated complications: From diagnosis to management. *Expert Rev Anti Infect Ther*. 2010;8(2):137–150.

12. Kumar V, Abbas AK, Fausto N, et al. *Robbins Basic Pathology*. 8th ed. Philadelphia, PA: Saunders Elsevier; 2007: 403–406.

13. Sultan FA, Moustafa SE, Tajik J, et al. Rheumatic tricuspid valve disease: An evidence-based systematic overview. *J Heart Valve Dis*. 2010;19(3):374–382.

14. Baltimore RS. Re-evaluation of antibiotic treatment of streptococcal pharyngitis. *Curr. Opin. Pediatr*. 2010;22:77–82.

15. Sheeler, RD, Houston MS, Radke S, et al. Accuracy of rapid strep testing in patients who have had recent Streptococcal Pharyngitis. *J. Am. Board of Family Med*. 2002;15(4).

16. Danchin M, Carlin J, Devenish W, et al. New normal ranges of anti-streptolysin O and antideoxyribonuclease B titres for Australian children. *J Paediatr Child Health*. 2005;41(11):583–586.

17. Boyanova L, ed. *Helicobacter pylori*. Norfolk, UK: Caister Academic Press; 2011.

18. Baldwin DN, Shepherd B, Kraemer P, et al. Identification of *Helicobacter pylori* genes that contribute to stomach colonization. *Infect Immun*. 2007;75(2):1005–1016.

19. Yamaoka Y. *Helicobacter pylori: Molecular Genetics and Cellular Biology*. Norfolk, UK: Caister Academic Press; 2008.

20. Stenström B, Mendis A, Marshall B. *Helicobacter pylori*—The latest in diagnosis and treatment. *Aust Fam Physician*. 2008;37(8):608–612.

21. Falsafi T, Favaedi R, Mahjoub F, et al. Application of Stool-PCR test for diagnosis of *Helicobacter pylori* infection in children. *World J Gastroenterol*. 2009;15(4):484–488.

22. Waris ME, Toikka P, Saarinen T, et al. Diagnosis of *Mycoplasma pneumoniae* pneumonia in children. *J. Clin. Microbiol*. 1998;36(11):3155–3159.

23. Thurman KA, Walter ND, Schwartz SB, et al. Comparison of laboratory diagnostic procedures for detection of *Mycoplasma pneumoniae* in community outbreaks. *Clin Infect Dis*. 2009;48:1244–1249.

24. Walker DH. Rickettsiae. In: Barron S et al., eds. *Barron's Medical Microbiology*. 4th ed. Galveston, Texas: University of of Texas Medical Branch; 1996.

25. Perlman SJ, Hunter MS, Zchori-Fein E. The emerging diversity of 'Rickettsia.' *Proceedings of the Royal Society B-Biological Sciences.* 2006;273:2097–2106.

26. Paris DH, Blacksell SD, Stenos J, et al. Real-time multiplex PCR assay for detection and differentiation of *rickettsiae* and *orientiae. Trans R Soc Trop Med Hyg.* 2008 Feb;102(2):186–93.

27. Pépin J, Saheb N, Coulombe MA, et al. Emergence of fluoroquinolones as the predominant risk factor for *Clostridium difficile*-associated diarrhea: A cohort study during an epidemic in Quebec. *Clin. Infect. Dis.* 2005;41:1254–1260.

28. Barth H, Aktories K, Popoff M, et al. Binary bacterial toxins: Biochemistry, biology, and applications of common Clostridium and Bacillus proteins. *Microbiol Mol Biol Rev.* 2004;68:373–402.

29. Murray PR, Baron EJ, Pfaller EA, et al., eds. *Manual of Clinical Microbiology.* 8th ed. Washington DC: ASM Press; 2003.

30. Pickering LK, ed. *Syphilis, Red Book.* Elk Grove Village, IL: American Academy of Pediatrics; 2006.

31. Kent ME, Romanelli F. Reexamining syphilis: An update on epidemiology, clinical manifestations, and management. *Ann Pharmacother.* 2008;42(2):226–336.

32. Eccleston K, Collins L, Higgins, SP. Primary syphilis. *IntJ STD AIDS.* 2008;19:145–151.

33. Mullooly C, Higgins SP. Secondary syphilis: The classical triad of skin rash, mucosal ulceration and lymphadenopathy. *Int J STD AIDS.* 2010; 21(8):537–545.

34. Dylewski J, Duong M. The rash of secondary syphilis. *CMAJ.* 2007;176:33–35.

35. Bhatti MT. Optic neuropathy from viruses and spirochetes. *Int Ophthalmol Clin.* 2007;47:37–66.

36. Stamm LV. Global challenge of antibiotic-resistant *Treponema pallidum. Antimicrob. Agents Chemother.* 2010;54:583–589.

37. Harris A, Rosenberg AA, Riedel LM. A microflocculation test for syphilis using cardiolipin antigen: Preliminary report. *J Vener Dis Inform.* 1946;27:159–172.

38. Maple, PAC, Ratcliffe D, Smit E. Characterization of *Treponema pallidum* particle agglutination assay-negative sera following screening by Treponemal total antibody enzyme immunoassays. CVI. 2010;17:1718–1722.

39. Montoya, PJ, Lukehart SA, Brentlinger PE, et al. Comparison of the diagnostic accuracy of a rapid immunochromagraphic test and the rapid plasma reagin test for antenatal syphilis screening in Mozambique. *Bull World Health Organ.* 2006;84:97–104.

40. Leslie DE, Azzato F, Karapanagiotidis T, et al. Development of a real-time PCR assay to detect *Treponema pallidum* in clinical specimens and assessment of the assay's performance by comparison with serological testing. *J. Clin. Microbiol.* 2007;45:93–96.

41. Wang G, van Dam AP, Schwartz I, et al. Molecular typing of *Borrelia burgdorferi* sensu lato: Taxonomic, epidemiological, and clinical implications. *Clin. Microbiol. Rev.* 1999;12:633–653.

42. Derdáková M, Lencáková D. Association of genetic variability within the *Borrelia burgdorferi* sensu lato with the ecology, epidemiology of Lyme borreliosis in Europe. *Ann Agric Environ Med.* 2005;12:165–172.

43. Wilske B. Epidemiology and diagnosis of Lyme borreliosis. *Ann. Med.* 2005;37:568–579.

44. Steere, AC. Lyme Borreliosis. In: Fauci A, et al. *Harrison's Principles of Internal Medicine.* 17th ed. New York, NY: McGraw-Hill Medical Publishing; 2008.

45. Smith RP, Schoen RT, Rahn DW, et al. Clinical characteristics and treatment outcome of early Lyme disease in patients with microbiologically confirmed erythema migrans. *Ann. Intern. Med.* 2002;136:421–428.

46. Puius YA, Kalish RA. Lyme arthritis: pathogenesis, clinical presentation, and management. *Infect. Dis. Clin. North Am.* 22:289–300, 2008.

47. Auwaerter PG, Aucott J, Dumler JS. Lyme borreliosis (Lyme disease): Molecular and cellular pathobiology and prospects for prevention, diagnosis and treatment. *Expert Rev Mol Med.* 2004;6:1–22.

48. Singh SK, Girschick HJ. Lyme borreliosis: From infection to autoimmunity. *Clin. Microbiol. Infect.* 2004;10:598–614.

49. Samuels DS, Radolf JD, eds. *Borrelia: Molecular Biology, Host Interaction and Pathogenesis.* Norfolk, UK: Caister Academic Press; 2010.

50. Bratton RL, Whiteside JW, Hovan MJ, et al. Diagnosis and treatment of Lyme disease. *Mayo Clin. Proc.* 2008;83:566–571.

51. Steere AC, McHugh G, Damle N, et al. Prospective study of serologic tests for Lyme disease. *Clin Infect Dis.* 2008;47:188–195.

52. Mogilyansky E, Loa CC, Adelson ME, et al. Comparison of western immunoblotting and the C6 Lyme antibody test for laboratory detection of Lyme disease. *Clin Diagn Lab Immunol.* 2004;11:924–929.

53. Centers for Disease Control and Prevention. Lyme disease data and statistics. http://www.cdc.gov/lyme/stats/index.html. Accessed May 25, 2012.

54. Workowski KA, Berman SM. Sexually transmitted diseases treatment guidelines. *MMWR Recomm Rep.* 2006;55:1–94.

55. World Health Organization. *International Travel and Health.* chap. 5 Infectious diseases of potential risk to travelers. http://www.who.int/ith/ITH2009Chapter5.pdf Accessed May 25, 2012. Accessed

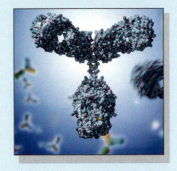

CHAPTER OUTLINE

20

Fungi and Parasites

■ OBJECTIVES—LEVEL I

After this chapter, the student should be able to:

1. Describe fungus, including cell description of yeast and mold forms.
2. List factors that appear to be linked to the worldwide increase in fungal infections.
3. Describe the patient information that is essential to the choice of laboratory tests in diagnosis of fungi and parasites.
4. Explain the use of serial serological tests in fungal infections.
5. Define the term *thermally dimorphic*.
6. Compare and contrast the different clinical pictures *Aspergillus* can cause.
7. Describe what causes blastomycosis, where it is important, and what part of the body is infected as well as its signs and symptoms.
8. Describe what antigens are used in blastomycosis diagnosis, and compare and contrast assays to diagnose it.
9. Describe *Candida* infections, and for each type, indicate who becomes infected and what can cause them.
10. Describe what cells protect against candidiasis infection.
11. Describe the tests that identify antibody to *Candida*.
12. Describe what causes coccidiomycosis, where it is important, and what part of the body is infected as well as its signs and symptoms.
13. Describe what antigens are used in coccidiomycosis diagnosis, and compare and contrast assays to diagnose it.
14. Describe the organism that causes cryptococcosis, where cryptococcosis is important, and what part of the body is infected as well as its signs and symptoms.
15. Describe what antigens are used in cryptococcosis diagnosis.
16. Describe the organism that causes histoplasmosis, where it is important, and what part of the body is infected as well as its signs and symptoms.
17. Describe what antigens are used in histoplasmosis diagnosis.
18. Describe *Pneumocystis jiroveci*, where *jiroveci* is important, and what part of the body it infects as well as its signs and symptoms.
19. Describe *Pneumocystis jiroveci* diagnosis.
20. Explain the reasons that parasites are more difficult for the immune response to fight, and list 5 ways parasites evade the host's defenses.
21. State and explain the 5 outcomes that may occur after parasitic infection.
22. Discuss the role of IgE in response to a parasite.
23. Describe the serological testing for *Cryptosporidium*.
24. Describe the etiology and epidemiology of *Cryptosporidium*.

■ OBJECTIVES—LEVEL I (continued)

25. Describe the treatment of *Cryptosporidium*.
26. Describe the serological testing for *Giardia*.
27. Describe the etiology and epidemiology of *Giardia*.
28. Describe the treatment of Giardial infections.
29. Describe the serological testing for *Toxoplasma gondii*.
30. Describe how an immunocompromised person or a pregnant woman can avoid toxoplasmosis infection.
31. Describe the etiology and epidemiology of *Toxoplasma gondii*.
32. Explain the signs and symptoms of toxoplasmosis in normal people, first-trimester fetus, congenitally infected newborns, and people who are immunocompromised.

■ OBJECTIVES—LEVEL II

After this chapter, the student should be able to:

1. Describe the ouchterlony for antibody testing and the sandwich enzyme immunoassay for antigen testing for *Aspergillus*.
2. Evaluate laboratory results to determine the cause of disease and whether the patient has an acute infection or whether one that has resolved.
3. Discuss the effect of various immunocompromised states on the outcome of laboratory analysis for fungal and parasitic infections.

KEY TERMS

allergic bronchopulmonary aspergillosis (ABPA)
aspergilloma
Aspergillus
Blastomyces dermatitidis
candidiasis
Coccidioides immitis
cryptococcosis
Cryptosporidium parvum
endemic
fungi

Giardia lamblia
high avidity antibody
histoplasmosis
hyphae
low avidity IgG antibody
mycelium
parasites
Pneumocystis jiroveci
thermal dimorphism
toxoplasmosis
yeasts

▶ INTRODUCTION TO FUNGI

Fungi are eukaryotic organisms; their cells contain membrane-bound structures, including a nucleus. They are higher organisms that are neither plants nor animals. They have a rigid cell wall made rigid by polymers of sugars called *chitin* and *glucan*. Fungi secrete enzymes that digest material in their surroundings and then the released nutrients are absorbed by the fungi. With this external digestion, the surroundings of fungi are equivalent to a stomach. Fungi can exist in a mold or yeast form. **Yeasts** are unicellular and multiply by budding, and the buds can easily be seen on the yeast cells; see Figure 20.1(a) ■. The mold form is a more complicated structure with long filaments of cells called **hyphae;** see Figure 20.1(b). The hyphae may be separated into individual cells by cell walls (*septate hyphae*) or may be multinucleated without divisions between the nuclei (*coenocytic hyphae*). A mass of hyphae is called **mycelium.** Fungi can reproduce asexually and form spores that are called either *conidiospores* (arthrospores and blastoconidia), *chlamydospores,* or *sporangiospores*. Microscopic identification of fungi relies on identification of asexual spores. Fungi can also produce spores sexually.

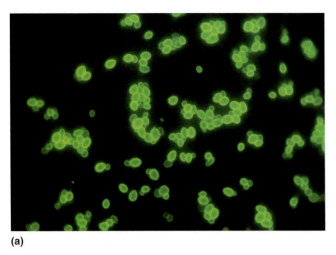

(a)

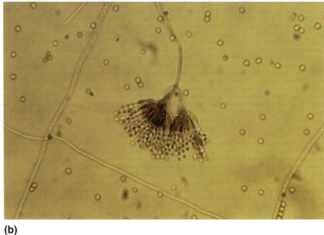

(b)

■ **FIGURE 20.1**   (a) Budding yeast cells (*Candida albicans*). *Source:* © CDC/ Maxine Jalbert, Dr. Leo Kaufman. (b) Mold from a penicillium fungus. *Source:* Biophoto Associates / Photo Researchers, Inc.

Hyphae reproduce asexually by forming conidia with conidiophores that end at conidiospores; see Figure 20.1(b). Some fungi exist in yeast form at one temperature and mold form at another temperature; these are said to exhibit **thermal dimorphism.** The thermal dimorphs are the fungi most often associated with disease. A fungal infection is called a *mycosis* (1, 2, 3, 4, 5, 6).

 Checkpoint! 20.1

Are fungi prokaryotic or eukaryotic? Are they plants, animals, or something entirely different?

The number of people in the world living in some kind of immunocompromised state has increased. These include cancer patients undergoing chemotherapy, transplant recipients, individuals treated with immunosuppressants for autoimmune disorders, individuals receiving broad spectrum antibiotics, and, of course, AIDS patients. All of these individuals have increased susceptibility to fungal infections, which rarely cause severe disease in healthy individuals. The increase in the number of susceptible individuals has led to an increase in the number of fungal diseases that are seen. However, certain fungal infections such as histoplasmosis, blastomycosis, and coccidiomycosis can infect and cause mild to severe disease even in healthy individuals (1, 2, 3, 4, 5, 6).

Phagocytic cell function and cell-mediated immunity are keys in preventing fungal infections. Fungi contain a number of pathogen associated molecular patterns (PAMPs) that the pattern recognition receptors (PRR) on phagocytic cells recognize. Cell-mediated immunity is important in anti-viral and anti-fungal responses, so defects in either phagocytic cells (neutrophils, macrophages, dendritic cells) or T cells

result in increased numbers and severity of fungal infections. Because fungal infections can be life threatening, early diagnosis is important. Currently, diagnosis includes analysis of the clinical situation, documentation of possible exposure, histology, culture and the nonculture analysis methods of PCR, and tests for antigens or immune response (1, 2, 3, 4, 5, 6).

To begin diagnosis, the clinical assessment of a patient suspected of having a fungal infection is important. This includes (1) the patient's possible exposure to the fungus, including travel history and occupational and hobby information (for gardening exposure, bird-dropping exposure), (2) the patient's immune status, and (3) the symptoms that the patient is experiencing. Laboratory diagnosis often involves histology and culture, antibody and antigen detection, and occasionally molecular techniques. Histology and culture are not possible with all infections because invasive procedures might be needed to obtain the samples. In addition, culture of fungi can be slow with identification often taking from 5 days to 4 weeks in some cases, during which time the patient's disease can rapidly progress. PCR has technical difficulties because the ubiquitous nature of fungi such as *Aspergillus* could lead to false positive results from spore contamination of the buffers. In addition, the half-life of fungal DNA needs to be studied so that the response of the disease to the patient's antifungal therapy is understood when using PCR to monitor the disease during treatment. Both of these problems will most likely be circumvented by further assay improvements (1, 2, 3, 4, 5, 6).

 Checkpoint! 20.2

What do you need to know about the patient to diagnose fungal infections?

Antibody testing for fungal diagnosis is not useful by itself for several reasons: many patients are immunocompromised and may not produce antibodies; individuals who are not currently infected can have antibodies, and in some cases, antibodies are produced only late in the disease. When antibody testing is utilized for diagnosis, it is often important to see a change in antibody titer. Due to the ubiquitous nature of these pathogens and the frequency of subclinical infections, the presence of antibodies may indicate only a previous infection unless a change in titer is seen. The detection of antigens has proven useful for some fungi, and the detection of antigen and antibody is sometimes used to increase the sensitivity of detection (1, 2, 3, 4, 5, 6).

ASPERGILLUS

Epidemiology

Aspergillus is a ubiquitous dimorphic fungus; it is found in soil, decaying matter, water, and air worldwide. Four species commonly cause disease: *Aspergillus fumigatus, flavus, niger,* and *terreus*. Infections occur after exposure to the spores of these species, and dusty environments can increase risk. *Aspergillus* infections include allergic bronchopulmonary aspergillosis, invasive aspergillosis, aspergilloma, sinus infections, cutaneous aspergillosis, and otitis externa (swimmer's ear) (7, 8, 9).

Allergic bronchopulmonary aspergillosis (ABPA) is usually diagnosed in people with cystic fibrosis or asthma, but can be diagnosed in healthy people as well. In ABPA, the patient shows signs of an IgE mediated disease, with wheezing and coughing evident. These patients have both IgE and IgG to *Aspergillus* (7, 8, 9).

An **aspergilloma** is a mass that looks like a fungal ball; it is caused by fungal growth either in a cavity in the lung, the brain, the kidneys, or other organs. The cavity that the aspergilloma fills in the lung usually is caused by another disease. Coughing up blood is a symptom seen in these patients (7, 8, 9).

Most people who contract an invasive *Aspergillus* infection are immunocompromised. Individuals who are at high risk for these infections include those who are undergoing cancer chemotherapy (which affects white blood cell counts), patients treated with immunosuppressant drugs (for autoimmunity or transplantation), bone marrow transplant recipients, subjects affected with chronic granulomatous disease (CGD), and those who are critically ill. The symptoms of invasive aspergillosis include fever, cough, difficulty breathing, and chest pain. Patchy and dense areas are visible by x-rays or CT scans (Figure 20.2 ■), or nodules are seen in the lungs. Invasive aspergillosis is seen primarily in severely immunocompromised individuals but can be seen in individuals that are not immunocompromised but who have pre-existing lung disease. The infection can spread from the lungs to the skin, brain, and bone. Invasive aspergillosis has a high mortality rate, so people who are immunocompromised and are at risk should avoid gardening and avoid dusty environments. In addition, they may want to use HEPA furnace filters for their homes and offices (7, 8, 9).

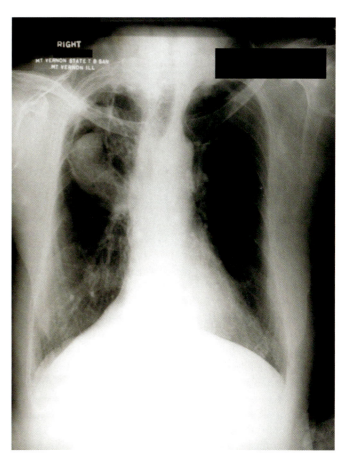

■ **FIGURE 20.2**   Aspergillosis fungal ball in the right lung. *Source:* © CDC/M. Renz.

Aspergillus sinusitis causes fever and sinus pain; these infections can be invasive or noninvasive, and invasive sinusitis infections can cause blindness in one eye and destruction of neighboring structures. Fungal sinus infections are now considered by some to be a major cause of chronic sinusitis even in immunocompetent individuals, but this remains controversial. Infection of the sinuses or skin can lead to disseminated infections in individuals who are immunocompromised (7, 8, 9).

Primary cutaneous *Aspergillus* infections can occur at IV insertion sites in compromised individuals, burn patients, and premature babies with AIDS, although the latter is rare. Cutaneous *Aspergillus* infections can occur, although also rarely, in immunocompetent individuals after an agricultural accident involving infection with a source of *Aspergillus*. Cutaneous aspergillosis infections can also occur secondarily to invasive aspergillosis. About 1 of every 8 cases of otitis externa (swimmer's ear) is fungal in origin, and 90% of them are caused by *Aspergillus* (7, 8, 9).

Diagnosis and Treatment

Often a patient with pulmonary symptoms and fever receives antibiotics for a bacterial infection, and when no improvement occurs, a fungal infection is suspected. This is because

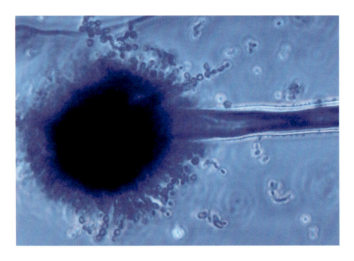

■ **FIGURE 20.3** *Aspergillus flavus* conidiophore. *Source:* © CDC/ Dr. Libero Ajello.

antibiotics will have no effect in the patient with invasive aspergillosis. Diagnosis of *Aspergillus* infections usually involves culture and microscopic identification (Figure 20.3 ■) but these tests can yield a false negative result, and culture can take up to 4 weeks. Antibody detection can be used in aspergilloma and ABPA, but in invasive aspergillosis, the patients are generally too immunocompromised to make antibodies. The primary method of antibody detection is by Ouchterlony, also known as *immunodiffusion precipitation reaction* (see Chapter 6). In this assay, the patient's serum is placed in a well opposite one containing *Aspergillus* antigens, and a control positive serum is placed in a third neighboring well. A reaction of identity must be seen for diagnosis. The positive control serum should show at least 3 bands in reaction with the *Aspergillus* antigens. Complement fixation tests have been utilized for antibody detection; these tests utilize the consumption of complement components by antibody bound to antigen as an indicator of infection and many controls are required. Complement fixation has, in general, been replaced by simpler methodologies. People with ABPA will also have elevated IgE levels (7, 8, 9).

Antigen detection can be utilized regardless of the patient's immune status. The antigens used in screening for *Aspergillus* infections are 2 carbohydrate antigens, galactomannan and β-glucan. A sandwich enzyme immunoassay is used for antigen detection and can detect down to about 0.5 ng/ml of the antigen. This level of detection yields an assay sensitivity of 95% and a specificity of 82 to 99%. PCR assay development shows promise and may be used with antigen tests for diagnosis. A chest x-ray or culture methods can be used to confirm disease when appropriate (7, 8, 9).

ABPA treatment includes the use of prednisone to decrease the allergic response, and some physicians use an antifungal such as itraconazole to decrease fungal burden. In the treatment of an aspergilloma, surgery may be required. For treatment of invasive aspergillosis, antifungal agents such as voriconazole, posaconazole, or amphotericin B should be used. Both azoles and amphotericin B affect the fungal plasma

membrane; *azole* is a class of drugs that inhibit synthesis of the fungal plasma membrane whereas amphotericin B forms a hole in the fungal plasma cell membrane (7, 8, 9).

BLASTOMYCES DERMATITIDIS

Epidemiology

Blastomyces dermatitidis is a thermally dimorphic fungi that causes the disease blastomycosis. Its symptoms develop 3 to 15 weeks after inhaling spores from disturbed organic matter in wooded areas. The disease is seen in farmers, forestry workers, campers, and hunters, both in healthy people and individuals who are immunocompromised. Blastomycosis can be cutaneous or systemic. About half of the infections due to inhaled spores have a slow-onset symptomatic illness; patients present coughing with fever and muscle and joint pain. This acute illness can progress to a chronic pulmonary disease or a disseminated disease, and the disease can become systemic either through pulmonary or cutaneous initial infection. The skin, bones, and urinary tract in disseminated disease can be affected. Meningitis can also occur. A granulomatous (macrophage-filled) response is seen. Blastomycosis is not transmitted from person to person. It is found in the U.S. Midwest as well as in south central and southeastern states. It can also be found in Africa and Central and South America (10).

Diagnosis and Treatment

Diagnosis can be made by microscopic analysis and/or culture of fluid or tissue from an infected site. The yeast form of *Blastomyces* is most often isolated from human tissue and fluids whereas the mold form results with culture at 25° C. Culture can be slow and is potentially hazardous because of the spread of spores, so it must be performed using biosafety conditions. False negative results can occur with culture. A complement fixation test was used for blastomycosis, but it had low sensitivity and specificity. An immunodiffusion assay is used in which patient antibody against the "A" antigen of *Blastomyces dermatitidis* is diagnostic. An indirect enzyme immunoassay has been developed to measure IgM and IgG antibody to fungal antigens from *Blastomyces dermatitidis*. Itraconazole can be used for treatment, but if the patient is immunocompromised or has severe disease, amphotericin B should be used first (10).

CANDIDIASIS

Epidemiology

Candidiasis infections (infections with the *Candida* organism; Figure 20.1) can be in oral, genitourinary, or invasive form. Oral candidiasis is also known as *thrush* and is usually seen as a white coating in the mouth and mucous membranes. Normally, a small number of these yeasts can be on both the skin and mucous membranes, but an imbalance or immunodeficiency can allow their overgrowth. Oral candidiasis (Figure 20.4 ■) is seen in infants, denture wearers, individuals using inhaled steroids, and other individuals who are immunocompromised. The white patches can be painless

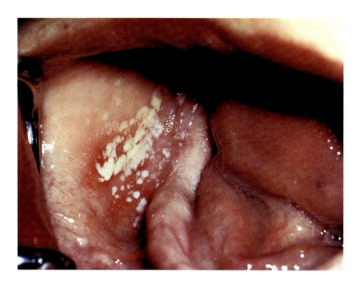

■ **FIGURE 20.4** Oral *Candida* in mouth of HIV patient. *Source:* © CDC.

or can cause soreness inside the mouth. Cracking and pain at the edges of the lips can also occur (11, 12).

Genital candidiasis is commonly called a "yeast infection." Women with this infection experience itching and burning at the site and can have a cottage cheese-like discharge that does not have a strong odor. About 75% of all women experience a yeast infection during their lifetime. Men with this infection can have an itchy rash on the penis; however, the infection is much more common in women than in men. It can be sexually transmitted but often occurs just because of an overcolonization of the person's own yeast from normal flora (11, 12).

In invasive candidiasis, the *Candida* organisms become bloodborne and cause fever, chills, and other nonspecific symptoms. These patients are usually first treated with antibiotics for the presumptive diagnosis of a bacterial infection but the antibiotics have no effect. If the bloodborne *Candida* infection is not treated properly, multiple organ infection can occur, resulting in damage to kidney, liver, and bones. Candidemia is the name of the disease caused by bloodborne *Candida* and is the fourth most common form of bloodborne infection in hospitalized patients. People at high risk for candidemia include low-birth weight babies, hospitalized individuals, people receiving intravenous fluids, people with indwelling catheters, injection drug users, and immunocompromised individuals including those receiving anti-TNF monoclonal antibody therapy (11, 12).

Diagnosis and Treatment

Oral candidiasis is diagnosed by appearance and by culture. Culture alone would not be diagnostic because *Candida* is part of the normal flora of the mouth. Treatment commonly involves an antifungal preparation such as nystatin and clotrimazole, which are swished around in the mouth and swallowed. Diagnosis of genital candidiasis is most often made microscopically. Treatment calls for an antifungal

cream or suppository, but oral fluconazole can also be used (11, 12).

Diagnosis of invasive candidiasis is usually through blood culture and microscopy, but sandwich immunoassays are under development which recognize either the β-(1–3)-D-glucan cell wall antigen (sensitivity 75 to 100% specificity 88 to 100%) or the surface mannan (sensitivity 31–90%). A latex agglutination inhibition test was on the market but had low sensitivity. Treatment can be with fluconazole, with the echinocandins, or other antifungals (11, 12).

✓ **Checkpoint! 20.3**

What disease is commonly called a yeast infection?

COCCIDIOIDES IMMITIS

Epidemiology

Outbreaks of coccidiomycosis (Figures 20.5 ■ and 20.6 ■) can occur after natural disasters such as earthquakes in semi-arid regions. The causative agent, the fungus ***Coccidioides immitis,*** lives in dry soil and is contracted by inhaling airborne dust containing the spores, although it is not spread from person to person. Coccidiomycosis is endemic in the southwestern United States, Mexico, and South and Central America (Figure 20.7 ■). The number of cases seen in the United States increased from the 1980s to 1993 and again from 1997 to 2006. Ten-fold higher rates of disseminated disease are seen in African-Americans and Filipinos, although the reason for this is not understood. People who work in dusty areas including construction workers, farm workers, and archeologists are more likely to be exposed and infected. Higher rates of severe infection occur in pregnant women and people who are immunocompromised. In addition, patients with HIV or organ transplants have increased risk of disseminated disease (13, 14, 15, 16, 17).

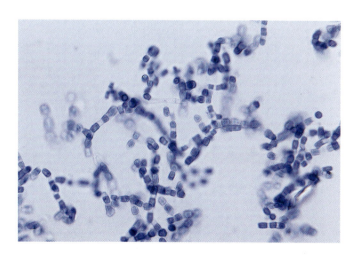

■ **FIGURE 20.5** Thick-walled barrel-shaped arthrospores on thin glass like hyphae; the room-temperature form of *Coccidioides immitis*. *Source:* © CDC/ Dr. Lucille K. Georg.

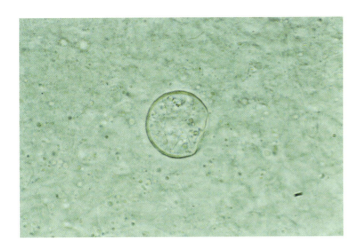

■ **FIGURE 20.6** Chlamydospore or spherule that occurs at body temperature. *Source:* © CDC/Dr. Gary Carroll.

In 60% of individuals, infections do not cause symptoms, but *Coccidioides immitis* can cause an acute disease with flu-like symptoms called *Valley fever* and also San Joaquin Valley fever, so named because high rates of infection are seen in the San Joaquin Valley. A temperature up to 104°F can occur with a dry cough, joint and muscle aches, and headaches. A lumpy red rash on the legs can appear. The severity of the infection depends on the individual's immune system and the number of spores inhaled. Most people recover in a few weeks to a few months after infection, but some develop a chronic lung infection, and a widespread disseminated infection can occur in some people. In the chronic lung infection, which can occur 20 or more years after the primary infection, lung abscesses filled with *Coccidiodes* can rupture, and the resulting fluid and pus can damage the lungs. The patient shows typical signs of pneumonia, and

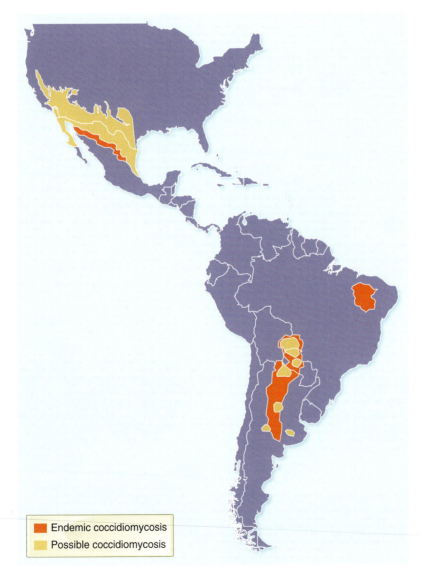

Endemic coccidiomycosis
Possible coccidiomycosis

■ **FIGURE 20.7**   Geographic distribution of coccidiomycosis.

treatment is needed for recovery. In widespread dissemination, meningitis, skin lesions, and bone and joint lesions can occur (13, 14, 15, 16, 17).

Coccidioides are thermally dimorphic with the mold form growing in the soil and the yeast form developing in the patient. The hyphae produce spores that have winglike structures that make them particularly likely to become airborne. Once inhaled, a yeastlike form called the *spherule* develops (Figure 20.8 ■). It is a sac that as it matures contains endospores (13, 14, 15, 16, 17).

Diagnosis and Treatment

Diagnosis of coccidioidomycosis is by microscopic examination of contaminated body fluids (sputum, tissue, or other body fluid), culturing a specimen from the same samples, or immunological analysis by detection of serum antibodies or a skin test. Arthroconidia are very infectious, so culture is potentially hazardous and must be done under biosafety conditions. Antibody testing uses Ouchterlony. In testing for *Coccidioides immitis,* the patient's serum is placed in a well across from another well containing the *Coccidioides immitis*

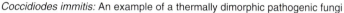

Coccidiodes immitis: An example of a thermally dimorphic pathogenic fungi

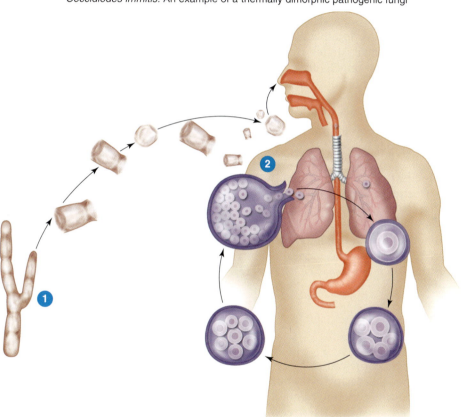

1 In dry sandy soil *Coccidioides imitis* grows as mycelia. When some of the cells in the mycelia die, the neighboring cells become spores. The spores easily become airborne as the dead cell fragments act as wings to help them take flight.

2 The spores are inhaled and become spherules or balls filled with smaller balls. The balls rupture and the smaller balls grow and in turn become filled with balls. Eventually these spherules can fill the lungs, causing inflammation and pneumonia.

High risk groups

• The immunocompromised: patients with HIV, lymphoma, transplants, and others on immunosuppressant therapy
• Diabetics
• Pregnant women
• African Americans, Filipinos

■ **FIGURE 20.8**   Life cycle of *Coccidioides immitis.*

antigens, and a positive control serum is placed in a well neighboring the patient's serum. A line of identity indicates that the patient is infected. Two different antigens, IDTP and IDCF, are utilized. Serial dilution and titration of the last positive dilution is performed, using the last dilution in which a line is seen as an endpoint. Immunodiffusion detection of antibodies, usually IgM antibodies, against the TP antigen indicates a recent infection whereas immunodiffusion detection of antibodies (usually IgG) against the F antigen indicates an infection within the past year. Latex agglutination and enzyme immunoassay tests have been developed; the latter is promising as a faster, more sensitive replacement for immunodiffusion. A skin test for a measure of T-cell-mediated immune response to the fungus has been utilized for diagnosis in immunocompetent individuals, but skin tests remain positive for life after an infection. A negative skin test that converts on repeat testing to a positive skin test is diagnostic, but because a positive skin test alone only indicates a current or a past infection, this test has been discontinued. Complement fixation tests for the antibody were also performed to detect patient antibody but they, too, have been largely discontinued. Complement fixation measures the utilization of complement after patient antibody has reacted with the antigen (13, 14, 15, 16, 17).

People who are mildly ill with Valley fever often recover without requiring any treatment. People who are immunocompromised and those who have disseminated disease should be treated with antifungals such as ketoconazole, itraconazole, and fluconazole. Intravenous therapy with amphotericin B is required for severe disease, and surgical removal of abscesses in the lungs, bones, or joints may be needed (13, 14, 15, 16, 17).

CRYPTOCOCCOSIS

Epidemiology

The disease cryptococcosis is primarily caused by *Cryptococcus neoformans*. This organism is associated with bird droppings with pigeons being the chief vector (Figure 20.9 ■). Cryptococcosis can also be caused by *Cryptococcus gattii*, which is associated with eucalyptus trees and the soil around them. Inhalation of either the yeast cells or the basidiospores causes cryptococcosis. *Cryptococcus neoformans* infections are usually seen in people who are immunosuppressed but can occasionally be seen in otherwise healthy individuals. The incidence in HIV-infected individuals was as high as 100 cases per 1000, but has dropped to about 7 per 1000 due to the effectiveness of HAART. The cases in the general population are usually around 0.4 to 1.3 cases per 100 000. *Cryptococcus gatti* infections are found in immunosuppressed individuals, and more often than *C. neoformans*, *C. gatti* infections are also found in individuals who are only mildly immunocompromised and in otherwise healthy individuals. A pulmonary infection with pneumonia-like symptoms, a skin infection with lesions, or a meningoencephalitis may be seen. The

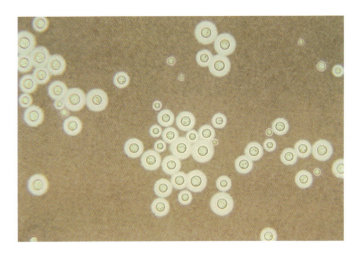

■ **FIGURE 20.9**   *Cryptococcus neoformans* with India ink stain.
Source: © CDC/ Dr. Leanor Haley.

incubation period from infection to disease is long: 2 to 14 months for *C. gatti;* however, the incubation period for *C. neoformans* is not known. Meningoencephalitis is most often seen in HIV patients; in the United States, the mortality from meningoencephalitis is 12%; in parts of Africa, it can reach 90%. A recent outbreak of *C. gatti* in the Pacific Northwest (60 cases from 2004–2010) showed infection in 9 of the 60 individuals with no risk factors, and 27 others who had conditions that indicated they were immunocompromised rather than severely immunosuppressed. Individuals who are immunocompromised included those with oral steroid use, diabetes, cancer, and other conditions that are not associated with severe immunosuppression. Although 60 is a small number of cases, this has caused concern about whether *C. gatti* will emerge as an infectious disease in the northwest United States (18, 19, 20, 21, 22).

Diagnosis and Treatment

Diagnosis of cryptococcosis is made by microscopic examination with India ink visualization of the capsule, with or without previous culture, or by an antigen assay on blood or cerebral spinal fluid. The antigen assay is a latex agglutination assay in which latex beads are coated with antibody to the *Cryptococcus* polysaccharide antigen, and the presence of this antigen will agglutinate the particles. An antibody detection agglutination assay is also available in which antigen-coated beads agglutinate in the presence of anti-Cryptococcus antibody in serum or cerebral spinal fluid (for infection of the central nervous system). A rapid lateral flow or sandwich immunochromatographic assay that tests for antigen (similar to the assay shown for the HCG pregnancy test in Chapter 7) has also recently become available. Complement fixation was previously performed to detect antibody to *Cryptococcus* but has been generally discontinued. Treatment is with amphotericin B with or without flucytosine. Flucanazole is used in HIV patients (18, 19, 20, 21, 22).

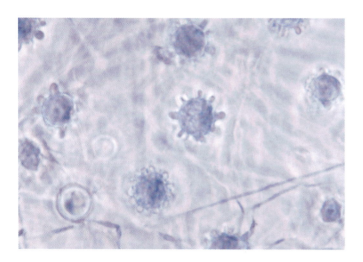

■ **FIGURE 20.10** *Histoplasma capsulatum* hyphae and macrocondia. *Source:* © CDC/Dr. Libero Ajello.

HISTOPLASMOSIS

Epidemiology

Histoplasmosis infections occur commonly throughout the world and in the United States are **endemic** in the Mississippi and Ohio River valleys. Skin testing showed that 80% of people in these areas had been infected by *Histoplasma capsulatum* (Figure 20.10 ■). Most of these individuals (99%) had a subclinical infection or a mild flulike disease. In individuals whose disease is apparent, either pulmonary disease (Figure 20.11 ■) or disseminated disease is seen. Like cryptococcal infections, histoplasma infections are associated with exposure to bird droppings. The disease does not spread from person to person. The very young and the very old are more likely to have symptomatic infections, and people who

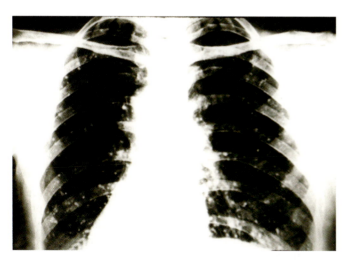

■ **FIGURE 20.11** Lungs showing appearance of acute histoplasmosis infection. *Source:* © CDC/ Dr. Lucille K. Georg.

are immunosuppressed are more likely to get disseminated disease. Pulmonary infections include fever, chest pains, and a nonproductive cough. Chronic lung disease, which is similar to that seen with a tuberculosis infection, can also occur, and occurs more frequently in patients with emphysema. The lung lesions heal but leave calcifications (23, 24, 25, 26, 27).

The fungus in disseminated histoplasmosis travels from the lungs to other organs in macrophages. This occurs only in people with defects in cell-mediated immunity and can result in a life-threatening disease. Disseminated disease is seen in people with HIV, hematologic malignancies, organ transplants, infants, and those receiving anti-TNFα therapy (Enbrel, Remicade, etc). Symptoms and physical signs of disseminated disease include fever, weight loss, pallor, malaise, lymphadenopathy and hepatosplenomegaly (23, 24, 25, 26, 27).

Diagnosis and Treatment

Diagnosis of *Histoplasma capsulatum* can include a urine test for antigens, an immunodiffusion test for antibody, or culture followed by a DNA probe. The urine test is a sandwich enzyme immunoassay that detects the *H. capsulatum* polysaccharide antigen. In disseminated disease, the sandwich immunoassay has a 95% sensitivity using urine and 86% sensitivity using serum. The sensitivity is lower in pulmonary disease with a range of 10 to 75%; however, the sensitivity increases with increasing severity of the disease. For antibody testing, immunodiffusion using the M and F antigens is most often utilized in a paired titer format; a 4-fold increases in titer is considered diagnostic. Tests for antibody are useful only in patients who are not immunosuppressed and thus are most useful in patients with acute pulmonary histoplasmosis that is not very severe. It is important to note that 2 to 6 weeks are necessary for paired titer testing so this would not be useful in patients with severe disease. Treatment is with itraconazole as the drug of choice, sometimes combined with amphotericin B, if the disease does not resolve by itself. Culture is potentially hazardous and must be done under biosafety conditions (23, 24, 25, 26, 27).

PNEUMOCYSTIS JIROVECI (FORMERLY KNOWN AS PNEUMOCYSTIS CARINII)

Epidemiology

Pneumocystis jiroveci, which causes an infection in AIDS patients, was formerly known as *Pneumocystis carinii,* but the name was changed when this organism, previously thought to be a parasite (a protozoa), was reclassified as a fungus using nucleic acid and biochemical analysis. In addition, *Pneumocystis jiroveci* infects only humans unlike the different organism, still known as *Pneumocystis carinii,* which was isolated from rats (28).

This fungus occurs commonly worldwide and causes pneumocystis pneumonia (PCP) in immunosuppressed individuals and in malnourished premature infants. This is a defining infection of AIDS and is the most common serious opportunistic infection in these patients. Symptoms of PCP are a nonproductive cough and a fever; as the disease progresses and is not treated, increasing lung involvement can ultimately lead to death (28).

Diagnosis and Treatment
Diagnosis of PCP is made by microscopic analysis of sputum, bronchial lavage fluid, or biopsy material. Microscopy is aided through the use of direct immunofluorescence with monoclonal antibodies to *Pneumocystis jiroveci*. Trimethoprim-sulfamethoxazole is used to treat this infection (28).

Checkpoint! 20.4
What is the name of the organism that causes Pneumocystis pneumonia? *Is it a fungus or a parasite?*

▶ INTRODUCTION TO PARASITES

Parasites are organisms that live at the expense of other organisms. The classification of parasites involves several features; the first is based on whether the parasite lives inside the host (endoparasites) or outside the host (ectoparasites). Endoparasites can be further categorized as either protozoans or helminths. *Protozoans* are unicellular organisms whereas *helminths* are multicellular (eg, worms). Ectoparasites include blood-sucking parasites such as mosquitos, but this term mostly refers to ticks, fleas, lice, and mites—the burrowing type of animals that remain attached to the host for some time. Protozoans are not visible to the naked eye, while helminths and ectoparasites are. Protozoans that cause human disease live in the blood, tissue, or the intestines. The word *helminth* is from the Greek for worm, and this group includes flatworms, thorny-headed worms, and roundworms (29, 30).

Parasites are complicated antigenically and immunologically. Evasion of the immune system occurs through antigenic modulation, where surface antigens that are targeted by the immune system are altered by the parasite; immune evasion can also occur through antigenic sequestration by which the parasite hides either inside a cell or deep within tissues and, therefore, does not stimulate an immune response. In addition, the parasite can cover itself in the host's antigens and thus become invisible to the host's immune system (29, 30).

Parasites can also shed their antigens, thus preventing an immune response from reacting with the parasites;

Checkpoint! 20.5
Which of the following parasites cannot be seen by the naked eye: protozoans, helminths, or ectoparasites?

furthermore, they can also secrete immunomodulating agents that can reduce an immune response. However, the immune system can counteract some of these evading mechanisms with the involvement and collaboration of the innate and the acquired immune systems and their many cells and molecules. These include neutrophils, eosinophils, basophils, and natural killer, macrophage, and mast cells as well as molecules such as gamma interferon and hydrogen peroxide. Complement activation, and the production of various chemokines and cytokines further enhance the immune response to these pathogens. The antibody response to parasites includes IgM, IgG, IgA, and IgE. In the response to helminths (worms), mast cells, eosinophils, and IgE all play a role. In fact, many of the physiological responses observed in IgE-mediated allergy, such as increased mucous production, and involuntary defecation, can actually help rid the patient of the parasite. Eosinophil degranulation can destroy helminths, and eosinophils can also kill a helminth by antibody directed cell-mediated cytotoxicity (29, 30).

Globally, parasitic infections are a major health problem with the disease malaria caused by parasites of the genus *Plasmodium*, resulting in more than 1 million deaths per year (31). Even in developed countries, the parasitic diseases discussed in this chapter cause a huge disease burden that has increased with the number of people with AIDS and other forms of immunodeficiencies. There are more than 300 000 cases of cryptosporidiosis 2 million cases of giardiasis 1.5 million cases of *Toxoplasma*, and 7.5 million cases of trichomoniasis in the United States each year. *Cryptosporidium*, *Giardia* and *Toxoplasma* are described here because they can be diagnosed with antigen and antibody testing and because of their frequency in the United States. Although it is also commonly found in the United States, trichomoniasis is not described because the clinical immunology laboratory rarely diagnoses it (29, 30).

CRYPTOSPORIDIUM PARVUM

Epidemiology
When students in the United States begin studying parasites, they may think that they will never encounter such a diagnosis, or if they do, it will be only in a patient who has recently traveled to another part of the world. If this has gone through your mind, please revisit the numbers in the previous paragraph. These infections are often seen in the United States and are diagnosed serologically. ***Cryptosporidium parvum*** is seen all over the world, and an outbreak in 1993 infected 400 000 people in Milwaukee, Wisconsin! *Cryptosporidium* causes a watery diarrheal disease 2 to 10 days after infection, and the diarrhea lasts for 1 to 2 weeks. This infection is spread by ingestion of contaminated food and water, is very stable, and is resistant to chlorine disinfection. Contaminated drinking and recreational water is most often the source of spread. People who are immunocompromised can suffer a severe illness that could be fatal.

Diagnosis and Treatment

Diagnosis of *Cryptosporidium* is made by using stool samples. These samples can be viewed microscopically with acid fast staining or via direct immunofluorescent staining using fluorescently labeled monoclonal antibodies to the parasite. Diagnosis can also be made with an antigen-capture enzyme immunoassay using diluted stool as a sample source (Figure 20.12 ■). PCR assays have been developed and used in some laboratories. Tests for *Cryptosporidium* are usually performed in specialty laboratories. The current test of choice is the direct immunofluorescence assay.

Replacement of fluids can be important in treatment. Nitazoxanide can be used for treating the symptoms in healthy people. Paromomycin is used for treatment of people who are immunocompromised, but this does not eliminate the parasite. Antiretroviral therapy may improve the immune systems of people with HIV enough to decrease the symptoms of *Cryptosporidium*.

GIARDIA LAMBLIA

Epidemiology

Giardia lamblia infects people worldwide via fecal-oral transmission. For the life cycle of *Giardia lamblia* see Figure 20.13 ■. Two percent of adults and 6% to 8% of children in developed countries as well as 33% of people in developing countries have had *Giardia*. It causes diarrheal disease 1 to 2 weeks after fecal-oral contamination and can survive outside the body for weeks to months after defecation (32).

Diagnosis and Treatment

Giardia is excreted intermittently, so microscopic examination of concentrated extracts of the stool may miss this parasite. See Figure 20.14 ■ for scanning electron microscope images of *Giardia* An assay kit for direct immunofluorescent detection of this parasite is available. Capture immunoassays for

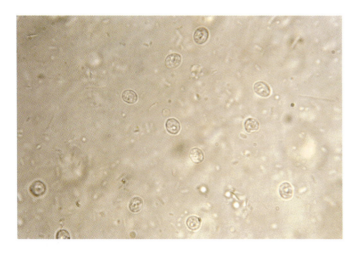

■ **FIGURE 20.12** *Cryptosporidium parvum* from stool. *Source:* © CDC/ Dr. Peter Drotman.

the antigen are also available and are superior to microscopic analysis. A rapid test has also been developed to identify this parasite. Molecular assays can be used to determine the subtype. Treatments can include metronidazole, tinidazole, or nitazoxanide (32).

 Checkpoint! 20.6

Why are concentrated stool samples sometimes negative for Giardia *even though the patient is infected?*

TOXOPLASMA GONDII

Epidemiology

Toxoplasmosis is caused by the protozoan parasite *Toxoplasma gondii*. It is transmitted to humans in several ways including the consumption of undercooked contaminated meat, especially lamb, pork, beef, and venison. For the life cycle of *Toxoplasma gondii* see Figure 20.15 ■ on page 360. This ingestion can occur by either the intentional consumption of the undercooked meat or its improper handling during preparation. *Toxoplasma gondii* is not absorbed through the skin, so handling raw meat is not a problem. However, accidental transmission can occur through the use of contaminated utensils or through hand-to-mouth contact after meat preparation (Figure 20.16 ■ on page 361). Cats are definitive hosts for this organism, so anything that is potentially contaminated with cat feces is also a source of infection; this can include not only the cat litter box but also garden soil. Another very important source of transmission, which can result in birth defects, is from a mother to child via congenital transmission. Finally, transmission can occur through organ transplant, but this is rare. In the United States, 22.5% of people over 12 have been infected whereas in other parts of the world (including Europe), up to 95% of the people have been infected. A woman who is infected at least 6 to 9 months before her pregnancy will develop immunity and will not pass *Toxoplasma gondii* to her baby. Because of this, the lower rate of infection in the United States actually has some negative ramifications: because few people are infected, pregnant women are at risk for a primary infection just before or during pregnancy (33, 34, 35).

In most people infection with *Toxoplasma gondii* is subclinical, yielding no signs or symptoms. Some people have symptoms that seem like a mild long-lasting flu or infectious mononucleosis. In people who are immunocompromised, the symptoms can be fever, retinal inflammation with blurred vision, headaches, confusion, and seizures. The immunocompromised people who are particularly severely infected include those with AIDS as well as those who have received an organ transplant, cancer patients receiving chemotherapy, and individuals taking immunosuppressant drugs. See Figure 20.17 ■ on page 361 for a photo of *Toxoplasma gondii* in the heart of an HIV patient. Half of the babies infected *in utero* are born prematurely, and their eyes, ears, nervous system, and skin

Giardiasis
(Giardia intestinalis)

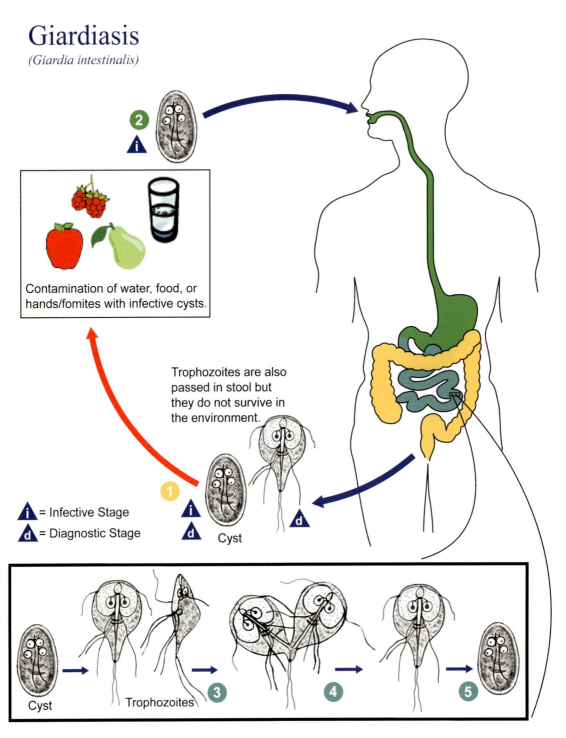

Contamination of water, food, or hands/fomites with infective cysts.

Trophozoites are also passed in stool but they do not survive in the environment.

▲i = Infective Stage

▲d = Diagnostic Stage

Cyst

Cyst   Trophozoites   ③   ④   ⑤

■ **FIGURE 20.13**   Life cycle of *Giardia. Source:* © CDC.

can be affected. Some of the babies will have obvious signs of infection at birth, but others who are more mildly infected will not show signs of infection until later. Almost all will develop some signs of infection, especially eye damage, by adolescence. Babies born with symptoms can have eye damage because of damage to the retina; in addition, they can have feeding problems, diarrhea and vomiting, hearing loss, enlarged liver and spleen, jaundice, skin rash, and low birth weight. The infection to newborns can be so severe that the measurement of a woman's immunity prior to or just after conception is now part of prenatal care. A set of assays used in detection of infectious diseases in pregnant women and newborns is called

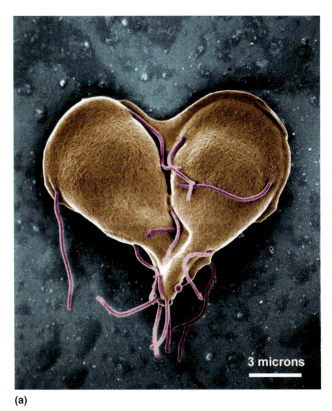

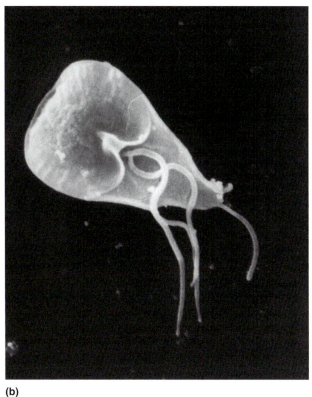

(a)   (b)

■ **FIGURE 20.14** (a) *Giardia lamblia* protozoan as it is replicating. *Source:* © CDC/Dr. Stan Erlandsen. (b) Scanning micrograph. *Source:* © CDC/Janice Haney Carr.

TORCH (*t*oxoplasmosis, *o*ther infections, *r*ubella, *c*ytomegalovirus, and *h*erpes simplex virus) (33, 34, 35). To prevent infection with toxoplasmosis in individuals who are immunocompromised or in pregnant women who do not show signs of immunity, the following guidelines are recommended:

1. Cook ground meat and pork to at least 160°F internal temperature except for ground chicken, which should be cooked to 165°F.
2. Cook veal, beef, lamb, and steaks to at least 145°F.
3. Cook whole poultry to 180°F and chicken breasts to 170°F.
4. Peel or thoroughly wash fruit before eating.
5. Wash cookware, countertops, and utensils with hot soapy water after they are used for raw meat.
6. Wash hands with hot soapy water after gardening or handling raw meat.
7. Have someone else change the cat litter box daily, keep cats indoors, and do not handle a stray cat or get a new cat while pregnant (33, 34, 35). (See Figure 20.16)

Diagnosis and Treatment

Diagnosis of a current infection with toxoplasmosis is made using a serological test in an indirect enzyme immunoassay for either IgM, low avidity IgG, or high titers of IgG. Testing

for IgG levels is performed in women prior to pregnancy when looking for immunity. Differentiating a primary infection of toxoplasmosis from a past infection serologically is complicated (33, 34, 35).

IgM levels are unusual in toxoplasmosis in that IgM remains detectable for up to 2 years following primary infection. IgA to *Toxoplasma* remains elevated for up to 4 years, and diagnosis with paired titer IgG levels can be difficult because the patient may already have high titers at the first blood draw. Measurement of the avidity of the IgG provides data that helps differentiate a present from a past infection. The avidity of IgG increases with time, and the avidity of the IgG antibody remains low in toxoplasmosis for the first few months. **Low avidity IgG antibody** is an indication that the patient has had toxoplasmosis within the last 8 months, and the presence of **high avidity antibody** indicates that the patient's infection occurred 5 or more months before testing. Past versus present infection is of key diagnostic importance when testing a pregnant woman. Avidity is assessed using 2 parallel enzyme immunoassays; in both tests, the serum is incubated with the antigen, then one is washed with a normal buffer, while one is washed with the buffer containing small amounts of urea. This urea will dissociate low avidity antibody, but high avidity antibody will remain attached to the antigen. The optical density of the set washed with urea

Toxoplasmosis
(Toxoplasma gondii)

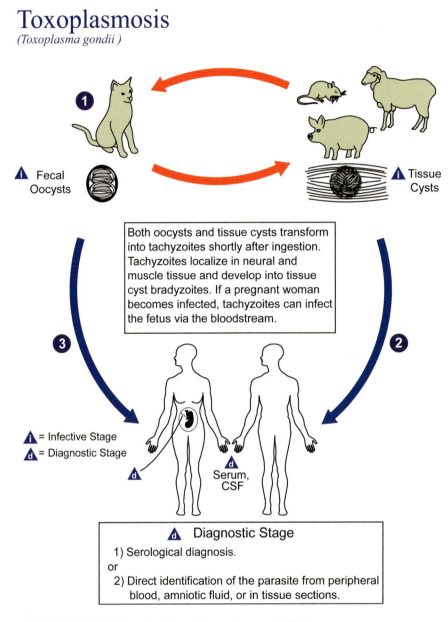

■ FIGURE 20.15   Life cycle of *Toxoplasma. Source:* © CDC.

is divided by the optical density of the set without it to give an avidity index. An avidity index of more than 0.25 indicates high avidity antibody is present. The Focus Diagnostic™ test kit performed this way demonstrates that 100% of recent infections show low avidity IgG whereas 100% of the past infections show high avidity IgG. A positive low avidity antibody test in a pregnant woman indicates that antimicrobials targeting *Toxoplasma gondii* should be used. Diagnosis can also be made by finding the parasite in cerebral spinal fluid (csf) or biopsy material, but this is rarely done. DNA testing can be performed on amniotic fluid to detect congenital transmission (33, 34, 35).

In most cases, toxoplasmosis in healthy individuals is too mild to need treatment, but a symptomatic patient can be treated with pyrimethamine and sulfadiazine, which can also be used in HIV patients and in fetal infection; leucovorin is added to treat infants for 1 year after birth (33, 34, 35).

Other parasites that are seen less frequently also may be diagnosed using antigen or antibody assays. Malaria, acquired by visiting endemic countries, occurs in about 1500 people in the United States each year. It is diagnosed classically using a Giemsa-stained thick blood smear for diagnosis and a thin smear to determine the species and

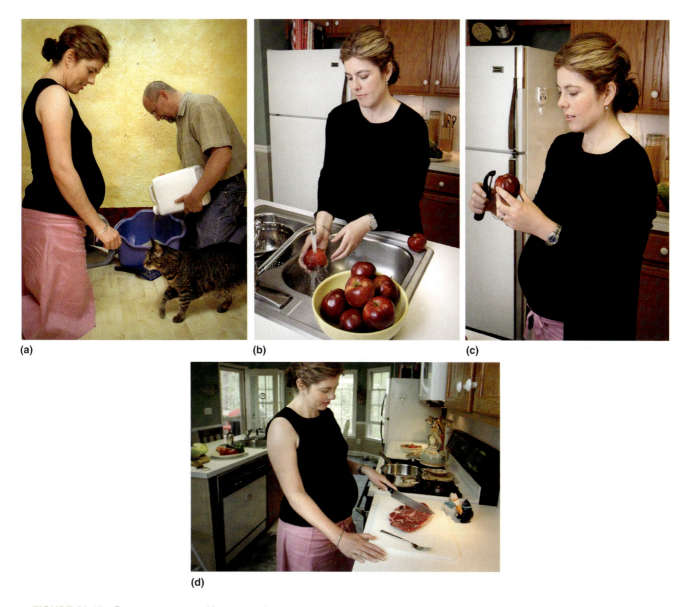

■ **FIGURE 20.16** Pregnant woman taking precautions to prevent a toxoplasmosis infection by (a) having someone else change the kitty litter box, (b) washing fruit before (c) peeling it and (d) cooking meat to the appropriate temperature. *Source (a)-(d):* © CDC.

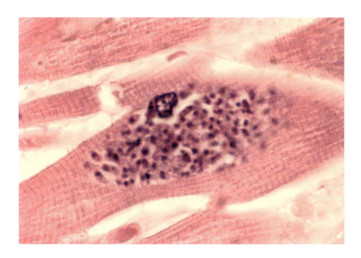

■ **FIGURE 20.17** *Toxoplasma gondii* in the heart of an HIV patient. *Source:* © CDC/ Dr. Edwin P. Ewing, Jr.

the degree or parasitemia. A new rapid diagnostic test (RDT) that is similar to the hCG immunochromatographic assay described in Chapter 7 is available; in this test, the malaria antigens bind labeled antibody and then travel to an area on the strip coated with a second capture antibody. This test may be more sensitive for most of the species of *Plasmodium* that cause malaria but may not detect some of the less common species. A negative RDT should be followed by microscopy, and a positive RDT is also followed by microscopy to speciate and determine the amount of parasitemia (33, 34, 35).

 Checkpoint! 20.7

Is it dangerous for a pregnant woman to handle raw meat?

CASE STUDY 1

Ariel, a 25-year-old woman who works in the lab with you has severe rheumatoid arthritis and is receiving anti-TNF monoclonal antibody therapy to immunosuppress her autoimmune response. Unfortunately, this therapy causes generalized immunosuppression. Ariel was gardening on Saturday and cleaned up the very back part of her yard that contained rotting apples and leaves that had been raked there the previous fall. She has developed a fever, cough, chest pain, and difficulty breathing. Her chest x-ray reveals patchy dense areas.

1. What disease do you think Ariel may have?
2. Can you test for antibody to diagnose Ariel's illness?
3. How can Ariel be treated? (*Hint:* Think deeply.)

CASE STUDY 2

Belle, a young Parisian foreign exchange student comes to the clinic; she is pregnant and has mild flulike symptoms. She has a cat and has recently heard that "something" can be transmitted from the cat to her if she changes the litter box and that this thing can infect her fetus. Sacre bleu! If only she had known about this, she never would have changed the nasty thing. She has had cats all her life and had never heard of such a thing before. It has always been her responsibility to change the litter box. If you can ease her mind, she will bring to you her famous steak tartare dish (raw meat) as a gift.

1. What organism is she thinking of?
2. What kind of organism is it?
3. What do you need to do to relieve her mind?
4. Why do you think that she probably need not worry?
5. What would have happened to the baby if she is infected?
6. Will you eat Belle's steak tartare?

SUMMARY

Fungi are eukaryotic organisms that can cause infection. The species that cause infection are often thermally dimorphic in the mold form in the environment, creating spores that can be inhaled, and once in the body, switching to the yeast form. Fungi that are important pathogens include *Aspergillus* species, *Blastomyces dermatitis, Candida albicans, Cryptococcus neoformans,* and *Cryptococcus gatti, Histoplasma capsulatum, Coccidioides immitis,* and *Pneumocystis jiroveci.* Phagocytic cell dysfunction, and/or T-cell dysfunctions lead to increased susceptibility to fungal infections. Histoplasmosis, blastomycosis, and coccidiomycosis are seen in healthy individuals and people who are immunocompromised, but most other fungal infections are seen in individuals who are immunocompromised. Culture, immunofluorescent analysis, antibody analysis, antigen analysis, and sometimes

molecular techniques are performed for diagnosis (1–28). Fungi are summarized in Table 20.1 ✪.

Aspergillus is a ubiquitous fungus transmitted by inhaling dust containing the spores. Different syndromes can occur after infection, including allergic bronchopulmonary aspergillosis, invasive aspergillosis, aspergilloma, *Aspergillus* sinus infections, cutaneous aspergillosis, and otitis externa. Of these disorders, invasive aspergillosis and cutaneous aspergillosis are seen primarily in individuals who are immunocompromised; the remaining infections can be seen in immunocompetent individuals as well. Antibody detection using an immunodiffusion can be used for diagnosis in immunocompetant individuals, and diagnosis with antigen detection using a sandwich immunoassay for the galactomannan antigen and the β-glucan antigen can be performed (7, 8, 9).

Blastomyces dermatitidis is also thermally dimorphic and transmitted by the inhalation of spores. It is found primarily in wooded areas in the midwest, south-central, and southeastern states of the United States, and it infects people who are in these areas and inhale the spores. Both healthy individuals and those who are immunocompromised can contract blastomycosis, which causes cough, fever, and muscle and joint pain. Disseminated infection and meningitis can also result. Antibody is diagnostic and is found by immunodiffusion or indirect enzyme immunoassay (10).

Candidiasis is seen as oral, genitourinary, and invasive disease. It is seen primarily in infants and in individuals who are immunocompromised with the exception of the genital form, which is a very common infection in women. It can be diagnosed by appearance or culture, but sandwich immunoassays that are under development will be useful for invasive candidiasis infections. The relevant antigens are the β-(1–3)-D-glucan cell wall antigen and the surface mannan (11, 12).

Coccidioides immitis, like *Aspergillus,* is thermally dimorphic and transmitted by the inhalation of spores in dust; *Coccidioides* is seen in dry regions and is endemic in the southwestern United States, Mexico, and South and Central America. The number of cases of this disease has been increasing. Many infected individuals show no signs or symptoms, but healthy individuals as well as individuals who are immunocompromised can become ill. The acute Valley fever flulike disease can develop; it includes a dry cough, joint and muscle pain, headaches, and a lumpy rash. A chronic infection or a disseminated infection can develop. It can be detected by using immunodiffusion, latex agglutination, or enzyme immunoassays for antibody (13, 14, 15, 16, 17).

Cryptococcal infections include infections by *Cryptococcus neoformans* found in bird droppings and *Cryptococcus gatti* found around eucalyptus trees. The disease is the result of inhalation of spores, and a pulmonary infection, a skin infection, or meningoencephalitis can be seen. Infections by both organisms are seen in individuals who are immunocompromised, but *C. gatti* is found more often than *C. neoformans* in healthy individuals as well. These infections are diagnosed with India ink visualization of the capsule or by using immunological techniques for antibody or antigen. Latex agglutination tests that detect either the antibody or the antigen have been developed; a rapid sandwich immunochromatographic assay has also been developed (18, 19, 20, 21, 22).

⊘ TABLE 20.1

Fungal Diseases

Fungus	Region	Dimorphic	Disease	Immunological Method of Analysis	Treatment	People Primarily Infected
Aspergillus	Ubiquitous	Yes	Allergic broncho-pulmonary aspergillosis	Immunodiffusion (ID) for antibody Elevated IgE Sandwich EIA for galacto-mannan and β-glucan	Prednisone and antifungals	People with cystic fibrosis, asthma Also healthy individuals
			Aspergilloma	Immunodiffusion (ID) for antibody Sandwich EIA for galacto-mannan and β-glucan	Surgery Antifungals instilled into fungal ball	Healthy individuals
			Invasive aspergillosis	Sandwich EIA for galacto-mannan and β-glucan	Voriconazole posaconazole or amphotericin B	Immunocompromised people People with lung disease
Blastomyces dermatitidis	Wooded areas Midwest, south central, and southeast United States Africa Central and South America	Yes	Acute Cutaneous or systemic Chronic pulmonary disease or dissemi-nated disease	ID antibody against the "A" antigen Indirect enzyme immunoassay	Itraconazole if immunocom-promised or severe disease Amphotericin B first	Farmers, forestry workers, campers, and hunters
Candida	Ubiquitous	Yes	Oral candidiasis	None	Nystatin Clotrimazole	Infants, denture wearers, inhaled steroids users, immunocompromised individuals
			Genitourinary candidiasis	None	Antifungal cream or suppository, oral fluconazole	75% of women, rarely men
			Invasive candidiasis	Sandwich immunoassays under development for the β-(1–3)-D-glucan cell wall antigen (sensitivity 75–100%; specificity 88–100%) or the surface mannan (sensitivity 31–90%)	Fluconazole, with the echino-candins or other antifungals	Low birth weight babies, hospitalized individuals, people on IV fluids, people with in-dwelling catheters, injection drug users, and people who are immunocompromised
Coccidioides immitis	Southwestern United States Mexico South and Central America	Yes	Valley fever Chronic lung infection	ID May be replaced by latex agglutination or EIA	Keto-conazole, itraconazole and fluconazole Intravenous therapy with amphotericin B for severe disease	People who work in dusty areas including construction workers, farm workers, and archeologists
			Disseminated disease			Severity depends on immune system and number of spores inhaled

✪ TABLE 20.1

Fungal Diseases *(continued)*

Fungus	Region	Dimorphic	Disease	Immunological Method of Analysis	Treatment	People Primarily Infected
Cryptococcus	Ubiquitous	Yes	Pulmonary infection Skin infection with lesions Meningoencephalitis	Latex agglutination assay or immunochromatographic assay for antigens Latex agglutination for antibody	Amphotericin B with or without flucytosine. Flucanazole is used in HIV patients	Immunosuppressed Occasionally in otherwise healthy individuals
Histoplasma capsulatum	Endemic in the Mississippi and Ohio River valleys in United States and throughout world	Yes	Subclinical infection or mild flulike disease Pulmonary Disseminated disease	Antibody testing ID Ab to M and F antigens (not in immunocompromised) Urine test for antigen is a sandwich enzyme immunoassay that detects the *H. capsulatum* polysaccharide antigen	Used with itraconazole as the drug of choice, sometimes combined with amphotericin B	Very young and the very old are more likely to have symptomatic infections Disseminated disease in people with HIV, organ transplants, hematologic malignancies, receiving anti-TNFα therapy (Enbrel, Remicade etc.), and in infants
Pneumocystis jiroveci	Ubiquitous	Yes	Pneumocystis pneumonia	Direct immunofluorescence	Trimethoprim-sulfamethoxazole	Immunocompromised HIV

Histoplasmosis is endemic in the Mississippi and Ohio River valleys and is associated with the inhalation of the spores from fungus that grows in bird droppings. Subclinical, mild flulike, pulmonary, or disseminated disease can develop. More severe disease is seen in individuals who are immunocompromised. The disseminated disease, which occurs only in people who are immunocompromised, can be life threatening. Urine sandwich enzyme immunoassays for the antigen, immunodiffusion for antibody, or culture followed by a DNA probe can be used for diagnosis. Culture is potentially hazardous (23, 24, 25, 26).

Pneumocystis jiroveci, formerly known as *Pneumocystis carinii*, occurs commonly worldwide and causes pneumocystis pneumonia (PCP), a defining infection of AIDS; it causes infection in other immunosuppressed individuals and in malnourished premature infants. Diagnosis of PCP by microscopic analysis is aided by direct immunofluorescence with monoclonal antibodies to *Pneumocystis jiroveci* (28).

Protozoan and helminths are parasites that cause disease in humans. Parasites are summarized in Table 20.2 ✪. Parasitic infections represent a major health problem, even in developed countries. *Cryptosporidium*, *Giardia*, and *Toxoplasma* can be diagnosed with antigen and antibody testing and are frequently found in the United States. *Cryptosporidium* occurs worldwide,

causing a watery diarrheal disease 2 to 10 days after infection, which lasts for 1 to 2 weeks. Spread by ingestion of contaminated food and water infection in people who are immunocompromised, *Cryptosporidium* can cause a severe illness that can be fatal. Diagnosis is made microscopically on stool samples with acid fast staining or with direct immunofluorescent staining. Capture enzyme immunoassays using diluted stool are also performed. PCR assays have been developed and used in some laboratories. *Giardia lamblia* infects people worldwide via fecal-oral transmission causing diarrheal disease. Microscopic examination and direct immunofluorescent detection of this parasite are used for diagnosis as are capture immunoassays for antigen. Toxoplasmosis is caused by the protozoan parasite *Toxoplasma gondii*. It is transmitted to humans by the consumption of undercooked contaminated meat, contamination with cat feces and congenital transmission and, rarely, through organ transplant. In healthy individuals, infection is usually subclinical, but may be seen as a mild, long-lasting flu; in people who are immunocompromised, the symptoms can be fever, retinal inflammation with blurred vision, headaches, confusion, and seizures. Babies infected *in utero* can be profoundly affected, and testing for toxoplasmosis is an important part of prenatal care (28, 29, 30, 31, 32, 33, 34, 35).

⊙ TABLE 20.2

Parasitic Diseases

Parasite	Region	Disease	Immunological Method of Analysis	Treatment	People Primarily Infected
Cryptosporidium parvum	World-wide	Watery diarrheal disease	Direct immuno-fluorescence on stool concentrate Capture enzyme immuno-assays using diluted stool as a sample source	Nitazoxanide for healthy people Immunocompromised paromomycin in HIV Antiretroviral therapy to improve immunity	Those who ingest contaminated food and water
		Severe illness in immuno-compromised that may even be fatal			Severe in immuno-compromised; defining disease in AIDS
Giardia lamblia	World-wide	Diarrheal disease	Direct immunofluorescence on stool concentrate Capture enzyme immuno-assays using diluted stool as a sample source Rapid test	Metronidazole, tinidazole, or nitazoxanide	2% adults and 6–8% of children in developed countries, and 33% of people in developing countries Fecal-oral contamination
Toxoplasma gondii	World-wide	Normals: Subclinical or infectious mononucleosis-like Immunocompromised Fever, retinal inflammation, headaches, confusion, and seizures. Babies: Born prematurely, and eyes, ears, nervous system, and skin can be affected	IgG for immunity Low avidity IgG for recent infection	Pyrimethamine and sulfadiazine normals and HIV In fetal infection, add leucovorin	In the United States, 22.5% of people over 12 In other parts of the world up to 95% of the people

REVIEW QUESTIONS

1. An AIDS patient who raised pigeons developed chest pains and headaches with dizziness. A sputum and a spinal tap were positive for yeastlike organisms, which is consistent with these findings?
   a. *Candida albicans*
   b. *Cryptococcus neoformans*
   c. *Toxoplasma gondii*
   d. *Coccidiodes immitis*

2. Which disease is also called San Joaquin Valley fever?
   a. *Crytococcus neoformans*
   b. *Candida albicans*
   c. *Toxoplasma gondii*
   d. coccidioidomycosis

3. Allergic reaction can play a big part in the pathology of which of the following infections?
   a. *Candida albicans*
   b. *Aspergillus*
   c. coccidioidomycosis
   d. cryptococcosis

4. An AIDS patient with a cat is experiencing headaches, fever, and chills, and after his CD4 count went to less than 100, he is diagnosed with cerebral toxoplasmosis. Like an exposed pregnant patient, his therapy should include
   a. penicillin
   b. erythromycin
   c. pyrimethamine and sulfadiazine
   d. mistletoe

5. Which of the following is associated with eating undercooked meat or changing the kitty litter box?
   a. CMV
   b. strep Group A
   c. EBV
   d. toxoplasmosis

REVIEW QUESTIONS (*continued*)

6. Which antibodies are found in an immune response to parasites?
   a. IgE only
   b. IgG, IgM, and IgA only
   c. IgG, IgM, IgA, and IgE
   d. IgG only

7. Bird droppings have been associated with the spread of
   a. *Cryptococcus neoformans*
   b. *Histoplasma capsulatum*
   c. *Coccidioides immitis*
   d. A and B

8. Laboratory professionals commonly look at feces for eggs to diagnose parasitic infections. However, serology can be important. For which of the following is(are) antibody or antigen detection important?
   a. *Giardia*
   b. *Cryptosporidium*
   c. toxoplasmosis
   d. all of the above

9. Most people infected with *Toxoplasma gondii* experience
   a. flatulence
   b. a mild flulike illness
   c. no symptoms
   d. hepatosplenomegaly

10. This parasite is in contaminated drinking water, causes watery diarrhea, and is resistant to chlorination. It is
    a. *Toxoplasma gondii*
    b. *Aspergillus niger*
    c. malaria
    d. *Cryptosporidium parvum*

11. Which parasitic disease is part of the TORCH testing for pregnant women
    a. *Cryptosporidium parvum*
    b. *Toxoplasma gondii*
    c. *Giardia lamblia*
    d. hepatitis C

12. In avidity testing,
    a. high avidity antibody stays attached with a wash containing urea
    b. high avidity antibody indicates a past infection
    c. high avidity antibody indicates a current infection
    d. A and B

13. Which of the following cell types are involved in the acquired antifungal immune response?
    a. neutrophils
    b. macrophage
    c. dendritic cells
    d. T cells

14. Pathogenic fungi are
    a. prokaryotic with hyphae and conidiophore
    b. eukaryotic and often thermally dimorphic
    c. eukaryotic monomorphic organisms that are always in the yeast form
    d. prokaryotic monomorphic organisms that are thermally dimorphic

15. A patient has just returned from a visit to an archeological dig in the southwestern United States. He is delighted to tell you the details of excavating Indian artifacts from the dusty soil. There was so much dust that he says dinner always just tasted of dust because he had inhaled so much. He has a temperature of 104°F with a dry cough, joint and muscle aches, and a headache. He has a lumpy red rash on his legs. Of course, testing must be done, but you suspect
    a. *Cryptococcus neoformans*
    b. *Histoplasma capsulatum*
    c. *Coccidioides immitis*
    d. *Aspergillus fumigatus*

REFERENCES

1. Erjavec Z, Verweij PE. Mini reviews. Recent progress in the diagnosis of fungal infections in the immunocompromised host. *Drug Resistance Updates*. 2002;5:3–10.

2. Doctorfungus. http://www.doctorfungus.org/thefungi/blastomyces.php. Accessed April 6, 2012.

3. Centers for Disease Control and Prevention. WHO Collaborating Center for the Mycoses. http://www.cdc.gov/ncidod/dbmd/mdb/index.htm. Accessed April 4, 2012.

4. Yeo SF, Wong B. Current status of nonculture methods for diagnosis of invasive fungal infections. *Clin. Microbiol. Rev.* 2002;15:465–484.

5. Jarreau PC. Serological Response to Parasitic and Fungal Infections. In Stevens C, ed. *Clinical Immunology and Serology: A Laboratory Perspective.* 3rd ed. Philadelphia, PA: F.A. Davis Company; 2010: chap 20.

6. Richardson MD, Warnock DW. *Fungal Infection: Diagnosis and Management.* Oxford, UK: Blackwell Publishing; Ltd. 2003.

7. Meridan Fungal Immunodiffusion System. http://www.meridian-bioscience.com/Content/Assets/Files/2.7%20Immunodiffusion%20Products/Package-Insert-Anti-Aspergillus-ID-CS.pdf. Accessed April 6, 2012.

8. Patient UK. Aspergillosis. http://www.patient.co.uk/doctor/Aspergillosis .htm. Accessed April 6, 2012.

9. Patient UK. Fungal ear infection (Otomycosis). http://www.patient .co.uk/showdoc/40001641/. Accessed April 6, 2012.

10. Centers for Disease Control and Prevention. National Center for Zoonotic, Vector-Borne, and Enteric Diseases Blastomycosis. http://www .cdc.gov/nczved/divisions/dfbmd/diseases/blastomycosis/. Accessed April 6, 2012.

11. Centers for Disease Control and Prevention. Division of Bacterial and Mycotic Diseases. http://www.cdc.gov/fungal/candidiasis/. Accessed April 6, 2012.

12. Centers for Disease Control and Prevention. Division of Bacterial and Mycotic Diseases. Invasive candidiasis. http://www.cdc.gov/fungal/ candidiasis/invasive/symptoms.html. Accessed April 6, 2012.

13. Immuno-Mycologics. Cocci LA/combination antibody system. http:// www.discovery-diagnostics.com/pdf/Immy-CI1001-package.pdf. Accessed April 6, 2012.

14. Immuno-Mycologics. Coccidioides. http://immy.com/?q=coccidioides. Accessed April 6, 2012.

15. Immuno-Mycologics. Latex agglutination. http://immy.com/?q=la. Accessed April 6, 2012.

16. Valley fever connections. http://www.valley-fever.org/valley_fever_ org_statistics.html. Accessed April 6, 2012.

17. Valley fever connections. Valley fever backgrounds. http://www .valley-fever.org/valley_fever_valley_fever_org_background.html. Accessed April 6, 2012.

18. Immuno-Mycologics. *Cryptococcus*. http://immy.com/?q=cryptococcus. Accessed April 6, 2012.

19. Immuno-Mycologics. Cr-Ag for the detection of cryptococcal antigen. http://www.immy.com/products/cryptococcal-antigen-lateral-flow-assay-lfa/. Accessed April 6, 2012.

20. Centers for Disease Control and Prevention. Division of Bacterial and Mycotic Diseases. Cryptococcus. http://www.cdc.gov/fungal/ cryptococcosis/_t.htm. Accessed April 6, 2012.

21. Centers for Disease Control and Prevention. Emergence of *Cryptococcus gattii*—Pacific Northwest, 2004–2010. *MMWR*. 2010;59(28);865–868.

22. MacDougall L, Fyfe M, Romney M, et al. Risk factors for *Cryptococcus gattii* infection, British Columbia, Canada. *Emerg Infect Dis* [serial on the Internet]. 2011. http://www.cdc.gov/EID/content/17/2/193.htm. doi: 10.3201/eid1702.101020. Accessed April 6, 2012.

23. Wheat LJ, Garringer T, Brizendinea E, et al. Diagnosis of histoplasmosis by antigen detection based upon experience at the histoplasmosis reference laboratory. *Diagn Micr Infec Dis*. 2002;43:29–37.

24. Centers for Disease Control and Prevention. Division of Bacterial and Mycotic Diseases. Histoplasmosis. http://www.cdc.gov/fungal/ histoplasmosis/. Accessed February 9, 2011.

25. Centers for Disease Control and Prevention. National Institute for Occupational Health and Safety. Histoplasmosis—Protecting workers at risk. http://www.cdc.gov/niosh/docs/2005-109/#c. Accessed April 6, 2012.

26. Centers for Disease Control and Prevention. Division of Bacterial and Mycotic Diseases. Histoplasmosis. http://www.cdc.gov/fungal/ histoplasmosis/definition.html. Accessed April 6, 2012.

27. Kauffman, CA. Histoplasmosis: A clinical and laboratory update. *Clin Microbiol Rev*. 2007;20(1): 115–132. doi: 10.1128/CMR.00027-06. http:// www.ncbi.nlm.nih.gov/pmc/articles/PMC1797635/?tool=pubmed. Accessed April 6, 2012.

28. Centers for Disease Control and Prevention. Laboratory identification of parasites of public health concern. http://www.dpd.cdc.gov/dpdx/ HTML/Pneumocystis.htm. Accessed April 6, 2012.

29. Centers for Disease Control and Prevention. Laboratory identification of parasites of public health concern: Diagnostic procedures. http:// www.dpd.cdc.gov/dpdx/HTML/DiagnosticProcedures.htm. Accessed April 6, 2012.

30. Centers for Disease Control and Prevention. Parasites. http://www.cdc .gov/parasites/about.html. Accessed April 6, 2012.

31. Centers for Disease Control and Prevention. Malaria. http://www.cdc .gov/malaria/diagnosis_treatment/rdt.html. Accessed April 6, 2012.

32. Centers for Disease Control and Prevention. Parasites: Giardia. http:// www.cdc.gov/parasites/giardia/index.html. Accessed April 6, 2012.

33. Centers for Disease Control and Prevention. http://www.cdc.gov/ parasites/toxoplasmosis/index.html. Accessed April 6, 2012.

34. Focus Diagnostics. Technical summary: Toxoplasmosis IgG avidity testing. http://www.focusdx.com/focus/techsheets/ToxplasmaAvidity .pdf. Accessed May 26, 2012.

35. PubMedHealth. Toxoplasmosis. http://www.ncbi.nlm.nih.gov/ pubmedhealth/PMH0001661. Accessed April 6, 2012.

Chapter written after consultation with:

Susan J. Wong, Ph.D., DABMLI.
Diagnostic Immunology Laboratory
Wadsworth Center, NYSDOH

Eileen M. Burd, Ph.D., DABMM
Director, Clinical Microbiology
Emory University Hospital
Associate Professor,
Emory University School of Medicine
Atlanta, GA

Susan E. Sharp, Ph.D. DABMM
Director of Microbiology
Kaiser Permanente
Portland, Oregon

Daniel Amsterdam, Ph.D. DABMM, FAAM, FIDSA.
Professor
Director, Department of Laboratory Medicine
Erie County Medical Center Healthcare Network
Buffalo, NY

Dr. Orrett
Sisters Hospital
Buffalo, New York

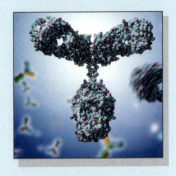

CHAPTER OUTLINE

PART 5
ADDITIONAL INFORMATION RELATED TO CLINICAL LABORATORY IMMUNOLOGY

21

Forensic Serology

Kristen Betker, Forensic Biologist III

■ OBJECTIVES—LEVEL I

After this chapter, the student should be able to:

1. Define *forensic serology.*
2. Describe a brief history of forensic science.
3. Define *forensic toxicology.*
4. Understand why forensic toxicology is important.
5. Explain how ELISA is used to detect drugs of abuse in biological specimens.
6. Define *forensic biology.*
7. Describe the principle behind tests used to identify blood.
8. Compare the ring precipitin and crossover electrophoresis methods for species identification.
9. Explain why the detection of semen is important in a sexual assault investigation.
10. Understand the principle of an immunoassay used to identify semen.
11. Discuss the methods available that can be used to identify saliva from items of evidence.
12. Understand the importance of forensic serology in criminal investigations.

KEY TERMS

agglutination
aspermic
biochip
blood
chain of custody
controlled substance
creatinine
crossover electrophoresis
drugs
extract
forensic biology
forensic science
forensic serology
forensic toxicology

hemoglobin
metabolite
oligospermic
poison
prostate-specific antigen (PSA or p30)
questioned stain
ring precipitin
saliva
salivary alpha amylase
semen
spermatozoa
urea
urine

► INTRODUCTION

Forensic serology is the branch of **forensic science** that deals with the identification of bodily fluids as well as foreign substances in the body through immunological procedures. The immunoassays used are based on the reactions that occur between antigens and antibodies (1). These reactions allow the forensic scientist to detect the presence of biological fluids such as blood, semen, and saliva on crime scene evidence. They also allow for the identification of various drugs and **poisons** in specimens collected from victims and suspects involved in criminal activity.

► HISTORY

Criminal investigations have relied on help from the sciences for hundreds of years. As early as 44 BC, medical evidence was used to suggest that only one of the 23 stab wounds in Julius Caesar was fatal (2). Modern forensic science is believed to have emerged from the works of Sir Arthur Conan Doyle, the author of the stories of Sherlock Holmes (3). These stories showed insight into the methods and procedures that would later become practice in the forensic science field. Some of the early forensic science methods focused on blood typing and toxicology.

One of the most influential people of early serology techniques was Dr. Karl Landsteiner. He was the first person to identify the blood group antigens, A, B, and O, and he published this discovery in 1901 (1). Dr. Landsteiner was awarded the Nobel Prize for Physiology or Medicine in 1930 for this achievement (4). Leone Lattes further advanced Landsteiner's findings by developing a procedure to test for the different blood groups (3). This procedure, based on **agglutination** principles, is still used today.

Another prominent individual in the field of forensic science was Mathieu Orfila who in 1813 published the first work regarding forensic toxicology. This work was a comprehensive book that classified and described everything known about poisons at that time. Based on his publications and other scientific accomplishments, Orfila is considered to be the "father of toxicology" (3).

With the scientific advancements that were being made in human identification and toxicology and the increased understanding of the value of using science to solve crimes, forensic laboratories began to emerge. A national forensic laboratory was organized in 1932 by the Federal Bureau of Investigation to assist with criminal investigations in the United States (3). It provided a facility for scientific testing that law enforcement officials could utilize to assist in solving crimes. Hundreds of state, local, and private forensic science laboratories exist in the United States today.

The entertainment value of forensic science that was seen with the publication of the Sherlock Holmes novels in the late 19th century continues today and has spread to a variety of television shows that portray this science in an exciting, if somewhat exaggerated, way. Although not all the information on television can be accomplished in the laboratory, the ability of the forensic laboratory to determine the events that occurred in a criminal act is remarkable. This chapter is limited to the immunological techniques in the forensic laboratory.

► CHAIN OF CUSTODY

A common early principle regardless of the type of analysis being done is that the chain of custody of evidence must be preserved. **Chain of custody** refers to the tracking of a particular piece of evidence from the time it was first discovered until the present time. It is a list of exactly who has handled the item and where it was located at all times. Chain of custody is important because it ensures that the evidence has not been compromised. This is especially imperative in a court of law to establish that the integrity of the evidence has been maintained.

► DRUG SCREENING USING SEROLOGICAL TECHNIQUES

Forensic toxicology involves the analysis of biological samples to detect the presence of **controlled substances,** alcohol, or other toxic material (2). Detection of foreign substances in biological specimens can aid in criminal investigations regarding events such as driving while intoxicated, drug-facilitated sexual assault, poisoning, and drug abuse. It can also help to determine the circumstances and cause of death, thus assisting in such investigations. A major responsibility of a forensic toxicologist is to screen for **drugs** in submitted samples and to interpret the results. Serological techniques are commonly used to accomplish this goal.

The presence of drugs in body fluids such as blood and urine can be detected with the use of immunoassays. Immunoassays are serological tests that can identify a drug or a **metabolite** of a drug in biological specimens from an individual. Antibodies specific for the particular molecule of interest are used to detect these substances by means of serological techniques. These techniques include enzyme-linked immunosorbent assays (ELISA), radioimmunoassay (RIA), and fluorescence polarization immunoassay (FPI). These techniques use an antibody or antigen that has been labeled with an enzyme, radioactive label, or fluorescent tag, respectively. The antigen-antibody reactions involving the labeled components ultimately cause a reaction that can be observed.

Modern techniques used in forensic toxicology laboratories to screen for drugs and poisons rely greatly on immunoassays for several reasons. Immunoassays are very sensitive and therefore, small quantities of the foreign substance can be detected (5). Also, the biological sample can be used directly because it is not necessary for any preliminary processing steps such as extraction. In addition, newer automated instruments that can decrease the amount of time and cost required to perform an analysis are available for forensic toxicologists.

Radioimmunoassay was the first method used in forensic toxicology to detect the presence of various drugs in biological specimens. As previously stated, radioimmunoassay utilizes the properties of a radiolabeled antibody to detect a particular drug or drug metabolite. This type of serological procedure has great sensitivity; however, issues arise in the safety of this assay because of the use of the radioactive isotope. Therefore, newer assays have been developed to provide alternative methods to the use of the radioactive label.

Currently, the most common assay type used for drug screening is ELISA. This serological technique is used in forensic toxicology laboratories to screen biological specimens for various drugs of abuse such as amphetamine, cannabinoids (the active ingredients in marijuana), opiates, oxycodone, and methylenedioxymethamphetamine (MDMA). ELISA provides

the forensic toxicologist a specific, sensitive, and relatively rapid means to detect drugs and toxins in specimens such as blood, urine, and oral fluid (6, 7).

The principle of the ELISA test kits that are commercially available is based on competitive binding of antigens to antibodies (6). Polyclonal antibody against the drug in question is fixed to a well of a microtiter plate (Figure 21.1 ■). The biological evidence sample to be tested is added to the plate well with kit supplied antigen that is labeled with an enzyme. The antigens in the evidence compete with the enzyme-labeled antigens to bind to the antibody fixed to the well. After stringent washing to get rid of any unbound antigen, a substrate is then added to the plate wells. This substrate reacts with the enzyme on the labeled antigens to produce a color. Color development is halted with a stop solution so that the results can be interpreted. The greater the intensity of the color, the more enzyme-labeled kit antigen is bound to the antibody in the well. Thus, a more intense color indicates that there are fewer antigens from the evidence bound to the antibody and, therefore, a smaller amount of drug present in the questioned sample.

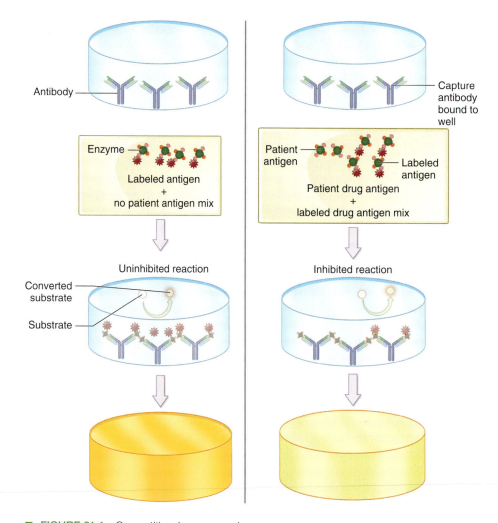

■ FIGURE 21.1   Competitive drug enzyme immunoassay.

Serological techniques are also used to test for the presence of illegal substances in hair (8, 9). A commercial kit is available to screen hair samples for drugs such as cannabinoids, opiates, cocaine, amphetamines, and MDMA (also known as *ecstasy*) (9). These test kits utilize the principles of the ELISA system as previously described. The sample is prepared by cutting the hair into fragments and then extracting the fragments in methanol overnight at 40° C. A portion of this extract is allowed to evaporate to dryness in the presence of methanol/hydrochloric acid and then is reconstituted in the diluent solution present in the kit. The prepared solution with the extracted hair sample is then subjected to analysis by the ELISA system of the kit.

Checkpoint! 21.1

Who commonly uses ELISA to detect the presence of controlled substances?

New techniques are being developed to make drug screening even more efficient. Increasing efficiency will consequently reduce the amount of time it takes to analyze forensic samples as well as the cost to perform that analysis. One advance being made in the field of forensic toxicology is the development of biochip array technology (10). This drug-screening technology is essentially ELISA performed on a biochip that is evaluated on an automated analyzer. A **biochip** is a solid substrate on which a collection of microsized test sites are present. These test sites are the tiny equivalent of a microtiter plate well with each test site having a different coating antibody and a reaction with a different drug. A major benefit of a biochip is that the multiple test sites permit the analysis of several drugs at the same time from a single sample. This greatly reduces testing time and as a result, high throughput analysis can be accomplished. Also, because of the high sensitivity of biochip array technology, only a small sample size is required.

Checkpoint! 21.2

What immunoassay also has the advantage of high sensitivity and was the first method used in forensic toxicology?

▶ OTHER FORENSIC ANALYSIS USING SEROLOGICAL TECHNIQUES

Forensic biology is the examination of items of evidence to identify biological fluid stains. Forensic biologists analyze evidence to detect the presence of biological materials on various items to ultimately link a suspect to the crime. Many of the tools forensic biologists use to identify biological stains

are immunology-based methods. These serological techniques aid in the detection of various biological fluids such as blood, semen, and saliva.

Once a particular body fluid is identified, it can be further characterized to a particular individual. This can be achieved through additional serological testing such as species identification and ABO blood typing. Results of these tests can establish investigative information for law enforcement officials to employ while trying to solve crimes.

BLOOD

Blood is the most common biological fluid encountered at a crime scene (11). Many crimes scenes have blood evidence and, therefore, the identification of blood can be vital to solving crimes such as homicides, assaults, and burglaries. Clothing from a suspect of a homicide can be examined for the presence of blood to find bloodstains matching the victim's blood. It may be deposited at the scene of an assault from the perpetrator with whom the victim struggled. A person committing a burglary can cut herself or himself at the crime scene, particularly at the point of entry, and leave blood evidence behind. These are just a few of the many examples of the usefulness of blood analysis in the criminal justice system. See Figure 21.2 ■ for a typical piece of bloodstained evidence.

Forensic scientists view potential bloodstains as dried or wet red stains at the crime scene. The first step of the analysis is to determine whether the red stain is actually blood or a different substance. Serological tests available to confirm whether the stain is blood are based on the presence of hemoglobin in the sample (12, 13). **Hemoglobin** is a protein in red blood cells that functions to transport oxygen throughout the body and remove carbon dioxide. To perform a hemoglobin test, an **extract** of the **questioned stain** is added to the sample well of a test kit (12, 13). A colloid-labeled

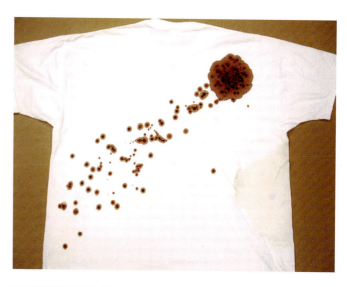

■ FIGURE 21.2   Bloodstained evidence.

immunochromatographic sandwich assay similar to the pregnancy assay described in Chapter 7 and pictured in Figure 7.3(a) is performed to determine whether hemoglobin is in the sample. Mobile antihemoglobin antibodies labeled with dye particles are present in the sample well and will bind any hemoglobin present in the extract to form a complex. This antigen-antibody complex travels through the test strip to the test area. At the test area, a second anti-hemoglobin antibody is fixed to the membrane. This secondary antibody binds the hemoglobin of the antigen-antibody complex. The collection of the antibody-antigen-antibody complexes at the test site forms a visible color line because of the dye particles attached to the first antibody. The formation of a colored line is a positive reaction for the presence of blood. This positive result is specific for human blood; however, the tests have demonstrated cross-reactivity with the blood of primates and ferrets (14).

Once it has been determined that the red stain is indeed blood, it may be necessary to know whether the blood originated from a human being or a different animal such as a dog, deer, or cow. When dog fighting is alleged, knowing whether the dried red stain present on weapons and restraints collected from the crime scene is in fact canine blood can be important. This information can confirm the investigators' assumption. Potential murder weapons found at food preparation facilities such as a meat market can contain the blood of different animals, thus requiring the need for species differentiation. In addition, persons of interest wearing bloody clothes have been apprehended and occasionally have claimed that they had just been out hunting and the blood on the clothing was from a deer. Determining whether the stains are deer blood or human blood is a crucial aspect of the investigation.

Two tests utilized for species identification are the ring precipitin test and crossover electrophoresis analysis (1, 15). The **ring precipitin** test is one of the oldest species identification tests that is still used today. This procedure involves adding a chosen antiserum to a test tube containing antibodies directed against antigens found on the cells of the species in question. For example, if the forensic scientist is trying to determine whether the dried red stain is human blood, then anti-human antiserum is used.

Following the addition of the antiserum to the test tube, an equal amount of extract of the questioned stain is then added carefully so as not to disturb the interface between the 2 layers. The extract contains the antigens of the animal species it originated from in the form of soluble proteins. Over the course of about 10 minutes, the antibodies present in the bottom layer of antiserum migrate upward, and the antigens present in the top layer of extract move downward until they meet at the interface. If the antigens in the extract are from the particular species for which the antibodies are specific, the antigens and antibodies combine at the interface to form a lattice structure that results in a white precipitin. This precipitin ring can be visually observed. The presence of a precipitin

ring at the interface is a positive test. Refer to Figure 21.3 ■ for a positive ring precipitin test for human blood. The white precipitin ring can be seen at the interface.

✓ Checkpoint! 21.3

How would a species of origin test be of assistance if a suspect in a homicide investigation claims that the blood on her or his shirt was from an injured animal that she or he was trying to help?

Crossover electrophoresis is another method that can be used to determine the animal species from which the bloodstain originated. The principle behind this method is the same as the ring precipitin test; however, with crossover electrophoresis, samples are added to wells that are punched into an agarose gel. Antiserum to the species in question is added to wells on the anode (+) side, and extracts of the questioned stain are placed in corresponding wells on the cathode (−) side. An electric field is then applied to the agarose gel. This electric current causes the antibodies and antigens to migrate toward each other. If the sample extract contained antigens of the animal species against which the antiserum was developed, a precipitin line of identity forms at the juncture where the antigens and antibodies meet. Figure 21.4 ■ is a photograph of a crossover electrophoresis gel following staining with Commassie blue. Positive reactions indicated by the lines of identity can be seen in between the wells on the left side of the gel.

Once the dried red stain has been identified as human blood, the bloodstains can be further differentiated by ABO blood typing. The presence or absence of the ABO antigens and antibodies forms the basis for the earliest forensic differentiation tests of human blood.

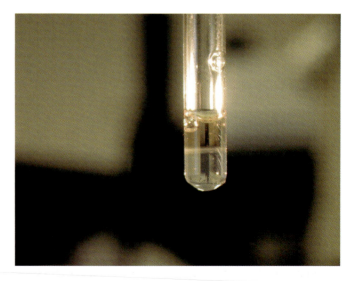

■ **FIGURE 21.3** Positive ring precipitin test.

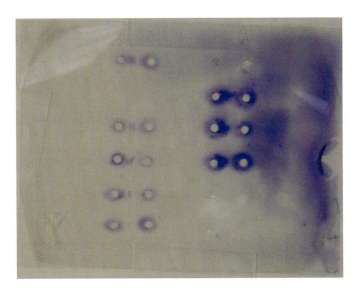

■ **FIGURE 21.4** Crossover electrophoresis.

 Checkpoint! 21.4

Who was the first person to identify the blood group antigens ABO?

Determining the ABO blood type of a stain isolated from crime scene evidence can narrow the number of possible contributors of that bloodstain or can eliminate a person of interest from being its source. This information can be very useful to piece together the crime that took place and help to identify the perpetrator. Although ABO blood typing is very beneficial, most forensic laboratories have replaced this method with DNA analysis, which can characterize a biological stain to a particular individual, thus identifying the source of that stain with scientific certainty.

SEMEN

Semen is a biological fluid produced by the male reproductive organs. It consists primarily of seminal fluid that includes several proteins and enzymes secreted from various glands. Examples of the constituents found in semen are albumin, acid phosphatase, organic acids, semenogelin, and prostate-specific antigen (16). Semen may also contain **spermatozoa,** the male reproductive cells.

The identification of semen can be a critical part of a criminal investigation, particularly one involving a sexual assault. When an individual states that he or she has been sexually assaulted, evidence is collected and submitted to the laboratory. Items that are collected include vaginal, anal, and oral specimens as well as bedding and clothes. A sexual assault kit and some of the components contained within the kit that are used to collect evidence from a victim of a sexual assault appear in Figure 21.5 ■.

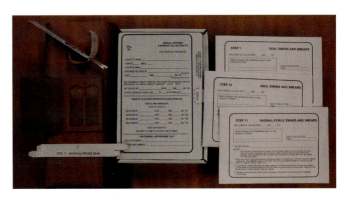

■ **FIGURE 21.5** Sexual assault evidence collection kit.

Upon receipt at the forensic laboratory, the submitted evidence is screened for the presence of semen. When a suspected semen stain is detected, the semen's identification must be confirmed by additional testing. One way to confirm this is to microscopically identify spermatozoa on the sample. The drawback to this is that semen does not always contain spermatozoa. This is especially true for **aspermic** or **oligospermic** males who have had a vasectomy or have an underlying medical condition in which little or no spermatozoa are produced. An alternative way to confirm a positive presumptive semen test is by performing a serological test to identify the **prostate-specific antigen (PSA or p30).**

PSA is a 30 000 dalton glycoprotein that was first described in the early 1970s (17). Although it is found in different biological material such as breast milk, female urine, and breast tissue, it is present in high concentrations in semen (18). Past methods used to detect PSA included electrophoresis, Ouchterlony, and enzyme-linked immunoassays. The method currently used in forensic laboratories is based on a serological assay. This process is carried out by the use of commercial gold red *colloid-labeled immunochromatographic sandwich assay* kits similar to the pregnancy test described in Chapter 7 and as described above for hemoglobin analysis (19, 20). An extract of the suspected semen stain is applied to the sample well. The sample well contains mobile gold-labeled anti-PSA monoclonal antibody that was produced in a mouse. This antibody specifically combines with any PSA that may be in the sample. This PSA-antibody complex then travels down the membrane. A second mouse anti-PSA monoclonal antibody is fixed on the membrane at the test area. As the PSA-antibody complex migrates toward the test area, it combines with the second anti-PSA monoclonal antibody. This gold-labeled anti-PSA, PSA, anti-PSA complex remains fixed at the test area. With the accumulation of the antibody-antigen-antibody complexes, a red line, which is a positive result, thereby indicating semen is present in the sample, appears at the test site.

Two additional red lines must also appear on the membrane for the test to be valid. Adjacent to the test area is an area of PSA that is fixed to the membrane at a concentration of 4 ng/μl. The excess gold-labeled anti-PSA monoclonal antibody from the sample well will bind to this fixed PSA to exhibit a red line. This allows for this method to be semi-quantitative. A test red line equal to the intensity of this line indicates the level of PSA in the sample being analyzed is 4 ng/μl. A test line with greater intensity indicates a higher concentration of PSA; a less intense line indicates a lower concentration.

An internal control area is adjacent to the fixed PSA on the membrane. At this area, anti-mouse polyclonal antibody is affixed to the membrane. As the samples move through the membrane, the excess mouse anti-PSA antibodies originally present in the sample well reaches the control area, binds with the anti-mouse polyclonal antibody, and forms a complex to reveal a red line. As in Figure 21.6 ■, a positive result for the prostate-specific antigen test is exhibited by the presence of 3 red lines as opposed to a negative result, which exhibits only 2 red lines.

 Checkpoint! 21.5

The presence of PSA indicates that the questioned stain is semen. What molecule indicates the presence of blood?

SALIVA

Saliva is another biological fluid that is frequently encountered in forensic science. It is a substance produced by the parotid, submaxillary, and sublingual glands in the mouth whose purpose is to aid in digestion (21). One type of crime in which saliva identification is important is a sexual assault

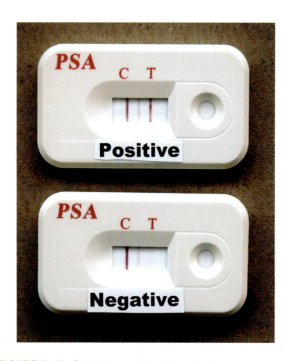

■ **FIGURE 21.6** Prostate-specific antigen test.

case. In such a case, the victim may claim that the perpetrator had oral contact with a part of his or her body. That area is then swabbed by a sexual assault nurse examiner and sent to the laboratory for analysis. Identifying saliva on the collected sample can be used to corroborate the victim's story and help to identify the suspect.

Saliva can also be found on various items left at a crime scene or associated with a crime. Examples include cigarette butts smoked by the perpetrator(s), cups or bottles that the perpetrator(s) drank from, envelopes that the suspect(s) licked to seal and send threatening letters, bite marks on an assault victim, or bite marks on partially consumed food left at the crime scene. An additional instance in which saliva identification is valuable occurs when crime scene investigators find what appears to be expectorant left at a crime scene. It is important for the forensic scientist to know whether the specimen is in fact saliva to determine whether the sample should be processed further for possible DNA evidence to associate the stain to a particular individual.

Various methods exist for the forensic identification of saliva. The target enzyme on which many saliva detection tests are based is **salivary alpha amylase,** a digestive enzyme found in saliva that is used to break down carbohydrates. It differs from pancreatic amylase, which is present in semen, urine, feces, and vaginal secretions. The digestive action of alpha amylase is the principle behind early saliva identification test methods (15, 21, 22).

One method to detect the enzymatic activity of alpha amylase, thus indicating the presence of saliva, is the starch iodine test. This is a radial diffusion test involving an agarose gel plate that contains nonhydrolyzed starch. Sample wells are punched into the agarose gel and an extract of the suspected saliva stain is added to the well. The extract is allowed to diffuse into the agarose gel by an overnight incubation at 37° C. An iodine solution is then added to the gel. Nonhydrolyzed starch stains a blue color with the addition of iodine. If alpha amylase is present in the extract, it diffuses outward from the sample well, hydrolyzing the starch present in the gel as it moves along. Hydrolyzed starch does not stain with iodine. Therefore, a clear zone surrounding the sample well indicates the presence of alpha amylase and hence saliva. See Figure 21.7 ■ for the results of a starch iodine test. The clear zone in the middle represents a saliva sample control. The diameter of the clear zone increases in size with increasing amounts of amylase.

The enzymatic action of alpha amylase is also the principle behind another test available to forensic laboratories to help identify saliva. This test involves dye particles attached to starch molecules that are fixed to filter paper (22). If alpha amylase is present in the questioned stain, it will digest the starch, thereby releasing dye particles. This event causes a blue color to form resulting in a positive test for alpha amylase.

Newer serological methods that exist for the detection of alpha amylase are serological assays that utilize monoclonal antibodies specific for human salivary alpha amylase. These

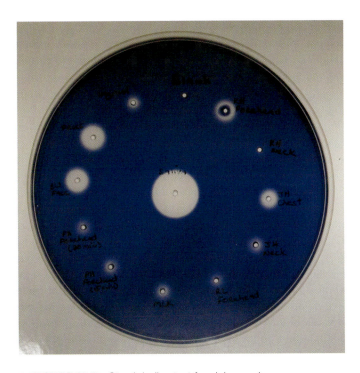

■ **FIGURE 21.7** Starch iodine test for alpha amylase.

procedures are performed using a colloid-labeled immuno-chromatographic sandwich assay test strip.

✓ **Checkpoint! 21.6**

What biological fluids other than saliva can be detected using a colloid-labeled immunochromatographic sandwich assay?

Sample extracts are added to the sample well of the test strip. The sample well contains free anti-human salivary alpha amylase monoclonal mouse antibodies conjugated to colloidal gold. When alpha amylase is present in the extract, it binds the gold-labeled antibodies in the sample well, and this complex migrates to the test line. At the test line, the second anti-human salivary alpha amylase monoclonal mouse antibody captures the alpha amylase-antibody complex, and a red line appears. Regardless of whether alpha amylase was present in the sample, the running buffer continues to flow to the control position, carrying with it free anti-human salivary alpha amylase monoclonal mouse antibodies from the sample well. Anti-mouse IgG antibodies are bound at the control position and capture the free mouse antibodies, forming a red line. This presence of the red line in the control area demonstrates that the test strip is working properly. Refer to Figure 21.8 ■ for the results of human salivary alpha amylase testing by this serological method.

The serological assays that involve the use of monoclonal antibodies have many advantages over the tests that rely on

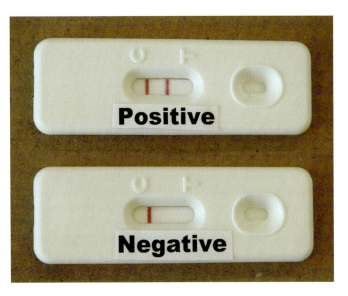

■ **FIGURE 21.8** Human salivary alpha amylase test.

the enzymatic activity of alpha amylase. Serological assays using monoclonal antibodies can be faster to perform, allowing the analyst to obtain results in a few minutes or less as opposed to the starch iodine test, which has to incubate overnight. Also, the monoclonal antibodies used in the test strips are specific for human salivary alpha amylase. Although the other tests do detect amylase, they are not specific for human salivary alpha amylase. Therefore, a positive result obtained with the immunologically based test strip method is a better indicator of the presence of human saliva than a positive result with the methods that depend on the enzymatic action of alpha amylase.

FUTURE

Forensic science is a continually advancing field. Much research is currently being performed to improve testing methods that can increase the efficiency, sensitivity, and specificity of the assays. Areas on which the characterization of biological stains focus involve the study of new antigens that antibodies can be produced against for use in a particular immunoassay. Examples of alternative antigens being evaluated to characterize biological fluids are molecules found in semen and urine.

Semenogelin is the predominant protein found in semen (23). It is primarily produced by the seminal vesicles and functions in the coagulation of semen (24). The detection of semenogelin through the use of immunoassays can provide a confirmatory test for the presence of semen. Studies show that semenogelin is not detectable in other secretions such as breast milk, urine, saliva, or vaginal secretions. This makes semenogelin a specific marker indicating the presence of semen, which makes it very useful in the forensic community.

A study was recently published identifying urine proteins that can be used to detect the presence of **urine** (25). To identify urine, forensic biologists currently perform presumptive testing to detect the presence of **urea** and **creatinine** (15). Although these methods are generally accepted as a presumptive identification for urine, they are not specific indicators of urine because urea and creatinine can be found in other body fluids such as sweat, blood, and amniotic fluid.

New urine detection markers have been investigated for use in forensic laboratories. These new markers include Tamm-Horsfall protein (THP), a major constituent of urinary protein, and uroplakin III (UPIII), a transmembrane glycoprotein found in the cells of urinary tract organs such as the ureter and bladder (25). Techniques evaluated for the detection of these markers include enzyme-linked immunoassays and immunohistochemical staining. The enzyme-linked immunoassays use sheep antibodies made against the human glycoprotein of interest and a secondary antibody that is rabbit antisheep antibody conjugated to horseradish peroxidase. Immunohistochemical staining is performed by adding a mouse monoclonal antibody made against the glycoprotein of interest to a specimen slide. This is followed by addition of biotin-conjugated goat anti-mouse antibody and then peroxidase-conjugated streptavidin and a substrate. Both processes result in a color change representing the presence of urine.

The semen and urine markers described show promise in the field of forensic biology for the characterization of these stains. Studies have demonstrated that immunoassays designed to detect these molecules have great specificity and sensitivity. Future forensic examination of evidence may rely on the use of these alternative markers.

✓ Checkpoint! 21.7

In addition to semen and urine, name 2 other biological fluids that are important in criminal investigations.

CASE STUDY

You have finished school and have decided to accept a job in a rural laboratory. You and your wife just bought a cool farmhouse from a man who mostly grew corn, but had a pig or 2. When you toured the house, he and his wife were arguing loudly. You hope bad karma does not come with the house.

When you move in, the man is there to wish you well but his wife is not there. He leaves and as you finish unpacking, you notice a pool of blood on the garage floor. Your wife is quite worried, but you feel that he must have slaughtered one of the pigs in the garage.

1. What will the forensic laboratory do to test to determine whether the fluid is blood?

2. What will the forensic laboratory do to test to determine whether the blood is human?

SUMMARY

Immunology plays an important role in the field of forensic science. Whether a biological stain needs to be identified or it is necessary to determine whether a collected sample contains drugs of abuse, serological techniques are a critical step in the process. The criminal justice system depends greatly on the results and conclusions that are obtained by the analysis of evidence at the forensic laboratories. The data generated by forensic laboratories as summarized in Table 21.1 ✪ provide a scientific basis to establish the criminal case to the criminal courts.

✪ TABLE 21.1

Summary of Forensic Toxicology and Forensic Biology

Field	Purpose	Uses	Assays Utilized	Anything New
Forensic toxicology	Detect the presence of controlled substances, alcohol, and other toxic material	Criminal investigations related to driving while intoxicated, drug-facilitated sexual assault, poisoning, and drug abuse	ELISA, radioimmunoassay (RIA), and fluorescence polarization immunoassay (FPI)	Biochip ELISA
Forensic biology	Identify biological fluid stains	Forensic detection of various biological fluids such as blood, semen, and saliva	Colloid-labeled immunochromatographic sandwich assay Ring precipitin tests Crossover electrophoresis	Alternative markers for semen and urine

REVIEW QUESTIONS

1. Who is known as the father of toxicology?
   a. Alphonse Bertillon
   b. Karl Landsteiner
   c. Mathieu Orfila
   d. Sherlock Holmes

2. Forensic toxicology involves the analysis of biological samples in order to detect what?
   a. drugs of abuse
   b. poisons
   c. alcohol
   d. all of the above

3. What is the most common assay type used for drug screening?
   a. ELISA
   b. agglutination
   c. electrophoresis
   d. radioimmunoassay

4. The principle of commercially available ELISA test kits is based on
   a. diffusion of antigens through an agarose gel
   b. oxidase activity of an enzyme
   c. competitive binding of antigens to antibodies
   d. migration of antigens through an electric field

5. The analysis of evidence to detect the presence of biological fluids such as blood, semen, and saliva is referred to as
   a. forensic odontology
   b. forensic biology
   c. forensic psychiatry
   d. forensic toxicology

6. Which of the following is the molecule that forensic scientists test for to identify the presence of blood?
   a. albumin
   b. bilirubin
   c. hemoglobin
   d. creatinine

7. Which method can be used to determine the species of origin of a bloodstain?
   a. ring precipitin
   b. crossover electrophoresis
   c. both A and B
   d. none of the above

8. Which of the following is *not* a component of semen?
   a. acid phosphatase
   b. hemoglobin
   c. prostate-specific antigen
   d. spermatozoa

9. Prostate-specific antigen (PSA) is important in the identification of
   a. blood
   b. semen
   c. saliva
   d. urine

10. Which of the following is *not* a method routinely used to detect saliva?
    a. ring precipitin
    b. starch iodine test
    c. procedures that test for the digestive activity of alpha amylase
    d. immunoassays that use monoclonal antibodies against human salivary alpha amylase

11. The presence of urea and creatinine is an indicator that the collected stain is
    a. blood
    b. semen
    c. saliva
    d. urine

12. Serological techniques are essential tools used in forensic science laboratories to aid in criminal investigations of
    a. sexual assaults
    b. homicides
    c. drug abuse
    d. all of the above

REFERENCES

1. Saferstein R. Forensic serology. *Criminalistics. An Introduction to Forensic Science.* 7th ed. Prentice Hall; Upper Saddle River, NJ; 2001: chap 12.

2. Anonymous. All about forensic Science.com. http://www.all-about-forensic-science.com. Accessed April 3, 2012.

3. Saferstein R. Introduction. *Criminalistics. An Introduction to Forensic Science.* 7th ed. Prentice Hall; Upper Saddle River, NJ; 2001: chap 1.

4. The Official Website of the Nobel Prize. http://nobelprize.org. Accessed April 3, 2012.

5. Saferstein R. Forensic toxicology. *Criminalistics. An Introduction to Forensic Science.* 7th ed. Prentice Hall; Upper Saddle River, NJ; 2001: chap 10.

6. Immunalysis. Direct ELISA Kit Product Inserts for Opiates, Cannabinoids (THCA/CTHC), and Oxycodone. http://www.immunalysis.com/elisa/elisa-for-forensic-matrices. Accessed April 3, 2012.

7. Laloup M, Tilman G, Maes V, et al. Validation of an ELISA-based screening assay for the detection of amphetamine, MDMA and MDA in blood and oral fluid. *Forensic Sci Int.* 2005;153:29–37.

8. Huestis MA, et al. Cannabinoid concentrations in hair from documented cannabis users. *Forensic Sci Int.* 2007;169:129–136.

9. Pujol ML, Cirmele V, Tritsch PJ, et al. Evaluation of the IDS One-Step ELISA Kits for the detection of illicit drugs in hair. *Forensic Sci. Int.* 2007;170:189–192.

10. Randox—The Complete Immunoassay Solution. http://www.randox.com/brochures/PDF%20Brochure/LT193.pdf. Accessed April 2, 2012.

11. Tobe SS, Watson N, Daéid NN. Evaluation of Six Presumptive Tests for Blood, Their Specificity, Sensitivity, and Effect on High Molecular Weight DNA. *J. Forensic Sciences.* 2007;52:102–109.

12. ABAcard® Hematrace® for the Forensic Identification of Human Blood. Abacus Diagnostics, Inc. Technical information sheet. http://www.abacusdiagnostics.com. Accessed April 3, 2012.

13. Seratec® HemDirect Hemoglobin Assay. Seratec®. User instruction sheet. http://www.seratec.com/docs/user_instructions/hbf07_en.pdf. Accessed April 3, 2012.

14. Misencik A, Laux DL. Validation study of the Seratec HemDirect Hemoglobin Assay for the forensic identification of human blood. *MAFS Newsletter.* Spring 2007:18–26.

15. Erie County Central Police Services Forensic Biology Manual. Effective date February 25, 2008. Erie County Central Police Services Forensic Laboratory, Buffalo, NY.

16. Duncan MW, Thompson HS. Proteomics of Semen and its Constituents. *Proteomics Clin. Appl.* 2007;1:861–875.

17. Laux DL, Tambasco AJ, Benzinger EA. Forensic detection of Semen II. Comparison of the Abacus Diagnostics OneStep ABAcard p30 Test and the Seratec PSA Semiquant Kit for the determination of the presence of semen in forensic cases. http://www.mafs.net/pdf/laux2.pdf. Accessed April 3, 2012.

18. Simich JP, Morris SL, Klick RL, et al. Validation of the use of a commercially available kit for the identification of prostate specific antigen (PSA) in semen stains. *J. Forensic Sciences.* 1999;44(6):1229–1231.

19. Seratec. PSA in Body Fluids—An Overview for Users of the Seratec PSA Semiquant Tests. Technical bulletin. http://ebookbrowse.com/gdoc.php?id=48295386&url=2cacddcc2ff1f7ab408601e9aa718b4d. Accessed April 2, 2012.

20. Seratec® PSA Semiquant. Seratec®. User instruction sheet. http://seraquant.seratec.com/instructions/PSA_EN.pdf. Accessed April 3, 2012.

21. Old JB, Schweers BA, Boonlayangoor PW, et al. Developmental validation of RSID™-saliva: A lateral flow immunochromatographic strip test for the forensic detection of saliva. *J. Forensic Sciences.* 2009;54:866–873.

22. Phadebas® Forensic. Forensic Examination of Items for the Presence of Saliva product insert. http://www.phadebas.com/data/phadebas/files/document/Instructions_Phad00ebas_Forensic_Press_Test.pdf. Accessed April 2, 2012.

23. Lilja H, Abrahamsson PA, Lundwall A. Semenogelin, the predominant protein in human semen. Primary structure and identification of closely related proteins in the male accessory sex glands and on the spermatozoa. *J. Biological Chemistry.* 1989;264:1894–1900.

24. Robert M, Gagnon C. Semenogelin I: A coagulum forming, multifunctional seminal vesicle protein. *Cellular and Molecular Life Sciences.* 1999;55:944–960.

25. Akutsu T, et al. Evaluation of Tamm-Horsfall protein and Uroplakin III for forensic identification of urine. *J. Forensic Sciences.* 2010;55:742–746.

PEARSON myhealthprofessionskit™

Visit www.myhealthprofessionskit.com to access the interactive Companion Website for this textbook. Simply select "Clinical Laboratory Science" from the choice of disciplines. Find this book and log in by using your user name and password to access additional learning tools.

22

Basic Laboratory Safety

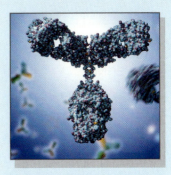

■ OBJECTIVES—LEVEL I

After this chapter, the student should be able to:

1. Describe the different types of general laboratory equipment designed for laboratory safety.

2. Describe the National Fire Protection Association (NFPA) diamond.

3. Describe a chemical fume hood and give details concerning flow rate.

4. Describe different types of personal protection equipment and their function.

5. Describe and perform proper hand-washing techniques

6. Describe the concept behind universal precautions.

7. Describe proper disposal of biological specimens, chemical waste, and radioactive waste.

8. Give examples of requirements dictated by the Occupational Exposure to Blood-borne Pathogen Standard.

9. Describe the purpose of the Needlestick Safety and Prevention Act.

10. Describe different examples of postexposure procedures.

11. List different exposure and risk codes for HIV-infected specimens.

12. List the precautions that laboratory workers and the general public should take to prevent exposure to HIV.

13. Understand the protective benefits of gloves in the event of a needle stick.

14. Describe in detail treatment after a needle stick, and explain what postexposure prophylaxis is.

15. Describe disinfectants used for biological samples.

16. Describe the risks involved in the use of liquid nitrogen.

17. Describe the best way to lift a heavy object.

18. Compare and contrast the risk after a needlestick from a patient with hepatitis B, hepatitis C, and HIV.

■ OBJECTIVES—LEVEL II

After this chapter, the student should be able to:

1. List postexposure treatments according to different exposure and risk codes for HIV-infected specimens.

KEY TERMS

biological containment hood
chemical fume hood
material safety
    data sheet (MSDS)
National Fire Protection
    Association (NFPA)
    diamond
Occupational Safety and
    Health Administration
    (OSHA)
personal protection
    equipment
universal precautions

▶ INTRODUCTION

Clinical laboratories, like any laboratory, can be the source of many different safety hazards; these can range from biological hazards, to chemical, radioactive, and physical ones and can include biological contamination, radioactive contamination, burns (from both chemical and heat sources), needlesticks, cuts from sharps, and other physical trauma. Therefore, safety equipment as well as safety precautions and practices are imperative for laboratory workers. In this chapter, we cover common equipment, practices, and regulations designed to prevent accidents from happening, and procedures that follow exposure to a particular hazard or the occurrence of an accident.

▶ SAFETY EQUIPMENT

Safety equipment varies greatly and can include standard laboratory items such as warning labels, containment hoods, emergency showers, eyewashes, first aid kits, waste disposal containers, and personal protection equipment. Warning labels are the most basic form of safety equipment; they are critical in identifying a potential hazard and can be found on laboratory doors, equipment, containers of chemicals, biological samples, and radioactive materials. Safety posters from the doors of 3 different research laboratories (Figure 22.1 ■) are examples of safety labels that are designed to inform the laboratory personnel and emergency responders of potential hazards specific to those laboratories. Safety posters differ based on the presence and nature of the hazards that may be encountered in a particular laboratory. The word CAUTION attracts attention to the information below about the type of hazard in the lab and the poster also contains the **National Fire Protection Association (NFPA) diamond** (1). This diamond indicates health risks (blue), flammability risks (red), reactivity risks (yellow), and special risks (white). The numbers in each of these colors indicate the level of risk; for example, 0 in flammability indicates nonflammable reagents whereas 4 indicates that material in the room will disperse in the air and readily burn at all temperatures. The signs also give information about whom to contact if there is any emergency or problem in the room.

✓ Checkpoint! 22.1

The following picture shows the warning label on a reagent bottle. What information can you derive from such a label?

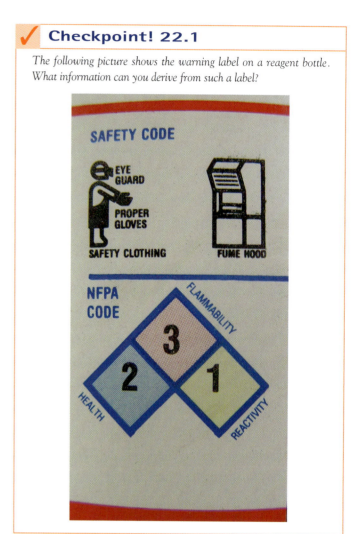

Containment hoods are designed to protect either the operator from a biological or chemical hazard or a particular specimen from contamination. Examples of containment hoods are chemical hoods (also commonly known as a *fume hood*) whose role is to contain chemicals that are flammable or may release flammable or toxic vapors (Figure 22.2 ■). The Occupational Safety and Health Administration (OSHA) defines a **chemical fume hood** as a device that is enclosed on 5 sides. This enclosed area has a partial covering or sash so that work can be done within the hood with only the technician's arms and hands inside the hood. A fan is installed to create a negative pressure so that air is drawn in from the laboratory and is exhausted into a separate air-handling system so that individuals in the laboratory are not exposed to fumes from the reagents within the hood. The National Research Council recommends that each person working with others in a fume hood have 2.5 linear feet of space. It also recommends that the flow should be high enough to ventilate 60 to 100 linear feet per minute but not high enough to cause turbulence. For safety reasons, laboratory hoods should be used as workspaces,

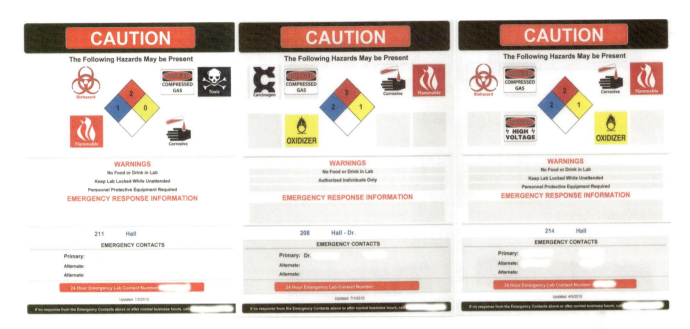

■ **FIGURE 22.1** Safety posters from different research laboratories.

not for storage. Clutter causes accidents and increases the chance of fire when working with flammable reagents.

Biological containment hoods, on the other hand, can be used to protect the operator and to avoid contaminating a particular sample or specimen. The air is filtered through a HEPA filter usually of 0.3 microns. A classical example of a biological containment hood is a laminar flow hood (Figure 22.3 ■) in which a sheet of forced air is constantly running downward at the opening of the hood to prevent any entry or exit of contaminating particles. Please note that these hoods can be designed to protect only the sample from outside contamination, not to protect the room from the sample. The hood can

also be maintained under sterile conditions by using germicidal ultraviolet lights on the inside of the hood, which are turned off when the operator handles the specimen. For appropriate airflow the biological safety cabinet should be placed where there are no drafts from doors, windows, or traffic.

To handle any operator contamination including large spills on a laboratory worker, clothing that may be set on fire by flammable chemicals or splashes of contaminants or chemicals into an operator's eyes, protective laboratory equipment includes emergency showers (Figure 22.4 ■) and eyewash stations (Figure 22.5 ■). Each of these pieces of equipment must be located so that a person who urgently needs treatment has

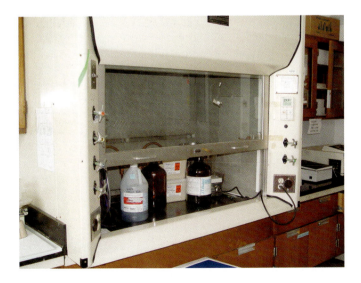

■ **FIGURE 22.2** Typical laboratory chemical hood.

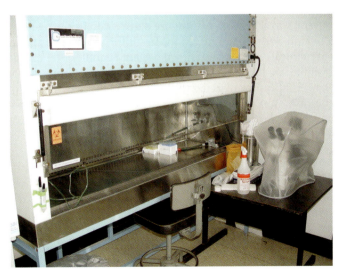

■ **FIGURE 22.3** Laminar flow hood.

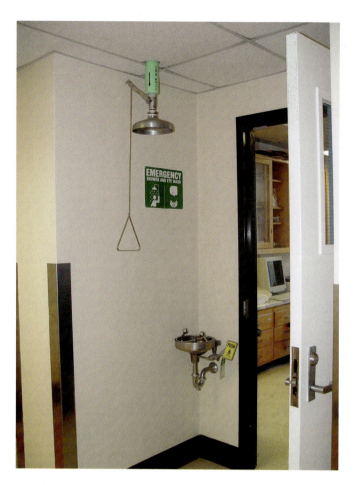

■ FIGURE 22.4 Typical laboratory emergency shower.

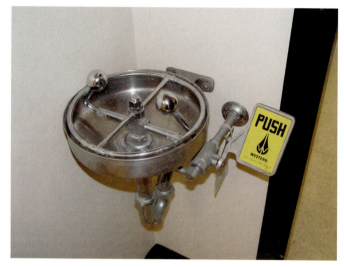

■ FIGURE 22.5 Emergency eyewash station.

be overfilled because an overfilled sharps container puts the laboratory technician at risk for injury (Figure 22.6 ■). Broken glass and other sharps such as surgical blades and glass slides must also be disposed of in appropriate puncture-proof containers (Figure 22.7 ■), which, depending upon need, can also be autoclaved. All biological materials must also be disposed appropriately; this is usually done in leak-proof, plastic bags that can be autoclaved, are clearly labeled with biohazard warning, and can be disposed of after autoclaving, in appropriately labeled biohazard disposal boxes (Figure 22.8 ■).

an unrestricted path to it and can reach it in 10 seconds or less. To achieve this, an injured person must have to travel 100 feet or less from the site of the injury. If strong acids or bases are used, the showers and eyewashes should be 10 feet or less away. Eyewash stations are designed to be operated by a person with impaired vision, from, for example, a splash of chemicals to the eyes; they have large handles that can be easily located and operated, and provide copious amounts of water that can be directed to the face and eyes. Two types of eyewash stations are available, the plumbed device permanently connected to the wall (Figure 22.5), and the one that dispenses fluid by gravity flow and contains either water or saline for a 15-minute wash (2). A preserved saline solution that is less irritating to the eye is sometimes used.

Other types of safety equipment include containers for the proper disposal of biological hazards, hypodermic needles and syringes, and glass and sharps. None of these materials can be discarded in conventional trash containers or bags but must be collected and processed accordingly. Hypodermic needles and syringes are usually disposed of in puncture-proof containers that can also be autoclaved. These containers are designed to have openings that prevent retrieval of materials after their disposal. It is important that these containers not

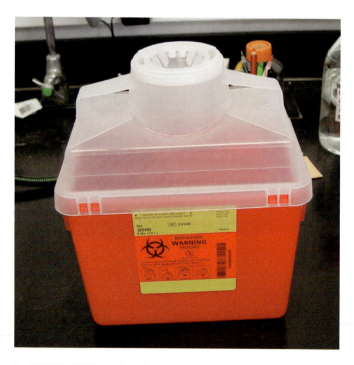

■ FIGURE 22.6 Typical disposal container for sharps such as needles.

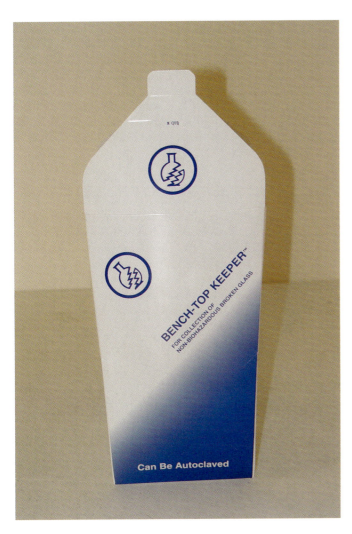
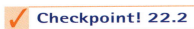

■ **FIGURE 22.7** Typical container for the disposal of broken glass or other sharps.

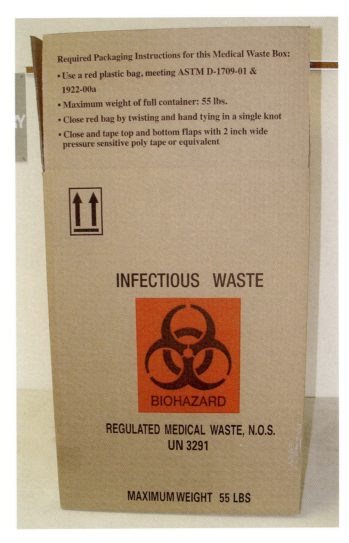

■ **FIGURE 22.8** Typical box used for the disposal of bagged, sealed, and autoclaved biological waste.

✓ **Checkpoint! 22.2**

What is the major difference between a chemical fume hood and biological containment hood?

▶ PERSONAL PROTECTION EQUIPMENT

Personal protection equipment is as important as laboratory safety equipment for the protection of the operator. It includes items such as goggles or face shields, laboratory coats or gowns, face masks, and gloves. See Figure 22.9 ■ for a typical set of personal protection equipment. Proper use of this equipment is just as important as the equipment itself.

LABORATORY COATS AND GOWNS

Designed to prevent contamination of the operator and his or her clothing by biological specimens (eg, body fluids including blood, urine, saliva, and excretions), laboratory coats and gowns should be fully buttoned and preferably fluid resistant and should have tight sleeves, which can fit beneath the gloves. Laboratory coats and gowns designed for multiple uses must be washed frequently, and single-use items such as gowns must be properly discarded immediately after each use.

GLOVES

Gloves come in different sizes and types from sterile surgical gloves to nonsurgical latex ones, to simple vinyl ones; in most cases nonsterile gloves are sufficient for the typical requirements of the clinical laboratory. As with the laboratory coats

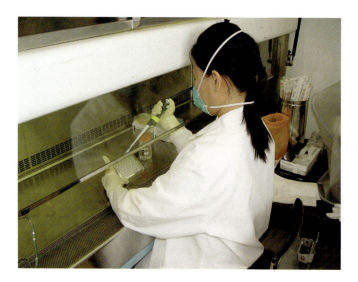

■ **FIGURE 22.9** Operator using personal protection equipment.

or gowns, gloves are designed to protect the operator from different biological specimens such as blood, body fluids, and excreta as well as potentially contaminated items that may have come in contact with these specimens. Gloves alone are not sufficient for complete protection, and hands must be washed thoroughly both before and after wearing gloves. Gloves must also be changed after seeing each patient and must be removed immediately after use and disposed of properly to avoid contaminating other items or personnel after they have been used for specimen handling.

The proper use of gloves ensures their effectiveness in preventing contamination. Gloves must be snug and well fitting; those that are too tight can impair hand movement and break from stretching; gloves that are too large can interfere with proper specimen handling by extending over the length of the fingers or by being too loose and affecting procedures that may need careful and precise hand coordination. Gloves must extend over the cuffs or sleeves of laboratory coats and gowns to prevent operator contamination. Again, gloves must be changed after seeing each patient and between samples, and hands must be washed between changes. Gloves should never be worn when leaving the laboratory or when changing from one station of the laboratory to another. They should never be worn while opening doors, touching environmental surfaces, or operating laboratory equipment that may be shared by different laboratory operators or when leaving the operating station.

Gloves made of latex, a natural product derived from fluid of the rubber tree, are the most commonly supplied ones in the laboratory, but some people have latex allergies and should not use these gloves (3). An allergic reaction to latex gloves can have many different manifestations. A type I hypersensitivity reaction can occur within minutes or many hours after exposure. These reactions range from red, itchy skin and hives to coughing and wheezing. Workers can be exposed to latex

allergens by wearing the gloves and by inhaling the latex-contaminated powder residue from powdered gloves. Because of the risk posed by inhaling latex-contaminated dust, individuals with latex allergies should avoid areas where people change their gloves. Latex dermatitis, a type IV hypersensitivity reaction, can also occur. It is a contact dermatitis and can develop as a T-cell response to the chemicals added in the synthesis of latex. Individuals with either of these reactions must use nonlatex gloves.

MASKS, GOGGLES, AND FACE SHIELDS

Masks, goggles, and face shields are designed to protect the operator from splashes from biological samples and from potentially airborne aerosols and pathogens. Such protective equipment is to be worn when manipulating any biological sample to prevent contamination of the mucosa in the mouth, nose, and eyes. As with other equipment, many forms of each are available, but all serve basically the same purpose. As an alternate to goggles or face shields, a laboratory bench shield may be used.

PERSONAL CARE

Long hair must be tied back to reduce the risk of contamination with biological fluids or chemicals and to reduce the risk of entrapment in moving equipment. Closed-toe shoes must be worn. People should not put anything in their mouth while in the laboratory; this is not the place to chew on a pencil.

VACCINATION

Since 1991, OSHA has required employers to offer hepatitis B vaccination without charge to any employee who might be at any risk for exposure. It also recommends that hospital employees, especially women of child-bearing years be vaccinated against rubella, mumps, measles, and influenza.

▶ SAFETY PROCEDURES AND UNIVERSAL PRECAUTIONS

All the safety equipment in the world can be ineffective if proper safety procedures are not followed. Some safety procedures are self-evident and based on common sense; others are dictated by various different guidelines and regulations. The most basic approach to sample handling is a set of guidelines introduced in the mid-1980s known as **universal precautions.** These guidelines state that all patients and their samples are to be considered potentially infectious and possible carriers of pathogens (4). Therefore, universal precaution guidelines recommend that personal protection equipment such as gloves, masks, and coats or gowns be worn whenever a worker collects blood or handles body fluids that may be contaminated with blood and when there is a possibility of blood splashing on mucosal surfaces. The universal precautions guidelines were later extended to other body fluids such as semen; vaginal secretions; and synovial, amniotic, cerebrospinal, pleural, peritoneal, and pericardial fluids. Universal precautions have additional guidelines for many aspects of working with patient samples. Guidelines recommend that workers wash their hands after removing gloves and never pipette by mouth, and that all samples be transported in containers that have a lid and are leakproof. Work surfaces are to be decontaminated after working with any blood or body fluid on them. Spills of biological material should be disinfected with a freshly made 1:10 dilution of bleach or a commercial disinfectant. Contaminated material must be decontaminated before disposal. Protective clothing should not be worn out of the laboratory.

HAND WASHING

Our hands are among our most versatile tools; as such, they can be the source, carrier, and target of contamination. Thus, hand washing is one of the most basic yet effective safety procedures an operator can employ. The proper way to wash hands includes using plenty of warm water and soap. Water that is too hot can damage the skin and increase the risk of infection, whereas water that is too cold does not effectively interact with the soap. The Association for Professionals in Infection Control and Epidemiology (APIC) and the Centers for Disease Control and Prevention (CDC) offer the following guidelines: (1) Use warm water to wet hands, (2) apply soap and spread over hands, (3) rub hands together for 20 seconds, rubbing all surfaces and under fingernails hard enough to generate friction, (4) rinse thoroughly, (5) dry with towels, and (6) use a towel to turn off the faucet. A clue suggested by the CDC for the length of time to wash your hands is to sing or hum the "Happy Birthday" song twice. Hands should be washed from the wrist area to the tips of the fingers and rinsed with the water flowing in a downward direction from wrists to fingers, to carry contaminated water away from the individual and into the sink. Hands should be washed any time contamination is suspected, before and after wearing gloves, between patients and between handling different samples, when gloves are changed, before leaving the laboratory, before any handling of food and drink, and after using restrooms (5).

✓ Checkpoint! 22.3

Why is washing your hands properly and often important if you are going to wear gloves anyway?

HANDLING BIOLOGICAL SAMPLES AND PATIENT-RELATED ITEMS

The best approach to handling biological specimens and patient-related items is to assume that every one of them is a source of contamination. The spread of infection follows a specific pattern: a source of the infection, a method of transmission of the infectious agent, and, of course, a host (5). Biological specimens are the most common source of infection in the clinical laboratory. In addition, any item that may have come in contact with either the specimen or the patient from which it originated can also be a source of infection; these include any clothing items, hospital and/or medical equipment (eg, a wheelchair), or laboratory equipment used to obtain or transport the specimen. Particular care must be taken with hypodermic needles and other sharps, such as scalpel blades, used in obtaining a particular specimen. The hypodermic needle in particular, is one of the common threats for the spread of bloodborne pathogens (see below about needlestick injuries) and should *not* be recapped by hand if possible because needlestick injuries are one of the most common ways for operators to be infected by a specimen (6). Modern hypodermic equipment that does not require manual recapping of needles is available: It ranges from needles that recap automatically, or needles that break off without operator assistance. Immediately after use needles should be discarded in a sharps container.

To protect themselves from infections, laboratory workers should refrain from certain activity in the laboratory. OSHA has developed directives for laboratory behavior that include no mouth pipetting, as well as no eating, drinking, smoking, applying cosmetics or lip balm, or handling contact lenses in the laboratory. In addition, no food or drink should be stored in laboratory refrigerators or laboratory bench tops where anything infectious could be present. To further protect from injury, chipped or broken glassware should not be utilized and should be discarded appropriately (7).

Occasionally during centrifugation, a tube of blood may break; this usually occurs when the centrifuge buckets are not properly balanced. This presents the danger that the sample may be aerosolized in the centrifuge. To remove the tube and clean the centrifuge, wait 20 minutes for the sample to settle, and clean up using a mask, gloves, and a lab coat.

▶ SAFETY AND THE LAW

Laboratory safety practices are not only dictated by common sense; they are also regulated by different governmental laws at both the local and federal levels. In 1991, the **Occupational Safety and Health Administration (OSHA)** issued a set of regulations, "Occupational Exposure to Bloodborne Pathogen Standard" (29 CFR 1910.1930) that became law. This set of regulations was designed to instruct millions of health workers about and protect them from exposure to bloodborne pathogens from human blood, human blood components, and products made from human blood. This set of rules covered everything from the development and implementation of an exposure control plan to providing health workers with free laboratory coats and gowns and other personal safety equipment described previously, including warning labels. The law prevented eating and drinking in the laboratory and required that laboratory workers receive free immunizations against hepatitis B and free laundering services or facilities for multiple-use items such as coats and other protective clothing. More importantly, the law required the maintenance of records of health workers' training and the establishment of well-defined procedures and follow-ups should a worker be exposed to a bloodborne pathogen, which OSHA defined as pathogenic microorganisms that are present in human blood and can cause disease in humans, including, but not limited to, hepatitis B virus (HBV) and human immunodeficiency virus (HIV) (8).

▶ NEEDLESTICK INJURIES

Injuries from needlesticks represent one of the most common forms of hazards encountered by health professionals and laboratory workers. It is estimated that several hundred thousand needlestick injuries occur in the United States every year, and that many of these are unreported. Because of this, Congress passed a Needlestick Safety and Prevention Act (9) in 2000. It required that by 2002, all hospitals and medical facilities must be in full compliance. The act requires employers to implement measures that prevent or, at least, minimize puncture wounds and cuts from contaminated needles or other sharps such as lancets or scalpel blades. Particular attention was given to contamination and infection by HIV and hepatitis viruses B and C. To comply with the act, employers must assess the safety of these devices and their proper disposal; they also must use the most recent safety devices that come with protection systems such as automatic needle retraction systems or built-in after-use sheaths.

Fortunately, the rates of infection from needlestick injuries are relatively low. It is estimated that only 0.3% of people who sustained a needlestick contamination from an HIV-infected individual become infected. This transmission rate decreases by 80% with postexposure prophylaxis. A 1999 report indicated that only 49 cases of HIV had been acquired in the United States because of needlesticks. The rate for transmission of hepatitis B by a needlestick from a contaminated individual to nonimmunized individuals is higher, ranging from 1 to 40%; immunization reduces this risk by almost 95%. The rate for hepatitis C ranges from 0 to 10%.

▶ POSTEXPOSURE TREATMENT

Although safety equipment, procedures, and regulations are successful in preventing the infection of health care workers and laboratories from contaminated samples, accidental exposure to such infectious items do occur. This may be the result of human error, for example, failure to follow universal safety precautions (Where are your gloves? Did you recap a needle manually?), use of equipment without safety features, or the use of equipment with a disabled safety feature. The risk is also increased by repeated performance of exposure-prone tasks. Thus, it is imperative that postexposure prophylaxis (PEP), treatments, and follow-up protocols be in place in both the clinical setting and the laboratory as required by OSHA 29 CFR 1910.1930 (8).

NEEDLESTICK INJURIES

Needlestick injuries require performing several steps. First and foremost is to *gently* squeeze a drop of blood out; "gently" is a critical term here: you do not want to treat the puncture area in a harsh manner because you don't want to draw white cells to the area, as these cells may become infected (remember, white blood cells are the cells that are infected by HIV). The area should then be carefully but thoroughly washed. The next step, which is just as important, is to report the incident immediately to the person's supervisor. Clinical and laboratory settings must have mechanisms in place for reporting and recording the incident. The worker should also go to the employee clinic where clinic personnel take a history to determine risk factors for HIV, hepatitis, and tetanus. The employee may also be asked about immunization records (hepatitis and tetanus), previous occupational exposure to body fluids, IV drug use, sexual history, body piercing or tattooing, receipt of blood or blood products, history of dialysis, and travel outside the United States within the last year. Clinic personnel may also perform a physical examination to determine baseline lung, liver, and lymph node status. Immediate care includes irrigating and cleaning the wound, giving a tetanus shot, hepatitis B prophylaxis if the person has not been immunized, and assessing HIV risk. Additional testing of the employee may include HIV, hepatitis B surface antibody (Did your vaccine work?), and hepatitis C antibody at baseline and then at 2 weeks, 4 weeks, and 8 weeks after exposure. With proper consent, the patient from whom the specimen comes from may also be tested for HIV, hepatitis B, hepatitis C, and aspartate aminotransferase/alanine aminotransferase (AST/ALT) and alkaline phosphatase levels.

HIV EXPOSURE AND RISK CODES

One of the major concerns in accidental exposures to infectious agents (either via needlestick or other means) is exposure to HIV-infected specimens. Therefore, well-detailed exposure

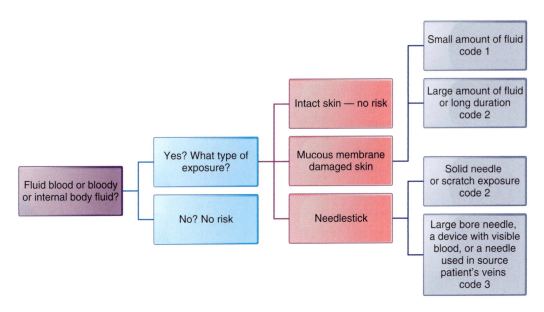

■ **FIGURE 22.10**   Different exposure codes for potential HIV infection.

and risk codes for HIV must be in place for proper postexposure prophylaxis (PEP) procedures to be considered. Refer to Figure 22.10 ■ for different HIV exposure codes.

Once an exposure code has been determined, a risk assessment of the patient from whom the sample was obtained is necessary. See Figure 22.11 ■ for the different risk codes for a patient. Various combinations of risk exposure and assessment codes then dictate different approaches for PEP. Different PEP approaches based on various exposure and risk assessment codes are given in Table 22.1 ✪.

If postexposure prophylaxis is warranted but before such therapy is initiated, the exposed health care worker is subjected to a pregnancy test (if this worker is female and in reproductive years), as well as tests for liver function (AST/ALT, alkaline phosphatase, bilirubin), kidney function (serum creatinine/BUN levels), urinalysis with microscopic analysis, and for general health status, a complete blood count. PEP includes anti-retroviral therapy (see also Chapter 16) whose

basic regime involves 4 weeks of treatment with zidovudine (AZT) and lamivudine (3TC), a nucleoside analog reverse transcriptase inhibitor. The expanded regime adds the use of indinavir (a protease inhibitor) in conjunction with nelfinavir (protease inhibitor) to the basic regime treatment. After the exposure, the health care worker should abstain from sex for 6 months or until a 3rd negative test; breast feeding and donating blood are discouraged during this time. Follow-up care should continue for 6 months to determine seroconversion status. Postexposure prophylaxis decreases seroconversion to HIV positive status by 80% but has many side effects and so should not be used unless there is true risk.

OTHER POTENTIAL PATHOGENS

Although HIV is of major concern in needlestick injury, this injury can transmit other pathogens. With hepatitis C, the average chance of seroconversion after a needlestick injury

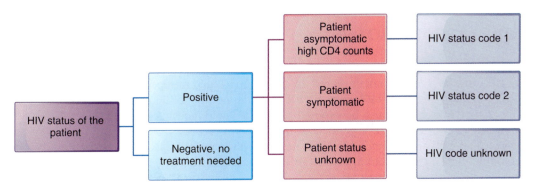

■ **FIGURE 22.11**   Risk assessment codes for an HIV-infected patient.

⊗ **TABLE 22.1**

Postexposure Prophylaxis (PEP) Modalities Based on Different Exposure and Risk Assessment Codes

Codes	Postexposure Prophylaxis
Exposure code 1+ HIV risk 1	Not a known risk; still an informed decision between health care worker and physician
Exposure code 1+ HIV status code 2	Negligible risk; recommend basic regime, use of PEP appropriate
Exposure code 2 HIV status 1	Basic regime; no increased risk observed but PEP appropriate
Exposure code 2 HIV status code 2	Expanded regime; increased risk for the person
Exposure code 3 HIV status code 1 or 2	Expanded regime; increased risk for the person
Exposure code 2 or 3 and unknown HIV status	If suggestion of HIV status, then PEP

is 1.8%. Health care workers and patients can be tested for anti-HCV antibodies; follow-up should be performed for 4 to 6 months looking for antibody or 4 to 6 weeks if testing for HCV RNA. Confirmatory tests are also recommended. In addition, although very rarely, other pathogens and/or conditions can be transmitted by needlestick injuries and can include:

- Blastomycosis
- Brucellosis
- Cryptococcosis
- Diphtheria
- Cutaneous gonorrhea
- Herpes
- Malaria
- Mycobacteriosis
- Mycoplasma caviae
- Rocky Mountain spotted fever
- Sporotrichosis
- *Staph. aureus*
- *Strep. Pyogenes*
- Syphilis
- Toxoplasmosis
- Tuberculosis

▶ CHEMICAL AND RADIOACTIVE HAZARDS

Although the most common hazards encountered in a clinical immunology laboratory are of biological nature, health care and laboratory workers can also be exposed to chemical hazards in the form of chemical reagents used in various laboratory procedures. Again, common sense dictates various safety procedures; these include avoiding contact with exposed skin, mucous surfaces, and clothing via the use of protective equipment such as laboratory coats, masks, face

shields, and gloves as previously discussed. Chemicals that can release flammable or toxic vapors should be handled inside a fume hood (Figure 22.2), and labels on reagent bottles should be read carefully to learn of potential hazards as well as proper handling instructions. Most reagents come with a **material safety data sheet (MSDS)** that provides information on the properties of that specific chemical described by that specific MSDS, including physical properties such as melting point, boiling point, flash point, reactivity, toxicity, and health effects. The MSDS also includes information of first aid procedures, requirements for specific protective equipment, and detailed instructions for storage, disposal, and procedures to handle spills (10). In the case of a spill onto a worker, the area affected should be washed immediately with copious amounts of water for 15 to 20 minutes followed by proper first aid if needed. All workers should also be aware of the location of emergency showers (Figure 22.4) and eye-washing stations (Figure 22.5) and practice reaching them quickly even under impaired conditions (because a spill can impair vision) to save time when an emergency occurs. To clean chemical spills on surfaces, the appropriate "spill kit" should be utilized. The MSDS for the material should suggest what absorbent or neutralizing material should be used for a spill.

An important chemical to consider in the laboratory is one that is often overlooked: liquid nitrogen. Many laboratories have liquid nitrogen tanks to preserve cells including bone marrow, stem cells, and sperm. If spilled on the skin, this material can cause a cold-contact burn. However, the most important risk is due to the fact that when exposed to room temperature conditions, liquid nitrogen quickly becomes a gas. The liquid-to-gas volume ratio for liquid nitrogen is 1:694, so the vaporization of the liquid quickly expands as a gas. Like any gas, liquid nitrogen can replace the oxygen in the room and thus can act as an asphyxiant in the air (11). When room oxygen levels are replaced such that the oxygen concentration is below 16% a dangerous situation may arise. Because of this, an area that is used for storage of liquid nitrogen should contain an oxygen sensor.

Clinical laboratory workers can also encounter radioactivity hazards because certain assays require the use of radioactively labeled reagents (for example, radioimmunoassay). The level of radioactivity used in routine clinical laboratory assays is usually very low and poses little risk of radiation exposure. However, exposure to radiation is to be limited because its effect can be cumulative with time. Radioactive materials are regulated by the Nuclear Regulatory Commission (NRC), which dictates the amount of radiation allowable in a particular laboratory, the different isotopes to be used for the assays, and monitors and tracks the disposal of radioactive materials. Laboratories using radioactive materials are required to keep records of the amount of radioactive materials used, the specific isotopes used, the disposal of radioactive waste, the purchase of such materials, and the disposal of unused materials; these records are usually kept in a book or binder provided by the radiation protection services of that particular laboratory or hospital. Workers using radioactive materials use personal protection such as gloves, masks, and gowns to avoid contamination; in many cases, they are also required to wear dosimeters, which are devices that record the amount of radioactivity to which a worker might be exposed. Dosimeters are assigned to a single individual user, can either be worn as badges or as rings, and are periodically monitored by the radiation protection services to measure the amount of radioactivity (if any) to which a worker had been exposed. Refer to Figure 22.12 ■ for a sample of a radioactive protection services record book, and two badge-type dosimeters.

Work with radioactive material is performed in specifically designated areas, whether a laboratory bench or a separate room; such areas are labeled for the use of radioactive materials and are monitored routinely (usually once a month) for contamination with periodic swab tests as mandated by local and NRC regulation, and the results of these swab tests are recorded in the radiation protecting services record book. Disposal of radioactive materials is also carefully regulated and monitored by both local regulation and the NRC, and it varies according to the type of materials (solid, liquids, volatile chemicals), the amount of radioactivity, and the radioisotopes involved.

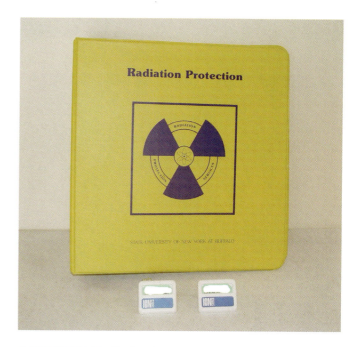

■ **FIGURE 22.12** Radioactive protection services record book and two badge-style dosimeters.

▶ GENERAL SAFETY

All people in the laboratory should be trained in the use of all safety equipment. Laboratory personnel should know the location of fire blankets, fire extinguishers, showers, eyewash stations, decontaminating solutions, spill kits, and first aid kits. Different fire extinguishers are used for different types of fire; it is important that individuals in a laboratory know the type of fire extinguisher that is in the lab and the material for which it can be used. The fire evacuation route should also be clearly understood. An evacuation meeting place should be designated so that a roll call can ascertain whether anyone was unable to leave the building.

To reduce the risk of electrical shock, electrical equipment should not be plugged into extension cords or "gang" plugs. Back injuries can occur in any job, not just in a laboratory, so they represent an important issue. To minimize back injury, get help to lift a heavy object. When lifting, bend your legs not your back or arms, and have your legs about 10 inches apart. Lift with the object close to you, not with your arms outstretched. Lift by straightening your bent legs.

 Checkpoint! 22.4

Why do operators who work with radioactive materials have to wear dosimeters even though the materials used in the average clinical laboratory have low levels of radioactivity?

CASE STUDY

1. What's wrong with pictures (a) through (e)?

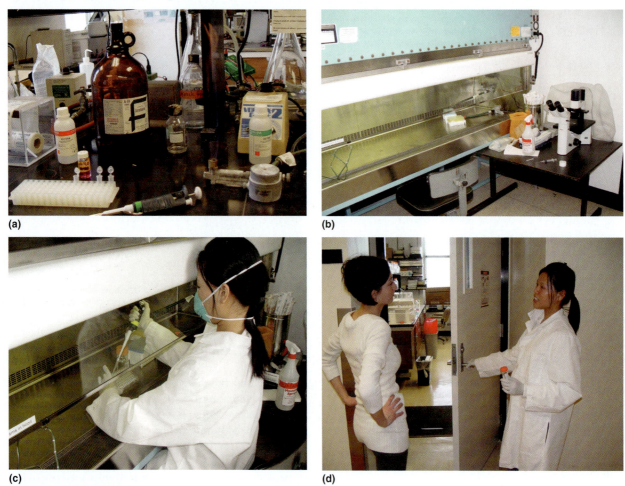

(a)

(b)

(c)

(d)

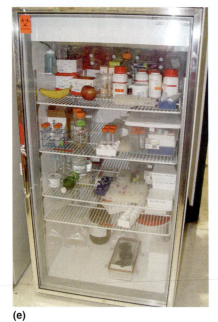

(e)

SUMMARY

Laboratories can present a wide variety of hazards—biological, chemical, radioactive, and physical, thus, laboratory safety is essential for the function of the laboratory and its personnel. Safety can be achieved by using laboratory items and equipment such as labels, fume hoods, biological containment hoods, emergency showers, eyewash stations, and safety containers for the proper disposal of dangerous items such as hypodermic needles, sharps, broken glass, and contaminated items. The use of personal protective equipment, such as laboratory coats or gowns, gloves, face masks, goggles, and face shields, can do much to ensure operator safety. Of course, proper safety procedures and proper use of safety equipment are just as important as the equipment itself.

Safety procedures should follow guidelines of universal precaution, which assume that all patients and their samples are to be considered potentially infectious and possible carriers of pathogens. Safety procedures should also dictate the proper use of all safety equipment, both personal and laboratory. Different regulations also control laboratory safety including the OSHA 29 CFR 1910.1930 and the Needlestick Safety and Prevention Act. Regulations also control the proper disposal of various chemicals, sharps, biologically contaminated materials, and radioactive materials. Should exposure to a hazard occur, post-exposure procedures must be in place; particular attention is given to those procedures and treatment when a laboratory employee has been exposed to specimens from HIV-infected individuals. These procedures are also regulated by laws such as the OSHA 29 CFR 1910.1930.

REVIEW QUESTIONS

1. What flow rate is appropriate for a chemical fume hood?
   a. 10–60 linear feet of air per minute
   b. 60–100 linear feet of air per minute
   c. 100–200 linear feet of air per minute
   d. 200–300 linear feet of air per minute

2. What concentration of bleach is used as a disinfectant?
   a. 100%
   b. 50%
   c. 40%
   d. 10%

3. A person should lift a heavy object
   a. with someone else
   b. by keeping the arms and back straight and bending the legs
   c. with the legs about 10 inches apart
   d. all of the above

4. The most dangerous thing about liquid nitrogen is the fact that it
   a. has an extremely explosive nature
   b. can cause cold-contact burns
   c. can replace room air and cause asphyxiation
   d. it is so toxic that a small amount on the skin can cause death

5. The degree of risk of infection after exposure to a patient's blood includes
   a. the type of exposure and whether on skin or mucosa or by a penetrating needlestick
   b. the amount of virus the patient has in her or his blood stream
   c. whether the patient also has influenza
   d. A and B only

6. The NFPA hazardous material symbol
   a. is a diamond composed of 4 diamonds indicating whether the material in the room is a health, fire, reactivity, or special hazard
   b. is a diamond separated into 3 parts indicating whether the material is a health, fire, or reactivity hazard
   c. is a diamond separated into 5 parts indicating whether the material is a health, fire, reactivity, biological, or special hazard
   d. none of the above

7. After a needlestick, every laboratory technician should
   a. get post-exposure prophylaxis
   b. wash hands and squeeze out 1 drop of blood
   c. pour 10% bleach on the hand(s)
   d. wash hands with water as hot as can be tolerated

8. In an emergency, you should be able to get to the emergency shower in
   a. 1 minute
   b. 5 minutes
   c. 30 seconds
   d. 10 seconds

9. In case of an eye exposure, how long should the eyewash be used?
   a. 1 minute
   b. 5 minutes
   c. 15 minutes
   d. 10 seconds

10. Hepatitis B, hepatitis C, and HIV
    a. are the only pathogens that can be transferred with a needlestick
    b. are extremely infectious with nearly 100% of the needlesticks resulting in seroconversion
    c. do not cause infections in people who are vaccinated
    d. None of the above

REFERENCES

1. National Fire Protection Association. http://www.nfpa.org/categoryList.asp?categoryID=124&URL=Codes%20&%20Standards. Accessed May 25, 2012.

2. Agriculture and Natural Resources Research and Extension Center. System Policy and Procedures Emergency Eyewash and Shower Placement/Design. http://safety.ucanr.org/files/2876.pdf. Accessed March 31, 2012.

3. Centers for Disease Control and Prevention. NIOSH Publications and Products. Latex allergy: A prevention guide. http://www.cdc.gov/niosh/docs/98–113. Accessed May 25, 2012.

4. Centers for Disease Control and Prevention. Update: Universal precautions for prevention of transmission of human immunodeficiency virus, hepatitis B virus, and other bloodborne pathogens in health-care settings. *MMWR*. 1988;37(24):377–382, 387–388.

5. Barrs AW Handwashing: Breaking the chain of infection. *Infection Control Today*. July 1, 2000. http://www.infectioncontroltoday.com/articles/2000/07/handwashing-breaking-the-chain-of-infection.aspx. Accessed May 25, 2012.

6. Canadian Centre for Occupational Health and Safety. http://www.ccohs.ca/oshanswers/diseases/needlestick_injuries.html. Accessed May 25, 2012.

7. U.S. Department of Labor Occupational Safety and Health Administration. Part 1910.1450(a) Occupational exposure to hazardous chemicals in laboratories. http://www.osha.gov/pls/oshaweb/owadisp.show_document?p_table=standards&p_id=10106. Accessed May 25, 2012.

8. U.S. Department of Labor Occupational Safety and Health Administration. Bloodborne pathogens. http://www.osha.gov/pls/oshaweb/owadisp.show_document?p_table=STANDARDS&p_id=10051. Accessed May 25, 2012.

9. Needlestick Safety and Prevention Act. http://www.osha.gov/needlesticks/needlefaq.html. Accessed May 25, 2012.

10. U.S. Department of Labor Occupational Safety and Health Administration. Material safety data sheet. http://www.osha.gov/dsg/hazcom/msds-osha174/msdsform.html. Accessed May 25, 2012.

11. Aristy-Reeyes G. Safety first: Working with liquid nitrogen in a laboratory setting. *LabQ Clinical Laboratory*. 2010;18.

PEARSON
myhealthprofessionskit™

Visit www.myhealthprofessionskit.com to access the interactive Companion Website for this textbook. Simply select "Clinical Laboratory Science" from the choice of disciplines. Find this book and log in by using your user name and password to access additional learning tools.

23

Molecular Biology Techniques

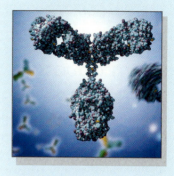

■ OBJECTIVES—LEVEL I

After this chapter, the student should be able to:

1. Describe the structure of DNA and RNA and the molecules required to convert from genes to proteins.
2. Describe the chemical relationship that allows complementarity among nucleic acids.
3. Define *hybridization* and describe its role in the function of nucleic acid probes.
4. Describe dot blot, Southern blot and Northern blot and the role of each in molecular diagnostics.
5. Describe the role of *in situ* hybridization.
6. Discuss the use of microarrays (gene chips) and their advantage over other techniques.
7. Describe single-strand conformational polymorphism (SSCP).
8. Describe the principle of target amplification using the polymerase chain reaction (PCR).
9. Discuss the different forms of PCR and their application.

■ OBJECTIVES—LEVEL II

After this chapter, the student should be able to:

1. Discuss the pros and cons of molecular biology techniques used in diagnostics.
2. Describe examples of non-PCR target amplification methods.

KEY TERMS

annealing
codon
deoxyribonucleic acid (DNA)
DNA replication
dot blot
gene

genetic code
hybridization
intron
restriction endonuclease
transcription
translation

▶ INTRODUCTION

The term *molecular biology* may appear somewhat vague, perhaps even self-evident, implying the description of the role of molecules in biological processes. Of course, every biological process involves molecules; water is a molecule; so is sodium chloride and, for that matter, insulin and hemoglobin. However, by convention, *molecular biology* has been used for many years to describe the study and/or analysis of nucleic acids such as DNA, RNA, and related molecules. Some have dubbed these nucleic acids the "blueprints of life"; as such, they can be used as powerful tools for the identification and recognition of the components for which they encode. These nucleic acids represent unique "fingerprints" for a variety of molecules, and, indirectly, tissues, cells, and microorganisms. In fact, throughout this book, we have mentioned various molecular biology techniques that have been used in laboratory tests, diagnostic approaches, and disease monitoring. In this chapter, we describe the role of nucleic acid and the principle and laboratory methodologies of commonly used molecular biology techniques. One can argue that these techniques are not "clinical immunology" techniques, that is, they may not necessarily involve immune components such as antibodies in their procedure, and, in fact, it is not within the scope of this chapter to cover every possible molecular biology technique used in diagnostics. However, the advent of modern molecular biology techniques has traditionally supplemented the immunological techniques and although molecular biology today may be conceptually separate from clinical immunology, we believe that covering some basic principles of molecular biology techniques routinely used in diagnosis would make this book more comprehensive.

▶ NUCLEIC ACIDS, TRANSCRIPTION, AND TRANSLATION

Although it is beyond the scope of this chapter to describe in detail the various biological processes that go from genes to proteins, a brief review of such processes can help in understanding the basic principles as well as the significance of the techniques described here. **Deoxyribonucleic acid (DNA),** is a complex of 2 separate strings, or chains, composed of repeating units called *nucleotides;* the 2 chains have carbohydrate backbones to which different bases are linked and run in opposite directions with respect to each other in an arrangement called *antiparallel.* Four types of bases are found in DNA: adenine, cytosine, guanine, and thymine. The 2 strands are connected to each other by the interaction of these bases in a defined pattern with adenine binding to thymine, and cytosine binding to guanine (1). See typical arrangement of bases in DNA in Figure 23.1 ■. The 2 strands are then arranged into a helical structure (Figure 23.2 ■) first described by Watson and Crick in 1953 (2). Within a cell, the DNA is arranged in

structures called *chromosomes,* which divide and make copies of themselves when the cell divides by a process called **DNA replication.** Other components, for example, chromatin proteins such as histones, play a role in packaging, organizing, and arranging the DNA (1).

The sequence of these different bases along the strands or backbone of DNA encodes the information for the basic building blocks of life (ie, amino acids and, subsequently, proteins). Such information is arranged in stretches of DNA called **genes;** within each gene are sequences that provide information not only for the physical structure of the final product (ie, the amino acid sequence of the protein that is encoded by the stretch) but also for various other regulatory functions of that gene and, thus, its product as well as certain noncoding sequences called **introns.** The creation of a protein from the information stored in DNA follows a **genetic code;** different sets of 3 nucleotide each, called **codons,** encode for a specific amino acid; thus, the sequence of a set of codons determines the sequence of different amino acids that, in turn, determines the protein encoded by that stretch of DNA. For example, the 3 nucleotides AAA in the gene sequence codes for the placement of lysine in the protein while the 3 nucleotides ACA code for the placement of threonine in the protein (1).

✓ **Checkpoint! 23.1**

How can a change in a single nucleotide within a DNA sequence affect the structure and function of the protein encoded by that sequence?

Proteins are not synthesized directly from the DNA sequence, and the sequence of DNA that encodes for the final product is often "interrupted" by other stretches of DNA such as the introns. The first step to bring the genetic material to protein production is that DNA is "copied" into another nucleic acid, ribonucleic acid, or RNA, by a process called **transcription.** RNA is arranged in a way similar to DNA with different bases providing the sequence information for the different codons; the genetic difference is that RNA has a base called *uracil* (Figure 23.3 ■) instead of thymine. In addition, RNA contains the backbone sugar ribose instead of the sugar deoxyribose. During transcription, the enzyme RNA polymerase "reads" a sequence of DNA along one of the DNA strands, and for each base read, an RNA base is attached to the DNA base, creating a complementary template of RNA following the pattern uracil-adenine, adenine-thymine, and guanine-cytosine. This involves various steps starting with the unwinding and "unzipping" of the 2 DNA strands, the pairing of DNA-RNA nucleotides, and the creation of a strand of RNA template followed by the separation of such strand from the DNA template, resulting in the production of a single strand of RNA (Figure 23.4 ■). This RNA "copy" represents a primary RNA transcript that

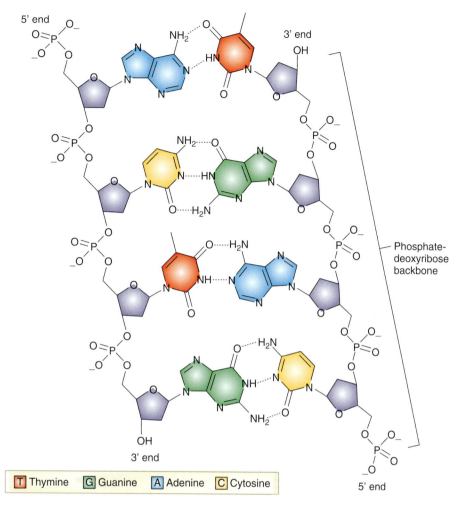

5' end

3' end

OH

Phosphate-
deoxyribose
backbone

3' end

| T | Thymine | G | Guanine | A | Adenine | C | Cytosine |

5' end

■ **FIGURE 23.1**   Chemical structure of DNA.

contains not only the coding sequence of the protein but also a copy of other parts of the gene, such as the introns. A splicing process removes the non-coding regions from the primary transcript; the resulting RNA is called *messenger RNA*, or *mRNA*.

Following the genetic code from this RNA, the information from the different codons is used to make the resulting chain of amino acids, which, in turn, make the final protein. This process is called **translation,** and other forms of RNA, namely ribosomal RNA (rRNA) and transfer RNA (tRNA), are

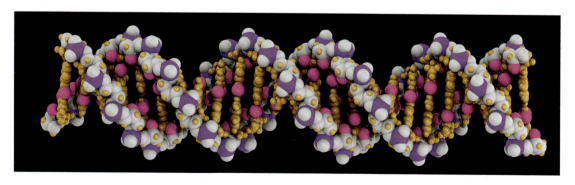

■ **FIGURE 23.2**   Three-dimensional model of DNA. *Source:* © Scott Camazine/Alamy.

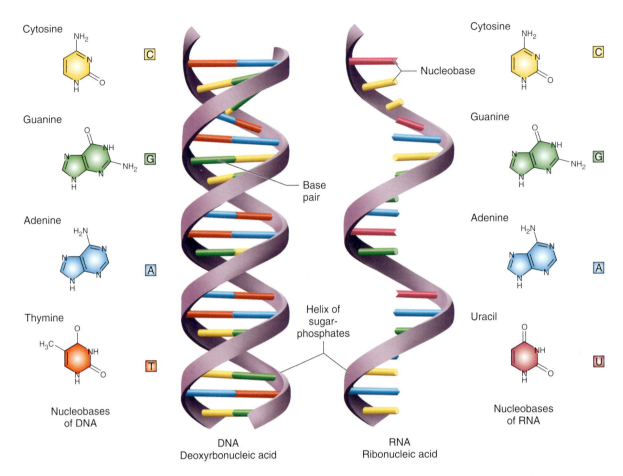

Cytosine

Guanine

Adenine

Thymine

Nucleobases
of DNA

Base
pair

Helix of
sugar-
phosphates

DNA
Deoxyrbonucleic acid

RNA
Ribonucleic acid

Nucleobase

Cytosine

Guanine

Adenine

Uracil

Nucleobases
of RNA

■ **FIGURE 23.3**   Comparison of a single-stranded RNA and a double-stranded DNA with their corresponding nucleobases.

now involved in this process. The mRNA, containing the coding sequence of the encoded protein, delivers this information to the ribosomes, which are components of the cell that are responsible for protein synthesis. The mRNA binds to the ribosomes to start the translation of proteins from the mRNA sequence. Translation is accomplished with the help of the tRNA, which has an anticodon sequence that matches a particular RNA codon specific for a particular amino acid. The

tRNA also has a binding site for that particular amino acid, so as the mRNA is "read" by the ribosomes, different tRNAs carrying different amino acids bind and add that amino acid to the growing protein chain. The assembly of a protein in the ribosomes is depicted in Figure 23.5 ■. The resulting chain of amino acids reflects the codon sequence of the mRNA, which was derived from the original sequence of the initial DNA (1). Refer to Figure 23.6 ■ for a diagram of this whole process (ie,

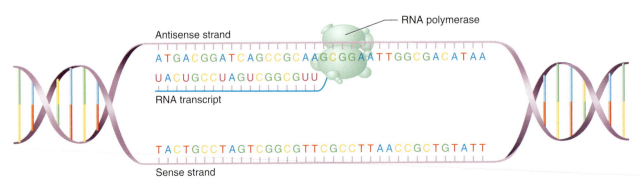

Antisense strand

RNA polymerase

ATGACGGATCAGCCGCAAGCGGAATTGGCGACATAA
UACUGCCUAGUCGGCGUU

RNA transcript

TACTGCCTAGTCGGCGTTCGCCTTAACCGCTGTATT

Sense strand

■ **FIGURE 23.4**   DNA transcription.

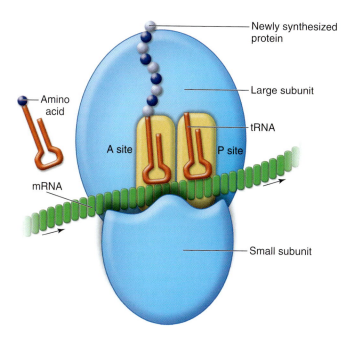

■ **FIGURE 23.5**   Diagram showing how the translation of the mRNA and the synthesis of proteins are carried out by the ribosome.

specific for that protein and thus can be used to either study, monitor, or identify such a protein product and, by default, other biological entities associated with that protein. So, for example, if a particular microorganism has a protein that is very unique to it, finding the DNA sequence of the protein can identify the organisms. DNA is a very sturdy molecule; it can survive unaltered for a very long time under very harsh conditions, so it is an ideal tool for laboratory tests, forensics, and diagnostics.

✓ **Checkpoint! 23.2**

If a gene encodes for a particular protein, why does it contain additional and unrelated sequences to the sequence that encodes for that protein's amino acid?

▶ **NUCLEIC ACID PROBES**

Based on the premise that a sequence of a stretch of DNA is highly specific for its final product (ie, a protein) and that nucleic acids interact with each other by the base pair relationships discussed in the preceding section, nucleic acid probes can be created to identify a particular stretch of DNA by synthesizing the "fishing" probe with a sequence that is complementary to the stretch of DNA of interest (1, 3). Think of the well-known childhood experiment that uses a magnet to bind to iron filings from an iron filing-sand mixture. Although this analogy may be overly simplistic, the basics are pretty much the same, that is, a nucleic acid probe with a

from DNA to protein). As the figure implies, control of protein synthesis can be regulated at any of the levels described from transcription to translation, although we do not discuss control of synthesis in this chapter.

The important message of this background is that the DNA sequence that encodes for a particular protein is uniquely

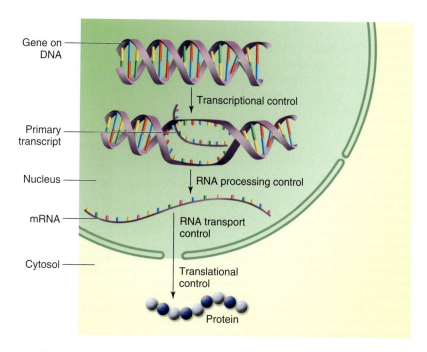

■ **FIGURE 23.6**   Sequence of events from DNA to protein.

particular sequence can be used to bind to and thus identify a complementary stretch of DNA. This approach called **hybridization** is a key process and the basis for several molecular biology techniques (1, 3). Obviously, the longer the probe, the higher the likelihood that it will be specific; in general, however, probes of at least 20 consecutive bases specific for a particular stretch of DNA have been shown to be highly specific for that stretch, and nonspecific binding of a 20+ bases probe to an unrelated stretch of DNA has been ruled extremely unlikely to occur. The first step in hybridization techniques is the denaturation (also called *melting*) of the DNA template with high temperature to break the hydrogen bonding between the complementary base pairs. Heat causes the separation of the two DNA strands by breaking all hydrogen bonds that hold the strands together; the temperature needed to achieve this varies depending on the particular sequence of DNA (for example, cytosine-guanine bonding with 3 hydrogen bonds is stronger than adenosine-thymine bonding with only 2 hydrogen bonds; therefore cytosine-guanine bonding requires more heat to be disrupted), the size of the DNA stretch to be denatured, and salt concentration. Boiling a DNA solution followed by quickly chilling it on ice (to avoid reannealing of the two strands) is often used to "unzip" the DNA strands and open them so that the probe can bind to its complementary sequence. Although hybridization can be carried in solution, the more common form of probe used in hybridization involves the use of a solid matrix to which the DNA to be analyzed is bound. DNA samples are attached to a solid matrix (eg, a membrane) and then are denatured by heat; specific nucleic acid probes labeled with either a radioactive or an enzyme label are then allowed to react with the denatured DNA. After washing the unbound material, the presence of radioactivity or the presence of the enzyme (by colorimetric methods after adding the appropriate substrate) is detected (3). The presence of the bound label indicates that the probe has hybridized to the sample DNA, which, in turn, reflects the presence of the specific DNA sequence in the sample. If the sample to be analyzed is on a tissue or cell, the hybridization technique is termed *in situ hybridization.*

▶ HYBRIDIZATION USING SOLID MATRICES

In its most basic and simplest form, solid matrix hybridization involves the application of a "dot" of a clinical sample to a membrane (for example, nitrocellulose) and the addition of a specific, labeled probe to the sample. After washing the unbound material, the dot is visualized by detecting the label on the probe. This **dot blot** assay is an all-or-none approach (ie, it is simply used to determine whether a particular sequence of DNA is present or absent in a sample). If the label is detected (either by radiographic or by colorimetric methods, depending on the type of label used), the probe has bound to the sample, indicating the presence of the DNA complementary to the probe in that sample (3).

Variations in DNA sequences can also be detected by a method called *restriction fragment length polymorphism* (RFLP) (4). In this method, DNA is first cut into smaller fragments using **restriction endonucleases,** which are enzymes that cut DNA at specific sequences. The fragments from this process are separated according to size by electrophoresis in an agarose gel in a similar manner to the separation of proteins by Western blotting (see Chapter 7). The size of the fragments (which can be labeled and thus visualized) obtained by such cutting depends on the DNA having the specific sequence where the specific endonuclease cuts. Knowledge of that sequence allows prediction of the size of the fragments; if a variation of such sequence should occur, the DNA would not be cut or the resulting fragments would be of different size. Consider an imaginary example: If we had a piece of DNA that is 1000 bases long and a particular enzyme cuts at base 850, such cutting should result in 2 pieces of DNA approximately 850 and 150 bases long, respectively. If the sequence of that DNA were different or altered (for example, in the case of a genetic disease that caused a mutation or an aberration at the site where a particular endonuclease cuts), the cutting by the endonuclease would either fail (ie, no cutting would occur) or result in pieces of different sizes than expected (ie, the sequence that the endonuclease recognizes is located at a different position). RFLP is not routinely used much anymore, but was an important tool in the mapping of various genes to detect genetic disorders and in evaluating genetic variations in a particular gene among different individuals. Refer to Figure 23.7 ■ for an example of an RFLP analysis of different genotypes using the HaeIII restriction endonuclease.

An additional development of solid matrix hybridization is a technique called *Southern blotting*. The name comes from Edwin Southern, the scientist who first described the technique (5). Using Southern blotting, high molecular weight DNA is first cut using restriction endonucleases into small fragments, which are then separated according to size by electrophoresis in an agarose gel. The separated components

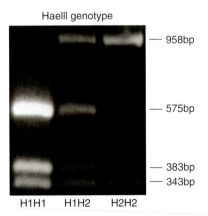

Haelll genotype

— 958bp

— 575bp

— 383bp
— 343bp

H1H1   H1H2   H2H2

■ **FIGURE 23.7** Restriction fragment-length polymorphisms showing different HaeIII genotypes in the β-fibrinogen gene in homozygous and heterozygous individuals.

are then transferred directly onto a nitrocellulose membrane, where they remain bound in the positions determined by the electrophoresis separation. Attachment to the membrane is achieved by treating it with high heat. The membrane is then "blocked," or treated with unrelated DNA (eg, DNA from fish sperm) to avoid nonspecific binding of the probe to the membrane. Labeled probes (either radioactive, enzyme, or fluorescent) specific for a particular DNA sequence are then allowed to react with the membrane, and if specific binding occurs, one or more fragments of the original DNA is labeled. The major difference between this technique and dot blotting is that Southern blotting determines whether a specific sequence is located only in one area of the DNA or is repeated on more than one fragment of that DNA.

As we described, gene expression results in the production of RNA; a hybridization method that can be used to detect specific RNA sequences is the *Northern blotting* method. The name is derived from the similarity of its method with Southern blotting: The only difference is that the target of analysis in Northern blotting is RNA rather than DNA (6). Once again, RNA is cut into small fragments using restriction enzymes, and the fragments are then separated by electrophoresis. After transferring the fragments onto a membrane, specific labeled probes are allowed to react with the membrane; specific RNA sequences are identified by the presence of the label on a particular fragment. Refer to Figure 23.8 ■ to see a sample radiograph of a Northern blot.

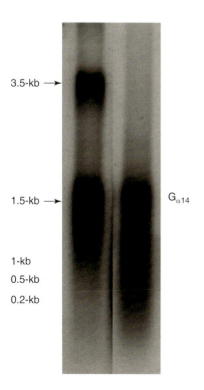

■ **FIGURE 23.8** Northern blot of the $G\alpha_{14}$ subunit in the salivary glands of a 1-week-old and a 4- to 6-week-old rat. *Source:* Dr. Olga J. Baker, University at Buffalo.

▶ *IN SITU* HYBRIDIZATION

In addition to identifying specific DNA sequences on DNA bound to an artificial solid matrix (such as a nylon or nitrocellulose membrane), nucleic acid probes can also be used to identify specific DNA sequences in a biological sample. This approach is called *in situ hybridization (ISH)* (3, 7). The principle is the same as that in other hybridization techniques; the source of the nucleic acid template just happens to be a biological specimen, either a piece of tissue or a cell, and the target could be either DNA or RNA. The first step in ISH is to treat the tissue or cell to fix the target nucleic acid and make it more accessible to the probe. Labeled probes (either DNA or RNA) are then allowed to react with the treated tissue or cell under high temperature to allow hybridization. The probes can be labeled with a radioactive, antigenic (for example, digoxigenin, or DIG, which can be visualized using a specific labeled antibody to it), biotin, or a fluorescent label. In the latter case, ISH using fluorescence is called, appropriately, *fluorescence in situ hybridization (FISH)* (3). A schematic representation of the methodology of FISH is shown in Figure 23.9 ■. ISH and FISH can be used to identify and localize either DNA or RNA in a particular tissue or cell, which in turn reflects the expression of the component encoded by that DNA or RNA in that particular tissue or cell. FISH can also be used to identify and study a particular gene in a particular chromosome. The availability of different types of labels (ie, radioactive, fluorescent, or enzymatic) allows the detection of different DNAs or RNAs within a particular tissue or cell. A picture of the use of FISH in interphase nuclei is shown in Figure 23.10 ■.

▶ SINGLE-STRAND CONFORMATIONAL POLYMORPHISM

Gene polymorphisms are alterations by which individuals may have variations in the same gene within the biological range. In a population, a genetic polymorphism is present when different forms of a gene at a given locus exist with a frequency of more than 1% to 2%. Single nucleotide polymorphisms (SNPs) are sites in the genome where the DNA sequence of many individuals differs by just a single base. About 10 million SNPs have been estimated in the human population with an estimated 2 common missense variations per gene. The great majority of SNPs are silent (ie, they do not cause any changes in the function of a particular gene or its product); however, in some cases, a SNP may be associated with an alteration (either structural or functional) of the molecule encoded by that gene. Therefore, studies of SNPs in different individuals or populations are important in both basic molecular biology and/or diagnostics. One technique used to detect SNPs is single-strand conformational polymorphism (SSCP) (8). Single base changes in a large fragment of DNA cannot be detected simply by gel electrophoresis because the difference

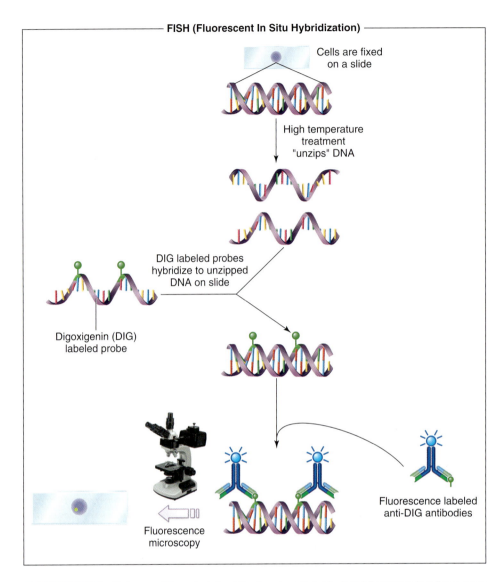

■ **FIGURE 23.9**   Scheme of the principle of the fluorescent *in situ* hybridization to localize a gene in the nucleus.

in the size of the dissimilar fragments from single base change is negligible. However, after being denatured, single-stranded DNA folds onto itself in a 3-dimensional structure during the renaturation process. The conformation of a single-stranded DNA depends on its DNA sequence, and any mutation even at a single nucleotide base can affect the 3-dimensional conformation of the strand. These single-stranded DNA molecules even with single nucleotide differences when separated by electrophoresis on a gel matrix under non-denaturing conditions migrate differently to keep their conformations intact. Therefore, genes of interest, for example, from individuals who are normal and disease suspects, can be amplified by PCR (described later in this chapter) and subjected to SSCP for diagnostic purposes. SSCP can indicate only that there is a difference between 2 fragments of DNA, and subsequent DNA sequencing is necessary to pinpoint the changes. SSCP is currently used in genotyping and in identifying different alleles

in homozygous and heterozygous subjects. It is also used in virology, especially in the study of viruses that have numerous and frequent genetic variations.

▶ MICROARRAYS

The techniques described in the preceding sections usually target a single DNA sequence, gene, or, at the most, a limited number of sequences or genes. However, in some situations, there is a need to analyze hundreds or even thousands of different DNA sequences or genes. This is where microarrays come into place. DNA microarrays, also known as *gene chips,* are solid matrices of various materials (eg, glass or silicone) to which hundreds, thousands, or even tens of thousands of different DNAs in minute quantities (either pieces of genes or specific sequences in picomole quantities) are

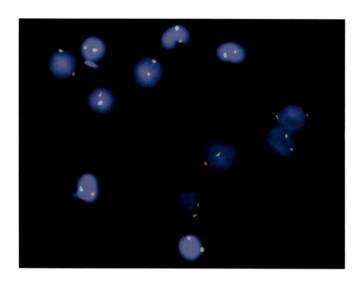

■ **FIGURE 23.10** Fluorescence *in situ* hybridization (FISH) is a cyto-genetic technique that is used to detect the presence or absence of specific DNA sequences on metaphase chromosomes or non-dividing (interphase) cells. FISH utilizes fluorescent DNA probes that bind to chromosomal regions with sequence complementarity. Shown here are interphase nuclei hybridized with probes for the repetitive sequences near the centromeres of the X (orange) and Y (green) chromosomes. The blue counterstain is used to identify nuclear material. *Source:* AnneMarie W. Block, PhD. Clinical Cytogenics Laboratory, Rosewell Park Cancer Institute.

chemically attached to different microscopic spots (9). Utilization of a microarray is a form of hybridization in which probes are attached to the matrix and the DNA sample to be tested is added to the matrix. Test samples of DNA (called *targets*) labeled with either fluorescent or chemiluminescent labels are then allowed to react with the probes on the chip; after washing the unbound material, the specific binding of the targets to a particular probe is evaluated. The binding strength of the particular target to its counterpart probe, in turn, depends on the target's complementarity to the probe. In other words, the closer the target sequence is to the complementary sequence of the probe, the more strongly the target binds to that probe. This, in turn, is a reflection of the homology of that target with the probe: the more similar the sequences between target and probe, the stronger is the binding. Such "strength" of binding results in a brighter fluorescence or chemiluminescence, which can be measured and quantitated by a machine. See Figure 23.11 ■ for the basic principle of a DNA microarray chip, Figure 23.12 ■ for a commercially available gene chip (Affymetrix), and Figure 23.13 ■ for a typical result obtained after target/probe reactions. Gene chips are used to detect different levels of expression of a particular DNA or RNA under different conditions, differences in sequence in a particular DNA segment or gene in health and disease, or in different individuals or to identify single-base differences known as *single nucleotide polymorphisms*.

▶ POLYMERASE CHAIN REACTION

In 1968, Kjell Kleppe and Gobing Khorana developed a method to amplify (ie, produce in large quantities) a specific DNA sequence. In 1983, Kary Mullis improved this method by which a particular piece or stretch of DNA could be "amplified" by making numerous (thousands to millions) identical copies of it (10). The advantage of this technique was the fact that having a large amount of the same stretch of DNA made its study and/or analysis easier. The technique requires deoxynucleotides (dNTP of the different DNA bases), a thermally stable DNA polymerase, short stretches of DNA called *oligonucleotide primers* (usually 10–30 base pairs long), and a thermal cycling machine (a thermocycler). The principle of the reaction is as follows: the area of the DNA that contains the sequence of interest is heated to "melt" or "unzip" the DNA; this is called the *denaturation step*. Specific oligonucleotide primers that flank the region to be amplified, one at the 3´ end of one of the DNA strands and the other at the 3´ end of the other antiparallel strand are then allowed to bind to their specific sequence on each "unzipped" strand. There is a "cooling" period when the primers are allowed to bind to the single strands of DNA; this is called the *annealing step* (3, 11). At this point, a temperature-stable DNA polymerase synthesizes a complementary DNA strand starting at the primers and using the open DNA strands as a template. The polymerase adds nucleotides, again following the sequence of the stretch of DNA that has been "unzipped." So, one strand is replicated in one direction and the other strand is replicated in the other direction, thus making a copy of each of the open strands in the *elongation step*. At this point, there are 2 copies of the DNA stretch: one for each strand. The entire process is then repeated by reheating the DNA, allowing the primers to bind to their specific sites again (which after the first cycle have now doubled), synthesizing 2 more copies of the DNA stretch (which, because they were doubled in the first cycle, now result in 4 copies of it), and then repeating the entire procedure of denaturating, annealing, elongating, and cooling numerous times to obtain exponential numbers of the DNA stretch to be amplified (3). The last step is to cool the entire reaction mixture to 5 to 15 degrees centigrade to store the final product for additional use. See Figure 23.14 ■ for a diagram of the principle of DNA amplification by PCR. The fragments of DNA obtained can then be visualized by staining them with ethidium bromide in an agarose gel (Figure 23.15 ■). PCR has many uses in molecular biology; for example, it can identify an organism that is difficult to grow in laboratory conditions or that is present in very low numbers. In Chapter 14, we mentioned the importance of genotyping for HLA components for selections of donor and recipients in transplantation; PCR plays a major role in this genotyping by identifying specific DNA sequences specific for a particular HLA genotype.

PCR can also be used to amplify stretches of RNA. The principle of amplification is the same except that in the case of RNA, an additional initial step is necessary before amplification. This involves the conversion of the target RNA into

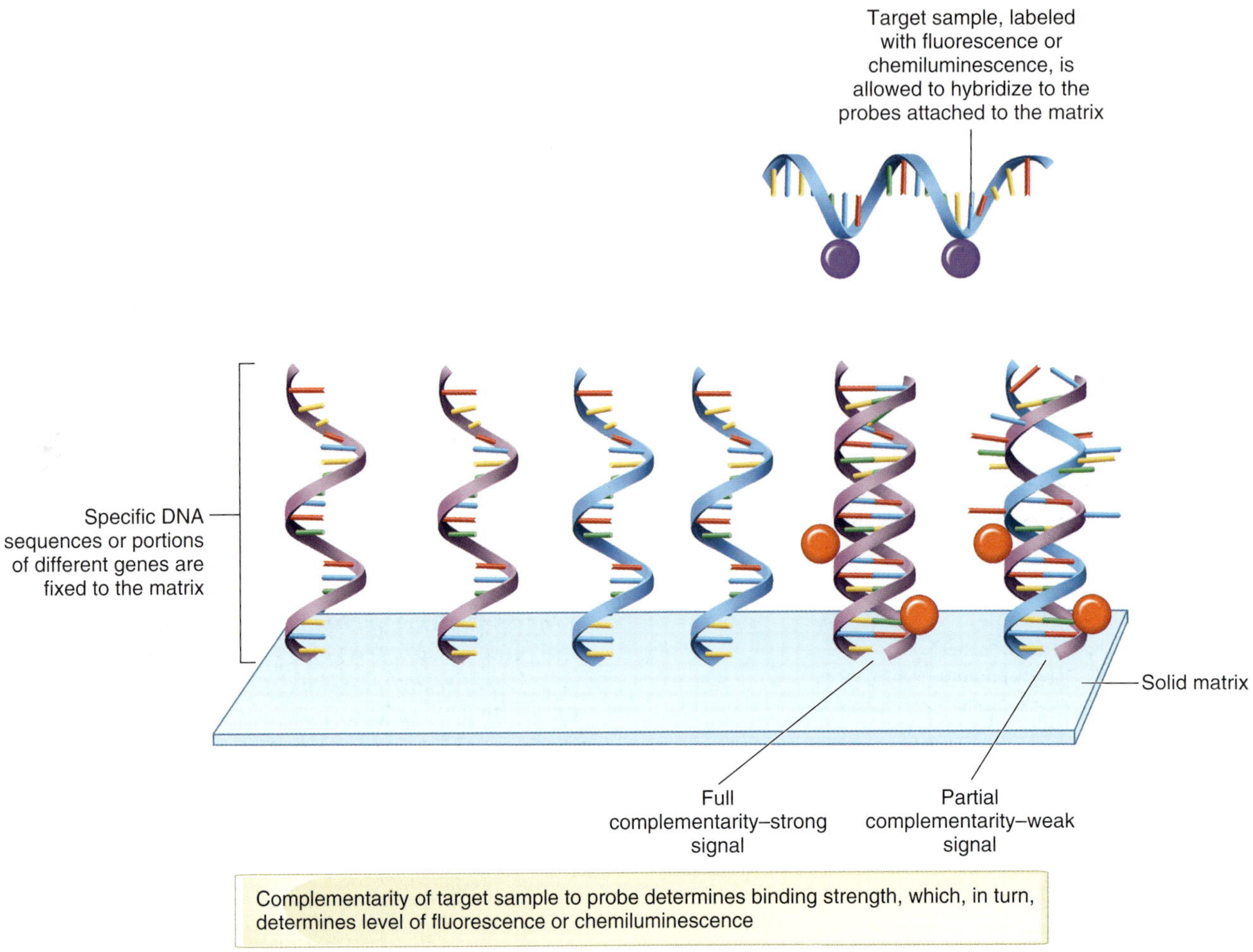

Target sample, labeled with fluorescence or chemiluminescence, is allowed to hybridize to the probes attached to the matrix
Specific DNA sequences or portions of different genes are fixed to the matrix
Solid matrix
Full complementarity–strong signal
Partial complementarity–weak signal
Complementarity of target sample to probe determines binding strength, which, in turn, determines level of fluorescence or chemiluminescence

■ **FIGURE 23.11** Basic principle of target-probe hybridization in microarray chips.

AFFYMETRIX
GeneChip®
Human Genome
U133 Plus 2.0

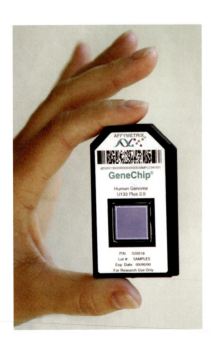

■ **FIGURE 23.12** An Affymetrix microarray gene chip. *Source:* Picture used with permission of Affymetrix, Inc., Santa Clara, CA.

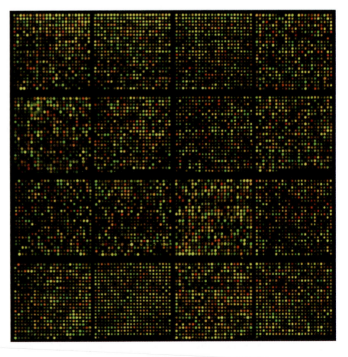

■ **FIGURE 23.13** Example of an approximately 37,500 probe-spotted oligo microarray. *Source:* National Cancer Institute.

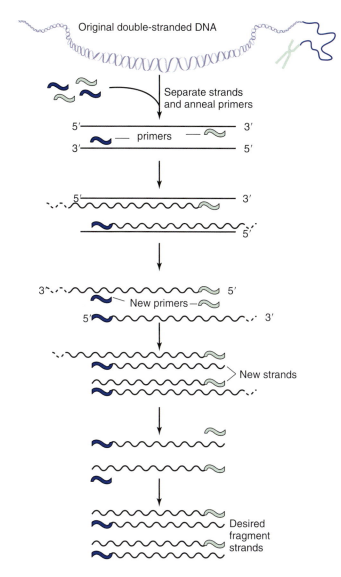

■ **FIGURE 23.14**   Principles of amplification of selected fragments of DNA by polymerase chain reaction cycling.

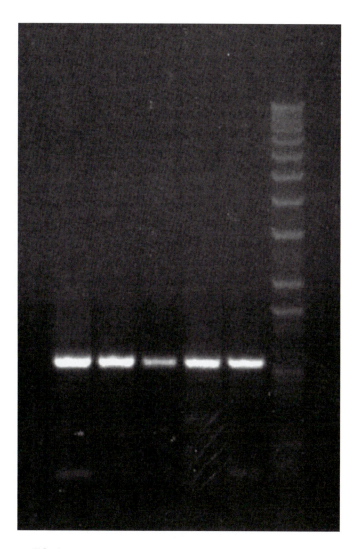

■ **FIGURE 23.15**   Simple amplification of 1kb DNA fragments by polymerase chain reaction.

DNA using reverse transcriptase, which is an enzyme that transcribes RNA into DNA. Thus, the technique is termed reverse transcriptase PCR, or RT-PCR (3,12). As we saw in Chapter 16, a classical example of the use of RT-PCR is the identification of viral RNA in HIV testing. RNA is extracted from an individual's plasma and allowed to react with a preparation of reverse transcriptase; this converts the viral RNA into cDNA. The polymerase chain reaction (PCR) is then used to amplify specific areas of the DNA that encode for specific viral genes. RT-PCR is also used to monitor gene expression because the production of RNA from the gene reflects the expression (in other words, the "turning on") of that particular gene. A more recent form of PCR is called the *"real-time" PCR,* which follows the same principles as conventional PCR; however, real-time PCR incorporates a fluorescent label into the amplified products so that the production of the products can be monitored and measured continuously in real time instead of waiting for the full number of thermal cycles to be completed. The amount of fluorescence detected is a reflection of the amount of product produced, which, in turn, can be quantitated. There are numerous variations of PCR, including asymmetric, allele-specific, nested, multiplex, overlap extension, intersequence-specific, and methylation-specific PCR, to name a few. It is not within the scope of this chapter to train the student in becoming an experienced molecular biologist; however, the interested reader can refer to the quintessential molecular biology manual, *Current Protocols in Molecular Biology* (3).

✓ **Checkpoint! 23.3**

A colleague in the lab wants to use a standard PCR to identify certain nucleic acid sequences from a retrovirus. You agree to the approach but suggest that RT-PCR be used instead. Why?

► NON-PCR AMPLIFICATION

Amplification techniques that can be carried out at constant temperatures are also available, and have the advantage of not necessitating a thermocycler. An example of such an approach is the nucleic acid sequence-based amplification (NASBA) (13, 14). NASBA is used to amplify sequences of RNA and can be performed at a constant temperature (41° C). NASBA shows results more quickly than PCR and in certain cases it can also be more sensitive. In NASBA, a specific primer is allowed to bind to the 3´ end of the RNA template to be amplified. Reverse transcriptase then synthesizes the complementary DNA sequence. At this point, an enzyme called *RNAse-H*, which degrades RNA but not DNA, is added to the RNA-DNA complex, resulting in a single DNA strand. A second primer, containing a binding site for T7 RNA polymerase, is then allowed to bind to the 5´ end of the DNA strand; T7 RNA polymerase is an enzyme that promotes the synthesis of RNA in a 5´ to 3´ direction. The addition of the second primer creates a double-stranded DNA that contains the binding site for T7 RNA polymerase. The addition of T7 RNA polymerase creates a complementary RNA sequence, which can then be used as a template like the original RNA template. The cycle is then repeated. NASBA is used in the diagnosis of various viral agents including influenza A, coronavirus, and HIV.

Another sensitive method often used in the detection of retroviruses such as HIV is the branched DNA test (bDNA) (15, 16) or Quantiplex bDNA test (see also Chapter 16). In this test, after viral particle disruption and the release of viral RNA, special oligonucleotides (label extenders and capture extenders) are added and bind to viral RNA and to certain oligonucleotides bound to the wall of a microtiter plate or vessel. This immobilizes the target RNA to the vessel; because the target RNA is immobilized against the vessel walls, washing unbound materials can be done easily to reduce false positive results. A different set of oligonucleotides is then added and bind at several locations to this RNA; then other oligonucleotides that bind at several locations to those previous oligonucleotides are added. This creates a large complex (ie, "branches") that amplifies the signal. Finally, enzyme-labeled oligonucleotides that bind to the last set of oligonucleotides are added; the presence and amount of the enzyme can be detected by a color reaction, which allows quantification of the viral RNA in the original sample.

► PROS AND CONS OF AMPLIFICATION TECHNIQUES

The advent of molecular biology techniques in the study of nucleic acids has been a milestone for both basic research and diagnosis. In particular, amplification techniques, both PCR based and not, have provided the ability to identify a very minute quantity of target nucleic acids, both DNA and RNA.

Unfortunately, because of their very nature, amplification techniques have been a double-edged sword because any potential contaminant nucleic acid, even in minute quantities, can be amplified by error and, thus, create false positive results. Contaminants can come from poor specimen handling, unrelated samples, or even from an operator. Therefore, very careful procedures and quality assessment must be observed in all cases. One must also remember that these techniques detect the presence of nucleic acids; the significance of the results are then conceptually extrapolated to the presence and nature of a particular microorganism and, in turn, a particular clinical condition. However, the mere presence of a minute amount of a nucleic acid in a sample may or may not necessarily indicate a live organism in that sample and, in turn, may or may not necessarily reflect an ongoing clinical condition. Finally, many clinical conditions associated with a particular microorganism may require a certain threshold or minimal number of such organisms for colonization and subsequent infection; because amplification techniques can detect very minute amounts of nucleic acids, even if those amounts are associated with live organisms, such organisms may be in such low numbers that they may not necessarily have biological relevance. Taking all aspects into consideration, however, molecular biology techniques have been a powerful tool for several years in both research and clinical laboratories.

 Checkpoint! 23.4

The same colleague in Checkpoint 23.3 is complaining that when carrying out a standard PCR on a patient's sample, she obtained an amplified DNA product even in the negative control tube (ie, no template DNA). You notice that the samples were not handled properly and she wasn't wearing any gloves. What do you suspect is the problem?

 CASE STUDY 1

Katie is an immunologist who is just learning molecular biology techniques. She is working at a police lab and is trying to design a technique to show that penetration in rape cases occurred. She has an idea that a probe for the Y chromosome could be used right on the cells from a vaginal swab to prove penetration by showing the presence of the Y chromosome. She wants to look up protocols about how to do this technique, but she cannot remember what this type of assay is called.

1. What test is she thinking about?

2. How is the technique for this test performed?

CASE STUDY 2

You work in a rural laboratory and until recently, the material for molecular techniques ordered for patient diagnosis was sent to a different laboratory. Your lab just received a thermocycler, so now you should be able to perform some of these tests in house after you develop skills need to use it.

1. What assays can you now perform because you have a thermocycler?

2. Name a clinical technique mentioned in this chapter that utilizes PCR.

3. Name a clinical technique mentioned in this chapter that utilizes RT-PCR.

SUMMARY

By their very nature of being blueprints for biological molecules, nucleic acids have been powerful tools in the identification and study of the molecules they encode, and, by extrapolation, the biological entities that are associated with those molecules. Because of the nature of the interaction among nucleic acids, nucleic acid probes can be used in a process called *hybridization* to find and/or identify stretches of DNA and/or RNA that are complementary to those probes. Several techniques follow this principle: in the simplest form, the dot-blot, labeled probes are used to detect the presence or absence of a particular stretch of nucleic acid in a sample. Southern blots allow the identification of a DNA stretch in a sample and the number of copies of that DNA stretch in a sample of DNA that has been broken into smaller pieces. This approach can also be applied to RNA by using a technique called Northern blot. Variation in sequences in DNA can also be detected using restriction fragment-length polymorphism; in this technique, specific endonucleases that cut at specific sequences are used to obtain fragments of DNA whose size can be predicted by the position at which a particular endonuclease cuts. Variations of sequences at that position result in different size fragments. Hybridization techniques with nucleic acid probes can also be performed directly on biological specimens such as tissues or cells. This approach is called *in situ hybridization,* and can be used to detect and monitor either DNA or RNA in that particular specimen. Hybridization techniques can also be performed on a very large scale by using thousands of different DNA probes to study a DNA sample. This approach is usually performed using microarrays or gene "chips" to which a very large number of DNA probes are attached in microscopic spots. The sample of DNA to be tested is then allowed to react with the different probes and, based on the complementarity of the sample to the probes, the "strength" of binding of the DNA to the probe can be quantitated. Gene chips are used to detect different levels of expression of a particular DNA or RNA under various conditions, differences in sequence in a particular DNA segment or gene in health and disease, and single nucleotide polymorphisms. Very commonly used techniques involve the amplification of a target DNA to obtain large quantities (many copies) of it. The quintessential DNA amplification method is the polymerase chain reaction, or PCR, which can also be used to amplify sequences of RNA using reverse transcriptase in a variation of technique called *RT-PCR.* PCR can also be monitored during the series of amplification reactions in real time by using a technique appropriately called *real-time PCR.* Amplification techniques can also be performed at constant temperatures, thus eliminating the need for a thermocycler. These include the nucleic acid sequence-based amplification (NASBA) and the branched DNA test. Although being powerful tools, amplification techniques can be prone to providing false positives because of the possible presence of minute amounts of contaminants. In addition, because amplification techniques detect the mere presence of a particular nucleic acid sequence, caution must be exerted in interpreting the real biological significance of such presence in a biological sample.

REVIEW QUESTIONS

1. The process of copying a sequence of DNA into RNA is known as
   a. translation
   b. transcription
   c. transition
   d. transformation

2. The generation of an amino acid sequence from a sequence of mRNA is known as
   a. transcription
   b. translation
   c. replication
   d. restriction

3. The groups of nucleotide triples encoding for a specific amino acid is called a
   a. intron
   b. codon
   c. exon
   d. histone

4. The binding of a nucleic acid probe to its complementary sequence on a target nucleic acid is a process called
   a. transition
   b. replication
   c. hybridization
   d. resolution

REVIEW QUESTIONS (*continued*)

5. The most basic and simplest form of solid matrix hybridization that does *not* require separation of different fragments of nucleic acids is the
   a. Northern blot
   b. dot blot
   c. Southern blot
   d. Western blot

6. An alteration in the nucleic acid sequence where specific restriction endonuclease cuts can be detected by using
   a. Western blot
   b. dot blot
   c. RFLP
   d. FISH

7. The identification of a particular sequence of nucleic acid on a solid biological sample such as a cell or tissue can be accomplished by the use of
   a. Northern blot
   b. RFLP
   c. FISH
   d. Southern blot

8. The major advantage of microarrays is that they allow
   a. detection of both DNA and RNA
   b. analysis of a very large number of target sequences
   c. identification of introns in a sample of genomic DNA
   d. separation of different fragments of nucleic acids according to their molecular size

9. The amplification of a target sequence to obtain large amounts of that sequence can be achieved by using
   a. Northern blot
   b. PCR
   c. FISH
   d. dot blot

REFERENCES

1. Alberts B, Johnson A, Lewis J, et al. *Molecular Biology of the Cell.* 5th ed. New York: Garland Science, Taylor & Francis Group. 2008; 538–539.

2. Watson JD, Crick FHC. A structure for deoxyribose nucleic acid. *Nature.* 1953;171(4356):737–738.

3. Ausubel FM, Brent R, Kingston RE, et al., eds. *Current Protocols in Molecular Biology.* New York: Wiley. 2011:1934–3639.

4. Saiki, RK, Scharf S, Faloona F, et al. Enzymatic amplification of beta-globin genomic sequences and restriction site analysis for diagnosis of sickle cell anemia. *Science.* 1985;230:1350–1354.

5. Southern EM. Detection of specific sequences among DNA fragments separated by gel electrophoresis. *J. Molec. Biol.* 1975;98:503–517.

6. Alwine JC, Kemp DJ, Stark GR. Method for detection of specific RNAs in agarose gels by transfer to diazobenzyloxymethyl-paper and hybridization with DNA probes. *Proc. Natl. Acad. Sci. U.S.A.* 1977;74:5350–5354.

7. Jin L, Lloyd RV. In situ hybridization: Methods and applications. *J. Clin. Lab. Analysis.*1997;11:2–9.

8. Kubo KS, Stuart RM, Freitas-Astúa J, et al. Evaluation of the genetic variability of orchid fleck virus by single-strand conformational polymorphism analysis and nucleotide sequencing of a fragment from the nucleocapsid gene. *Arch Virol.* 2009;154:1009–1011.

9. Schena M, Shalon D, Davis RW, et al. Quantitative monitoring of gene expression patterns with a complementary cDNA microarray. *Science.* 1995;270:467–470.

10. Bartlett, Stirling. A short history of the polymerase chain reaction. *Methods Mol Biol.* 2003;226:3–6.

11. Rychlik W, Spencer WJ, Rhoads RE. Optimization of the annealing temperature for DNA amplification in vitro. *Nucleic Acids Res.* 1990;18:6409–6412.

12. Bustin SA. Absolute quantification of mRNA using real-time reverse transcription polymerase chain reaction assays. *J. Mol. Endocrinol.* 2000;25:169–193.

13. Compton J. Nucleic acid sequence-based amplification. *Nature.* 1991;350:91–92.

14. Kievits T, Van Gemen B, Van Strijp D, et al. NASBA isothermal enzymatic in vitro nucleic acid amplification optimized for the diagnosis of HIV-1 infection. *J Virological Met.*1991;35:273–286.

15. Collins ML, Irvine B, Tyner D, et al. A branched DNA signal amplification assay for quantification of nucleic acid targets below 100 molecules/ml. *Nucleic Acids Research.* 1997;25:2979–2984.

16. Murphy DG, Gonin P, Fauvel M. Reproducibility and performance of the second-generation branched-DNA assay in routine quantification of human immunodeficiency virus type 1 RNA in plasma. *J Clin Microbiol.* 1999;37:812–814.

PEARSON myhealthprofessionskit™

Visit www.myhealthprofessionskit.com to access the interactive Companion Website for this textbook. Simply select "Clinical Laboratory Science" from the choice of disciplines. Find this book and log in by using your user name and password to access additional learning tools.

ANSWERS TO REVIEW QUESTIONS

✔

CHAPTER 1
1. b
2. b
3. a
4. b
5. d
6. b
7. b
8. d
9. d
10. c
11. c
12. d
13. d
14. c
15. b
16. d

CHAPTER 2
1. a
2. a
3. d
4. c
5. a
6. d
7. c
8. a
9. d
10. d
11. a
12. c
13. b
14. b
15. c
16. c
17. b
18. b
19. a

CHAPTER 3
1. c
2. d
3. a
4. d
5. d
6. b
7. a
8. d
9. a
10. c
11. c
12. a
13. b
14. c
15. d

CHAPTER 4
1. b
2. d
3. a
4. a
5. b
6. a
7. c
8. d
9. b
10. a
11. d

CHAPTER 5
1. c
2. c
3. b
4. d
5. c
6. a
7. a
8. c
9. a
10. d
11. a
12. b
13. a
14. c
15. a
16. c
17. b
18. b
19. d
20. a
21. b
22. d
23. b

CHAPTER 6
1. b
2. b
3. b
4. d
5. a
6. b
7. c
8. b
9. b
10. c
11. b
12. a

CHAPTER 7
1. d
2. b
3. b
4. c
5. a
6. c
7. c
8. d

9. c
10. a

CHAPTER 8
1. d
2. c
3. a
4. b
5. c
6. c
7. a
8. d
9. b
10. c
11. d

CHAPTER 9
1. b
2. d
3. b
4. b
5. a
6. b
7. b
8. d
9. b
10. d

CHAPTER 10
1. c
2. a
3. c
4. b
5. d
6. d
7. b
8. d
9. c
10. d

CHAPTER 11
1. d
2. c
3. d
4. b
5. b
6. d
7. b
8. a
9. a
10. d
11. c
12. d

CHAPTER 12 ✕
1. b
2. c
3. d
4. a

5. b
6. c
7. d
8. d
9. a
10. b
11. c
12. b
13. d
14. a
15. d
16. b
17. d
18. a
19. d
20. d

CHAPTER 13
1. d
2. d
3. b
4. d
5. c
6. a
7. a
8. d
9. a
10. d

CHAPTER 14
1. a
2. b
3. b
4. c
5. d
6. d
7. b
8. a
9. b
10. a
11. b

CHAPTER 15
1. b
2. d
3. c
4. b
5. d
6. c
7. c
8. b
9. b
10. b

CHAPTER 16
1. b
2. b
3. d
4. a

5. b
6. d
7. c
8. a
9. a

CHAPTER 17
1. b
2. a
3. c
4. d
5. b
6. a
7. b
8. a
9. d
10. b
11. d
12. c

CHAPTER 18
1. b
2. d
3. b
4. a
5. d
6. c
7. d
8. c
9. d
10. c
11. a
12. a
13. d
14. c
15. d
16. d
17. d
18. b
19. d
20. d

CHAPTER 19
1. T
2. T
3. T
4. T
5. F
6. b
7. b
8. d
9. d
10. d
11. d
12. a
13. a
14. d
15. a
16. b

17. d
18. d
19. d
20. d

CHAPTER 20
1. b
2. d
3. b
4. c
5. d
6. c
7. d
8. d
9. c
10. d
11. b
12. d
13. d
14. b
15. c

CHAPTER 21
1. c
2. d
3. a
4. c
5. b
6. c
7. c
8. b
9. b
10. a
11. d
12. d

CHAPTER 22
1. b
2. d
3. d
4. c
5. d
6. a
7. b
8. d
9. c
10. d

CHAPTER 23
1. b
2. b
3. b
4. c
5. b
6. c
7. c
8. b
9. b

ANSWERS TO CASE STUDIES

CHAPTER 1

1. skin
2. inflammation
3. neutrophils first and then macrophage

CHAPTER 2

1. IgG
2. The baby was infected with respiratory syncytial virus.
3. IgA
4. IgE

CHAPTER 3

1. The component used for the vaccination may share some antigenic determinants (epitopes) with components of the participant's red blood cells, causing a cross-reactive reaction, which, in turn, causes cellular damage of these cells.
2. The antibody response obtained is probably generated to a linear determinant of the component of the organism. This determinant may be exposed after biochemical treatment (boiling and detergent treatment) of the component but may not be exposed in the entire live organism (ie, may be hidden in a folded form of the protein from which it is derived) and thus is not accessible to antibodies generated against the denatured peptide.
3. An immunologic adjuvant can only increase the response to a component that, by itself, is immunogenic (ie, one that can induce an immune response in a host). An adjuvant cannot make a nonimmunogenic component immunogenic. In this case, the compound used is probably too small (in terms of molecular size) and not chemically complex enough to be immunogenic.
4. One possibility is to link the hapten compound covalently to a large, immunogenic component (carrier) such as a large protein and use that as the immunogen. The host animal will make antibodies to various different antigenic determinants of the protein as well as to the compound itself. Once that occurs, the antibodies specific for the small compound can then be isolated and used for the development of the kit.

CHAPTER 5

1. It appears that my serum did not contain a good source of complement.
2. The classical pathway
3. By using a CH50
4. By using an AH50
5. C1, C4, or C2
6. Radial immunodiffusion

CHAPTER 6

1. After the antigen-coated beads are added to the patient's serum, you can add anti-human immunoglobulin to cross-link the human antibody bound to the antigen on the beads.
2. The pH of the reaction is important because it affects the charge. The charge on the particle is the particle's zeta potential. Decreasing the charge or zeta potential would increase the apparent titer because it would take less immunoglobulin to hold these less charged particles together. To improve binding of charged particles (1) use low ionic strength media to decrease charge (LISS), (2) use increased viscosity media to decrease the water of hydration, (3) alter the temperature to improve antibody binding, (IgM antibodies agglutinate best between 4° and 27° C, and IgG antibodies agglutinate best at 37° C.) (4) treat the red cells with enzymes to decrease surface charge, and (5) add agitation or centrifugation to increase interaction.

CHAPTER 7

1. The patient may have rheumatoid factor. This antibody would bind the first antibody which captures IgM, and then although it did not bind the antigen, it bound the Fc of the enzyme labeled IgG to the pathogen. Then the enzyme reacted with the substrate and gave a positive result.
2. The patient's serum could be diluted with a solution that contains IgG that does not react with the pathogen. In this case, the rheumatoid factor would bind to the IgG in solution and would not become involved in the solid-phase assay.

CHAPTER 8

1. For Test A, 98% sensitive means that of every 100 people tested who were positive, 2 people test negative even though they are positive.

   For Test B, 90% sensitive means for every 100 people tested who were positive, 10 people test negative even though they are positive.

   Both tests are 99.9% specific, which means that for every 1000 people who are not pregnant, 1 tests positive.

   Now that you know what this means you can decide which to purchase.

CHAPTER 9

1. Type I hypersensitivity
2. Lauren may need epinephrine because she has just been exposed to something to which she has a severe allergy.

3. It would probably be less because an immune reaction to parasites involves the production of IgE; because of the large number of parasites that have infected Lauren, her IgE levels against them are high. This, in turn, translates into fewer IgE binding sites on mast cells that are available to bind IgE generated against the food allergen. This, in turn, results in a less severe reaction. However, each allergic reaction can result in increases in the amount of IgE produced and could also play a role, so she should make sure to have the epinephrine pen handy!

CHAPTER 10

1. The ANA testing should be repeated on serial dilutions of this sample to determine the titer. Positivity at higher titers would decrease the likelihood that this was a false positive reaction.

   If clinical signs and symptoms exist and the titer is relevant to further testing, the serum should be screened to determine with which antigen the serum reacts. A speckled pattern can result from reactivity to either saline-extractable antigens, Sm, SS-A, SS-B, SCl-70, or RNP. Enzyme immunoassays should be performed against these antigens. Reactivity with saline extractable antigens or Sm indicates that your professor has SLE, reactivity with SS-A, SS-B indicates Sjogrens Syndrome, whereas reactivity with SCl-70 indicates that she has progressive systemic sclerosis, and finally reactivity with RNP would indicate that she has mixed connective tissue disease or SLE.

CHAPTER 11

CASE STUDY 1
1. Myasthenia gravis
2. Antibody to the acetylcholine receptor
3. Treatment should be with acetylcholinesterase inhibitors to increase the concentration of acetylcholine within the neuromuscular junction. Patients can be treated with immunosuppressive drugs, such as glucocorticoids. In severe generalized myasthenia gravis, particularly with respiratory failure, plasmapheresis is performed to decrease acetylcholinesterase receptor antibody titers.

CASE STUDY 2
1. Graves disease
2. Hashimoto's disease
3. Your husband should be checked for thyroid-stimulating immunoglobulin (TSI). You should be checked for thyroglobulin and thyroperoxidase antibodies.

CHAPTER 12
1. CEA
2. CEA
3. The lymph nodes did not show any CEA staining.
4. Breast, lung, pancreas, stomach, and ovarian
5. No

CHAPTER 13

CASE STUDY 1
1. MGUS
2. Mr. Grime's risk of subsequently developing multiple myeloma should be explained to him and he should be told the signs and symptoms of multiple myeloma so that he can monitor his progression if necessary. He should also have a checkup periodically to determine whether progression has occurred.
3. Individuals who are at least 80 years of age are more likely to have MGUS because the incidence increases with age. Individuals who are male and who are black are also more likely to have this disease.

CASE STUDY 2
1. Hodgkin's lymphoma
2. Reed-Sternberg cells
3. There is a good prognosis, with about a 90% survival rate for stage I or II patients.

CHAPTER 14

1. First, Mr. Stearn's ABO type should be identified; his HLA should be typed using PCR, and he should be tested for antibodies to other HLA antigens by multiplexing. CMV reactivity should also be determined.
2. General health clearance should be performed of the possible donors to determine whether they are healthy enough to donate and their kidneys healthy enough to be donated. Infectious disease testing for hepatitis B, hepatitis C, HIV, Human T Lymphotropic Virus (HTLV), and West Nile virus (WNV) should be performed. Following these "background" tests, ABO and HLA typing and then cross-matching should be performed.

CHAPTER 15

1. They probably had X-linked agammaglobulinemia (also called Bruton agammaglobulinemia).
2. He would not have any tonsils.
3. You could determine the presence or absence of serum immunoglobulin.

4. This is an X-linked recessive disease, so the architect has a 50% chance of being a carrier. If the architect is a carrier and has a son, there is a 50% chance that he would have the disease. Further, if the architect is a carrier and has a daughter, the daughter would have a 50% chance of being a carrier also but would not have the disease.

5. He could receive passive transfer of immunoglobulin and antibiotics when he was sick.

CHAPTER 16

1. A screening test for anti-HIV antibody should be performed.

2. The CDC recommends that a positive ELISA test should be confirmed by a second and third identical ELISA test on the same individual. If two of the three test results are positive, a confirmatory test must be performed

3. HIV-infected individuals develop anti-HIV antibodies within 30 to 60 days after exposure, and almost 100% of infected individuals show antibodies to HIV 3 months after infection. Therefore, the women who had their last potentially infectious relationship more than 3 months prior to the testing do not need to be tested again unless they have other experiences that put them at risk. The two women who had this high risk exposure between 1 and 3 months ago should be retested until 3 months have passed between their encounter and the testing. The woman with the exposure this morning could receive prophylactic treatment to reduce her risk of seroconversion.

4. A Western blot should be used as a confirmatory test. The CDC has suggested that reactivity against *2* of the following viral components can be considered a positive confirmatory test: p24, p31, gp41, and gp120/160. If the test shows less than these requirements, it is considered intermediate and should be repeated later.

5. Monitoring the CD4+ count is essential in determining both the level and course of HIV infection as well as the development of AIDS. The CDC uses CD4+ T-cell counts as one of the major parameters in its classification system for HIV-infected individuals.

6. Quantitative nucleic acid testing can be used to determine whether the antivirals are working.

7. Genotyping of targeted mutations in the genes of viral components that have been associated with resistance of the virus to antiviral drugs can be performed to select the best therapy. Examples of mutations targeted are M41L, K103N, V108I, and T215F for reverse transcriptase and Q58E, L63P, V77I, and L90M for protease.

CHAPTER 17

1. She ate undercooked seafood in an area associated primarily with hepatitis A and hepatitis E, which are both fecal-oral associated. In addition, because she worked with blood and body fluid samples in a clinical laboratory scientist program, she could have been exposed to either hepatitis B or C bloodborne virus. However, Meghan does not remember any incident in the laboratory in which she had body fluid exposure.

2. Assays for IgM anti-HAV, IgM anti-HBcAg, HBsAg, and anti-HCV should be performed.

3. Individuals with known exposure to hepatitis A virus can receive either an injection of immune globulin; exposed individuals who are 1 to 40 years old can receive the hepatitis A vaccine. The vaccine is the preferred choice because it would also protect the individual from any subsequent exposure. The groups who should receive the postexposure prophylaxis include household and sex contacts of individuals with confirmed cases of hepatitis A and those who have close personal contact such as child care workers and physical attendants. So, you should receive the vaccine. This is a nationally reportable disease and should be reported. Meghan should rest and be observed to determine whether she will need hospitalization. She should also complete her hepatitis B series.

CHAPTER 18

CASE STUDY 1

1. Yes, she does: There is agglutination in the presumptive well and the well after guinea pig kidney absorption but no agglutination after absorption with bovine erythrocytes.

2. You may have had a mild infectious mononucleosis infection when you were young, and then you would be immune and not be sick now. Many U.S. children have relatively mild EBV infections early in life. Even when people are infected with EBV during the teenage years or early adulthood, infectious mononucleosis instead of mild or asymptomatic disease develops in only 35% to 50% of the cases.

CASE STUDY 2

1. Mumps

2. Patients are contagious 1 to 2 days before the swelling begins and up to 5 days after the swelling is apparent, so Sally was contagious when she gave you the rest of her sundae and you used her spoon. Although you were vaccinated when you were a baby and when you were 4, the protection after one vaccination is estimated to be 61% to 91% and after two injections, it is 76% to 95%. There are slight antigenic variations in different strains of mumps, and although they all are antigenically similar and protection usually occurs, slight differences may yield less than complete vaccine efficacy.

CHAPTER 19

CASE STUDY 1

1. Her mother thought she had strep throat.

2. Her mother thought that Anna could get rheumatic fever if she did not receive treatment.

3. Two throat swabs should be performed, one for culture and one for use in a rapid strep test. The culture can take up to 48 hours. The rapid strep test is an immunological assay in which the antigens of the streptococcus are extracted, bind to an antibody labeled with a colored colloid, and travel up the chromatography strip to be bound to a capture antibody that will yield a positive line. This rapid test often takes only 3 minutes.
4. Anna should receive erythromycin to treat her infection.

CASE STUDY 2

1. *Helicobacter pylori*
2. Damage to the stomach can result from a combination of bacterial products, inflammatory responses, and fluctuations of gastric acid levels.
3. Assessing IgG antibodies against *H. pylori* in an infected individual can be performed by different immunological methods, including ELISA, latex bead agglutination, immunodot blot, and quick tests using flow-through immunomembrane technology. However, the most common method is ELISA. Because *H. pylori* is antigenically variable, several antigens from a wide variety of different *H. pylori* strains are used as targets. Common antigens against which infected individuals produce antibodies are vacuolating cytotoxin A (VacA) and CagA protein.
4. Treatment involves the use of proton pump inhibitors and antibiotic regimens until the organism is eradicated.

CASE STUDY 3

1. *Clostridium difficile*
2. Enzyme-linked assays are now available for the detection of both Toxin A and Toxin B from *C. difficile*. ELISA testing is also used to monitor the elimination of the toxins from the stools, to evaluate the effectiveness of treatment. Rapid immunochromatography assays are also available for these toxins. Real-time PCR can be used as can "loop-mediated isothermal DNA amplification" (LAMP).

CASE STUDY 4

1. The rash was a "bull's-eye rash" called erythema migrans.
2. Lyme disease analysis is performed using the third generation ELISA in which a single peptide is used as coating antigen which represents the immunodominant region of a Borrelia protein.

CHAPTER 20

CASE STUDY 1

1. Invasive aspergillosis
2. Invasive aspergillosis patients are generally too immunocompromised to make antibodies, but antigen detection can be utilized regardless of the patient's immune status. The antigens used in screening for *Aspergillus* infections are two carbohydrate antigens, galactomannan and b-glucan. A sandwich enzyme immunoassay is used for antigen detection and can detect to about 0.5 ng/ml of the antigen.

3. For treatment of invasive aspergillosis, antifungal agents such as voriconazole, posaconazole, and amphotericin B should be used. Because Ariel is immunosuppressed due to the anti-TNF therapy, it would be reasonable to discontinue the immunosuppressive treatment until the infection is eliminated.

CASE STUDY 2

1. *Toxoplasmosis gondii*
2. A protozoan parasite
3. Toxoplasmosis is diagnosed with a serological test in an indirect enzyme immunoassay measuring avidity of antibody and IgM levels or by observing a high titer of IgG when looking for a current infection and by testing for IgG levels when looking for immunity. Serologically differentiating a primary infection of toxoplasmosis from a past infection is complicated. IgM levels are unusual in toxoplasmosis in that IgM remains detectable for up to 2 years following primary infection. IgA to toxoplasma remains elevated for up to 4 years, and paired titer IgG levels can be difficult because the patient may already have high titers at the first blood draw. Measurement of the avidity of the IgG provides data that help determine a present from a past infection. The avidity of IgG increases with time, and in toxoplasmosis, the avidity of the IgG antibody remains low for the first few months. Low avidity IgG antibody indicates that the patient has had toxoplasmosis within the last 8 months, and the presence of high avidity antibody indicates that the patient's infection was 5 or more months before testing. Past versus present infection is of key diagnostic importance when testing a pregnant woman. Avidity is assessed using two parallel enzyme immunoassays; the serum in both is incubated with the antigen, one is washed with a buffer, and one is washed with the buffer containing small amounts of urea. This urea will dissociate low avidity antibody, but high avidity antibody will remain attached to the antigen. The optical density of the set washed with urea is divided by the optical density of the set without urea to give an avidity index. An avidity index of more than 0.25 indicates that high avidity antibody is present. The Focus Diagnostic™ test kit performed this way demonstrates that 100% of recent infections show low avidity whereas 100% of the past infections show high avidity. A positive low avidity antibody test in a pregnant woman would indicate that antimicrobials targeting *Toxoplasma gondii* should be used.
4. Toxoplasmosis is transmitted to an infant *in utero* only by a primary infection. Belle probably had been infected earlier with risk factors including her European origins, her responsibilities in changing the litter box throughout her life, and her love of the steak tartare dish made with raw meat.
5. Half of the babies infected *in utero* are born prematurely, and their eyes, ears, nervous system, and skin can be affected. Some of the babies will have obvious signs of infection at birth, but others who are more mildly infected will not show signs of infection until later.

Almost all will develop some signs of infection, especially eye damage, by adolescence. Babies born with symptoms can show eye damage as the result of damage to the retina; in addition, they can have feeding problems, diarrhea and vomiting, hearing loss, enlarged liver and spleen, jaundice, skin rash, and low birth weight.

6. This is up to you, but definitely not if you are pregnant because toxoplasmosis can be acquired from raw meat.

CHAPTER 21

1. It will perform a test for hemoglobin, probably using a colloid-labeled immunochromatographic sandwich assay.

2. Two tests utilized for species identification are the ring precipitin test and crossover electrophoresis analysis. The antiserum chosen will contain antibodies directed against antigens found on the cells of the species in question. For example, if the forensic scientist is trying to determine whether the dried red stain is human blood, anti-human antiserum is used. In this case, anti-pig antiserum would also be used. Crossover electrophoresis is another method that can be used to determine the animal species from which the bloodstain originated from.

CHAPTER 22

1. (a) Cluttered work surfaces should be avoided; more importantly, extreme care must be taken to avoid open flames, such as the one in the picture, near flammable chemicals such as acetone. (This picture was taken using an empty and well-rinsed acetone bottle partially filled with water.)

   (b) Hypodermic needles and related equipment should never be left uncapped or unguarded and should be disposed of immediately after use.

   (c) Laboratory coats or gowns should have sleeves that can be cuffed underneath the gloves to avoid

operator contamination or interference with particular procedures.

   (d) Gloves should be removed and discarded immediately after use and should not be worn when touching surfaces, such as the door handle in the picture, unrelated to the particular laboratory procedure performed while wearing them.

   (e) Laboratory refrigerators or freezers should *never* be used to store food or other laboratory-unrelated items.

CHAPTER 23

CASE STUDY 1

1. Fluorescence *in situ* hybridization. (FISH)

2. The first step in ISH is to treat the tissue or cell in such a way as to "fix" the target nucleic acid and make it more accessible to the probe. Labeled probes (either DNA or RNA) are then allowed to react with the treated tissue or cell under high temperature to allow hybridization. The probes can be labeled with a radioactive label, an antigenic label (for example, digoxigenin, or DIG, which can be visualized using a specific labeled antibody to it), biotin, or a fluorescent label. In the latter case, ISH using fluorescence is called, appropriately, fluorescence *in situ* hybridization, or FISH.

CASE STUDY 2

1. You can perform any of the many types of polymerase chain reactions: PCR, RT-PCR, real-time PCR, asymmetric PCR, allele-specific PCR, nested PCR, multiplex PCR, overlap extension PCR, intersequence-specific PCR, and methylation-specific PCR, to name a few. Of course, you will also need a method of detecting the amplified nucleic acid.

2. Genotyping by identifying specific DNA sequences specific for a particular HLA genotype for transplantation

3. A classical technique that utilizes RT-PCR is the identification of viral RNA in HIV testing.

ANSWERS TO CHECKPOINTS

Chapter 1

Checkpoint! 1.1
innate—the response was immediate and non-specific

Checkpoint! 1.2
a macrophage

Checkpoint! 1.3
pattern recognition receptors

Checkpoint! 1.4
the gamma peak

Checkpoint! 1.5
T helper cells and T regulatory cells.

Checkpoint! 1.6
GALT and RALT

Chapter 2

Checkpoint! 2.1
Pepsin

Checkpoint! 2.2
IgM and IgA

Checkpoint! 2.3
Immunoglobulin light chains

Checkpoint! 2.4
memory

Checkpoint! 2.5
antigen-independent random recombinational events of DNA gene segments
    antigen-independent clonal deletion of self-reactive B cells
    antigen-independent somatic mutation and affinity maturation

Checkpoint! 2.6
myeloma cell

Chapter 3

Checkpoint! 3.1
autoantigen; less

Checkpoint! 3.2
the protein because it is more antigenic than a carbohydrate. However, the protein would have to be accessible for the antibody to react with.

Checkpoint! 3.3
Cross reactivity

Checkpoint! 3.4
MHC class I molecules

Chapter 4

Checkpoint! 4.1
T cells play a major role in B-cell activation by providing a feedback signal to B cells that have presented antigen peptides to the T cell; in fact, a strong antibody response by a B cell is dependent on a T cell feeding back to that B cell once the T cell has recognized the antigen peptide presented by the B cell. If the T cell that can recognize that particular antigen peptide is not present, this feedback mechanism cannot occur, and the B cell does not continue in its activation against that antigen. Thus, lack of T-cell help against self-antigens (because of the elimination of self-reactive T cells by central tolerance) plays a major role in B cell tolerance against that self-antigen

Checkpoint! 4.2
All nucleated cells, including antigen-presenting cells, express MHC class I molecules because MHC class I molecules are involved in the presentation of endogenous antigens such as altered self-components or a viral component expressed by a virally infected cell. Because *all* nucleated cells can be potentially infected or altered and, thus, need to be eliminated by cytotoxic T cells, antigen-presenting cells also express MHC class I molecules.

Checkpoint! 4.3
8. To help remember which molecule presents to which cell, the answer is 8. That is MHC class II present to CD4 cells, 2 times 4 is 8, and MHC class I molecules present to CD8 cells, so 1 times 8 is also 8.

Checkpoint! 4.4
As in any highly complex system, redundancy is key for that system's proper and efficient function. Should a particular component of that system fail, a redundant component can take over and achieve the same function. In addition, many different functions of the immune system are modulated by very carefully controlled "blends" of different cytokines, often in a synergistic approach.

Checkpoint! 4.5
Cytokines can simulate cells to release other cytokines and can downregulate the production of other cytokines from cells. Certain cytokines can recruit cells at a particular site and induce those cells, in turn, to release their own cytokines locally. In addition, cytokines can modulate the expression of cytokine receptors on other cells, thus affecting the response of those cells to the cytokines for which they have receptors.

Chapter 5

Checkpoint! 5.1
The classical pathway because C1 requires calcium to stay together and C4b forms a Mg++ dependent complex with C2, and the lectin pathway because Mg++ is required for C4b complex with C2 in this pathway as well.

Checkpoint! 5.2
C3 and the membrane attack complex of C5-C9

Checkpoint! 5.3
C4a

Checkpoint! 5.4
C1q

Checkpoint! 5.5
Immune complex clearance is facilitated by complement through opsonization followed by phagocytosis and by CR1 on platelets and red blood cells binding of C3b-coated complexes to bring the complexes to the spleen and liver for clearance

Checkpoint! 5.6
C1INH

Checkpoint! 5.7
a functional assay

Chapter 6

Checkpoint! 6.1
Repeat the assay with diluted serum to see whether the first reaction was negative because of a prozone reaction.

Checkpoint! 6.2
Fahey method

Checkpoint! 6.3
yes

Checkpoint! 6.4
A and D

Checkpoint! 6.5
1. B
2. A
3. C

Chapter 7

Checkpoint! 7.1
Ruth Yalow in 1959

Checkpoint! 7.2
radioactivity

Checkpoint! 7.3
Heterogeneous, the chromatography along the membrane, separates bound from free.

Checkpoint! 7.4
No, it would not because each patient's immunoglobulin would have to be purified prior to labeling. This would be costly, and in purification steps some antibody would be lost, decreasing sensitivity. In addition, variations in the purification steps from patient to patient would yield erroneous results.

Checkpoint! 7.5
the way the antibody is labeled and the way the label is measured, the rest of the steps are the same

Checkpoint! 7.6
No, a lattice structure does not form for the labeled assays; a plateau may be seen with high amounts of antibody, but an apparent negative result would not occur.

Chapter 8

Checkpoint! 8.1
$$\frac{1}{10} = \frac{x}{4} \quad 10x = 4 \quad x = \frac{4}{10}$$

$$X = 0.4$$

serum and 4ml total -0.4ml serum = 3.6 ml of diluent is needed

Checkpoint! 8.2
The following is one of several ways to do this. A 1:10 000 dilution can be made by making the same dilution twice:

$$\frac{1}{100} \times \frac{1}{100} = \frac{1}{10\ 000}$$

So the way to make two 1/100 dilutions with 2 ml of buffer is

$$\frac{1}{100} = \frac{x}{1\ ml}$$

$$100x = 1$$

$$x = 0.01\ \text{or}\ 10$$

microliters into 1ml of buffer (minus 10 microliters) and mix and then 10 microliters from this tube into the second tube containing 1 ml (minus ten microliters).

You could quickly make a 1/100 dilution and then make a 1/100 dilution from it.

Checkpoint! 8.3
You have more:
0.1 milligrams = 100 micrograms = 100 000 nanograms.

Chapter 9

Checkpoint! 9.1
Remember the mnemonic ACID

Type I	**A**naphylaxis
Type II	**C**ell or surface bound antibody
Type II	**I**mmune complex mediated
Type IV	**D**elayed type hypersensitivity

Checkpoint! 9.2
Remember types I, II, and III involve antibody, while type IV involves a cell mediated response.

Checkpoint! 9.3
The subject could be tested for elevated levels of total IgE, which would suggest a type I hypersensitivity reaction also known as an *immediate type hypersensitivity reaction.* Exposure to agents such as latex, poison ivy, skin creams, fragrances, cosmetics, thimerosal can cause type IV hypersensitivity. A type I hypersensitivity reaction rash looks different from a type IV hypersensitivity rash (Figure 9.4 versus Figure 9.15). The type I hypersensitivity rash pits with pressure while the type IV hypersensitivity rash does not. The type IV hypersensitivity rash may also blister and ooze (Figure 9.15). Skin testing for the type I allergen or patch testing for a type IV allergen can be performed. *In vitro* testing for IgE to the type I allergen can be performed using chemiluminescence. *In vitro* testing measuring T cell proliferation in response to the type IV allergen can also be performed.

Checkpoint! 9.4
IgE antibodies, which are circulating throughout the body on mast cells, are responsible for type I hypersensitivity. As soon as the antigen binds to the IgE on the mast cell, the IgE becomes cross-linked and sends a signal to the mast cell to degranulate. These released products cause an immediate effect. In delayed type hypersensitivity, the effector mechanism is the accumulation of specific reactive T cells followed by other cells. These specific T cells have to actually travel from wherever they are in the body and migrate to the site of the allergen to cause the effector response. Cytokines that they release will bring other cells to the area.

Chapter 10

Checkpoint! 10.1
A vaccine involves immunizing a host with an antigen that immunologically mimics a particular infectious organism so that when the real organism is introduced into the host, the host responds with a strong secondary immune response. In choosing such an antigen for the vaccine, one must be careful not to introduce antigenic determinants that may cross-react with the host tissues, potentially causing an autoimmune reaction in the host.

Checkpoint! 10.2
The clinical symptoms of SLE are numerous and diverse. They can differ in individuals, and many mimic the symptoms of other diseases. In addition, many of the symptoms can be erratic in appearance and timing, thus increasing the difficulty in making a diagnosis.

Checkpoint! 10.3
One of the factors that is suspected to contribute to autoimmune reactions is an abnormality in the clearance of dead cells and the resulting debris from these cells. Sunlight, through UV light, can cause the death of many cells, supplying additional antigens for immune complex formation. with the antibodies to nuclear antigens that are circulating in the patient.

Checkpoint! 10.4
A superantigen activates T cells nonspecifically, resulting in their polyclonal activation and an enormous release of different inflammatory molecules. This happens because the superantigen can bind simultaneously to MHC class II components and T-cell receptors but bypasses the antigen-specific presentation mechanism described in Chapter 4. By bypassing the unique specificity of the antigen-binding pockets of the MHC and TCR, superantigens can activate a large number of different (antigen specificity-wise) T cells, thus resulting in their massive response.

Chapter 11

Checkpoint! 11.1
TSI are biologically active causing upregulation of thyroid function.

Checkpoint! 11.2
measurement of elevated ACTH

Checkpoint! 11.3
both autoantibodies and T-cells

Checkpoint! 11.4
direct immunofluorescence

Checkpoint! 11.5
functional studies

Chapter 12

Checkpoint! 12.1
Fred has a sarcoma and Velma has an adenocarcinoma.

Checkpoint! 12.2
The increased growth rate of cancer cells can result in increased cellular acidity because of a higher metabolic rate.

Checkpoint! 12.3
oncofetal and carcinoembryonic antigens

Checkpoint! 12.4
1. A, D
2. C
3. B

Chapter 13

Checkpoint! 13.1
1. multiple myeloma

Checkpoint! 13.2
1. Replacement of the normal cells of the bone marrow with these malignant plasma cells results in decrease in the production of normal blood cells.

2. A compensatory increase in plasma volume to reduce the viscosity of the serum. This increase in plasma volume results in a decrease in the number of RBCs, white cells, and platelets per ml of blood and thus causes the anemia to worsen.

Checkpoint! 13.3
1. C
2. B
3. A

Checkpoint! 13.4
The bands would be closer together, and the total distance from the first band to the last would be less because with less charge, the current would not carry the molecules as far.

Checkpoint! 13.5
The bands would be closer together, and the total distance from the first band to the last would be less because the current had had less time to carry the proteins along the gel.

Checkpoint! 13.6
The bands would be sharper.

Chapter 14

Checkpoint! 14.1
Group O individuals have neither the A or B antigens on the surface of their red blood cells, so their red blood cells will not react with antibodies against either A or B potentially present in a recipient's serum. On the other hand, because individuals with AB blood group have *both* antigens on the surface of their red blood cells, they will not produce antibodies against either antigen and therefore can receive red blood cells from a donor regardless of the donor's blood group.

Checkpoint! 14.2
Hematopoietic stem cells are self-renewing and pluripotent, which means that they can proliferate and make a large number of daughter cells and, under the influence of various different blends of cytokines, they can differentiate into many different types of blood cells. Because of this, stem cells can be used to replace a particular population of cells that is defective and/or missing or to restore a defective immune system.

Checkpoint! 14.3
If the graft happens to be made of a variety of immune cells, it acts as a "minihost" with its own "immune system" and sees the recipient of the graft as "foreign," just as the recipient's immune system in other types of transplants may see the graft.

Checkpoint! 14.4
Corneas are anatomically located in what is known as an *immunologically privileged site,* which is isolated from the lymphatic system. Because of this, immune cells' ability to get to such site is limited. In addition, several active mechanisms inhibit inflammatory reactions to an

antigen in immunologically privileged sites. These include production of cytokines that downregulate an immune response (eg, TGF-β), decreased expression of class I MHC molecules, and downregulation of the complement system. The lack of lymphatic drainage and the presence of these downregulatory mechanisms prevent an inflammatory reaction against a foreign antigen in these sites.

Chapter 15

Checkpoint! 15.1
Upon encountering an antigen, a B cell can initially produce antibodies with minimal T-cell participation. However, further activation of a B cell depends on the interaction of that B cell with a helper T cell and on receiving secondary signals from that T cell. This is necessary for further B-cell differentiation, isotype switch, subsequent antibody production, and the development of memory B cells. A dysfunction in T cells thus affects these additional steps in B-cell activation.

Checkpoint! 15.2
The β_2-integrins are expressed on a variety of cells, including lymphocytes, monocytes, macrophages, neutrophils, and natural killer cells, thus affecting both their cell-to-cell interactions as well as their locomotion. Because so many cell types and their functions are affected, it is easy to understand why this disease has such dire consequences.

Checkpoint! 15.3
Most immunodeficiencies are recessive; that is, the disease manifests itself only when two copies of the recessive gene(s) associated with the disease are inherited. Inbred populations do not have the genetic diversity of outbred populations; interbreeding among family members (eg, cousin-to-cousin marriages) increases the chances that an offspring will inherit two copies of a recessive gene.

Chapter 16

Checkpoint! 16.1
The proper function of neutrophils requires energy, which is tied in part to carbohydrate metabolism. Altered carbohydrate metabolism may thus affect protein glycosylation, the formation of certain radicals during phagocytosis, and the nitric oxide-cyclic guanosine 3'–5' monophosphate pathway, resulting in alterations of normal neutrophil function.

Checkpoint! 16.2
No, unlike some pathogens and related diseases whose life cycle includes an insect vector (eg, malaria), HIV does not survive in such insect vector and therefore cannot be transmitted that way.

Checkpoint! 16.3
HIV does not survive on environmental surfaces, nor is it transmitted by exposure to such surfaces even after an HIV-infected individual has been in contact with them.

Checkpoint! 16.4
The fact that the vaccine can generate an antibody response in a laboratory animal has little significance because real-life HIV also generates a strong initial antibody response in infected individuals. However, in the long term, this response is only partially effective and does not prevent the eventual development of AIDS. In addition, because of the great antigenic variation of the virus, the vaccine may not be effective against all the antigenic variations of the virus that an individual may encounter.

Chapter 17

Checkpoint! 17.1
Hepatitis is any inflammation of the liver and the AST/ALT, so bilirubin levels could be elevated because of alcohol, drugs toxins, or autoimmunity if the viral causes have been ruled out.

Checkpoint! 17.2
Antibody to HBeAg indicates that the patient is recovering from the infection. Antibody to HBsAg can be measured after the disappearance of HBsAg and indicates recovery because this antibody provides protective immunity.

Checkpoint! 17.3
In the EIA-3, a positive result is repeated in duplicate and if these are positive (the serum is repeatedly reactive), one of two protocols can be used. Positive results are tested either by RIBA for antibody confirmation or by a molecular technique for viral RNA. If the molecular test is done first, and is positive, this molecular result is reported and indicates that the patient is currently infected whereas a negative molecular result is reflexed to the RIBA. If the antibody tests are positive but the if molecular tests are negative this indicates that this patient may be one of the 25% of the hepatitis C patients who cleared the infection. However, the molecular test should be repeated because the patient can be transiently negative for viremia. If the RIBA was performed first and is positive, a molecular assay is performed. If the molecular assay is positive the patient is currently infected. If the signal-to-cutoff ratio is used and the signal from the EIA was high, there is a high signal-to-cutoff ratio with the cutoff value being the reading at which a patient's sample would be considered negative. The sample can be confirmed with a molecular test for hepatitis C RNA without a RIBA. A positive EIA, which had a low signal-to-cutoff ratio would be followed by a RIBA; if it is positive, it would be followed by a molecular assay.

Chapter 18

Checkpoint! 18.1
Epstein-Barr virus (EBV), Cytomegalovirus (CMV), Herpes Simplex 1 (HSV1) and 2 viruses (HSV2) and Varicella Zoster Virus (VZV).

Checkpoint! 18.2
Toxoplasmosis, **o**ther infections, **r**ubella, **c**ytomegalovirus, and **h**erpes simplex virus

Checkpoint! 18.3
All cause a lifelong infection with a latency period.

Checkpoint! 18.4
measles, mumps, and rubella (mmr) vaccine

Checkpoint! 18.5
HIV, hepatitis B, hepatitis C, West Nile virus

Chapter 19

Checkpoint! 19.1
The M protein can interfere with a host's ability to fight off *S. pyogenes;* for example, it can prevent opsonization by complement components, thus interfering with a phagocyte's ability to ingest the organism. In addition, the M protein can have cross-reacting epitopes that mimic host epitopes, thus causing autoimmune responses against the host.

Checkpoint! 19.2
H. pylori produces urease, an enzyme that ultimately causes the generation of bicarbonate, which neutralizes the stomach acids. In addition, *H. pylori* can sense different pH gradients and can move to areas of higher pH.

Checkpoint! 19.3
Being obligate intracellular parasites, *Rickettsiae* can survive and replicate only within a host's cell. This makes their study difficult because their growth requirement are fastidious and they can be cultured only in live tissues.

Checkpoint! 19.4
Vaccines are generated against various immunogenic components of a particular microorganism, often proteins on the surface of the organism. *T. pallidum* does not grow in culture and *T. pallidum* lacks many surface proteins found in many other microorganisms; this lack has made the production of a vaccine very difficult. In addition, the antibodies formed to *T. pallidum* have not been found to be protective, individuals can be infected more than once.

Checkpoint! 19.5
The transmission of the microorganism from tick to host requires the tick to remain attached to the host and feed on it for a long time. Someone who is bitten by an adult tick will probably remove it before it has a chance to infect the person. However, at the nymphal stage, the ticks are very small and can go undetected. At this stage, they also feed for a long time, thus increasing the chance of transmission.

Chapter 20

Checkpoint! 20.1
They are eukaryotic and are neither plants nor animals.

Checkpoint! 20.2
The patient's possible exposure, immune status, and symptoms are important for diagnosis.

Checkpoint! 20.3
genital candidiasis

Checkpoint! 20.4
Pneumocystis jiroveci, a fungus

Checkpoint! 20.5
protozoans

Checkpoint! 20.6
Giardia are shed only intermittently, so concentrated stool samples are sometimes negative.

Checkpoint! 20.7
Toxoplasmosis cannot infect through the skin, so it is not dangerous for a pregnant woman to handle raw meat.

Chapter 21

Checkpoint! 21.1
forensic toxicologists

Checkpoint! 21.2
radioimmunoassay

Checkpoint! 21.3
It can determine whether the blood is human in origin or from a specific animal, thus disproving or corroborating her or his story.

Checkpoint! 21.4
Karl Landsteiner

Checkpoint! 21.5
hemoglobin

Checkpoint! 21.6
blood and semen

Checkpoint! 21.7
blood and saliva

Chapter 22

Checkpoint! 22.1
The chemical (isopropyl ether) is highly volatile and flammable; it has a medium level of health hazard and can be somewhat reactive. Its safe handling requires the use of a chemical fume hood and protective equipment such as protective clothing, gloves, and goggles for the operator.

Checkpoint! 22.2
Both can protect the operator from contamination (chemical/biological) from a sample, but a biological containment hood can also protect the sample from contamination from the operator and the surrounding environment.

Checkpoint! 22.3
Wearing gloves is only one level of contamination prevention. Hands must be washed before handling the gloves themselves (putting them on/removing them), which can contaminate the gloves and/or the hands, thus rendering their wearing ineffective.

Checkpoint! 22.4
The effect of radiation on an individual can be cumulative with time, so frequent and/or long-term exposure to even low levels of radioactivity must be monitored carefully.

Chapter 23

Checkpoint! 23.1
A change in a single nucleotide can change the particular codon that nucleotide is part of, which, in turn, can result in a different amino acid in that sequence. In certain situations, a different amino acid because of its particular properties and features can change the shape of the backbone of the protein and, in turn, affect its structure and/or function.

Checkpoint! 23.2
A protein needs not only to be synthesized but also to be regulated. For example, a cell making a specific protein can make that protein after receiving specific signals, so the gene that encodes for that protein must be able to respond to such signals and be turned on or off, depending on a particular situation. Portions of the gene that are not part of the coding sequence are usually related to these regulatory functions.

Checkpoint! 23.3
The genome of retroviruses are made of RNA instead of DNA, so RT-PCR is indeed the technique of choice when dealing with RNA.

Checkpoint! 23.4
The samples were contaminated by unrelated DNA, possibly even the colleague's own. Because you need very minute quantities of template DNA and the procedure amplifies a particular sequence enormously, even a very small amount of contaminants (eg, from the operator's hand) can give erroneous results.

GLOSSARY

2-fold serial dilution a series of tubes set up to yield a 1:2 dilution from one tube to the next with the same amount of diluent in each. The resultant dilutions are 1:2, 1:4, 1:8, 1:16 and so on.

Acquired immune system response that is specific, has a large scope, can discriminate, and has a memory.

Acute HIV syndrome flulike symptoms including headaches, nausea, sore throat, fever, diarrhea, and enlargement of the lymph nodes associated with early HIV infection.

Acute leukemia a cancer in which many immature tumor leukocytes are in the blood.

Acute phase protein (also called *acute phase reactant*) protein whose concentrations change with an inflammation and can either be increased or decreased by the inflammation.

Acute phase reactant protein whose concentrations change with an inflammation and can either be increased or decreased by the inflammation.

Acute phase response inflammatory response that is the result of macrophage activation via surface PRRs of PAMPs on pathogens with the release of IL-1, IL-6, and TNF-α.

Acute rejection the activation of CD4+ and CD8+ recipient T cells against the graft from an allogeneic donor.

Adaptive immune system system that produces responses that are specific, have a large scope, can discriminate, with a memory component.

Adenocarcinoma a tumor arising from epithelial cells that formed glandular structures.

Adenosine deaminase deficiency condition characterized by the toxic buildup of deoxyadenosine and S-adenosylhomocysteine, affecting immature B and T cells.

Adhesin family of proteins involved in cell-to-cell attachment; plays a major role in cell-to-cell interactions and in cell locomotion.

Adjuvant chemical that when mixed with an immunogen enhances the immune response to that immunogen.

Affinity measure of the strength of the binding of one Fab with its corresponding epitope on the antigen.

Agammaglobulinemia immunodeficiency that results in a lower than normal level(s) of one or more of the different immunoglobulins.

Agglutination cross-linking of particulate antigen (bacteria, cells, or latex particles) by antibody to form larger complexes that are also visible.

AH50 assay test that utilizes the fact that rabbit red blood cells (RBCs) can directly activate the alternative pathway of complement. In this test, rabbit RBCs are mixed with the serum to be tested, and the amount of hemoglobin released by the cells is proportional to the amount of alternative pathway activity.

Alanine aminotransferase (ALT) a liver enzyme that is elevated with hepatitis.

Allergen a harmless antigen that can specifically stimulate an IgE response, causing a reaction that can create pathologic effects.

Allergy refers to two of the four forms of hypersensitivity, type 1 hypersensitivity (also called *immediate hypersensitivity*); and type 4 hypersensitivity (also called *delayed type hypersensitivity*). In allergy the effector mechanisms that the immune system selects to defend the host from a perceived threat are more damaging to the host than the innocuous antigen itself.

Allergic bronchopulmonary aspergillosis (ABPA) allergic lung reaction in which patients who have both IgE and IgG to *Aspergillus* show signs of an IgE-mediated disease with wheezing and coughing evident.

Alloantigen antigen from other members of the same species as the host.

Allograft a graft transplanted between two genetically different individuals of the same species.

Allorecognition immune response of a recipient against a donor allograft.

Allotypic antigen substance (such as an immunogen or a hapten) inherited from parents that is different in different members of the same species.

Alpha-1 acid glycoprotein an acute phase reactant which is a plasma protein produced by the liver whose primary function may be the inhibition of progesterone and other drugs.

Alpha 1-fetoprotein (AFP) a tumor marker that is elevated in non-seminomatous testicular cancers and liver cancer (hepatoma) and some rare germ cell tumors.

Alternative pathway complement pathway that is initiated by activator surfaces such as lipopolysaccharide-containing bacterial cell walls, fungi, viruses, and some parasites including trypanosomes, endotoxins, and aggregated IgG2, IgA, IgE. C3w and C3b, factors B, D, and properdin are utilized to activate C3.

Amyloidosis when a protein is abnormally folded and thus is insoluble and precipitates in organs and tissues causing pathology.

Analytical ultracentrifugation a high-speed ultracentrifuge that has optics so that the sedimentation coefficient can be determined.

Anaphylactic severe allergic reaction belonging to the type I hypersensitivity reactions.

Anaphylatoxin small peptide that causes histamine release from mast cells and results in smooth muscle contraction and increases in vascular permeability.

Aneurysm a blood-filled bulge or swelling in a blood vessel often associated with a weakening of the vessel at the area of the bulge; rupture can cause devastating damage.

Annealing the pairing of DNA or RNA to a complementary sequence by hydrogen bonding.

Anorexia lack or loss of appetite for food.

Antigen molecules that the immune system recognizes as foreign. Important characteristics include (a) foreignness, (b) molecular size, and (c) chemical complexity.

Antigenic determinants   (also called *epitopes*) are restricted portions of a molecule that are involved in the actual binding with the combining site of a particular antibody.

Antigen presentation   process by which a macrophage, dendritic cell, B cell, or neutrophil shows antigen to a T cell in a MHC class II molecule, also that process in which any nucleated cell shows antigen to a T cell in an MHC class I molecule.

Antigen-presenting cell   cell that takes up antigens, biochemically processes them, and then presents components of those antigens in MHC molecules to a T cell.

Antigen processing   a mechanism that comprises a series of essential cellular and biochemical events that activate CD4+ and CD8+ T cells after an accessory or antigen-presenting cell binds a particular antigen, internalizes it, processes it biochemically, and then presents it to the T cell.

Anti-human immunoglobulin   antibody made in another species, usually rabbit or goat that reacts with human immunoglobulin. It is used to detect human immunoglobulin in indirect immunoassays. It can either react with all classes of immunoglobulin or be specific for one class of immunoglobulin.

Antimicrobial peptide   peptide produced in the body and skin and by neutrophils and natural killer cells. These are less than 100 amino acids in length, bind to the cell wall of the microbe and increase the membrane permeability to ultimately cause death of the pathogen. Two major families of antimicrobial peptides in humans are defensins and cathelicidins.

Antinuclear antibody (ANA)   a group of antibodies that react to different nuclear, nucleolar, or perinuclear antigen such as nucleic acids, histones, chromatin, and nuclear and ribonuclear proteins.

Arthus reaction   a reaction characterized by localized swelling, redness of the skin, localized increased blood flow, and in more severe cases, tissue necrosis and ulceration. It is caused by immune complexes generated by IgG that has infiltrated the tissues combining with an antigen that has been injected intradermally.

Aspartate aminotransferase (AST)   a liver enzyme that is elevated with hepatitis.

Aspergilloma   is a mass that looks like a fungal ball; caused by fungal growth either in a cavity in the lung, brain, kidneys, or other organs.

Aspergillus   ubiquitous dimorphic fungus found in soil, decaying matter, water, and air throughout the world that causes infections such as allergic bronchopulmonary aspergillosis, invasive aspergillosis, aspergilloma, sinus infections, cutaneous aspergillosis and otitis externa (swimmer's ear). Four species commonly cause disease: *Aspergillus fumingatus, flavus, niger,* and *terreus.*

Aspermic   the absence of spermatozoa in semen.

Ataxia   the loss of full control of bodily movements.

Autoantigen   self-antigen (ie, part of the host).

Autocrine effect   a cytokine or hormone that acts on the cell that produced (secreted) it. Also called *autocrine response.*

Autocrine response   a cytokine or hormone that acts on the cell that produced (secreted) it. Also *autocrine effect.*

Autograft   graft obtained from an individual and transplanted in a different anatomical part of that same individual.

Avidity   number of binding sites times the affinity.

 B

Basophil   rarest of the granulocytes whose function is not completely defined but it plays a role in inflammation and allergy; has blue-black stained granules after Wright staining, which indicates that the granule is basic.

Bence-Jones protein   immunoglobulin light chain found in the urine of patients with multiple myeloma.

Benign tumor   noncancerous tumors that do not grow into other tissues or spread to other parts of the body; and usually not life threatening.

Beta-2 microglobulin   component of the class I molecule; serum levels elevated in and used in diagnosing multiple myeloma, chronic lymphocytic leukemia, and some lymphomas.

Bexxar   iodine-labeled antibody to CD20 that is used in the radioimmunotherapy of B cell non Hodgkin lymphomas.

Bilirubin   breakdown product of heme, usually from red blood cells; water insoluble pigment in bile.

Biochip   solid substrate on which a collection of microsized test sites is present.

Biological containment hood   an area enclosed on 5 sides which can be used to protect the operator and/or to avoid contaminating a particular sample or specimen. The air is filtered through a HEPA filter usually of 0.3 microns. A classical example of a biological containment hood is a laminar flow hood used for tissue culture.

Blastomyces dermatitidis   thermally dimorphic fungi that causes blastomycosis disease occurring after inhaling spores from disturbed organic matter in wooded areas; causes coughing, fever, and muscle and joint pain; disseminated disease can affect skin, bones, and urinary track and cause meningitis.

Blood   is a fluid substance that flows throughout the body carrying oxygen and nutrients to tissues while helping to remove waste products.

Bone marrow   primary lymphatic organ in which B cells mature.

BRCA1   caretaker gene that produces a protein that can repair DNA, a mutation in this increases susceptibility to breast cancer.

BRCA2   caretaker gene that produces a protein that can repair DNA, a mutation in this increases susceptibility to breast cancer.

Bruton's disease   also called *X-linked agammaglobulinemia (XLA)*, it is a condition involving impaired B-cell development, lack of mature B cells, and low or lacking levels of immunoglobulins of all isotype.

 C

CA 15-3   tumor marker that measures an epitope on the MUC-1 molecule which is used in monitoring breast cancer.

CA 19-9   tumor marker used to monitor the course of disease in pancreatic cancer and hepatobiliary cancer.

CA 27-29   tumor marker that measures an epitopes on the MUC-1 molecule which is used in monitoring breast cancer.

CA 125   tumor marker used to follow the response to surgery and therapy of women with ovarian cancer.

Cancer group of diseases that begin with the abnormal and uncontrolled proliferation of one cell.

Candidiasis infection with *Candida albicans*; can cause an oral form, genital-urinary form (yeast infection), or an invasive form.

Carcinoembryonic antigen (CEA) oncofetal antigen elevated in the serum of patients who have colorectal breast, lung, pancreas, stomach, and ovarian cancer; used for monitoring colorectal cancer patients.

Carcinoma tumors that arises from epithelial tissue.

Cathelicidin a family of antimicrobial peptides produced by epithelial cells and phagocytes; provides protection from outside attacks at all the epithelial surfaces from mouth to anus.

CD45 cluster of differentiation molecule found on white blood cells, tumors of hematopoietic origin (leukemias, lymphomas, myelomas) present on normal white blood cells.

Central nervous system cancer cancer arising in either the brain or the spinal cord.

Central tolerance the process by which developing thymocytes are selected by their ability to recognize self-MHC components while not reacting to self-antigens.

CH50 assay test of total function of complement initiated through the classical pathway that begins with antibody-coated sheep red blood cells to determine the ability of the patient's serum to lyse the red blood cells; requires C1, C2, C4, C1INH, and the complement components C3 and C5-9. Hemoglobin released from these cells is used as a measure of lysis.

Chain of custody chronological documentation that tracks a particular piece of evidence from the time it was first discovered until the present time.

Chancre painless ulceration characteristic of early stages of syphilis. It contains white blood cells, and often contains the infectious agent.

Chemical fume hood a device which is enclosed on 5 sides. This enclosed area has a partial covering or sash so that work can be done within the hood with the technician's arms and hands only inside of the hood. A fan is installed which creates a negative pressure so that air is drawn in from the laboratory and is exhausted into a separate air-handling system, so that individuals in the laboratory are not exposed to fumes from the reagents within the hood. The air flow should be high enough to ventilate 60 to 100 linear feet per minute but not high enough to cause turbulence.

Chemiluminescence emission of light as the result of a chemical reaction that produces no heat.

Chemokine peptide mediator that attracts chemotactic cells to a particular site; regulates the recruitment and movement of a variety of different cells.

Chemotactic factor chemicals that attracts cells to the site.

Chemotaxis the process in which a chemical causes movement of cells to a site.

Cholestasis a condition characterized by decreased or interrupted flow of bile from the liver.

Chronic granulomatous disease (GCD) a variety of hereditary diseases characterized by an aberration of phagocytes' ability to form the reactive oxygen species needed for intracellular killing of ingested microorganisms.

Chronic leukemia a cancer with excess mature tumor white cells in the blood and sometimes in the bone marrow.

Chronic rejection inflammatory mechanism that leads to the deterioration of the vasculature of a graft, often months or years after transplant, causing vascular damage, atherosclerosis, narrowing of the vessels, decreased blood supply to the graft, and graft death.

Circumoral pallor white masklike pattern around the mouth often seen in scarlet fever.

Classical pathway first complement pathway discovered. It is initiated by antibody bound to antigen; activated by classes of antibody including IgM and the IgG subclasses, IgG3, IgG1, and IgG2; antibody binds to antigen and a conformational change occurs revealing a site on the antibody molecule that binds the C1q molecule. Activated C1q splits C4 is split to C4a and C4b, C4b lands on the surface next to C1 and converts C2 to C2a and C2b, C2b floats away, and C2a joins C4b on the surface to become a C3 convertase.

Clinical latency asymptomatic period between decreased viremia and the onset of clinical symptoms.

Coccidioides immitis pathogenic fungus that does not cause symptoms in 60% of individuals but can cause fever with a dry cough, joint and muscle aches, headaches, and lumpy red rash on the legs as well as an acute disease with flulike symptoms called *San Joaquin Valley fever* or simply *Valley fever.*

Codon sequence of 3 nucleotides that encodes for a specific amino acid.

Cold agglutinin autoantibody in *M. pneumoniae* infection thought to be generated by cross-reactive antigens on the microorganism; agglutinates red blood cells at lower than body temperatures (thus the name "cold"); exhibited by only about half of infected individuals, making it unreliable for diagnosis, especially considering that other microorganisms including some viruses can also cause the production of it.

Colloid particle tiny particulate substance that contains one substance dispersed in another substance; allows visualization of the reaction in colloid immunoassays.

Common variable immunodeficiency (CVID) variety of different immunodeficiency conditions all resulting in low levels of immunoglobulins of different isotypes.

Competitive immunoassay assay in which a test kit analyte competes for limited reagent with the analyte in the patient's sample.

Complement protein one of about 35 proteins involved in pathogen lysis, opsonization, immune complex clearance, chemotaxis, and vascular permeability changes.

Complement system involves 3 pathways of activation: alternative, lectin, and classical, which differ in the formation of C3 convertase; after this step, pathways the same with a cascade of proteins activating other proteins and so on until pathogen lysis occurs. Plays a role in lysis, opsonization, chemotaxis, leukocyte activation, immune complex and apoptotic cell clearance, coagulation, and memory of the immune system.

Complementary determining regions (CDRs) area in the variable region that binds the epitope and forms a complementary shape and charge.

Compound dilution process of making 2 or more dilutions to achieve desired final dilution to avoid requirement of large volume of diluent and extremely small volumes of solute.

Confirmatory diagnosis analysis used to confirm what other tests or physical features have indicated.

Conformational epitope area on an antigen which interacts with the immune components in a way that depends on the antigen's 3-dimensional structure.

Congenital rubella syndrome pathology caused by the fetus's infection while *in utero*; includes mental retardation, cataracts, deafness, heart malformations, and spleen and liver damage.

Contact dermatitis localized type IV hypersensitivity reaction usually initiated by small substances acting as allergens that contact the skin and penetrate it.

Controlled substance drug or chemical whose use and possession is regulated by state and federal laws.

C-reactive protein (CRP) sensitive indicator of inflammation so named because it reacts with the C-polysaccharide of *Streptococcus pneumonia*.

Creatinine molecule produced as a result of muscle metabolism, molecule that is a waste product carried to the kidneys through the bloodstream where it is filtered out and excreted in the urine.

Crossover electrophoresis serological technique that utilizes an electric field and an antibody and antigen reaction to determine the species of origin of a bloodstain.

Cross-reactivity is the reaction of an antibody with an antigen other than the one that induced its formation. Sometimes cross-reaction occurs because the molecules contain the exact same epitope but different areas elsewhere on the molecule; at other times something can cross-react because it contains an area very similar to the epitope.

Cryptococcosis infection caused by inhalation of either yeast cells or basidiospores from *Cryptococcus neoformans* (associated with bird droppings, primarily pigeons) and *Cryptococcus gatti* (associated with eucalyptus trees and the soil around them).

Cryptosporidium parvum infection that causes a watery diarrheal disease for 1 to 2 weeks beginning 2 to 10 days after infection; is spread by ingestion of contaminated food and water, is very stable, and resists chlorine disinfection.

Cytokeratin marker used to identify carcinomas; also occurs on normal epithelial cells.

Cytokine peptide mediators that allows communication among different cells, cells signal by secreting a certain cytokine, that, in turn, binds to specific receptors on the surface of the cell receiving the signal.

Cytomegalovirus (CMV) member of the Herpesviridae family that can cause asymptomatic infection which includes sore throat, fatigue, fever, and swollen glands, all symptoms similar to those seen in infectious mononucleosis.

Cytopathic effect degenerative change in cells in tissue culture usually the result of the action of certain microorganisms or their toxins.

Cytotoxic T cell CD8+ subset of T cells that can kill target cells infected by endogenous antigen such as a virus.

▶ D

Davidsohn differential (also called *Mono-Diff*) was used as a differential test to distinguish between infectious mononucleosis, serum sickness, or Forssman antibody in individuals with a positive presumptive test. Utilizes absorption with bovine erythrocyte stroma and guinea pig kidney to differentiate the reactivities.

Defensin family of antimicrobial peptides produced by epithelial cells and phagocytes; provide protection from outside attacks at all epithelial surfaces from mouth to anus.

Dendritic cells are named for the long branching processes that they project. They express CD11c and are found in an immature state in the bloodstream and in a mature state in tissues. The concentration of these cells are very low, but they are very active and efficient in immune processes including phagocytosis and antigen presentation.

Deoxyribonucleic acid (DNA) complex of 2 separate strings, or chains, composed of repeating units called *nucleotides*.

Diapedesis process by which white blood cells squeeze through the cells of the intact blood vessel walls.

DiGeorge syndrome condition caused by a deletion in chromosome 22 that affects many organs and body parts resulting in, among other pathologic effects, failed development of the thymus, thus affecting T-cell function.

Diluent buffer solution that dilutes the solute.

Dilution contains the *solute* and the *diluent*. The solute is the material being diluted and the diluent is the solution in which it is diluted.

Direct agglutination the agglutination of particles that naturally have the antigen on their surface.

Direct antiglobulin test (DAT) measures whether antibody is present on an individual's red blood cells. Anti-human immunoglobulin is added directly to red cells from the patient and the cells are observed for agglutination.

Direct immunoassay process that utilizes a labeled antibody binding to an antigen or vice versa to detect an antigen in a cell preparation or biopsy sample.

DNA replication process by which cells divide and make copies of themselves beginning at the level of DNA.

Domain a 110-amino acid area that forms a globular structure on the antibody molecule.

Dot blot the most basic and simplest form of solid matrix hybridization, involving the application of a "dot" of a clinical sample to a membrane and the addition of a specific labeled probe to the sample.

Double diffusion gel precipitation also known as *ouchterlony analysis*, both the antibody and the antigen diffuse through agar or agarose, and where they meet at equivalence form a lattice structure. It is a qualitative technique.

Double negative thymocyte stage of development in the production of T cells in which the cells does not express CD4 or CD8 molecules.

Double positive thymocyte stage of development of T cells in which the cell expresses both CD4 and CD8 molecules.

Drug chemical substance that affects organisms by altering bodily functions; can be used in the prevention, diagnosis, and treatment of diseases.

▶ E

Echtyma a form of impetigo involving deep tissues.

Eclipse phase a period of time during which viral components are not easily detectable in a subject's blood.

Efficiency   the efficiency of a test (that is, the total number of times the test obtained the correct results) can be calculated: true positives + true negatives ÷ total analyzed; the total analyzed is the true negatives plus the true positives plus the false negatives plus the false positives.

Endemic   description indicating that an infection is in the population and stays in it without the need for any external input of the disease.

Endocarditis   inflammation of the inner layer of the heart.

Endocrine effect   action on cells far away from the cell that produced them.

Endocrine response   result of interaction with a molecule produced far away.

Endogenous antigen   foreign entity, such as fragment from foreign protein after the cell has been infected by an organism (such as a virus or an intracellular bacteria) that replicates intracellularly, from within a cell.

Eosinophils   contains red stained granules after Wright staining, which indicates that the granules are acidic. These cells are involved in anti-parasitic responses and allergic reactions.

Epitope   restricted portion of a molecule involved in actual binding with the combining site (paratope) of a particular antibody.

Epstein-Barr virus (EBV)   is the causative agent for infectious mononucleosis and is associated with Burkitt's lymphoma and nasopharyngeal carcinoma.

Equivalence   when the antigen and antibody meet at a concentration in which the number of paratopes (antibody binding sites) approximately equals the number of epitopes; this part of the precipitation curve is where large complexes called *lattices* are formed.

Erythroblastosis fetalis   condition in which pregnant mother makes antibodies against the red blood cells of her fetus because of incompatible blood antigens between mother and fetus. Also known as *hemolytoc disease of the fetus and newborn (HDFN)*.

Estrogen receptor   marker on the tumor tissue indicating that tumor is likely to respond to endocrine therapy.

Exogenous antigen   is an antigen that comes from the outside (ie, extracellularly; for example, from an infectious microorganism or a foreign protein) and that has been engulfed by an antigen-presenting cell.

Exophthalamos   the protruding or forward bulging of the eye from its orbit.

Extract   substance of interest when removed from the substrate on which it was originally collected.

Exudate   fluid from the circulation leaking into tissues or areas of inflammation.

 F

Fab   the antigen-binding fragment result of treatment of IgG with papain; amino terminal end of the immunoglobulin molecule; composed of one of the light chains and about half of the heavy chain.

F(ab')$_2$ the amino terminal end of the immunoglobulin molecule composed of all of 2 light chains and slightly more than half of both heavy chains as the result of the treatment of IgG with pepsin; is divalent binding 2 epitopes.

Factor XIIa   the Hageman factor, a serine protease involved in coagulation, that activates factor X and prekallikrein. It can activate C1q.

Fahey method   radial immunodiffusion method plotted using semi-log paper with diameter on the arithmetic axis and concentration on the y-axis. In an antibody-antigen precipitation reaction that allows diffusion to proceed for 18 hours; diameter is proportional to the log of the concentration.

False negative   a result that indicates that a disease is not present in a person who is infected.

False positive   a result that indicates that a disease is present in a person who is actually not infected.

Fc (fragment crystallizable)   part of the antibody molecule after it has been cleaved by papain; crystallizable nature indicates that this part of the antibody molecule is homogeneous regardless of which antigen the antibody molecule binds. This contains the carboxy terminal end of the antibody molecule.

Fibrinogen   an acute phase reactant involved in clot formation.

First-set rejection   the immune reaction upon first encounter with an allograft.

Flocculation   process by which particles come out of suspension to form flakelike structures that can be seen microscopically or macroscopically.

Flow cytometry   instrumental method for analyzing individual cells that pass single file through a laser beam to measure the amount of forward scatter (related to size), side scatter (related to granularity), and fluorescent tag.

Fluorescence   the emission of light from a substance that has absorbed light energy at a high wavelength to be emitted at a lower wavelength.

Fluorescence polarization immunoassay   a homogeneous assay that places a fluorescent label on a small molecule that is the analyte; because small molecules rotate freely in solution, plane-polarized light as an excitation wavelength for the fluorochrome attached to these small molecules results in the emission of the fluorescent light in a variety of directions, so that, due to the free rotation, the light is no longer in 1 plane. However, if this small molecule has been bound by a relatively large antibody molecule, the rotation is retarded, and the emission remains polarized. The polarized emission can be measured utilizing an appropriately placed detector.

Follicle   a small sac-shaped secretory cavity or gland.

Foreignness   amount of difference from self.

Forensic biology   involves the analysis of evidence to detect the presence of biological fluid stains and characterizing that stain to a particular individual.

Forensic science   application of science to the law.

Forensic serology   use of antigen and antibody reactions for the legal identification of bodily fluids and foreign substances in the body using immunoassays based on the reactions that occur between antigens and antibodies.

Forensic toxicology   involves the analysis of biological samples to detect the presence of controlled substances, alcohol, and other toxic material.

Forssman antigen   heterophile foreign substance present on sheep red blood cells, horse red blood cells, guinea pig kidney, and some normal healthy people have antibody to this. Antibody to this yields positive results in a mono-spot or presumptive assay for infectious mononucleosis but negative results after absorption with guinea pig kidney.

Framework regions   area present on the variable regions and areas between the hypervariable regions.

Free to total PSA   the percentage of PSA that circulates as a free molecule rather than complexed to protease inhibitors; lower in cancer patients with a cutoff of 25%.

Fungi   are eukaryotic organisms whose cells contain membrane-bound structures, including a nucleus and can exist in a mold or yeast form; are higher organisms that are neither plants nor animals.

▶ **G**

Gardasil   vaccine used to prevent human papilloma virus (HPV)-associated cervical cancer.

Gell and Coombs classification   descriptive division of hypersensitivity reactions based on the molecular and immunological mechanisms involved in such reaction.

Gene   distinct sequence of nucleotides forming part of a chromosome.

Genetic code   nucleotide triplet that carries genetic information in living cells.

Giardia lamblia   a parasite that causes diarrheal disease 1 to 2 weeks after fecal-oral contamination, and can survive outside the body for weeks to months after defecation.

Glomerulonephritis   acute kidney inflammation.

Grade   the change in cellular differentiation that is a tool for the clinical evaluation of the tumors.

Graft   transplanted organ or tissue.

Graft-versus-host disease (GVHD)   the immune reaction of a graft against recipient cells and tissues.

Granuloma   round mass of immune cells including granulocytes that wall off antigenic substances of organisms when they are not able to completely eliminate them from the host.

Gumma   a soft, noncancerous form of granuloma often seen in tertiary syphilis.

▶ **H**

Haplotype   a set of alleles from a particular chromosome that are transmitted together.

Haptens   small compounds able to combine with elements of the immune system such as antibodies but unable to stimulate an immune response unless they are linked to a much larger immunogenic molecule called a *carrier*.

Haptoglobin   an acute-phase protein that removes free hemoglobin that has been released through injury.

HBc   nucleocapsid of hepatitis B is composed of this core protein.

HBeAg   between the nucleocapsid and the lipoprotein envelope of hepatitis B virus. Measurements for this become positive shortly after

HBsAg, the presence of this antigen indicates that the patient is highly infectious.

HBsAg   hepatitis B surface antigen (HBsAg) is a protein in the lipoprotein envelope of the hepatitis B virus. This antigen is produced in excess and exists in particles called *Australian antigen*. HBsAg presence is one of the first measurable signs of infection, it disappears within 4 to 6 months if the patient is recovering but stays elevated if chronic hepatitis B develops.

Heavy chain   polypeptide chain of the immunoglobulin molecule that on the amino terminal end is involved in antigen binding and at the carboxy terminal end is involved in the biological function of the molecule; governs the class or isotype of the immunoglobulin molecule.

Heavy chain disease   cancer caused by an uncontrolled proliferation of plasma cells with production of immunoglobulin heavy chain only, this heavy chain is not usually full length.

Helper T cells   the CD4+ subset of T cells that modulate and coordinate an immune response, usually via the secretion of selected cytokines.

Hematuria   the presence of red blood cells in the urine.

Hemoglobin   protein in red blood cells that transports oxygen throughout the body; used for the forensic detection of blood.

Hemolysis   the breakdown of blood.

Hepatitis   any inflammation of the liver.

Hepatitis A   single-stranded positive strand RNA virus in an icosahedral capsid in the Picornaviridae viral family that causes acute hepatitis after fecal-oral contamination and an incubation period of about 28 days.

Hepatitis B   DNA virus with partially double-stranded circular DNA attached to a polymerase protein and surrounded by a nucleocapsid that is surrounded by a lipoprotein envelope of the cell from which the virus budded; causes acute hepatitis after approximately 90 days after infection (60 to 150 days) through contact with infectious blood or body fluids via mucosal contact or through breaks through the skin (percutaneous).

Hepatitis C   spherical and enveloped single-stranded RNA virus member of the Flaviviridae family. Six main genotypes of hepatitis C virus exist with more than 50 subgroups of these genotypes; causes an acute infection 6 to 7 weeks after infection although most people are not symptomatic with the acute infection.

Hepatitis D   virus also called *hepatitis delta* that has small circular single-stranded RNA and is the only known animal virus with circular RNA; is defective so that it can co-infect only with the hepatitis B virus to replicate.

Hepatitis E   fecal-oral form of hepatitis that is a single positive strand RNA virus with an icosahedral capsid.

Hepatotropic viruses   liver cell–seeking viruses including hepatitis viruses A, B, C, D (also called *delta*), and E.

Herceptin   monoclonal antibody used in passive immunotherapy of a percentage of breast cancer patients that reacts with HER-2 antigen.

Hereditary angioedema (HAE)   genetic defect in the plasma component C1-inhibitor resulting in changes in vascular permeability, vascular leakage, and edema.

Herpes simplex virus 1 (HSV1)   organism that causes oral herpes ("cold sore") at the mouth.

Herpes simplex virus 2 (HSV2)   organism most often associated with genital herpes.

Herpesviridae family   viruses that contain ds DNA and have a latency period, include Epstein-Barr virus (EBV), cytomegalovirus (CMV), herpes simplex 1 (HSV1) and 2 viruses (HSV2), and varicella zoster virus (VZV).

HER-2 marker   measured to determine whether tumor will be susceptible to monoclonal antibody treatment with the anti-HER-2 antibody Herceptin and indicates susceptibility to anthracycline therapy.

Heteroantigen   are antigen from a species different from the host, for example, a different animal, a plant or a microorganism.

Heterogeneous assay   are immunoassays that require a step to separate the bound from free antigen and antibody.

Heterophile antibody   an antibody that reacts with antigens from 2 or more species in a pattern without evolutionary relatedness, usually IgM antibodies, and are found to often react with carbohydrate antigens.

High avidity antibody   antibody that indicates a past infection because there has been time since the primary infection for the B cells to undergo somatic mutation to create an antibody that binds the antigen better.

Highly active antiretroviral therapy (HAART)   combination of 3 synergistic anti-HIV drugs from at least 2 functional antiviral drug categories.

Hinge region   proline rich area on the IgG, IgA, and IgD that allows flexibility. It is between the Fab and Fc regions and between C_H1 and C_H2.

Histoplasmosis   caused by *Histoplasma capsulatum* and is associated with bird droppings. Subclinical infection or a mild flulike disease, a pulmonary disease or disseminated disease are seen. Disseminated disease is seen in people with HIV, organ transplants, hematologic malignancies, people receiving anti-TNF-α therapy (Enbrel, Remicade, etc), and in infants. Symptoms and physical signs of disseminated disease include fever, weight loss, pallor, malaise, lymphadenopathy, and hepatosplenomegaly.

Hodgkin's disease   a lymphoma characterized by the presence of Reed-Sternberg cells which generally has a good prognosis.

Homogeneous assays   are immunoassays that do not require a separation or washing step to separate the bound from the free. These assays can be accomplished because the binding of antigen to antibody affects the activity of the label in such a way as to cause a measureable change.

Human anti-mouse antibody (HAMA)   a special type of heterophilic antibody that is produced by the immune response of a patient that has been treated with therapeutic or diagnostic mouse monoclonal antibody. It can interfere with immunoassays, especially capture immunoassays.

Human chorionic gonadotropin (hCG)   a tumor marker that is elevated in nonseminomatous testicular cancer, gestational trophoblastic and germ cell tumors. It is also elevated in pregnancy.

Humoral   the fluid phase of blood, when clotting has been allowed to take place it is called *serum*, when an anticoagulant has been use it is called *plasma*.

Hybridization   the binding of a strand of a nucleic acid to another complementary strand following a specific pattern of base pairs coupling.

Hybridoma cells   a cell formed by the joining of 2 different cells; for example, a cell formed by the fusion of a spleen cell making the desired antibody and a myeloma cell having the property of immortality. The result of this is a clone of cells that makes monoclonal antibody.

Hyperacute rejection   antibody-induced inflammatory responses and thrombus formation that blocks the blood vessels of the graft resulting in the deprivation of blood to the graft, causing its death. This is caused by antibody that is already present in the patient prior to the transplant.

Hyper-IgM syndrome   a group of different immunological malfunctions which result in elevated levels of IgM.

Hyperpigmentation   a condition where there is a darkening of an area of the skin, usually caused by overproduction of melanin.

Hypersensitivity   reactions which are immune reactions that are overtly injurious to the host often in response to an innoucuous antigen. They occur in subjects previously exposed to an antigen and who have developed an immune response to that antigen (sensitization). The clinical manifestations observed in hypersensitivity reactions are dependent upon the host's response and not upon the nature of the antigen.

Hypervariable regions   three regions on the light chain and three regions on the heavy chain which bind the epitope of the antigen, they are also called *complementary determining regions*.

Hypervolemia   excess accumulation of fluid in the blood.

Hyphae   are long filaments of cells in molds.

 I

Identity   the name of the arched reaction line which occurs when, in double diffusion gel precipitation reactions the antigens in the 2 wells are the same.

IgA   the immunoglobulin that has a primary role in secretions, and in secretions is a dimer.

IgD   the immunoglobulin that serves a differentiation role on B cells, and no other known function.

IgE   the immunoglobulin that plays a primary role in allergy and in fighting parasites.

IgG   the primary immunoglobulin in serum and is transferred from the mother to the fetus.

IgM   the first immunoglobulin produced in an immune response. The largest immunoglobulin.

Immune system   the mechanism by which the individual is protected from non-self. Composed of two general components; the innate immune system and the acquired immune system.

Immunity   the discrimination between self and non-self and the subsequent protection from non-self.

Immunochromatographic sandwich assay   an assay in which the bound antigen and labeled antibody is separated from free by migration along a chromatographic membrane, where it binds the capture antibody forming the labeled antibody-antigen-capture antibody sandwich.

Immunofixation electrophoresis   serum protein electrophoresis followed by immunoprecipitation with an overlay by monospecific antisera.

Immunogen   compound that is capable of eliciting an immune response in a host.

Immunoglobulin superfamily   a large group of different proteins sharing structural similarities that are involved in a variety of different functions. Members of the group include T-cell receptors, antibodies, adhesins, and MHC components.

Immunoglobulin supergene family   (also called *immunoglobulin superfamily*) a family of related molecules that have globular domains of about 110 amino acids which came from a common ancestral gene. This family includes immunoglobulin, the T-cell receptor, MHC class I and class II molecules, and CD markers including CD4, CD8, and CD19.

Immunolocalization   involves the intravenous injection of radio-labeled monoclonal antibody followed by patient imaging to allow determination of the presence or absence of tumor metastasis.

Immunological cross-reactivity   the reaction of an antibody with an antigen other than the one that induced its formation. The sharing of antigenic determinants between 2 different antigens.

Immunological tolerance   state of unresponsiveness specific for a particular antigen.

Immunologically privileged site   an area of the body that is physically isolated from the immune system, such as brain, eye, and testes.

Immunology   the study of the reaction when the host encounters a foreign substance.

Immunoproliferative disease   a malignant growth of lymphocytes resulting in a lymphoma, a leukemia, or a plasma cell dyscrasia including multiple myeloma, Waldenstrom macroglobulinemia, light chain deposition disease, and heavy chain disease.

Indirect antiglobulin test (IAT)   looks for presence of patient antibody to red blood cells. The patient's serum is added to the red blood cells and after incubation and washing anti-human immunoglobulin is added. The cells are centrifuged and observed for agglutination.

Indirect immunoassay   utilizes an unlabeled antigen, an unlabeled antibody and a labeled antiglobulin to detect the reaction of the initial antibody and antigen complex. This is usually done to measure a patient's antibody titer to a known antigen.

Infectious mononucleosis   involves the familiar clinical symptoms of malaise, sore throat, enlarged tonsils, fever, and swollen glands. Antibody to heterophile antigens used in its diagnosis.

Inflammation   the response to harmful stimuli and the hallmarks are redness, pain, heat, swelling, and sometimes loss of function.

Influenza   is an Orthomyxoviridae virus and as such has single-stranded negative sense RNA that is segmented in 8 segments. The surface of the virion contains a hemagglutinin (H) which binds to surface sialic acid and a neuraminidase (N) which cleaves sialic acid for virus exit from the cell.

Innate immune system   includes elements that are available quickly, and are not specific to the pathogen in question. This includes skin, the acid ph of bodily fluids, normal flora, ear wax, mucous, the sneeze and cough response, phagocytic cell types, pattern recognition receptors and the internal and external components.

Integrase   enzyme that mediates the incorporation of the viral DNA into the genome of the infected cell.

Integrins   a group of proteins belonging to the adhesins family.

Intron   a segment of a nucleic acid that does not code for proteins and interrupts the sequence of a gene.

Invariant chain (Ii)   a protein involved in the processing of exogenous antigens via the MHC class II antigen processing pathway. The invariant chain prevents class II molecules from binding peptides derived from endogenous antigens.

Isograft   a graft transplanted between 2 genetically identical individuals.

Isotypic determinants   epitopes related to what class the immunoglobulin is.

 J

Jarisch-Herxheimer reaction   a reaction due to the massive release of toxins from bacteria that are killed in large numbers by antibiotic treatment.

 K

Knockout mice   a mouse that has been genetically manipulated to have a particular gene deleted from its genome.

 L

Lancefield serotyping   classification of Beta-hemolytic Streptococci based on differences in carbohydrates composition of the components of the cell wall.

Lattice   name of the cross-linked structure of antibody and antigen that forms in equivalence in either precipitation or agglutination assays.

Lectin   molecules which specifically bind to carbohydrates.

Lectin pathway   as complement pathway that begins with carbohydrates on the pathogen binding with carbohydrate binding protens of phagocytic cells.

Leukemia   is a cancer of the white blood cells of either the myeloid or lymphoid lineage, that starts in the bone marrow.

Leukocyte adherence deficiency (LAD)   an autosomal recessive genetic defect in the gene that encodes for CD18, a molecule shared by the β_2-integrins, that play a critical role in the adhesion and emigration of leukocytes to extravascular sites.

Light chains   the polypeptide chains of the immunoglobulin molecule that on the amino terminal end are involved in antigen binding. There of 2 of these chains in an IgG molecule. The molecular weight of this chain is close to half of the weight of the heavy chain and is 22 000 daltons.

Light chain deposition disease   is a cancer caused by an uncontrolled proliferation of plasma cells with production light chain only. Bence-Jones proteins can be found in the urine, and renal damage can occur due to accumulation of light chain in the kidney.

Linear epitopes epitopes based on the actual amino acid sequence of a particular antigen; they are not affected by the 3-dimensional structure of the antigen in space.

Low avidity IgG the first IgG antibody produced after the class switch from IgM occurs. Produced before somatic mutation results in the production of high affinity antibody. Its presence indicates a current infection. This antibody binds antigen in a normal buffer, but not when low concentrations of urea are added, so the amount of low affinity versus high affinity IgG can be measured.

Lymphoid cells are progeny of the common lymphoid precursor, and become either the B cells, T cells and NK cells.

Lymphoma is a cancer of the white blood cells that arises from mature lymphocytes in the organs of the lymphoid system.

▶ **M**

Macrophages CD14+ and are the largest white blood cell, they are called *monocytes* in the blood, and when they travel to tissues, they are called *macrophages*. Are active in phagocytosis.

Major histocompatibility complex (MHC) region formed by genetic loci that plays a central role in both humoral and cell-mediated immunity; it is composed of a family of a large number of genes on chromosome 6.

Malignant tumors cancerous tumors that can invade and grow into other organs and spread throughout the body.

Mancini method (also called *end-point method*) radial immunodiffusion method in which the reactants are allowed to come to equilibrium (24–72 hrs) and the square of the diameter is directly proportional to the concentration of the antigen.

Mantoux test a test determining the possibility that an individual has been exposed to *Mycobacterium tuberculosis*.

Mast cells mast cells have a surface receptor that binds IgE with a high affinity, and this relates to their primary role in allergic and anti-parasitic reactions. Mast cells contain granules of histamine and heparin and are the cell responsible for most of the effects in allergic reactions. Mast cells are found in tissues, in connective tissues and near mucosal surfaces.

Material safety data sheet (MSDS) forms that provide information on the properties of the chemical including physical properties such as melting point, boiling point, flash point, and others of that chemical, as well as its reactivity, toxicity, and health effects. Includes information of first aid procedures, requirements for specific protective equipment, and detailed instructions for storage, disposal, and procedures to handle spills.

Measles is also known as rubeola. It is a member of the Paramyxoviridae family of viruses as are mumps and respiratory syncytial virus. These viruses are single-stranded negative strand RNA viruses. Both measles and mumps are preventable by the MMR vaccine. Measles is the leading cause worldwide of deaths in children.

Megaloblastic anemia an anemic condition that results from a decrease or inhibition in the synthesis of DNA during the production of red blood cells.

Membrane attack complex (MAC) composed of the complement components C5, C6, C7, C8, C9, and also C5-9. These components are common to all 3 complement pathways and drill a hole into the membrane of the pathogen.

Metabolite is a breakdown product of a substance. In the field of toxicology, it can be detected in the biological specimens to indicate the consumption of a particular drug.

Metastasize the ability to spread throughout the body.

MHC restriction the ability of a host to react with a particular antigen only when components of that antigen, after processing, are presented to T cells in combination with that individual's MHC.

Microsome part of the endoplasmic reticulum and associated ribosomes.

Molecular mimicry an instance in which 1 set of molecules looks enough like another set that an immune response formed to one reacts with the other.

Monitoring following the patient's therapeutic response using serum levels of markers.

Monoclonal antibody antibody that is made by a clone of cells, with each molecule identical. Naturally produced by a tumor type called *myeloma*, also produced as a result of a laboratory process in which a hybrid is formed by a spleen cell and a myeloma cell that does not make antibody.

Monoclonal gammopathy of undetermined significance (MGUS) when monoclonal antibody is present but no tumor appears to be present.

Monoclonal immunoglobulin tumor marker for myeloma.

Mono-Diff test is used as a differential test to distinguish between infectious mononucleosis, serum sickness, or Forsmann antibody in individuals with a positive presumptive test. Utilizes absorption with bovine erythrocyte stroma and guinea pig kidney to differentiate the reactivities.

Monospot test was used as a presumptive to diagnose infectious mononucleosis. These tests utilized the fact that a heterophile antibody developed during infectious mononucleosis that reacted to srbc. Does not rule out serum sickness or Forsmann antibody that could be present in normals.

M protein a major virulence factor of *S. pyogenes*.

Multiple myeloma cancer caused by an uncontrolled proliferation of plasma cells with production of either monoclonal IgG, IgA or rarely monoclonal IgD or IgE. The plasma cells grow in the bone and bone marrow and create lesions in the bone.

Multiplexed fluorescent microbead assays multiple analyte assays, in which color-coded beads have been prepared that have a discreet fluorescent color code associated with a particular surface antigen. These different color beads have been prepared bound with different surface antigens. The patient's serum is added, incubated and the beads are washed. Next a fluorescently labeled anti-human immunoglobulin is added, and the beads are washed. Analysis is in a Luminex instrument that uses flow cytometric methodology. The bead internal fluorescence and surface flourescence due to fluorochrome conjugated anti-human antibody binding are measured to determine multiple reactions at once.

Mumps is a Paramyxovirus, having single-stranded negative strand RNA as its nucleic acid. It causes swollen parotid salivary glands, and the submaxillary and sublingual salivary glands may also be enlarged.

The immunity to mumps created by the MMR vaccine after 2 immunizations protects only 76 to 95% of those vaccinated, so after exposure some vaccinated people can get infected.

Myalgia   general medical term to describe muscle pain.

Mycelium   a mass of hyphae.

Myeloid   indicates that the cells are of the lineage of common myeloid progenitor cell, and this includes monocytes, granulocytes, mast cells, red blood cells, and platelets.

Myeloma   cancer of plasma cells that produce IgG, IgA, or less commonly IgD and IgE.

Myocarditis   inflammation of the heart muscle.

 N

National Fire Protection Association (NFPA) diamond   a symbol indicating different levels of health risks (blue), flammability risks (red), reactivity risks (yellow), and special risks (white).

Natural immune system   (also called the *innate immune system*) hallmarks are that it is *available quickly* and is *not specific* to the pathogen in question.

Natural killer (NK) cells   are nonantigen specific lymphocytes that have an antiviral and anti-tumor role.

Negative predictive value   the percent of time a negative value was truly negative for the disease in question for a certain population.

Negative selection   process in the development of thymocytes in which self-reacting thymocytes are deleted from the T-cell repertoire of the host.

Nephelometry   uses optical analysis methods to acquire and analyze antibody and antigen lattice formation. Scattered light is measured at a 10 to 90° angle from the light source, usually at 70°.

Neutralizing antibodies   antibodies that target functional viral components such as envelope proteins involved in viral entry.

Neutrophils   are the most abundant granulocyte, and they contain neutrally staining granules, that is, their granules do not stain when Wright stain is utilized. Fifty to 70% of the white blood cells in the blood are neutrophils. The nucleus of a neutrophil is irregular in shape with multiple lobes, also called *polymorphonuclear leukocyte*, with the shortened names or either "polys" or "PMNs" used. Increases in acute infection, first phagocytic cell to appear at the site of inflammation.

Non-Hodgkin's lymphoma   diagnosed with the general clinical symptoms of weight loss, fever, and night sweats that are found with fast growing lymphomas. Reed-Sternberg cells are not present.

Nonidentity   is the name of the 2 crossed reaction lines when, in double diffusion gel precipitation reactions the antigens in the 2 wells are different.

 O

Occupational Safety and Health Administration (OSHA)   organization that regulates components of workplace safety.

Oligodendrocyte   type of brain cell of the neuroglia group that acts as insulation for the axons of neurons.

Oligospermic   semen with a low concentration of spermatozoa.

Opsonin   is a compound that binds to the foreign particle and increases phagocytic cell uptake of the particle.

Optical immunoassays   special adaptations of the peroxidase enzyme immunoassay and are visualized based more on a property of the solid phase of the reaction than on the substrate. They are based on the change in the color of light reflected from the solid phase polymer membrane when antigen and antibody are bound in comparison to the color when antigen and antibody is not bound.

 P

Pannus   a general medical term for an abnormal flap of tissue, usually granulation tissue.

Paracrine effect   (also called *paracrine response*) the action of a cytokine or hormone on a nearby cell or tissue.

Paracrine response   (also called *paracrine effect*) the action of a cytokine or hormone on a nearby cell or tissue.

Paramyxoviridae family   single-stranded negative strand RNA viruses, and includes measles, mumps, and respiratory syncytial virus.

Parasites   are organisms that live at the expense of the other organisms.

Paratope   an area on the immunoglobulin molecule that binds the epitope of the antigen.

Partial identity   the name of the arched reaction lines with a spur that forms when, in double diffusion gel precipitation reactions the antigens in the 2 wells are share an epitope, but one of the antigens has an additional epitope. The "spur" points to the simpler antigen.

Particle-counting immunoassay (PACIA)   an instrumentation enhanced agglutination method in which residual nonagglutinating particles are counted.

Particle-enhanced turbidometric inhibition assay (PETINA)   an instrumentation enhanced agglutination method in which drug linked to particles and antibody to the drug cause increased turbidity of the solution when added to the particles. When the patient serum containing the drug is added to this mixture it will inhibit the cross-linking of the particles by the antibody.

Passive agglutination   an agglutination reaction using particles that have been coated with the antigen. Latex particles are most often used.

Pathogen-associated molecular patterns (PAMPs)   the pattern on groups of microorganisms recognized by the innate immune system.

Pattern recognition receptors (PRRs)   the molecules of the innate immune system that recognize pathogen-associated molecular patterns.

Paul-Bunnell antigen   antigen on the sheep red blood cells that reacts with the infectious mononucleosis serum.

Pericarditis   inflammation of the fibrous sac surrounding the heart.

Peripheral tolerance   process that downregulates potentially self-reacting immune cells that may have bypassed central tolerance.

Personal protection equipment   equipment that directly protects the operator from contamination by a biological sample. Examples include goggles or face shields, laboratory coats or gowns, face masks, and gloves.

Phagocytosis the engulfment and digestion of foreign cells and particles.

Phylogenetic the relatedness of 2 different species in term of genetic sequence. In other words, the evolutionary relatedness among groups of different organisms.

Plasma the fluid component of blood that is separated from the cells when an anticoagulant is used.

Plasma cell dyscrasias these include the cancers multiple myeloma, Waldenström macroglobulinemia, light chain deposition disease and heavy chain disease and the benign monoclonal gammopathy of undetermined significance.

Plasmapheresis the removal of plasma from an individual by drawing blood, separating it into plasma and cells, then replacing the cells back into the bloodstream.

Pleiotropic the ability of an entity to have multiple functions. For example, a single cytokine can activate different cells or different biological mechanisms.

Pleuritis inflammation of the pleural cavity surrounding the lungs.

Pneumocystis jiroveci a fungi that causes Pneumocystis pneumonia in AIDS patients and was formerly known as *Pneumocystis carinii*.

Poison is a toxic substance that causes injury, illness, or death.

Polymorphonuclear leukocyte a neutrophil. The nucleus is irregular in shape with multiple lobes. Increases in acute infection, first phagocytic cell to appear at the site of inflammation.

Polyarthritis a type of arthritis involving 5 or more joints.

Porins proteins that act as molecular holes in cellular membranes though which different molecules can diffuse.

Positive predictive value the percent of time there is a true positive result of the obtained positive results for a certain population.

Positive selection process in the development of thymocytes in which the MHC restriction of the immune repertoire of the host is achieved.

Postsynaptic membrane the membrane on the side of a cell such as a muscle cell or neuron that receives a signal from a synapse.

Postzone exists when the amount of patient antibody is low so that each antibody is bound by 2 antigen molecules, resulting in no bridging of 2 antibody molecules by the antigen, so little or no precipitation occurs.

Precipitation the cross-linking of soluble antigen to create an insoluble precipitate that is visible.

Primary adrenal insufficiency a condition in which damage to the adrenal glands results in the impaired production of steroid hormones from such glands.

Progesterone receptor marker on tumor tissue indicating that the tumor is likely to respond to endocrine therapy.

Prostascint antibody to prostate specific membrane antigen (PSMA). It is used in radioimmunolocalization after prostatectomy to look for distant metastasis.

Prostate-specific antigen (PSA) a tumor-associated antigen, present in low amounts in the serum in normal men. PSA concentration is used in screening and monitoring, and PSA velocity and free and complexed PSA are also used in screening measurements. It is also used for the forensic identification of semen.

Protease enzyme that cleaves viral proteins into different components.

Proteinuria the presence of excess amounts of serum proteins in the urine.

Provenge a new prostate cancer vaccine in which antigen-presenting cells are loaded with a tumor antigen called *prostatic acid phosphatase*. After amplification they are returned to the patient and stimulate the patient's T cells to make a response.

Provirus viral DNA integrated into the host genome.

Prozone is when, in a precipitation reaction, there is too much antibody, so that there are 2 antibodies bound to every bivalent antigen and there is no need for bridging of 2 antigen molecules by an antibody molecule. In this situation little or no precipitate would form, that makes it appear that the patient does not have antibody to the antigen, when, in fact, they have too much antibody for the reaction to occur.

PSA velocity the amount of increase in the PSA levels from the previous year.

Purine nucleoside phosphorylase deficiency (PNP) a condition causing accumulation of deoxy-GPT that is toxic for T cells and results in impaired cell mediated

 Q

Quasi-elastic light scattering method (QUELS) an instrumentation enhanced agglutination method in which light scattering changes are measured.

Questioned stain a sample in which the identity of the stain is unknown.

 R

Radial immunodiffusion (RID) single diffusion of the antigen into a gel that already contains the antibody throughout. It is a quantitative technique.

Radioallergosorbent test (RAST) test that evaluates levels of IgE specific for a particular allergen.

Radioimmunosorbent test (RIST) test that evaluates total serum levels of IgE, regardless of its antigen specificity.

Radioimmunotherapy the transfer of radiolabeled antibody at a level high enough to have a therapeutic effect on the tumor.

Raynaud phenomena is pain in hands and feet due to decreased blood supply

Recombinant immunoblot assay (RIBA) a strip immunoblot which has some but not all of the characteristics of a Western blot. A nitrocellulose strip is prepared by the manufacturer that has multiple viral antigens placed onto it, and an indirect enzyme immunoassay is performed by the clinical laboratory on the strip, testing for patient's antibody to the different antigens on the strip and comparing it to the control.

Redundant action that can be achieved by different entities to result in the same function. For example, different cytokines can activate the same cell or the same biological mechanism.

Regulators of complement   components that decrease or turn-off complement functions. These include soluble and membrane bound components. Membrane bound components include CR1 and DAF. Soluble inhibitors of complement include C1INH, C4BP, and factor H and I.

Regulatory T cells   subset of T cells that act as regulator of the immune response. They also play an important role in immunological tolerance.

Restriction endonuclease   an enzyme that cuts DNA at specific sequences along the DNA.

Reticular dysgenesis   condition characterized by low lymphocyte counts and the lack of blood monocytes and neutrophils.

Reverse passive agglutination   an antibody rather than antigen is linked to the particles, this method was developed to detect antigen in patient's fluids.

Reverse transcriptase   enzyme that converts viral RNA into DNA.

Reyes syndrome   is associated with the combination of aspirin and chicken pox. It is a very severe disease of children affecting the brain and the liver.

Rheumatoid factor   present in most patients with rheumatoid arthritis, is defined as antibody to the Fc region of the IgG immunoglobulin. It is usually, but not always of the IgM class.

Ribonucleic acid RNA   this is the molecule that DNA is "copied" to by a process called *transcription*. RNA is arranged in a similar way as DNA, with different bases providing the sequence information for the different codons; the genetic difference is that RNA has a base called uracil instead of thymine. In addition ribonucleic acid contains the backbone sugar ribose instead of the sugar deoxyribose.

Ring precipitin   serological technique used to determine the species of origin of a bloodstain.

Rituximab   an antibody used in cancer therapy to CD20 that is on the cell surface of B cell lymphomas.

Rubella   is in the Togaviridae family. It is also called *3 day measles* or *German measles*. It causes a mild infection with a rash, but is clinically important because it can cause severe birth defects.

▶ **S**

Saliva   a secretion of the glands of the mouth area that aids in digestion.

Salivary alpha amylase   a digestive enzyme found in high concentrations in saliva that is used to break down carbohydrates.

Sandwich assay   this assay usually captures antigen between 2 molecules of antibody, 1 antibody captures the antigen to a solid phase and the other antibody is labeled and is used to visualize the reaction, sometimes antigen can capture antibody and labeled antigen is used to visualize the reaction but this is rarely used.

Sarcomas   cancers that arise from supportive or connective tissue such as muscle, bone, cartilage, fat, and blood vessels.

Screening   testing for cancer in a population when no symptoms of the cancer exist, to allow for earlier diagnosis.

Secondary lymphatic organ   organs in which lymphocytes meet antigen, proliferate, and undergo somatic mutation as the response matures.

Second-set rejection   subsequent encounter, and quicker response to a graft from the same allogeneic individual.

Selective IgA deficiency   most common of the agammaglobulinemias, resulting in decreased levels of IgA.

Self-reactivity   ability of an immune response to react against self-antigens.

Self-tolerance   mechanism that prevents the immune system from reacting to self-antigens.

Semen   secretion of the male reproductive organs.

Sensitivity   gives us a measure of how often the assay will diagnose the disease or condition in question in a group of patients that have the disease or condition. This is the number of tested positive results divided by the number of positive individuals analyzed. The number of positive individuals analyzed = the number of tested positive + the number of false negatives.

Sepsis   the presence of harmful microorganisms within the blood, for example through a wound or other source of infection.

Serial dilution   a series of logarithmic dilutions that relate to each other and represent a way to prepare multiple dilutions of the patient's serum to test for antibody.

Seroconversion   the time at which antibodies to a virus or bacteria are detected in a person's bloodstream.

Serology   is the study of serum components of the blood. This science deals mostly with the *in vitro* measurement of antibody and antigen reactions in serum or plasma.

Seronegative   the absence of detectable antibodies to a particular antigen in a person's serum.

Seropositive   indicates that the patient has antibody for the antigen in question.

Serum   the liquid portion of the blood after coagulation has taken place.

Serum amyloid A   An apolipoprotein that is associated with high density lipoprotein (HDL) in the blood stream. It is involved with the transport of cholesterol to the liver, and it also is involved in induction of extracellular matrix degrading enzymes that are involved in repair after infection induced tissue damage and it is a chemoattractant, bringing cells of the innate and acquired immune systems to the site of the infection.

Serum sickness   immune complex-mediated immune response of type III hypersensitivity seen after the administration of large amounts of serum into a recipient, resulting in a systemic reaction characterized by fever, chills, generalized rash, arthritis and, sometimes, kidney damage.

Serum sickness antigen   heterophile antigen that is present on sheep red blood cells, horse red blood cells, and guinea pig kidney and bovine erythrocytes. Antibody to this antigen will yield positive results in a Mono-spot or presumptive assay for infectious mononucleosis, but will be negative after absorption either with guinea pig kidney or with bovine erythrocytes.

Severe combined immunodeficiencies (SCID)   number of different conditions that can affect one of more components of the immune system resulting defective development and/or function of T and B cells.

Single nucleotide polymorphism   variation in DNA sequence involving a single base pair**.**

Solute   material being diluted.

Specificity   is the percentage of time in which there is a true negative test result divided by the number of total true negatives when the total negatives equal tested true negatives plus false positives. This gives us a measurement of the assay's accuracy in terms of how often a true negative sample will yield a negative test result. The higher the percentage of specificity, the less likely we are to tell a patient who does not have the disease in question that he or she does have it. The higher the specificity the fewer the number of false positives.

Specificity   percent of time there is a true negative test result divided by the number of total negatives. Where total negatives = tested true negatives + false positives.

Spectrophotometer   the instrument used to make a quantitative measurement at a specific wavelength of the amount of light that is transmitted through a solution. Used with Beer's law to quantitate substances.

Spermatozoa   male reproductive cells.

Stage   determination of how far the tumor has grown and spread. Three letters are used, T for tumor size, N for number of lymph nodes involved and M for whether or not distant metastases are found.

Steric hindrance   when the size or shape of the molecule interferes with the interaction. In antibody binding to antigen this occurs when the antigen is too large for the epitopes to be bound by 2 neighboring paratopes. In IgM reactions this can result in less than 10 antigens being bound, often with steric hindrance the binding ability of IgM is decreased to 5 epitopes.

Superantigen   one of a class of antigens that causes nonspecific activation of T-cells resulting in polyclonal T cell activation and massive cytokine release.

Synergistic   combined action of 2 entities is greater than the sum of their actions as a single entity.

Synovitis   inflammation of the synovial membranes.

 T

T cells   are one type of cell of the acquired immune system.

T-cell receptor   member of the immunoglobulin superfamily used by T cells to recognize peptides from an antigen that has been processed and presented by an antigen-presenting cell.

Thermal dimorphism   is when a fungi exists in yeast form at 1 temperature and mold form at another temperature.

Tissue typing   HLA histocompatibility matching between a graft donor and a graft recipient.

Titer   reciprocal of the last dilution that yields a positive test in the assay.

Tolerization   repeated administration of antigen to downregulate the immune response to that antigen.

Toll-like receptors (TLR)   important set of cell surface PRR, 12 different Toll-like receptors in this family of molecules each binds to a different PAMP.

Toxoplasmosis, other infections, rubella, cytomegalovirus, and herpes simplex virus (TORCH)   a group of infectious agents which cause congenital infections and birth defects. The acronym stands for **t**oxoplasmosis, **o**ther infections, **r**ubella, **c**ytomegalovirus, and **h**erpes simplex virus. Infants are tested for these infections at birth.

Toxoplasmosis   caused by the protozoan parasite *Toxoplasma gondii*. It is transmitted to humans in several ways consumption of

under-cooked contaminated meat, especially lamb, pork, beef, and venison, can transmit the infection as can accidental ingestion of cat feces. An important source of transmission is mother to child transmission which can result in birth defects.

Transcription   the process of copying genetic information from DNA into RNA.

Translation   the process of converting genetic information in the form of codons into amino acids and, subsequently, proteins.

Transplacental passage   the passage of molecules or cells from mother to fetus through the placenta.

Tumor   a benign or a malignant abnormal growth of cells.

Tumor-associated antigens   substances which are expressed more in the tumor than in normal tissue. These substances can be used in screening, diagnosis, monitoring, localization, and therapy of the cancer patient.

Tumor immunology   the study of (1) the antigens associated with the tumor, (2) the patient's immune response to the tumor, (3) the use of the immune system to destroy the tumor, and (4) the effect of the tumor on the patient's immune status.

Turbidometry   turbidometry uses optical analysis methods to acquire and analyze antibody and antigen lattice formation. Light is measured directly opposite the light source.

 U

Universal precautions   care taken using the assumption that all patients and their samples are potentially infectious and possible carriers of pathogens.

Urea   breakdown product of proteins that is carried through the bloodstream to the kidneys where it gets excreted out of the body in urine.

Urine   secretion of the kidneys containing waste products of metabolism.

▶ **V**

Vasculitis   process involving the inflammatory destruction of blood vessels.

Varicella zoster virus (VZV)   member of the Herpesviridae family. It causes chicken pox and shingles.

Vimentin   marker used in immunohistochemistry to stain mesenchymal tumors (tumors of melanocyte, muscle fibrous, endothelium, nerve, paraganglioma, synovium, cartilage origin).

Viremia   presence of virus in the bloodstream.

▶ **W**

Waldenström macroglobulinemia   cancer caused by an uncontrolled proliferation of plasma cells with production of monoclonal IgM. The plasma cells grow lymphoid tissue and this is similar clinically to lymphoma.

West Nile virus (WNV)   is a Flavivirus and as such has single-stranded positive sense RNA which is enveloped and icosahedral. It is transmitted by mosquitoes and normally infects birds. Most cases are asymptomatic, or develop a mild disease called *West Nile fever*. About 1 out of 100 of infected individuals develop meningitis or encephalitis. Because it can be transmitted through blood transfusion and organ transplantation, blood and tissue testing prior to transfusions and transplantation is needed.

Western blot an adaptation of an enzyme immunoassay. This technique begins with electrophoretic separation of proteins utilizing a sodium dodecyl sulfate polyacrylamide gel electrophoresis (SDS-PAGE) which separates proteins by their molecular weight. The next step utilizes a transfer of these separated proteins to nitrocellulose, which is a suitable solid phase for the final step of a direct or an indirect enzyme immunoassay.

Window period the time between infection and when the clinical assay detects some changes that are associated with the infection.

 X

Xenograft graft transplanted between different species.

X-linked agammaglobulinemia (XLA) the condition involving impaired B-cell development, lack of mature B cells, and low or lacking levels of immunoglobulins of all isotypes. This is linked to the X chromosome and is recessive so it occurs almost exclusively in boys.

X-linked immunodeficiencies recessive deficiencies associated with the X chromosome and, therefore, affect primarily males.

 Y

Yeast form of fungi that is unicellular, and multiplies by budding. The buds can easily be seen on the yeast cells.

 Z

Zeta potential the charge on the particle involved in the agglutination reaction.

Zevalin an Indium labeled antibody for imaging and ^{90}Yttrium labeled antibody for therapy. It targets CD20 and is used in the radioimmunolocalization and radioimmunotherapy of B cell non-Hodgkin lymphomas.

INDEX

hematuria, 159
hemoglobin, 371
hemolysis, 319
hemolytic anemia, 139t, 146
hemolytic disease of fetus and newborn
    (HDFN), 145, 146, 147f
hepatic disease, 183–184
hepatitis
    autoimmune, 183–184, 184t
    bloodborne, 282–289
    defined, 278
    fecal-oral, 279–282
hepatitis A
    diagnosis of, 279, 280f
    epidemiology of, 279
    geographic distribution of, 280f
    postexposure prophylaxis, 281
    vaccine, 281
hepatitis B
    chronic, 284f
    diagnosis of, 283–285
    epidemiology of, 282–283
    geographic distribution of, 284f
    incidence of, 283f
    recovery, 284f
    treatment of, 285
    vaccine, 285–286
    virus structure, 283f
hepatitis C
    accidental exposure to, 387–388
    diagnosis of, 287–289, 288f, 289, 290
    epidemiology of, 286–287
    sources of infection, 287f
    treatment of, 289
    virus structure, 287f
hepatitis D
    diagnosis of, 286
    epidemiology of, 286
    virus structure, 285f
hepatitis E
    diagnosis of, 282
    epidemiology, 281–282
    geographic distribution of, 281f
    vaccine, 282
hepatotrophic viruses, 279
Herceptin, 208
hereditary angioedema (HAE), 250, 250f
HER-2 marker, 207
herpes simplex 1 and 2, 301–303
Herpesviridae family, 295–305
heteroantigens, 44
heterogenous assay
    defined, 105
    labels for, 116–118
    steps of, 111t
    types of, 106–115
heterophile antibody, 296
high avidity antibody, 359
highly active antiretroviral therapy (HAART),
    267–268, 268t
hinge region, 27, 28f
histamine, 141t
histocompatibility, 231–232, 231f, 232f
Histoplasma capsulatum, 355
histoplasmosis, 355
HIV (human immunodeficiency virus), 262f
    accidental exposure to, 386–387, 387f
    acute syndrome in, 263, 264f

AIDS classification, 265
antibody tests, 270–271
attachment by, 261f
cell entry by, 261f
classification system for infected individuals,
    265t, 266t
clinical characteristics of, 263–265
clinical latency of, 263
confirmatory tests for, 272
eclipse phase of, 262
enzymes in, 259
flow cytometry of CD4/CD8 cells in, 20, 20f
highly active antiretroviral therapy for,
    267–268, 268t
immune responses and, 261–262
infection, 259–269
laboratory tests for, 269–273
life cycle, 262f
neutralizing antibodies and, 261
pathogenesis of, 262–263
postexposure prophylaxis, 388t
provirus, 260
replication of, 260–261
screening, 271
seroconversion, 271
staging, 267t
statistics, 259t
structure of, 260f
symptoms of, 263–265
time course of infection, 263f
treatment, 265–268, 268t
vaccine prospects, 268–269
viral component tests, 272–273
virology of, 259–260
Western blot in diagnosis of, 111–112
window period for testing of, 269
HLA. *See* human leukocyte antigen (HLA)
Hodgkin disease, 216t
homogenous assay
    defined, 105
    types of, 118–119
hood
    biological containment, 381, 381f
    fume, 380, 381f
host defense mechanisms, for bacteria, 318–319
HSC. *See* hematopoietic stem cells (HSCs)
human anti-mouse antibody (HAMA), 120, 300
human chorionic gonadotropin (hCG),
    204–205, 210t
human heterophilic antibodies, 119–120
human leukocyte antigen (HLA), 156, 156t,
    231–232, 231f, 232f
human leukocyte antigen (HLA) typing, 235–236
humoral, 5
humoral immune system, 14f
hybridization
    defined, 397–398
    fluorescence *in situ,* 206–207, 399, 400f, 401f
    using solid matrices, 398–399
hybridoma cells, 37, 38f
hyperacute graft rejection, 233
hyperimmunoglobulin-M syndrome, 245t,
    246, 253t
hyperpigmentation, 178
hypersensitivity reactions
    classification of, 139t
    defined, 138
    delayed-type, 148–151

overview of, 138
type I, 139–145
    antigen allergenicity in, 142–143
    clinical manifestations of, 140–142
    individual susceptibility to, 142
    molecular mechanisms of, 140–142
    prophylaxis, 144–145
    skin testing for, 143–144
    testing for, 143–144
    treatment, 144–145
type II, 145–146
type III, 147–148, 148f
type IV, 148–151, 149f
hypervariable regions, 26
hypervolemia, 323
hyphae, 347

I

IAT. *See* indirect antiglobulin test (IAT)
IBD. *See* inflammatory bowel disease (IBD)
identity, 88, 89f
IgA. *See* immunoglobulin A (IgA)
IgD. *See* immunoglobulin D (IgD)
IgG. *See* immunoglobulin G (IgG)
IgM. *See* immunoglobulin M (IgM)
Ii. *See* invariant chain (Ii)
IL-2. *See* interleukin-2 (IL-2)
immediate hypersensitivity, 139–145
    antigen allergenicity in, 142–143
    clinical manifestations of, 140–142
    individual susceptibility to, 142
    molecular mechanisms of, 140–142
    prophylaxis, 144–145
    skin testing for, 143–144
    testing for, 143–144
    treatment, 144–145
immune system
    acquired, 4t, 12–14
        antibodies in, 12–13
        cells in, 12
        cellular arm of, 13, 14f
        diversity in, 34–37
    adaptive, 3
    bacterial, 3f
    cellular, 14f
    defined, 3
    humoral, 14f
    innate, 3, 4–12, 4t
        cells of, 5–7, 6f, 7t
        external components of, 4–5, 5f
        internal components of, 5–12
        molecules of, 8–9, 9t
        process of, 10–12
    natural, 3
    specificity, 3, 51–54
immunity, defined, 3
immunochromatographic sandwich assay, 108f,
    109
immunodeficiency(ies)
    diagnostic tests for, 252–254
    primary, 244, 244t
    treatment of, 254
    X-linked, 244, 244t
immunodiffusion techniques, 87–92
immunofixation electrophoresis, 223–224, 224f
immunogen, 45
    adjuvants and, 45

immunogenicity
  addition of immune-enhancing
    agents and, 45
  complexity and, 44
  foreignness and, 44
  nature and, 44–45
  requirements for, 44–45
  site and, 45
  size and, 44
  state and, 45
immunoglobulin A (IgA), 27t, 28–30, 30f, 219, 245–246, 253t
immunoglobulin D (IgD), 27t, 32, 32f
immunoglobulin E (IgE), 27t, 32–33, 32f, 33f, 139
immunoglobulin G (IgG), 25f, 26f, 27–28, 27t, 28f, 28t
immunoglobulin M (IgM), 27t, 30–32, 30f, 31f, 32f, 219
immunoglobulin quantitation, 224
immunoglobulins. *See also* antibody(ies)
  binding-site diversity in, 35f
  classes of, 26–34
  deficiencies, 244–247, 245t
  functions of, 29
  monoclonal, 204
  overview of, 12
  structure of, 25f
  subclasses of, 26–34
  weight of, 24–25
immunoglobulin superfamily, 61
immunoglobulin supergene family, 26
immunohistochemistry, 206–207
immunolocalization, 207–208
immunological cross-reactivity, 46
immunologically privileged sites, 156
immunological tolerance, 59–60
immunology
  defined, 3
  tumor, 201
immunoproliferative disease, 215f
  defined, 214
  laboratory analysis of, 220–224
  leukemia, 214
  lymphoma, 214–217
  plasma cell dyscrasias, 218–220
  risk factors, 214
immunosuppressive therapy, 239
immunotherapy, for tumors, 208
impetigo, 322, 322f
indirect antiglobulin test (IAT), 97
indirect immunoassay, 107
infection, autoimmunity and, 156
infectious mononucleosis, 296, 297f. *See also* Epstein-Barr virus (EBV)
inflammation, 10f
  defined, 10
inflammatory bowel disease (IBD), 180t, 182–183, 182f
influenza virus, 309–310, 311f
innate immune system, 3, 4–12, 4t
  cells of, 5–7, 6f, 7t
  external components of, 4–5, 5f
  internal components of, 5–12
  molecules of, 8–9, 9t
  process of, 10–12
in situ hybridization (ISH), 206–207, 399, 400f
integrase, 259

integrase inhibitors, 268t
integrins, 61
integumentary system, autoimmunity and, 184–187
interferons, 9t, 65. *See also* cytokine(s)
interleukin-2 (IL-2), 66. *See also* cytokine(s)
interleukin-7 (IL-7) receptor, 249f
interleukins, 9t, 64–65. *See also* cytokine(s)
intestinal autoimmune disease, 179–180, 180t, 181f
introns, 394
invariant chain (Ii), 51
ISH. *See in situ* hybridization (ISH)
isograft, 231
isotypic determinants, 33f–34
-itis, 10

▶ **J**

Jarisch-Herxheimer reaction, 335
jaundice, 278f

▶ **K**

Kaposi's sarcoma, 265f
kidneys, autoimmune disease in, 190, 191t
kilo-, 128t
knockout mice, 155
Koplik spots, 308f

▶ **L**

laboratory coats, 383
laboratory dilutions, 124–126
  compound, 124
  diluent in, 124
  serial, 124, 125f
  solute in, 124
  2-fold serial, 124, 125f
laboratory gowns, 383
laboratory safety
  chemical hazards and, 388–389
  equipment, 380–384
  general, 389
  law and, 385–386
  needlestick injuries and, 386
  overview of, 380
  personal protection equipment in, 383–384
  posters, 381f
  procedures, 384–385
  radioactive hazards and, 388–389
  universal precautions and, 384–385
LAD. *See* leukocyte adherence deficiency (LAD)
LAK. *See* lymphokine-activated killer (LAK) cells
laminar flow hood, 381, 381f
Lancefield serotyping, 319–320
Landsteiner's experiment, 53, 369
lattice, 88
law, lab safety and, 385–386
lectin pathway, 73, 74f, 76, 78f, 78t
lectins, defined, 3
leukemia, 199, 214, 215f
leukocyte adherence deficiency (LAD), 251–252, 253t
leukotrienes, 141t
light chain deposition disease, 214
light chain disease, 219
light chain quantitation, 224

light chains, 25, 25f, 26–34, 26f
linear epitope, 45, 46f
liver anatomy, 278f
liver disease, 183–184, 291f. *See also* hepatitis
low avidity IgG antibody, 359
low sperm count
  antigen in, 175t
  assays for, 175t
  clinical effects of, 175t
  diagnosis of, 175t
Lyme disease, 337–341
lymph nodes, 14, 16, 16f
lymphoid leukemias, 214
lymphoid organs, 14–17
lymphoid tumor, 216t
lymphokine-activated killer (LAK) cells, 5–7, 6f, 7t
lymphoma, 199, 206–207, 214–217, 216t, 217f
lysosome, 11f
lysozyme, 4

▶ **M**

MAC. *See* membrane attack complex (MAC)
macroglobulinemia, 216t, 219–220
macrophages, 5–7, 6f, 7t
major histocompatibility complex (MHC), 13, 46–49, 231–232, 231f, 232f
  class I, 50t, 51, 52f
  class II, 50t, 51, 52f
  haplotype, 58
major histocompatibility complex (MHC) genes, 47, 48f
malignant tumor, 198. *See also* tumor(s)
malnutrition, acquired immunodeficiency and, 258
MALT. *See* mucosa-associated lymphoid tissue (MALT)
mammogram, 202f
Mancini method, 92
mannose-binding lectin (MBL), 78f, 78t
Mantoux test, 150, 151f
masks, 384
mast cells, 5–7, 6f, 7t, 140f, 141t, 142f
material safety data sheet (MSDS), 388
MBL. *See* mannose-binding lectin (MBL)
M cells, 17, 18f
measles, 307–308, 307f, 308f
megaloblastic anemia, 181
melanoma, 206–207
membrane attack complex (MAC), 77, 79f
meningoencephalitis, 354
messenger RNA, 397f
metabolite, 369
metastasis, 198, 199f, 200f
metric prefixes, 128t
MGUS. *See* monoclonal gammopathy of undetermined significance (MGUS)
mHA. *See* minor histocompatibility antigens (mHA)
MHC. *See* major histocompatibility complex (MHC)
MHC restricted, 58, 58t
mice, knockout, 155
micro-, 128t
microarrays, 400–401, 402f
microcytotoxicity test, 235